ASSESSMENT OF ADDICTIVE BEHAVIORS

Assessment of
ADDICTIVE
BEHAVIORS

SECOND EDITION

Edited by
DENNIS M. DONOVAN
G. ALAN MARLATT

THE GUILFORD PRESS
New York   London

© 2005 The Guilford Press
A Division of Guilford Publications, Inc.
72 Spring Street, New York, NY 10012
www.guilford.com

Printed in the United States of America

This book is printed on acid-free paper.

Last digit is print number: 9 8 7 6 5 4 3 2 1

Library of Congress Cataloging-in-Publication Data

Assessment of addictive behaviors / edited by Dennis M. Donovan and G. Alan
Marlatt. – 2nd ed.
     p. cm.
   Includes bibliographical references and index.
   ISBN 1-59385-175-8 (alk. paper)
   1. Compulsive behavior—Diagnosis.   2. Compulsive behavior—
Treatment.   3. Substance abuse.   4. Psychodiagnostics.   I. Donovan, Dennis M.
(Dennis Michael)   II. Marlatt, G. Alan.
   RC533.A86 2005
   616.86—dc22

                                                                    2005000901

About the Editors

Dennis M. Donovan, PhD, was affiliated with the Addictions Treatment Center at the Seattle Department of Veterans Affairs Medical Center for over 20 years, while engaging in clinical, administrative, training, and research activities. During that time he was also instrumental in the development of, and served as the Associate Director of, the first Center of Excellence in Substance Abuse Treatment and Education (CESATE) within the national Department of Veterans Affairs. He currently serves as the Director of the University of Washington's Alcohol and Drug Abuse Institute and holds the faculty ranks of Professor in the Department of Psychiatry and Behavioral Sciences, and Adjunct Professor in the Department of Psychology at the University of Washington in Seattle. He has written over 120 journal articles, 30 book chapters, and 3 books in the area of alcoholism and addictive behaviors, with emphases on social learning theory and biopsychosocial approaches to the etiology, maintenance, and treatment of addictions; the clinical assessment process and assessment measures; treatment entrance and engagement; evaluation of treatment process and outcome; relapse prevention; and patient–treatment matching. Dr. Donovan's research has been funded by the National Institute on Alcohol Abuse and Alcoholism (NIAAA), the National Institute on Drug Abuse (NIDA), and the Center for Substance Abuse Treatment (CSAT). He has served as Associate Editor and as a member of the editorial boards for the *Journal of Studies on Alcohol, Psychology of Addictive Behaviors*, and *Addiction*. He has also been a member of the Clinical and Treatment Research Review Committee of NIAAA and the Behavioral AIDS Research Review Committee of NIDA. Dr. Donovan is a member of a number of national professional organizations and served as President of the Society of Psychologists in Addictive Behaviors. He has also been elected a Fellow of Division 50 (Division on Addictions) of the American Psychological Association.

G. Alan Marlatt, PhD, Director of the Addictive Behaviors Research Center and Professor of Psychology at the University of Washington, is renowned for his innovative theoretical and clinical work in the addictions field. Over the past two decades, he has made significant advances in developing programs for both relapse prevention and harm reduction for a range of addictive behaviors. In addition to coediting the first editions of *Relapse Prevention: Maintenance Strategies in the Treatment of Addictive Behaviors* (1985) and *Assessment of Addictive Behaviors* (1988), Dr. Marlatt is the editor of *Harm Reduction: Pragmatic Strategies for Managing High-Risk Behaviors* (1998), coeditor of *Changing Addictive Behavior: Bridging Clinical and Public Health Strategies* (1999), and coauthor of *Brief Alcohol Screening and Intervention for College Students (BASICS): A Harm Reduction Approach* (1999), all published by The Guilford Press. He is a Fellow of both the American Psychological Association and the American Psychological Society, and is a former president of the Association for Advancement of Behavior Therapy. He served as a member of the National Advisory Council on Drug Abuse at the National Institute on Drug Abuse from 1996 to 2002, and served on the National Advisory Council on Alcohol Abuse and Alcoholism Subcommittee on College Drinking from 1998 to 2001. Dr. Marlatt currently holds a Senior Research Scientist Award from the National Institute on Alcohol Abuse and Alcoholism, and received the Innovators Combating Substance Abuse Award from the Robert Wood Johnson Foundation in 2001. Previously, he was presented with the Jellinek Memorial Award for Alcohol Studies (1990), the Distinguished Scientist Award from the American Psychological Association's Society of Clinical Psychology (2000), the Visionary Award from the Network of Colleges and Universities Committed to the Elimination of Drug and Alcohol Abuse (2002), and the Distinguished Researcher Award from the Research Society on Alcoholism (2004).

Contributors

Samuel A. Ball, PhD, Department of Psychiatry, Yale University School of Medicine, New Haven, Connecticut

Arthur W. Blume, PhD, Department of Psychology, University of Texas at El Paso, El Paso, Texas

Kathleen M. Carroll, PhD, Department of Psychiatry, Yale University School of Medicine, New Haven, Connecticut

R. Lorraine Collins, PhD, Research Institute on Addictions, University at Buffalo, State University of New York, Buffalo, New York

Ned L. Cooney, PhD, Department of Psychiatry, Yale University School of Medicine, New Haven, Connecticut, and VA Connecticut Heathcare Center, West Haven, Connecticut

Jessica M. Cronce, BS, Department of Psychology, Yale University, New Haven, Connecticut

Berenice García de la Cruz, MA, Department of Special Education, University of Texas at Austin, Austin, Texas

Dennis M. Donovan, PhD, Alcohol and Drug Abuse Institute and Department of Psychiatry and Behavioral Sciences, University of Washington School of Medicine, Seattle, Washington

Christopher R. Freed, MPhil, MA, The Graduate Center, The City University of New York, New York, New York

William H. George, PhD, Department of Psychology, University of Washington, Seattle, Washington

Maureen Hillhouse, PhD, UCLA Integrated Substance Abuse Programs, Department of Psychiatry and Behavioral Sciences, David Geffen School of Medicine, Los Angeles, California

Ronald M. Kadden, PhD, Department of Psychiatry, University of Connecticut School of Medicine, Farmington, Connecticut

Jason R. Kilmer, PhD, Evergreen State College, Olympia, Washington, and Saint Martin's College, Lacey, Washington

Kristen P. Lindgren, MS, Department of Psychology, University of Washington, Seattle, Washington

Carmen L. Masson, PhD, Department of Psychiatry, University of California, San Francisco, San Francisco, California

Osvaldo F. Morera, PhD, Department of Psychology, University of Texas at El Paso, El Paso, Texas

Rebekka S. Palmer, PhD, Department of Psychiatry, Division of Substance Abuse, Yale University School of Medicine, New Haven, Connecticut

Richard A. Rawson, PhD, UCLA Integrated Substance Abuse Programs, Department of Psychiatry and Behavioral Sciences, David Geffen School of Medicine, Los Angeles, California

Lina A. Ricciardelli, PhD, School of Psychology, Deakin University, Burwood, Victoria, Australia

Roger A. Roffman, DSW, School of Social Work, University of Washington, Seattle, Washington

William G. Shadel, PhD, Department of Psychology, University of Pittsburgh, Pittsburgh, Pennsylvania

Howard J. Shaffer, PhD, CAS, Division on Addictions, Harvard Medical School, Boston, Massachusetts

Saul Shiffman, PhD, Department of Psychology, University of Pittsburgh, Pittsburgh, Pennsylvania

Jane M. Simoni, PhD, Department of Psychology, University of Washington, Seattle, Washington

Ruthlyn Sodano, BA, Department of Psychology, University of Albany, State University of New York, Albany, New York

James L. Sorensen, PhD, Department of Psychiatry, University of California, San Francisco, San Francisco, California

Howard R. Steinberg, PhD, Yale University School of Medicine, New Haven, Connecticut

Kari A. Stephens, MS, Department of Psychology, University of Washington, Seattle, Washington

Robert S. Stephens, PhD, Department of Psychology, Virginia Polytechnic Institute and State University, Blacksburg, Virginia

David A. Wasserman, PhD, Department of Psychiatry, University of California, San Francisco, San Francisco, California

James Westphal, MD, Department of Psychiatry, University of California, San Francisco, San Francisco, California

Jennifer G. Wheeler, PhD, Sex Offender Treatment Program, Monroe Correctional Complex–Twin Rivers Unit, Monroe, Washington

Tina M. Zawacki, PhD, Department of Psychology, University of Texas at San Antonio, San Antonio, Texas

Preface

Over a decade and a half ago, the introductory chapter for the first edition of this book dealt with the then "emergent" biopsychosocial model of addictive behaviors and its implications for their assessment. Much has happened in the addictions field since that time. We have a clearer and more thorough understanding of the genetic, biological, cognitive, psychological, and social factors that contribute to the development of addictive behaviors. We have a better understanding of how neurotransmitter systems and behavioral reinforcement principles interact and contribute to the experience of craving that motivates engagement in addictive behaviors and fosters the development of dependence. We have a better understanding of those behavioral and pharmacological interventions, used independently or in combination, that are effective in helping individuals achieve either abstinence-based or harm reduction goals. The biopsychosocial model has emerged and matured as an explanatory model that capably integrates this broad range of newly acquired knowledge about addictive behaviors and their treatment.

And yet, despite the many advances made over the past decade and a half, relapse continues to be one of the defining features of addictions and continues to occur at relatively high rates. The goal of treatment, regardless of its orientation, regardless of whether pharmacological or behavioral, is to reduce the likelihood of relapse and minimize the harm associated with a relapse if one does occur. Assessment of the individual's coping skills, cognitive expectations about the behavior and its perceived positive benefits and negative consequences, and situations that represent a high risk for relapse continue to serve as the cornerstone of treatment planning and relapse prevention. It is this latter point, in the broader context of the biopsychosocial model of addiction, that led to the development and organization of this revised and updated edition of *Assessment of Addictive Behaviors*.

A number of significant changes have been made in the present edition of this book. One of the most notable changes is the much more explicit focus on the relationship between assessment and relapse prevention processes and procedures. Assessment issues are now addressed in the context of relapse prevention. This new edition is designed to be used in conjunction with the second edition of our companion volume, *Relapse Prevention: Maintenance Strategies in the Treatment of Addictive Behaviors* (Marlatt & Donovan, 2005). Originally published in 1985 by Marlatt and Gordon, the new edition of the relapse prevention book contains chapters that are matched with content area covered in the revised assessment book. The same authors were invited to provide both the assessment and relapse prevention chapters, so as to enhance congruence of coverage and cross-referenced materials.

A second change from the previous edition is the greater breadth of coverage of the addictive behaviors. The revised edition has expanded beyond the "traditional" addictions (e.g., alcohol, opiates, cocaine, marijuana, tobacco) and other "consumptive" addictions such as obesity/eating disorders, and includes a number of new drug classes (e.g., methamphetamine, "club drugs," hallucinogens, inhalants, and steroids) and other non-substance-related addictive behaviors, including gambling disorders, sexual offending, and sexually risky behaviors. The inclusion of these "nontraditional" addictions is consistent with broadened working definitions of addictive behaviors used in this edition. A new chapter also discusses the issue of cultural relevance and sensitivity in the process of assessment when working with different ethnic populations.

A third difference between the previous and current editions is found in the chapter organization. In the original book, three chapters that dealt with biological, cognitive, and behavioral factors were devoted to each addictive behavior. In the current edition there is only one chapter per addictive behavior, each of which incorporates and integrates the associated biological, cognitive, and behavioral factors. Further, each chapter also uses a heuristic model of relapse precipitants, developed by Saul Shiffman, as a means of organizing information. This model focuses on three levels of precipitants based on their proximity in time to and presumed influence on relapse. These include relatively stable distal factors, fluctuating intermediate variables, and proximal factors found within high-risk relapse situations. Factors at each level for each of the covered addictive behaviors are presented and their relationship to one another and to relapse is discussed.

A final difference between the two editions is the inclusion of suggested instruments to assess each of the addictive behaviors. As clinicians and researchers, it is often frustrating to read a discussion about important constructs to assess but not know what measures are available to assist in this process. Our goal was to minimize this frustration by making readers aware of such measures.

Addictive behaviors are complex disorders and relapse is a complex process. The chapters in this volume focus on the application of the heuristic framework that the recently revised model of relapse (Witkiewitz & Marlatt, 2004) provides for the assessment of addictive behaviors. This model incorporates and elaborates on the dynamic interplay of factors from the biopsychosocial model, from distal to proximal. Each chapter provides both a general overview of the assessment issues and process with a particular addictive behavior, and more specific information about measures that have been developed to assess different aspects of the biopsychosocial model as related to relapse prevention. The goal is to provide a companion volume that interfaces with the application of relapse prevention techniques outlined in the revised *Relapse Prevention*. Used together, these books will provide information to conduct a targeted assessment of relapse risk factors for a given addictive behavior and to develop an appropriate individualized treatment plan meant to prevent relapse from occurring and to minimize harm if relapse does occur.

We would like to conclude by extending our sincere thanks and gratitude to our many colleagues who have contributed in important ways to the material presented in this book. First and foremost, we would like to thank the authors who contributed their time and efforts in writing chapters for our two books. We are delighted that we were able to include writings by the leading contributors and experts in each of the topic areas. As such, we feel we have included authors who are all at the "cutting edge" of their respective fields of expertise. We would also like to extend our sincere thanks and gratitude to two of our graduate students here at the University of Washington, Katie Witkiewitz and Ursula Whiteside, who provided extensive reviews and editorial suggestions for all chapters. They also provided us with a "motivational intervention" to move us from the "contemplation" to the "action" stage of behavior change—were it not for them, it might have taken yet another decade for us to complete these books! Thanks, too, to The Guilford Press for its continued support of our work, with special gratitude extended to our editor, Jim Nageotte, and to our production editor, Jeannie Tang. It has been a long haul and they have been with us all the way.

REFERENCES

Marlatt, G. A., & Donovan, D. M. (Eds.). (2005). *Relapse prevention: Maintenance strategies in the treatment of addictive behaviors* (2nd ed.). New York: Guilford Press.

Witkiewitz, K., & Marlatt, G. A. (2004). Relapse prevention for alcohol and drug problems: That was zen, this is Tao. *American Psychologist, 59*(4), 224–235.

Contents

CHAPTER 1

Assessment of Addictive Behaviors for Relapse Prevention

DENNIS M. DONOVAN

Over a decade and a half ago the introductory chapter for the first edition of this book dealt with the then "emergent" biopsychosocial model of addictive behaviors and its implications for their assessment (Donovan, 1988; Donovan & Marlatt, 1988). While this model had its early proponents (Ewing, 1977, 1980; Galizio & Maisto, 1985; Pattison, 1980; Spittle, 1982; Wallace, 1989, 1993; Zucker & Gomberg, 1986), it had not yet assumed a prominent role in conceptualizations of addictive behaviors or their treatment. The theoretical and clinical addictions landscape was filled with a number of single-factor models that promoted a particular theoretical orientation or clinical approach, often with little or no collaboration or interaction across disciplines or across proponents of differing models (Donovan & Marlatt, 1993; Siegler, Osmond, & Newell, 1968). However, it was becoming increasingly clear that no single approach was sufficient in and of itself to explain or ameliorate addictive behaviors, and that integrative models held the greatest likelihood of more effectively preventing relapse (Llorente, Fernandez, & Gutierrez, 2000). As Wallace (1993) noted, neither a naive disease model nor a naive behavioral concept (the most prominent models of the time) can explain addictive behaviors fully. Rather, multidimensional, interactive, biopsychosocial models are necessary for continued progress in understanding and altering these disorders. As Moos (2003), reflecting on advances made in the field of addictions over the past 30 years, recently stated:

> We have formulated conceptual models, measured key constructs, examined salient theoretical issues, and made substantial progress in understanding the ebb and flow of addictive disorders. An integrated biopsychosocial orientation and a theoretical paradigm of evaluation research have supplanted earlier adherence to

an oversimplified biomedical model and reliance on a restrictive methodological approach to treatment evaluation. And yet, in an ironic way, more remains to be done than before, in part because of our increased knowledge and in part because of new clinical perspectives and treatment procedures and the evolving social context in which we ply our trade. (p. 3)

This represents the current context in which the assessment of addictive behaviors must be viewed and understood.

Consistent with Moos's perspective, Shaffer (1997) has also suggested that addictions is yet an emerging scientific field in its relative developmental infancy and is in need of further conceptual clarity. Explanatory models are developed in order to provide a theoretical framework within which to explain the etiology, natural history, and consequences of a disorder (Meyer & Babor, 1989). The biopsychosocial model, an integrative model, which posits that addictive behaviors are complex disorders multiply determined through biological, cognitive, psychological, and sociocultural processes, can provide such needed clarity to the field.

There has been considerable progress since the first edition of this book appeared (Donovan & Marlatt, 1988). The biopsychosocial model is no longer "emergent"; rather, it has emerged. There is evidence of its application in research and practice in smoking behavior, alcohol and drug dependence, eating disorders, gambling, and sexual addictions. There is a better understanding of the biological, psychological, and sociocultural contributors to the addiction process. There has been continued development of an interdisciplinary approach to such addictive behaviors, with the realization that addictions are multiply determined and require a range of expertise to address them. This latter point is exemplified by the recent trend within the National Institutes of Health (NIH) promoting "transinstitute" research; that is, researchers who previously had traditionally worked within the "boundaries" of one of NIH's institutes that best reflected their expertise have crossed over these institute boundaries to work collaboratively on a common problem. An example of this was a recently convened NIH Special Emphasis Review Group that I chaired in response to a transinstitute request for applications (RFA), entitled "Maintenance of Long-Term Behavior Change." It was particularly gratifying to see researchers, both applicants and reviewers, from different academic disciplines, and with particular "institute identities," realize that they shared common behavioral principles and approaches to prevent relapse across a wide variety of apparently disparate behaviors such as maintaining a "five-a-day" fruit–vegetable diet; using sunscreen; continuing a regular exercise regimen; stopping tobacco, alcohol, and illicit drug use; and refraining from sexual behaviors having a high risk for HIV infection. Clearly, the reviewers came away with a new appreciation of what researchers from other disciplines have to offer in dealing with addictive behaviors and behavioral health issues.

Despite the many advances that have been made in the area of addictive behaviors over the past decade and a half, there is considerable room for continued improvement. This point was underscored recently by a report from the Centers for Disease Control and Prevention (CDC) that focused on "actual causes" of death in the United States (Mokdad, Marks, Stroup, & Gerberding, 2004). This term refers to major external (nongenetic) factors that contribute to death. The focus was on those categories of causes of death that are preventable. In most cases these actual causes reflect modifiable risk factors related to lifestyle patterns and their associated behaviors. Five of the nine most common actual causes of death in 2000 were addictive behaviors that are covered in this book and in the second edition of *Relapse Prevention* (Marlatt & Donovan, 2005). The top three most common actual causes of death were the result of tobacco use (435,000, 18.1% of total U.S. deaths), poor diet and physical inactivity (400,000 deaths, 16.6%), and alcohol consumption (85,000 deaths, 3.5%). Also among the top nine causes of death were risky sexual behaviors (20,000 deaths) and use of illicit drugs (17,000 deaths). Furthermore, it was projected that if the current rates continue, actual deaths attributable to poor diet and physical inactivity will surpass those attributable to smoking.

The public health implications of such findings are clear (Mokdad et al., 2004; Tucker, Donovan, & Marlatt, 1999): There is a continued need for prevention efforts targeting these behaviors and lifestyles. The rates of such behaviors have remained relatively high despite efforts at prevention, and most have high rates of relapse. Given this, it is important to develop efficacious treatments that can help individuals change these addictive behaviors and lifestyles, and assist them in maintaining long-term behavior change and preventing relapse.

The purpose of this chapter is to provide updated information on the biopsychosocial model of additive behaviors and its component factors as they relate to relapse and interventions aimed at preventing relapse. This is done within the context of this model's application to the assessment process that serves as a prelude to and guide for clinical interventions. It also provides an overview of assessment issues in the context of relapse prevention (see Marlatt & Donovan, 2005). More detailed information on specific approaches to and instruments to use in the assessment process can be found elsewhere (e.g., Carroll & Rounsaville, 2002; Donovan, 1998, 2003a, 2003c; Rotgers, 2002), as well as in the remaining chapters of this book.

WORKING DEFINITION OF ADDICTIVE BEHAVIORS

An important first step in dealing with relapse is to have a common concept of what constitutes an "addictive behavior." In this volume and in the second edition of *Relapse Prevention* (Marlatt & Donovan, 2005), this term is applied to a wide range of behaviors, including what are often traditionally thought of as addictions: dependence on alcohol, opiates, cocaine, and other stimulants, such as methamphetamines, marijuana, club drugs, and tobacco.

In addition to other shared features such as the potential for the development of tolerance and dependence, and potential underlying genetic and neurochemical underpinnings, these behaviors have often been viewed as similar because they involve ingestion of some type of substance. Consistent with this, they have been grouped together as substance use disorders in diagnostic systems such as the fourth edition of the *Diagnostic and Statistical Manual for Mental Disorders* (DSM-IV; American Psychiatric Association, 1994). In the developing revisions of the DSM system, these behaviors are categorized as forms of chemical abuse or dependence (DSM-IV-TR; American Psychiatric Association, 2000). However, we have also included non-chemical-related behaviors, including gambling, eating disorders, and sexual behavior, in our working conceptualization of additive behaviors.

The inclusion of these "nontraditional" addictions, which were not included in the original edition of this book, is consistent with broadened working definitions of addictive behaviors provided by Goodman (1990) and Smith and Seymour (2004), and their similarities with chemical dependencies (Lesieur & Blume, 1993; Schneider & Irons, 2001). Both of these definitions appear to apply comparably to substance-related and non-substance-related addictive behaviors. Goodman (1990) has proposed that addiction is a process whereby a behavior that can function both to produce pleasure and to provide escape from internal discomfort is employed in a pattern characterized by (1) recurrent failure to control the behavior and (2) continuation of the behavior despite significant negative consequences. To this definition Smith and Seymour (2004) add a third element: compulsive use or engagement in the behavior. They further suggest that all addictive behaviors attempt to meet one or more of three motives: (1) psychic rewards, or achieving a desired change in moods; (2) recreational rewards, or increasing sociability and having fun with others in mutually enjoyable activities; and (3) instrumental achievement rewards, or attempts to enhance performance with accompanying increases in a sense of success, mastery, and well-being. These broader definitions of addictive behaviors are similar to that previously used by Donovan and are consistent with the view inherent in a biopsychosocial conceptualization of addictive behaviors (Donovan, 1988).

While there are a number of common features across addictive behaviors (e.g., rates, timing, and precipitants of relapse) (Bradley, 1990; Goodman, 1990; Hayletta, Stephenson, & Lefevera, 2004; Marks, 1990; Patkar et al., 2004), each also has features that are unique to the particular substance or problem area. In order to prevent or to treat such disorders successfully, it is necessary to incorporate these multiple factors into a unified approach. If progress is to be made, it will be necessary to begin bridging the gap across addictions and disciplines, with an effort to work collaboratively and interactively toward a common goal, namely, the prevention and treatment of addictive behaviors. It is of note that nearly 35 years ago, Hunt, Barnett, and Branch (1971), in first bringing attention to the similar time–course and rates of relapse across alcohol, opiates, and tobacco, indicated then that those who work in the different areas of addiction might benefit from more interaction. This recommendation has contributed to the cross-addictions and interdisciplinary work that has been generated by the biopsychosocial model and relapse prevention. Furthermore, it will be necessary to bridge the gap between researchers and clinicians to develop and implement effective treatments in community-based clinical practice (Lamb, Greenlick, & McCarty, 1998).

RELAPSE PREVENTION: AN OVERVIEW

Before discussing assessment issues related to relapse in addictive behaviors, it is important to have a working knowledge of relapse prevention, its theoretical underpinnings, and its clinical application. This information is a prerequisite for identifying relevant assessment domains. An important component of rehabilitation and treatment planning with individuals attempting to change an addictive behavior is relapse prevention. Staying clean and sober or refraining from engaging in a particular behavior is one of the biggest challenges that individuals face after completing a treatment program or self-change. Although addictive behaviors represent a complex of genetic, physiological, sociocultural, and psychological components, and there are a number of models of the relapse process that give differing weights to biomedical and cognitive-behavioral constructs (Connors, Maisto, & Donovan, 1996; Donovan & Chaney, 1985), relapse prevention can be conceptualized as essentially a problem-solving process and a reorientation of life attitudes and values (Giannetti, 1993). Marlatt and colleagues (Larimer, Palmer, & Marlatt, 1999; Marlatt & Donovan, 1981; Marlatt & George, 1984; Marlatt & Gordon, 1980, 1985) have presented a model of relapse that has stimulated both clinical research and application.

"Relapse prevention" is a generic term that refers to a wide range of cognitive and behavioral strategies designed to prevent relapse in the area of addictive behaviors and that focus on the crucial issues of helping people who are changing their behavior to maintain the gains they have made during the course of treatment or self-change. The goals of relapse prevention strategies are twofold: (1) to prevent an initial lapse back to drinking, drug use, or other addictive behavior and (2) to prevent an initial lapse, if it does occur, from becoming more serious and prolonged by minimizing the physical, psychological, and social consequences of the return to use.

While the relative emphasis will vary depending on the program, a number of common elements are involved in relapse prevention. First, it is important to educate the individual about the relapse process. Despite having relapsed previously, many individuals are not familiar with the range of factors that trigger their actions; they feel that their relapses just come "out of the blue" in a very unpredictable way. A goal is to educate them about a number of predictable events that lead to relapse and the feelings that come after a relapse.

A second important part of the prevention process is to help the patient identify high-risk situations—thoughts, feelings, people, places, and social activities that have been repeatedly associated with past alcohol and drug use. Over time, through their repeated pairing with drinking, drug use, or a particular addictive behavior, these situations may come to serve as classically conditioned stimuli. Exposure to these internal cues (e.g., thoughts, feelings, physical states) or external stimuli (e.g., people, places, activities) may threaten one's abstinence or moderation goals, an increased experience of craving and selectively thinking about the "good old days," when one was able to use or drink without negative consequences. The most common situations related to relapse, across both individuals and addictive behaviors, include (1) peer or social pressure to use, either directly or more subtly by returning to the "old haunts" where they used to drink or use and are in ongoing social contact with their former using friends or drinking buddies; (2) a desire for social inclusion and the experience of positive interpersonal benefits of the behavior; (3) negative emotional states that include depression, loneliness, boredom, and lack of time structure; and (4) anger and resentment that typically result from some form of interpersonal conflict.

Not all individuals attempting to change an addictive behavior are subject to relapse, and all who do relapse do not have the same precipitants; that is, not all people will experience the same situations as equally risky. Thus, a crucial step in the treatment process is to help the individual identify personal "warning signs." These may include cognitive warning signs, such as "euphoric recall" (e.g., thoughts about the positive aspects of past use), justifications for relapse (e.g., "I owe myself a drink" or "One won't hurt"), dreams about drugs that lead to craving upon awakening, and rationalizations for discontinuing recovery activities. A second area includes emotional warning signs, such as positive emotional states (e.g., excitement, arousal, celebration), as well as negative affective states (e.g., depression, loneliness, anger, boredom). A third area represents behavioral warning signs, such as compulsive or impulsive behaviors previously related to drinking, drug use, or another addictive behavior, spending time with drug users or drinkers, and returning to secondary drug use (e.g., "Cocaine is my problem, so it's OK if I drink or smoke dope"). The occurrence of any of these warning signs may increase the risk of relapse. One way to identify these personal warning signs is to review past relapses, since specific relapse patterns often repeat themselves.

Once these areas of high risk for relapse have been identified, attention is turned to helping individuals develop practical ways to deal with such situations. This involves developing and practicing behavioral and cognitive coping strategies. While a goal may be to help the individual develop general coping skills, the more immediate goal is to help him or her learn skills that are related directly to avoiding or reducing alcohol-, drug-, or specific addictive behavior-related risks. These include ways to deal with craving and urges to drink, use, or engage in an addictive behavior; to manage thoughts about the addictive behavior; to develop problem-solving skills that can be applied to a range of potentially risky situations; to refuse offers to drink, use drugs, or engage in the behavior; to develop an emergency plan to minimize the chance of relapse if confronted by a risky situation; to anticipate and plan how to handle a slip if it does occur; to reframe relapse as not being the "end of the world" if it does occur; and to learn that a number of emotions (e.g., anger, disappointment, depression, embarrassment) are likely to occur following a relapse, that these are predictable, and that the individual can cope with them.

Early on in the skills training process, the focus should probably be concrete; as the person develops greater skill and confidence, a shift might be made from more behaviorally oriented approaches toward more cognitive ones. An important clinical consideration in the skills training process is to provide ample opportunity for the individual to learn these new skills, not just be exposed to them; that is, enough practice and behavioral rehearsal should be provided, through modeling, role playing, feedback, and homework, to ensure that patients have acquired the new skill and can actually apply it. The goal of such interventions is not only to give individuals specific skills to increase their coping abilities and be able to use alternative behaviors or thoughts that can help them either avoid or confront risky situations, but also to provide an increased sense of confidence, self-efficacy, and personal control.

There has been an increased focus on the use of empirically supported interventions in the addictions (McCrady, 2000). Relapse prevention and coping skills training, its major intervention approach, have demonstrated efficacy with a number of addictive behaviors (Carroll, 1996; Donovan, 2003b; Dowden, Antonowicz, & Andrews, 2003; Irvin, Bowers, Dunn, & Wang, 1999; Miller & Wilbourne, 2002; Monti, Gulliver, & Myers, 1994; Witkiewitz & Marlatt, 2004). Relapse prevention approaches are highly flexible and can be adapted to a range of treatment settings and a variety of addictive behaviors. They can be incorporated into inpatient, outpatient, or aftercare programs; delivered in individual, group therapy (Graham, Annis, Brett, & Venesoen, 1996), or couple formats (McCrady, 1993); integrated with motivational enhancement approaches (Baer, Kivlahan, & Donovan, 1999; Rohsenow et al., 2004); and combined with medications (Annis, 1991; Feeney, Young, Connor, Tucker, & McPherson, 2002; O'Malley et al., 1992; Schmitz, Stotts, Rhoades, & Grabowski, 2001). An advantage of relapse prevention is that it can be incorporated into programs with a variety of different clinical and philosophical approaches, including those with moderation goals (Larimer & Marlatt, 1990). It also should be incorporated into a broader context of change in the person toward a more balanced overall lifestyle. Individuals are also encouraged to develop peer and support groups that share the goal of a clean and sober lifestyle. Together, the increased support for being clean and sober and the availability of specific coping skills to deal with high-risk situations as they arise will reduce the chances of relapse.

From the standpoint of assessment, the task is to identify the potential precipitants of relapse and the individual's unique high-risk situations, and to determine the deficits and strengths in coping skills, the degree of self-efficacy, and the expectancies the person has about the anticipated outcomes from engaging in the addictive behaviors.

ASSESSMENT ISSUES
IN THE CONTEXT OF RELAPSE PREVENTION

The model of relapse developed by Marlatt and colleagues (Cummings, Gordon, & Marlatt, 1980; Larimer et al., 1999; Marlatt & Gordon, 1985) has provided an important heuristic framework within which to describe, understand, and, potentially, predict and prevent relapse. It has also stimulated a great deal of clinical research and the integration of relapse prevention into clinical programs for the treatment of addictive behaviors. An important component in this model is the assessment of those characteristics of the individual and of the situational context that would allow the prediction and classification of a relapse episode after a period of abstinence. This section provides a brief overview of issues involved in the process of assessment related to the classification and prediction of relapse (Donovan, 1996a).

Operational Definitions of "Lapse" and "Relapse"

Addictive behaviors are often described as chronic relapsing disorders. They are also characterized by high rates of relapse. In reviewing the relapse process and relapse prevention approaches, Einstein (1994) listed a number of critical issues that were as yet unresolved, the most prominent of which was the way "relapse" is defined: "At what point is a return to a defined pattern of single/ multiple substance use RELAPSE as well as what are the coping/adaptational and treatment implications of the definition(s)?" (p. 409). At first glance, it would seem that defining relapse would be straightforward: The person has either resumed or not resumed drinking or drug use, or is once again engaging in the addictive behavior following a period of abstinence or acceptable behavior. However, it is not as simple as it appears. Clearly, the term "relapse" connotes or denotes meaning that extends well beyond a simple dichotomous outcome. As the subtitle of an article by Miller (1996) suggests, there are at least "fifty ways to leave the wagon."

The complexity of this issue is demonstrated by the multiple meanings connoted by the term "relapse" in the literature. Litman, Stapleton, Oppenheim, Peleg, and Jackson (1983), Miller (1996), Saunders and Allsop (1987, 1989), Chiauzzi (1991), Wilson (1992), and others have presented a number of differing definitions. Miller (1996) suggests at least three possible meanings. These include the descriptive presence or absence of the behavior, the behavior exceeding a certain threshold, and a judgment about the behavior relative to standards of what is acceptable either to the individual or to society more broadly. Other definitions have included the following: (1) a process that gradually and insidiously leads to the initiation of substance use or engagement in the behavior after a period of abstinence (e.g., "apparently irrelevant decisions"); (2) a discrete event that is defined by the return to an initial use of the substance (e.g., a "lapse"); (3) a return to the same intensity of substance use (e.g., a "relapse"; Marlatt has made a conceptual distinction between a "lapse," which involves the initial use of a substance after a period of abstinence, and a "relapse," which involves continued use after this initial slip); (4) daily use for a specific number of sequential days (e.g., "hazardous drinking"); and (5) a consequence of substance use resulting in the need for subsequent treatment (e.g., "recidivism") (Donovan, 1996a). There have also been a number of multidimensional composite indices of outcome/relapse that take into account both return to limited versus more extensive engagement in the addictive behavior and the presence versus absence of related problems (e.g., Zweben & Cisler, 2003). Such multidimensional measures, which go beyond the binary classification of abstinence–relapse, are well suited for evaluating program outcomes in general and, more specifically, harm reduction programs that have nonabstinence goals (Marlatt & Witkiewitz, 2002).

Clearly, the definition arrived at in response to the question "What is relapse?" has a number of possible implications. Two implications, for instance, include (1) different estimates of the rates of relapse based on different definitions, and (2) different conceptual and methodological approaches involved in assessment and prediction models depending on the definition of relapse. Maisto, Pollock, Cornelius, Lynch, and Martin (2003) investigated the impact of differing definitions among adolescents following treatment. They used four definitions of relapse: (1) at least 1 day of drinking any amount after at least 4 consecutive days of abstinence; (2) at least 1 heavy (five standard drinks for boys, four for girls) drinking day after 4 abstinent days; (3) at least 1 day of drinking any amount, with associated problems, after 4 abstinent days; and (4) at least 1 heavy drinking day, with associated problems, following 4 abstinent days. They found that both the rates of relapse and the "time to relapse" varied greatly depending on the definition used. The relapse rates ranged from 50.0% to 73.9% of the sample, and the time to relapse ranged from 26 to 90 days. The different definitions of relapse during the 6-month posttreatment period also predicted different aspects of outcome during the 7- to 12-month period. The presence of any drinking (definitions 1 and 3) during the first 6 months posttreatment was predictive of having a current substance use disorder diagnosis during the subsequent 6 months. On the other hand, the definitions involving heavy drinking (2 and 4) were predictive of the average number of drinking occasions per month and drinks per drinking day.

The findings relative to differing lengths of time to relapse raise an important point both conceptually and methodologically. In the first edition of this book, Curry, Marlatt, Peterson, and Lutton (1988) described the application of survival analysis to the study of relapse. This procedure determines the length of time to a relapse, however defined, and the percent of a sample that are survivors at a given point in time. If one meets the criterion for relapse, one is no longer considered a survivor. A limitation in this approach is that it does not map onto the naturalistic course of addictive behaviors and the relapse process. Individuals move into and out of periods of use and abstinence, often evidencing a gradual change in use or behavior before the emergence of a more stable use or abstinence pattern. However, survival analysis is based on the use of a dichotomous outcome (relapsed or not). More recent approaches allow one to look at the occurrence of multiple events, such as the time to first use, the time to and length of the subsequent period of abstinence, and the time to a subsequent return to use (Wang, Winchell, McCormick, Nevius, & O'Neill, 2002). It is also possible to look at the predictors of each of theses events. Multiple event analyses can accommodate any definition of relapse.

The definition of relapse also has an impact on the conceptual and clinical approach to assessment. If relapse is viewed as a discrete event, then a static assessment model can be used; that is, information collected at some baseline point, incorporating information concerning prior relapse events and other drinking, social, psychological, and demographic information, can be used and should be sufficient for the prediction of relapse in the future. This approach has been used fairly frequently in treatment outcome studies in which an attempt is made to predict posttreatment status from intake information (Miller, Westerberg, Harris, & Tonigan, 1996). Alternatively, while still viewing relapse as a discrete event and employing a static assessment model, it might be argued that focusing on the immediate precipitants of that event to "capture the moment" of a relapse would be more appropriate than historical information collected at baseline. This has been the focus of studies that attempt to determine the precipitants that may be predictive of a lapse or relapse versus a a high-risk situation that is handled well (Moser & Annis, 1996). As might be expected, Miller et al. (1996) found that more proximal variables accounted for a substantially greater amount of variance in subsequent outcome than the more distal intake variables. Also, not surprisingly, the availability and use of adequate coping skills and higher levels of self-efficacy have been associated with preventing a crisis situation from turning into a relapse (Miller et al., 1996; Moser & Annis, 1996; Noone, Dua, & Markham, 1999; Vielva & Iraurgi, 2001).

Marlatt and Gordon (1985) and others (Litman, 1986) have described relapse not as a discrete event, but rather as the return to drinking, substance use, or other addictive behaviors at the end point of a process or the culmination of a series of related events. Within this framework, assessment models need to be dynamic, not static, in order to assess temporal variations in and among important elements of the process (Donovan, 1996a; Hufford, Witkiewitz, Shields, Kodya, & Caruso, 2003; Shiffman et al., 2000; Witkiewitz & Marlatt, 2004). Assessments must be taken periodically with some degree of regularity across time to capture the process as it unfolds. Consistent with this, Shiffman and colleagues (2000) found that while baseline levels of self-efficacy predicted an initial return to smoking, day-to-day fluctuations in strength of self-efficacy predicted the transition of an initial lapse into relapse.

A number of recent developments in the use of telephone-based, interactive voice response technology (Mundt, Bohn, King, & Hartley, 2002) has allowed the assessment of variables more proximal to the occurrence of a relapse, while ecological momentary assessments based on the use of palm-sized computers allow nearly real-time assessment of potential relapse precipitants in high-risk situations (Collins et al., 1998; O'Connell et al., 1998). Ecological momentary assessment procedures have been used to determine the precipitants of and reaction to relapse crises and actual lapses in smoking, drinking, and dieting (Carels, Douglass, Cacciapaglia, & O'Brien, 2004; Collins et al., 1998; Stone et al., 1998). Clearly, being able to assess adequately and accurately the relative strength of such variables and their dynamic interactions across time is quite challenging; however, it may be necessary in order to gain a clearer picture of the relapse process as it plays out across time and in the moment of crisis (Hufford et al., 2003; Witkiewitz & Marlatt, 2004).

Prospective versus Retrospective Assessment of Relapse Precipitants

An issue related to and confounded with the timing of assessments in the relapse process is the degree to which prospective versus retrospective approaches are used to identify relapse precipitants. The use of ecological momentary assessment techniques provides an opportunity for prospective assessment, in that ratings of possible precipitants are measured in near real time sometime prior to exposure to a high-risk situation. Similarly, such momentary assessments also can provide an opportunity to examine moods and cognitions shortly after a relapse, allowing an investigation of the abstinence violation effect (AVE; Shiffman, Hickcox, et al., 1996).

While providing a better perspective on the relationship between precipitants and relapse, ecological momentary assessments are beyond the scope of many, if not most, clinical programs.

As a result, most research in this area has been retrospective (McKay, 1999). Typically, individuals are asked at some point following treatment completion to provide a retrospective assessment of the events and emotions that occurred prior to a lapse episode during the follow-up period. There are a number of concerns about relying on such retrospective self-reports of relapse episodes, their precipitants, and their aftereffects (McKay, Rutherford, & Alterman, 1996). The first is a possible lack of awareness or insight into the reasons for a relapse episode. Furthermore, the acute effects of alcohol and drugs, as well as the "rush" that accompanies the recurrence of other addictive behaviors, may lead to reduced information processing, narrowed perception of most immediate internal and external stimuli, and distorted recollection of events. Shiffman and colleagues (1997) evaluated the correspondence between information about the same smoking lapse collected by ecological momentary assessment and retrospective recall. They focused on the recall of mood, activity, triggers or precipitants, and the AVE associated with the lapse. The momentary assessment of the relapse was recorded in an average of less than 10 minutes following its occurrence; the retrospective recall occurred approximately 3 months after the episode. Few individuals (23%) provided the correct date of the lapse, with recalled estimates about 14 days off the date. Similarly, there was a high rate of discrepancy between the momentary assessment and retrospective recall concerning the factors associated with the lapse. The average correlations between the two approaches in the measurement of the domains of mood, activities, triggers/precipitants, and AVE were .36, .24, .28, and .34, respectively. The lack of correspondence was also found on specific elements thought to be theoretical components of the relapse process: only 45% agreement on coping, and 32% agreement in the recall of the single most important trigger. Recalled mood showed only modest correspondence with real-time data. Although the focus of the study was on smoking lapse, alcohol consumption was the most accurately recalled variable, with 83% of participants correctly recalling drinking. These discrepancies occurred despite the fact that the participants reported having relatively high confidence in their ability to recall their prior lapse episode.

Of note, Shiffman et al. (1997) found that neither the degree of confidence in their participants' recall nor the length of the recall interval was related to accuracy. This is in contrast to findings by McKay et al. (1996) with cocaine abusers. These investigators found that reports of the experience of unpleasant affect, positive experiences, interpersonal problems, and self-help group involvement prior to relapse did not appear to be influenced to a significant degree by the amount of time that elapsed between the relapse and interview. As such, McKay et al. suggest that there is little need for concern about time effects when reports of experiences in these areas are used in clinical work, such as in relapse prevention. On the other hand, clinicians and researchers should take into consideration that the cocaine abusers tended to report more social pressure to use drugs and sensation seeking prior to relapse when a longer period of time elapsed between the relapse and interview.

Potential Attributional Biases in Retrospective Assessment

There are a number of other potential difficulties and attributional biases inherent in retrospective assessment (McKay, O'Farrell, Maisto, Connors, & Funder, 1989; Walton, Castro, & Barrington, 1994). Each of these factors may contribute independently or interactively to an inaccurate identification of "true" relapse precipitants (e.g., "false positives"). These factors include (1) a tendency to attribute failure to external factors and success to internal factors; (2) a tendency to "catastrophize" or "cry in one's beer" when intoxicated, which may lead to a distorted attribution of events to internal states and negative emotions; (3) coloring by the emotional overlay of depression, guilt, and other emotional reactions hypothesized to accompany the AVE associated with relapse; and (4) based on the original conceptualization of the AVE, a tendency to blame oneself (personal attribution) as the cause of relapse. Based on these possibilities, different mechanisms operative in retrospective assessments may contribute to incorrectly attributing relapse precipitants to either external or internal factors, depending upon the circumstances and the context in which the person finds him- or herself.

The influence of such factors was noted in the study of momentary versus retrospective assessment of precipitants to smoking lapses by Shiffman and colleagues (1997) described earlier. They reasoned that since one's experiences after an event can color recall concerning it, participants' smoking status at the time of the follow-up interview might bias their recall of their relapses. Furthermore, they assumed that AVE variables might be particularly vulnerable to recall bias given that smoking experience after an initial lapse is hypothesized to affect attributions for the lapse episode. For AVE assessment, participants were asked to characterize their reactions to the lapse, reporting whether they felt encouraged, their confidence to continue abstaining, whether they felt guilty, whether the episode was their fault, and whether they felt like giving up their efforts to abstain. They also rated their attributions for the cause of the episode on three dimensions: internality (outside me–inside me), controllability (controllable–uncontrollable), and stability (changing–unchanging). They examined the relationship between recall bias (i.e., retrospective recall vs. momentarily recorded AVE values) and smoking status at recall. In their retrospective recall, participants overestimated their negative affect and the number of cigarettes they had smoked during the lapse. Furthermore, their recall was influenced by current smoking status. As hypothesized, participants who had more smoking days exaggerated in retrospect how much the lapse had made them feel like giving up their quit effort; however, it was not related to bias of recall for any other individual AVE items. The findings suggest caution in the use of recall in research and intervention.

Single versus Multiple versus Interactive Precipitants

Another issue is whether one is attempting to determine the influence of a single precipitant or a set of multiple and interactive precipitants as factors in relapse. As originally developed, Marlatt's relapse taxonomy system (1996b) only allowed one precipitant to be identified for a lapse, namely, that which was most proximal in time to the lapse could be identified as *the* precipitant for the episode. Marlatt's broader model of the relapse process (Marlatt & Gordon, 1985), however, suggests that the relative risk of relapse is a function of the individual's immediate and recent emotional state; the social and interpersonal context of the situations to which the person is exposed; the availability and effectiveness of, and access to emotional and/or cognitive coping strategies; and the individual's sense of personal efficacy or confidence not to drink, use drugs, or engage in an addictive behavior in those situations appraised as high risk.

The more limited taxonomic approach is consistent with a reductionistic tendency to look at a relapse episode in an attempt to "capture the moment," by focusing on what happened immediately prior to the event. This is consistent with the perspective of the ecological assessment process. However, focusing only on factors immediately prior to a relapse is likely to be insufficient. It may lead to a false assumption that those variables (or in Marlatt's original taxonomy, the one variable) immediately preceding a relapse, because of their temporal proximity and relative influence, are the "real reasons," without looking beyond the immediate time frame at other potential contributing factors suggested in the model of the relapse process. Conversely, it further may lead to the erroneous conclusion that other variables more distant in time exert little or no influence on the occurrence of a relapse (e.g., "false negatives"). The need to take contextual factors into account is consistent with the use of retrospective assessment and the use of a functional behavioral analysis to identify both precipitants and consequences of the relapse.

Shiffman (1989) has suggested that multiple layers of assessment may be needed to predict relapse, and that one cannot focus only on a single level exclusive of the others. This suggests the use of a multivariate, multidimensional assessment process that takes into account a variety of stages and levels of variables (Donovan, 1988). An expanded model of Marlatt's relapse precipitant taxonomy has been recommended (Donovan, 1996b; Stout, Longabaugh, & Rubin, 1996). It would allow the inclusion of multiple variables exerting differential levels of influence across a range of time varying in proximity to the relapse event. A number of these recommendations have been incorporated recently into a reconceptualized cognitive-behavioral model of relapse that focuses on the dynamic interactions between multiple risk factors and situational determinants (Witkiewitz & Marlatt, 2004). When such an expanded model of assessment is used, it appears that multiple reasons, in combination and interaction, not just one, are rated by subjects as being important in the relapse process (Heather & Stallard, 1989; Miller et al., 1996; Zywiak, Connors, Maisto, & Westerberg, 1996).

Static versus Continuous Assessment

The previous discussion addresses in part another issue, namely, the appropriateness of a static versus continuous model of assessment. Given the multiple and interactive nature of these risk factors and situational determinants, and their likely fluctuation across both more distal and proximal time frames prior to a relapse, the ability to predict accurately a given relapse category without relatively continuous assessment is exceedingly difficult (Donovan, 1996a, 1996b; Marlatt, 1996a). This latter point was noted by Hodgins, el-Guebaly, and Armstrong (1995). In a prospective assessment condition, subjects were called weekly to provide mood ratings. For subjects in this condition who subsequently relapsed, the average length of time from the most recent assessment prior to the relapse episode was 2.4 days. Hodgins et al. noted that even this relatively short time frame may be too distant to capture adequately the rapidly fluctuating moods associated with relapse. Also, in the absence of both more proximal measures of the situation and other elements of the relapse model (coping skills, self-efficacy, etc.), it may be inappropriate to attempt to rely only on prior relapse episodes to predict subsequent relapses.

Clearly, it appears that a single baseline assessment at, for instance, the beginning or end of a treatment experience is likely to be insufficient to predict subsequent relapse. Rather, inherent in both Marlatt's definition of relapse as a process and in Shiffman's multivariate, multilevel model of precipitants is the need for periodic assessment across multiple domains. The assessment function will vary depending on where the individual is in the treatment/recovery process. At the point of treatment entry, the focus is on identifying individualized triggers/precipitants and high-risk situations to guide goal setting and treatment planning. During the course of treatment, the focus is on the acquisition of coping skills necessary to deal with these situations and the attendant self-efficacy that develops along with skills acquisition. Following treatment, the focus is on the degree to which the individual is confronted by high-risk situations, the degree of temptation experienced, the level of self-confidence and self-efficacy, and the frequency and nature of coping skills used. Periodic follow-up assessments may not only provide information about clients' clinical status but also may serve a therapeutic function that may help avert relapse or intervene more rapidly if a relapse has occurred (Breslin, Sobell, Sobell, Buchan, & Kwan, 1996; Stout, Rubin, Zwick, Zywiak, & Bellino, 1999).

Broad versus Specific Dimensions of Assessment

A final issue is the degree of specificity needed in the assessment process; that is, is it necessary to identify the individual's relapse precipitants with the degree of specificity found in Marlatt's original taxonomy versus surveying the broader context in which relapses occur? Marlatt's relapse taxonomy focuses on both broad dimensions of precipitants (e.g., interpersonal, intrapersonal) and much more specific precipitants within each of these dimensions (e.g., coping with interpersonal conflict–anger and/or frustration, coping with intrapersonal negative emotional states–anger and/or frustration). It is often assumed that the more specific the identified precipitant, the greater the utility in predicting future relapses. However, results from the Relapse Replication and Extension Project (RREP; Lowman, Allen, & Stout, 1996) suggest that the greater the specificity of the precipitants, the less reliable their classification (Longabaugh, Rubin, Stout, Zywiak, & Lowman, 1996).

A number of measures of relapse precipitants based on Marlatt's taxonomy, such as the Inventory of Drinking Situations (IDS; Annis, Graham, &

Davis, 1987), have been developed across a number addictive behaviors. Factor-analytic studies utilizing such self-report questionnaires, which involve relatively specific items reflecting relapse precipitants, have typically found a smaller number of broad categories of precipitants that accounted for the majority of the variance. For example, Litman et al. (1983) derived three factors from the Relapse Precipitants Inventory (RPI): unpleasant mood states (e.g., depression, anxiety, social anxiety), external events and euphoric states, and lessened cognitive vigilance. Similarly, both Cannon, Leeka, Patterson, and Baker (1990) and Isenhart (1991, 1993) found three primary factors for the IDS (Annis et al., 1987): negative affective states, positive affective states combined with social cues to drink, and attempts to test one's ability to control one's drinking.

Zywiak and colleagues have examined the dimensions of relapse precipitants using different assessment instruments in a number of samples of alcoholics. Zywiak et al. (1996) evaluated Marlatt's relapse taxonomy as assessed by the Reasons for Drinking Questionnaire (RFDQ). A factor analysis resulted in three factors, the first of which was characterized by negative emotions, including anger, depression, and anxiety. The second factor consisted of direct and indirect social pressure and positive emotions. The third factor consisted of physical withdrawal, craving, substance-related cues, and urges to drink. Each of the 13 categories in the Marlatt taxonomy loaded on one of the three factors. Zywiak et al. (2001) found a similar set of factors from the Relapse Questionnaire used in Project MATCH. Zywiak, Westerberg, Connors, and Maisto (2003), in a subsequent study in which participants were followed every 2 months for a year, examined the relationship of these three factors and subsequent relapses. They found that relapses were most likely to occur in the first 2 months, with comparable relapses occurring across the three reasons. Also, relapses due to craving and substance-related cues appeared to extinguish after the sixth month, while negative affect and social pressure relapses still occurred during months 7 through 12. If an individual had an initial relapse, there was a high risk for a subsequent relapse; however, there was no evidence that the subsequent relapse occurred within the same category of reasons as the initial episode. Negative affect relapses and craving–cued relapses were found to be more severe than social pressure relapses.

While Marlatt and colleagues (Cummings et al., 1980) have found considerable overlap across addictive behaviors, each has its own set of relatively specific relapse precipitants. As an example, Hodgins and el-Guebaly (2004) found that the two most highly endorsed reasons for relapse among pathological gamblers were optimism about winning and a need for money. Both positive and negative moods were related to gambling relapse, unlike substance abuse, in which relapses tend to be attributed to negative affect. Grilo, Shiffman, and Wing (1989) found that reasons for relapse among obese individuals with diabetes clustered into three groups: mealtime, low-arousal, and emotional upset situations. It is important to keep in mind that individuals with co-occurring psychiatric conditions may also have unique relapse precipitants that are related to the experience or exacerbation of their psychiatric disorder (Bradizza & Stasiewicz, 2003; Weiss, Najavits, & Greenfield, 1999). This population also presents unique challenges in assessment more generally (Carey & Correia, 1998). It has been recommended that treatment for individuals with co-occurring substance use and psychiatric disorders should include both general and substance-specific coping skills training as a means of reducing posttreatment substance use and improving the psychological functioning in this population (Moggi, Ouimette, Moos, & Finney, 1999).

DOMAINS OF ASSESSMENT

Shiffman (1989) presented a heuristic model of a multivariate, multilevel approach to assess potential relapse predictors. Three levels of assessment need to be considered in order to describe adequately and predict the likelihood of relapse. They differ along a continuum of time prior to a relapse episode and exert differing levels of influence on the individual and on the likelihood of relapse. The first level includes distal personal characteristics that are relatively long-standing, enduring, stable, and unchanging. The second level involves intermediate or background variables that fluctuate over time, but do so relatively gradually, and may somehow contribute to an increased probability of relapse. The third level involves very proximal precipitants that occur at or immediately prior to the lapse; these are relatively transient and occur within the context of a high-risk situation. These levels are comparable to those incorporated into the recent expansion of Marlatt's model of the relapse process and the dynamic interplay among factors from these levels (Witkiewitz & Marlatt, 2004). A category not mentioned by Shiffman (1989) but one that is important in a model that hypothesizes the probability of movement from lapse to relapse, includes transitional variables. These occur after an initial use of a substance or recurrence of an addictive behavior and either promote continued engagement in the behavior or lead to postlapse cessation, thus mediating the transition from lapse to relapse.

This heuristic assessment model is presented in Figure 1.1 (Donovan, 1996a) as a funnel to reflect the assumption that as one moves from the more distal factors, through the intermediate and proximal factors, to the point of a possible lapse, the influence of variables at each of these levels becomes less diffuse, more focused and intense, and narrowed or funneled more within the emergent situational context of the potential relapse setting. Table 1.1 presents variables within each of the assessment domains of this model. It is not clear in some cases where a variable fits best; furthermore, it is not clear that a variable falls into only one category, since there appear to be occasions in which there may be shifting across categories and interactions among variables in different categories. This reflects the clinical reality of multiple, interactive sets of precipitants contributing to relapse.

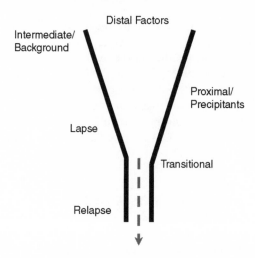

FIGURE 1.1. A heuristic framework for conceptualizing the levels of assessment involved in Shiffman's model of relapse predictors. From Donovan (1996a, p. 532). Copyright 1996 by Blackwell Publishing. Reprinted by permission.

TABLE 1.1. Assessment Domains Related to Relapse

Distal personal factors

- Family history of alcoholism
- "Type" of alcoholism
- Nature/severity of concurrent psychiatric disorders
- Nature/severity of concurrent substance use disorders
- Presence of cognitive impairment or reduced problem-solving abilities
- Severity of alcohol dependence
- Conditioned reactivity to alcohol-related cues

Proximal precipitating factors

- High-risk situations
- Cognitive vigilance and internal dialogue
- Emotional states
- Temptation-coping skills
- Situational response efficacy
- Conditioned cue reactivity
- Salience of expected/desired substance effects
- "Craving"
- Commitment to abstinence

Intermediate background factors

- Enduring life strain
- Everyday life problems
- Social and environmental supports
- Stress coping skills/anticipatory coping skills
- General sense of personal efficacy
- General expectancies concerning the effects of substance
- Motivation for self-improvement

Transitional factors

- Abstinence violation effect
  - Emotional states
  - Attributional tendencies
- Restorative coping skills
- Reaction of support system
- Commitment to return to abstinent state

Note. From Donovan (1996a, p. 533). Copyright 1996 by Blackwell Publishing. Reprinted by permission.

Distal Personal Factors

An important element in the prediction of behavior is what the individual brings into the situation, in his or her hereditary makeup, personal background characteristics, and behavioral competencies. Such distal personal background variables may lead to patterns of behavior that expose the individual to a greater risk of alcohol, drugs, or involvement in other addictive behaviors initially, to increased problems in these areas, and to subsequent relapse. These distal background variables develop through both genetic–biological factors and social learning processes.

One distal background variable that has a demonstrated impact on the acquisition of addictive behaviors and their subsequent course is family history. For example, there appears to be differential responsivity to alcohol among individuals with or without a family history of alcoholism (Schuckit, 1994); that is, sons of alcoholic fathers, and possibly daughters (Schuckit et al., 2000), tend to demonstrate less intense responses to low-to-moderate amounts of alcohol with respect to their physiological reactivity, psychomotor function, and subjective experiences of intoxication. This reduced response to alcohol is correlated with more severe alcohol use diagnoses and is predictive of self-reported drinking practices and the subsequent development of alcohol dependence (Mundt, Perrine, & Searles, 1997; Schuckit, 1994, 1998). A low level of response to alcohol at age 20 was associated with a fourfold greater likelihood of future alcoholism in the sons of alcoholics (Schuckit, 1994). Fifty-six percent of the sons of alcoholics with the lesser alcohol response developed alcoholism during the subsequent decade, compared to 14% of the men in this group who had highly sensitive alcohol responses (Schuckit, 1994).

Consistent with the apparent familial lineage of this response, recent research has begun to identify the genetic mechanisms of this phenomenon (Schuckit et al., 2001; Wilhelmsen et al., 2003). Similar familial and, presumably, genetic influences have also been found to increase the vulnerability to the development of drug dependence (Merikangas et al., 1998), including marijuana and cocaine dependence and habitual smoking (Bierut et al., 1998), and gambling (Eisen et al., 1998). It is thought that these genetic predispositions may be manifested in alterations in neurotransmitter systems, particularly the dopaminergic and serotonergic systems, which are thought to underlie craving, sensation seeking, impulsivity, and antisocial behavior (Hill et al., 2002; Hill, Stoltenberg, Burmeister, Closser, & Zucker, 1999; Limosin, Loze, Rouillon, Ades, & Gorwood, 2003; Noble, 1998). Although there appears to be no such thing as an "alcoholic personality," these traits and temperament variables have been among the most consistent predictors of subsequent alcoholism (Mulder, 2002).

Similarly, there appear to be different subtypes of substance abusers that have more or less genetic heritability and the manifestation of certain predisposing behavioral components. Subtypes can be characterized in terms of general severity of problems and multidimensional risk factors for developing an addiction, or in terms of differences in temperament (Henderson & Galen, 2003). Most of the empirically derived typologies have been based on a combination of family history, age of onset of drinking or drug use and dependence, personality or temperament factors, such as impulsiveness and risk-taking, and acting-out behavior (Cloninger, 1987; Epstein, Labouvie, McCrady, Jensen, & Hayaki, 2002; Mulder, 2002). As an example, Babor et al. (1992) and Cloninger (1987) have developed somewhat similar typologies of alcoholics. Those alcoholics classified as Type B in Babor's system and as Type II in Cloninger's system are characterized by a high level of genetic heritability and premorbid vulnerability. They are more likely to be males; to report greater alcohol consumption; to have an earlier onset of alcohol use, problems, and dependence (typically before the age of 25); and to have more alcohol-related antisocial behavior, more severe alcohol dependence, and a higher prevalence of comorbid depression and psychopathology; they also tend to have poorer treatment outcomes (Babor et al., 1992; Carpenter & Hasin, 2001; Driessen, Veltrup, Wetterling, John, & Dilling, 1998). A similar pattern of findings applies to comparable typologies among individuals dependent on cocaine (Ball, Carroll, Babor, & Rounsaville, 1995) and opiates (De, Mattoo, & Basu, 2003), and among obese individuals (Allison & Heshka, 1993).

These typologies not only have significantly more severe substance dependence and poorer treatment outcomes, but they also appear to be associated with differences in coping strategies and behaviors. Chung, Langenbucher, Labouvie, Pandina, and Moos (2001) found that Type B alcoholics used more avoidance coping strategies, such as wishful thinking or venting negative feelings, to manage stressors than did Type A alcoholics. Avoidance coping has been found in previous research to be associated with negative outcomes, including the development of alcohol problems. Lower levels of reliance on cognitive avoidance coping (e.g., daydreaming) predicted fewer alcohol, psychological, and interpersonal problems. Higher levels of behavioral approach coping (e.g., taking action) were associated with lower severity of alcohol problems. Type B alcoholics have been found to benefit differentially more in coping skills training group therapy than do Type A alcoholics (Litt, Babor, DelBoca, Kadden, & Cooney, 1992).

Individuals who have a positive family history and fall into categories such as Type B and Type II are those in whom the preponderance of metabolic, physiological, electrophysiological, and neurobiological deviances are found, consistent with these factors contributing to the predisposition toward alcoholism, drug dependence, and addictive behaviors. Consistent with this, these groups also appear to have differential responses to pharmacotherapies that affect neurotransmitter systems associated with craving and dependence (Chick, Aschauer, Hornik, & Group, 2004; Kranzler, Burleson, Brown, & Babor, 1996; Pettinati et al., 2000). Kranzler and colleagues (1996) reported that Type B alcoholics showed less favorable drinking outcomes in response to treatment with fluoxetine, a serotonin reuptake inhibitor, than with placebo.

This medication effect was not seen in Type A alcoholics, who have lower risk–severity of alcoholism and psychopathology. Johnson and colleagues (2000) found that early-onset alcoholics who received odansetron, a medication that affects the serotonergic system, had significantly better treatment outcomes (e.g., more time abstinent and fewer drinks per drinking day) than those receiving placebo or late-onset alcoholics. Johnson et al. found that odansetron was associated with significant reductions in craving (Johnson, Roache, Ait-Daoud, Zanca, & Velazquez, 2002) and in depression, anxiety, and hostility (Johnson, Ait-Daoud, Ma, & Wang, 2003) among early-onset but not late-onset alcoholics. It was thought that the reduction in craving and mood disturbances, and the more positive outcomes among early-onset alcoholics treated with odansetron were mediated by its ameliorating serotonergic abnormalities in this subtype.

The risk of substance use and substance-related problems is further increased if there is a history of psychiatric disorders in the biological parents. For example, the probability of offspring developing drug dependence is greater among adoptees who had a parent with both substance abuse and antisocial personality disorder when compared to adoptees with a parent having only one of these disorders, or to adoptees in which neither disorder was present in either biological parent (Langbehn, Cadoret, Caspers, Troughton, & Yucuis, 2003). Similarly, Read et al. (1990) found that a combined family history of alcoholism and an additional co-occurring psychiatric disorder were associated with an earlier onset of problem drinking, a more severe course of alcohol dependence, and a greater heterogeneity of psychopathology among first-degree relatives. Langbehn et al. (2003) suggest that the observed biological associations found in the increased vulnerability among individuals with a family history of both substance abuse and psychiatric disorders are broadly consistent with a generalization to Cloninger's Type II or Babor's Type B alcoholism subtypes.

There is also a relatively high rate of co-occurring personality disorders, Axis I psychiatric disorders, and/or concurrent substance abuse or dependence associated with addictive behaviors (Driessen et al., 1998; Havassy, Alvidrez, & Owen, 2004; Lehman, Myers, Thompson, & Corty, 1993). Such individuals represent a challenge to assess (Carey, 1997) and to treat (Drake, Mueser, Brunette, & McHugo, 2004; Kranzler & Rosenthal, 2003). They also experience unique challenges in their own recovery process (Laudet, Magura, Vogel, & Knight, 2000). There appears to be a relative lack of effective treatments for individuals with such co-occurring disorders (Cornelius, Bukstein, Salloum, & Clark, 2003; Watkins, Burnam, Kung, & Paddock, 2001). The presence and severity of concurrent psychiatric and/or substance use problems appear to contribute to poorer treatment outcomes, suggesting that they may serve as potential contributors to relapse risk. Such individuals appear to experience a number of unique, high-risk relapse situations associated with the occurrence or exacerbation of their psychiatric symptomatology, in addition to those associated with their substance dependence (Bradizza & Stasiewicz,

2003). Impaired interpersonal or cognitive problem-solving abilities are also common among this population (Tapert, Ozyurt, Myers, & Brown, 2004). Each of these conditions, independently, creates a backdrop against which alcohol, drugs, tobacco, food, or other behaviors, such as gambling, may be seen as a means of trying to cope with the problems that accompany such disorders.

Another important individual-difference distal factor is the severity of alcohol or substance dependence (Langenbucher, Sulesund, Chung, & Morgenstern, 1996), which may lead to differences in reactivity to substance-related cues and/or in the number and range of cues to which they are conditioned. There is clear evidence that stimuli in the person's environment, as well as interpersonal and intrapersonal cues, can become conditioned stimuli through classical conditioning from repeated pairings of theses cues and drinking, drugs use, or smoking (Drummond, 2000; Glautier & Drummond, 1994b; O'Brien, Childress, Ehrman, & Robbins, 1998; Rohsenow, Niaura, Childress, Abrams, & Monti, 1990–1991). Individuals with more severe levels of dependence, and also greater mood disturbances, appear to develop greater reactivity to such cues (Glautier & Drummond, 1994a; Litt, Cooney, & Morse, 2000). Furthermore, it appears that individuals who drink, use drugs, or smoke have an attentional bias that differentially focuses their attention on these conditioned cues (Bradley, Field, Mogg, & De Houwer, 2004; Field, Mogg, & Bradley, 2004a; Field, Mogg, Zetteler, & Bradley, 2004; Waters, Shiffman, Bradley, & Mogg, 2003). Studies with smokers indicate that stronger attentional biases are associated with more repeated unsuccessful attempts at abstinence (Bradley, Mogg, Wright, & Field, 2003) and a greater likelihood of having a lapse shortly following achieving abstinence (Waters, Shiffman, Sayette, et al., 2003). The bias appears stronger following periods of deprivation or abstinence and also appears to lead to increased reports of craving and the perceived pleasantness of smoking-related cues (Field, Mogg, & Bradley, 2004b).

An additional factor contributing to the risk of developing addictive behaviors, and also subsequently enhancing the likelihood of relapse, is the set of cognitive expectancies that individuals develop about the expected outcomes associated with such behaviors. A large body of literature has developed around such expectancies (e.g., Brown, Christiansen, & Goldman, 1987; Goldman, 1994; Oei & Baldwin, 1994), known as outcome expectancies. As noted in the working definition of addiction, underlying motives for engaging in addictive behaviors include both a desire to change one's mood and to increase sociability (Smith & Seymour, 2004). Individuals who develop problems with an addictive behavior typically have developed a set of expectancies that anticipate positive outcomes from engaging in the behavior, serving as a source of motivation to engage in it. Such expectancies appear to develop at a relatively young age and become solidified over time. Miller, Smith, and Goldman (1990; Dunn & Goldman, 1998) found that children as young as 6 years old had already developed alcohol-related expectancies, although they

were somewhat undifferentiated compared to those of older children and adolescents. Children held increasingly positive expectancies as they grew older,
with the greatest increases occurring in the third and fourth grades. These
findings are consistent with those of Gustafson (1992), who found that positive expectancies for alcohol were already relatively well established by the
age of 12 (e.g., sixth grade), before most of the children had any extensive personal drinking experience; these early expectancies developed further in a positive direction between the ages of 12 and 15. Such outcome expectancies are
shaped by an individual's past direct and indirect experience with the addictive behavior, including vicarious learning through the modeling they see dis-
played by parents and peers (Brook et al., 2003; Brown, Tate, & Goldman,
1999; Chassin, Pitts, & Prost, 2002; Connors & Maisto, 1988; Sale, Sambrano, Springer, & Turner, 2003).

A number of expectancy domains have been identified. In early work in
this area with alcohol and drug use, Brown (1985, 1993; Brown et al., 1987)
delineated six factor-analytically derived domains. Drinking and drug use
were anticipated to produce (1) positive global changes in experience, (2) sexual enhancement, (3) social and physical pleasure, (4) social assertiveness, (5)
relaxation/tension reduction, and (6) arousal/interpersonal power. Cooper,
Russell, Skinner, and Windle (1992) derived three primary dimensions that
constituted reasons or motives for drinking: to enhance positive affect, to cope
with negative affect, and to enhance social interaction and social activity with
friends. To the extent that these expectancies are activated and accessible to
the individual in high-risk situations, they appear to determine the anticipated
outcomes from engaging in the addictive behavior and to mediate subsequent
behavior (Kilbey, Downey, & Breslau, 1998; Palfai & Ostafin, 2003; Rather
& Goldman, 1994; Stacy, 1997; Stacy, Leigh, & Weingardt, 1994; Stacy,
Newcomb, & Bentler, 1995; Weingardt, Stacy, & Leigh, 1996). Given the
attentional bias of substance abusers toward substance-related cues and the
association of such cues and the enhanced salience of outcome expectancies
and craving, the likelihood of a lapse is markedly increased (Marlatt, 1990).

Shiffman (1989) suggests that a model focusing only on such distal personal background factors is able to predict who will relapse but not when relapse will occur. Such an approach is based on an assumption of a constant
risk or relapse proneness. Individuals with certain risk-enhancing characteristics have an elevated likelihood of relapse; however, this potential for relapse
may never be actualized unless other events occur. Thus, the background
characteristics of the person must interact with situational variables to determine behavior. The assessment model associated with an approach focusing
on distal personal characteristics requires only a single assessment at some
baseline point, since these relatively stable background variables are thought
to serve as predictors. As noted previously, models based solely on distal factors are typically less robust in predicting future behavior than ones that incorporate such distal factors with others in closer proximity to a relapse situation.

Intermediate Background Factors

Shiffman (1989) suggests that distal personal factors and intermediate background factors operate together to "set the stage" or predispose the individual for relapse to occur. The effects of intermediate factors are hypothesized to be cumulative, with their intensity and influence in the person's life ebbing and flowing contextually during the period of maintaining abstinence. Variables in this category include relatively infrequent major life events that usually require some immediate reaction, as well as more enduring life strain and daily problems. Repeated or continuous exposure to such intermediate background variables leads to increasing levels of stress, with its attendant emotional and behavioral manifestations; at some point, a critical threshold is reached, beyond which a return to the addictive behavior is highly likely. Brady and Sonne (1999) have noted that stress and the body's response to it most likely play a role in the vulnerability to initial alcohol and substance use and dependence, and in seeking treatment for substance abuse and relapse. Brown, Vik, Patterson, Grant, and Schuckit (1995) found that alcoholics experiencing highly threatening or chronic psychosocial stress following treatment were more likely to relapse than were abstaining individuals not experiencing such stress. Improved psychosocial functioning following treatment, in particular, increased levels of coping, self-efficacy, and social support, enhanced the ability of these individuals to remain abstinent despite severe stress. These life strains may reflect issues of the individual's lifestyle, including the imbalance between "wants" and "shoulds" that Marlatt has described as increasing a sense of deprivation that leads to an increased desire to indulge, increased levels of craving, and an increased risk of relapse (Larimer et al., 1999; Marlatt & Gordon, 1985).

One cannot measure the occurrence or magnitude of such intermediate variables in isolation; rather, they must be viewed in relation to the individual's social and environmental supports, general sense of efficacy or perceived control, and the ability to anticipate, avoid, and/or cope with the resultant stress. At the point that the stress level exceeds the individual's ability to cope, the perceived and anticipated positive benefits of the addictive behavior are likely to be more salient, and the risk of relapse may be potentiated into actual use.

The assessment of coping, in general (Moos & Holahan, 2003), and more specifically in relation to relapse, is no easy task (Shiffman, 1987, 1989; Shiffman & Wills, 1985). However, this construct plays a central role in the conceptualization of relapse and relapse prevention. This model views the individual as having deficits in his or her coping skills, both general and addiction-specific, and that the individual drinks, uses drugs, or engages in other addictive behaviors as a means of trying to deal with emotional distress and other high-risk situations in the absence of appropriate or effective coping skills. Consistent with this, Carpenter and Hasin (1999) found that drinking to cope was associated with the development of alcohol dependence.

Holahan, Moos, Holahan, Cronkite, and Randall (2001) investigated a form of avoidance coping, drinking to cope with emotional distress, in a large community-based sample of adults who were followed prospectively over a 10-year period. They found that a measure of drinking to cope at the initial baseline assessment predicted alcohol consumption and the development of problem drinking across the ensuing 10-year period. Initial drinking to cope also was found to mediate the relationship between emotional distress and drinking behavior. Furthermore, increases in drinking to cope over the 10-year period were associated with increases in drinking behavior, and decreases in drinking to cope were linked to decreases in drinking behavior.

Moos and Holahan (2003) distinguish between two general types of coping. The first is a relatively stable, trait-like coping style or dispositions that characterizes the individual's typical and habitual manner of interacting with the environment. The components of these dispositions involve relatively stable and enduring personality, attitudinal, and cognitive characteristics that represent the psychological context for coping. These include factors such as defensive style and general problem-solving abilities. This concept of coping style appears to fall into Shiffman's (1989) category of distal factors.

The second type involves the cognitive and behavioral coping responses or skills that the individual employs to manage specific stressful encounters. These skills are context- and situation-specific. Perspectives that emphasize coping styles versus coping skills reflect contrasting assumptions about the underlying determinants of the coping process. Stylistic or dispositional approaches assume that relatively stable, person-based factors underlie habitual coping efforts. Contextual approaches assume that more transitory, situation-based factors shape individuals' cognitive appraisals and their choice of specific coping responses. Schwartz, Neale, Marco, Shiffman, and Stone (1999) compared typical methods of assessing trait coping by using retrospective, summary questionnaires, with data from multiple, momentary reports of the use of the same coping cognitions and behaviors. They found that approximately 15–30% of the variability in momentary reports of how people are coping with a current stressor was attributable to consistent interpersonal differences in coping. Two types of coping, escape–avoidance coping and use of religion, exhibited stronger trait-like properties. Thus, while there appears to be evidence of a more stable coping style, successful coping may require the ability to deal with the stresses or temptations embedded in a specific high-risk situation. Consistent with this, Shiffman (1989) found a degree of consistency of behavioral coping strategies used across different relapse situations, whereas cognitive coping showed no cross-situation consistency.

It is of interest to note that short-term (within 48 hours) retrospective reports of the types of coping used to deal with stressful events do not correspond well with reports done using ecological momentary assessment close in time to when the stressor occurred (Stone et al., 1998). From an assessment perspective, such findings suggest that trait-like measures of coping style may not provide an accurate or sufficient picture of how the person will behave in high-risk situations. To the extent that one is able to get near-real-time assessments via ecological momentary assessment procedures or through the use of behavioral observations of how an individual handles simulated high-risk situations, prediction to actual high-risk situations will be improved (e.g., Drobes, Meier, & Tiffany, 1994; Monti et al., 1993).

As noted previously, Marlatt's relapse model is based on the premise that the individual is deficient in those skills necessary to cope with general stress and the more immediate demands of high-risk relapse situations. Considerable data support this tenet of the relapse prevention model (Miller et al., 1996). Therefore, it is important to assess the relative strengths and deficits in the individual's repertoire of coping abilities and skills (Monti et al., 1994; Monti & O'Leary, 1999). It is also important to assess the individual's ability to use or to deploy available coping strategies (Saunders & Allsop, 1987). In many instances, individuals appear to have the necessary coping abilities, yet they may not use them. It is important to determine the cognitive, psychological, and/or behavioral barriers that lead such individuals to resume drinking, drug use, or engagement in an addictive behavior rather than to use those skills available to them to prevent a relapse.

A number of different dimensions of coping need to be considered in the assessment process. These are presented in Table 1.2. First is the general domain in which the coping response occurs: affective, behavioral, and/or cognitive. In some of the earliest work on coping and alcohol dependence, Litman (Litman, 1986; Litman, Stapleton, Oppenheim, Peleg, & Jackson, 1984) identified a number of behavioral and cognitive strategies that protect against relapse. These appear to operate somewhat sequentially, from the point of initiating abstinence to more prolonged maintenance. Individuals who successfully avoided relapse initially appeared to have relied on behavioral avoidance of potential high-risk situations and, if they encountered such situations, sought out social support for continued sobriety. With longer periods of abstinence,

---

TABLE 1.2. Dimensions of Coping to Be Considered
in the Assessment of Relapse Risk

- Types of coping strategies
  - Behavioral
  - Cognitive
  - Affective
- Availability, strength, and deployability of coping skills
- Frequency of use versus effectiveness when used
- Stress-coping versus temptation-coping
- Static versus dynamic nature of coping skill
- Stages of coping
  - Anticipatory
  - Immediate
  - Restorative

Note. From Donovan (1996a, p. 534). Copyright 1996 by Blackwell Publishing. Reprinted by permission.

there appears to be a transition from predominantly behavioral strategies toward a greater reliance on cognitive coping. These cognitive strategies include thinking about the negative consequences of drinking in the past and, subsequently, thinking about the positive benefits derived from having achieved and maintained abstinence.

A number of studies across addictive behaviors have investigated the role of the type of coping strategies used and the likelihood of relapse. Breslin et al. (1996) evaluated the coping behaviors (cognitive or behavioral; active or avoidant) that problem drinkers reported using to avoid relapsing in high-risk situations. The proportion of cognitive coping responses (e.g., thinking through the consequences) was positively related to posttreatment improvement. Chung et al. (2001) looked at the relationship between changes in coping and drinking behavior over a 12-month period following treatment. They found that cognitive appraisal of threat showed a trend toward predicting avoidance coping at 6- and 12-month follow-ups. Decreased cognitive avoidance coping (e.g., daydreaming) predicted fewer alcohol, psychological, and interpersonal problems. Increased behavioral approach coping (e.g., taking action) predicted lower severity of alcohol problems.

Litman's (1986) results suggest that individuals with a greater diversity or range of available coping abilities, and the flexibility to shift adaptively among them as needed, are more likely to maintain sobriety. Related to this, Allsop and Saunders (1989) suggested that a restricted coping repertoire is thought to increase the likelihood of relapse. Moser and Annis (1996) found that survival of a relapse crisis among drinkers was most strongly related to the number of coping strategies used. Shiffman, Paty, Gnys, Kassel, and Hickcox (1996) found that smokers were 12 times more likely to report that they had coped in high-risk situations that they survived than those in which they lapsed. Myers and Brown (1990) found that adolescents with the poorest drug use outcomes following treatment reported use of significantly fewer problem-solving coping strategies and less self-efficacy in general high-risk relapse situations. However, only cognitive (vs. behavioral) coping strategies were effective. Bliss, Garvey, Heinold, and Hitchcock (1989) found that the successful survival of a relapse crisis by smokers was most strongly related to the number of coping strategies used, with no differences in the relative effectiveness across cognitive and behavioral coping strategies. Similarly, Grilo, Shiffman, and Wing (1993) examined dieters' attempts to cope with dietary relapse crises among obese subjects with type II diabetes. Performance of some form of coping response when confronted by the risk of relapse resulted in surviving the immediate crises without a lapse. However, there were no differences in outcome based on the specific type of cognitive or behavioral coping employed. Stoffelmayr, Wadland, and Pan (2003), analyzing information about nearly 3,000 smoking urge/lapse situations and the coping that occurred in these, found that the number of coping responses rather than number of high-risk situations encountered was related to more successful treatment outcome, and that the more coping responses discussed during treatment, the better the treatment outcome.

In addition to the type of coping strategies and the frequency with which they are used, their relative effectiveness must also be determined. Individuals may persist in using coping strategies that were effective at one point in the past or in certain situations but may no longer be appropriate or effective. The continued use of such inadequate strategies may contribute to a decreased sense of self-efficacy. Litman (1986) found that the rated effectiveness of the behavioral and cognitive coping strategies employed by the individual was more strongly related to avoiding relapse than was the absolute number of coping strategies employed. Those individuals who at intake described themselves as having more effective coping skills in general, and those who reported using behavioral avoidance and positive thinking about the anticipated benefits of sobriety, were more likely to have remained abstinent following treatment. Similarly, Connors, Longabaugh, and Miller (1996), based on results from the RREP, found that the availability of coping skills was a potent protective factor, and that the use of ineffective coping was a consistent predictor of relapse. Different coping strategies may be more or less effective depending on the target of their application. Some strategies that may be appropriate and effective in dealing with generalized stress may be less effective in dealing with temptation and craving in specific high-risk situations. It may be inappropriate to assume that an effective general coping strategy will generalize to and be equally effective in dealing with drinking-related temptations.

Two other considerations include the extent to which coping skills are static or dynamic and the role or function they serve in a potential relapse process. Coping appears to be a dynamic process (Marlatt, 1996a; Witkiewitz & Marlatt, 2004). Relapse prevention approaches work toward increasing skills in those areas in which the individual is deficient and toward increased use of effective strategies. Increases in these skills have been associated with improved outcomes across a variety of addictive behaviors. Litman (1986) found that while relapsers and nonrelapsers did not differ with respect to their coping abilities at intake to treatment, those who did not relapse showed significantly greater increases in their use of positive thinking and decreases in the use of behavioral avoidance from intake to the end of treatment. Increases in coping skills over time and treatment have been associated with better outcomes (Brown et al., 1995; Holahan et al., 2001; Kadden, 1995, 1999; Monti, Abrams, Kadden, & Cooney, 1989; Monti, Rohsenow, Colby, & Abrams, 1995).

The role or function of coping also changes depending on the stage in a potential relapse process (Shiffman, 1989). Anticipatory coping allows the individual to attempt to anticipate stresses or high-risk situations and, if unable to do so, to develop plans to avoid them and/or deal with the resultant stresses. Immediate coping strategies, needed while in the midst of a relapse crisis, deal much more with specific aspects of high-risk situations, temptation, and craving. Restorative coping strategies may be used after a lapse. They function to minimize the affective and cognitive components of the AVE, and to minimize the transition of a lapse into a more prolonged and serious relapse.

The results of research on the AVE as a theoretical construct and the specific elements that are thought to comprise it have been mixed (Birke, Edelmann, & Davis, 1990; Borland, 1992; Curry, Marlatt, & Gordon, 1987; Dohm, Beattie, Aibel, & Striegel-Moore, 2001; Grilo & Shiffman, 1994; Hudson, Ward, & Marshall, 1992; Mooney, Burling, Hartman, & Brenner-Liss, 1992; Ross, Miller, Emmerson, & Todt, 1988–1989; Schmitz, Rosenfarb, & Payne, 1993; Shiffman, Hickcox, et al., 1996; Stephens, Curtin, Simpson, & Roffman, 1994; Ward, Hudson, & Bulik, 1993). However, the role of restorative coping has been evidenced. Grilo et al. (1993) found that among women dieters who had a lapse, restorative behavioral coping was elicited as a response to overeating, while restorative cognitive coping seemed to be elicited by the negative thoughts and feelings that sometimes accompany lapses or temptations. Dohm et al. (2001), also working with dieters, found that those who were able to reduce their weight and maintain it, in contrast to those who were unable to maintain their reduced weight, were more likely to use direct coping and less likely to seek help. Shiffman, Hickcox, et al. (1996) found that smokers who attempted restorative coping were less likely to progress to another lapse on the same day. The pattern of such results leads to a conclusion similar to that of Dohm et al. (2001), who indicated that the most useful variables for differentiating between successful and unsuccessful weight loss maintainers may involve how individuals respond to a dietary lapse. The same appears to hold for other addictive behaviors as well.

An important element in determining the likelihood of relapse is the individual's commitment to or motivation for self-improvement (Donovan & Rosengren, 1999). Often individuals find themselves in stressful situations for which they have the prerequisite coping strategies, yet their commitment to self-improvement may be insufficient to lead them to use them. Allsop and Saunders (1989) and Baer and colleagues (1999) indicated that any analysis of relapse needs to examine the interaction between commitment and coping skills. Even well-developed coping abilities will not prevent relapse if the individual's commitment is weak; conversely, strong commitment may be insufficient in the absence of adequate coping skills. Thus, it is important to assess this commitment and motivation to change. Prochaska, DiClemente, and Norcross (1992) have suggested that this variable, like other intermediate background variables, also ebbs and flows. This suggests the need for repeated assessments in order to monitor periodically the relative strengths of the intermediate factors that either contribute to or protect against the likelihood of relapse as they vary in intensity across time. Also, it appears that certain interventions may be appropriate for individuals at different stages of readiness (Connors, Donovan, & DiClemente, 2001). Rohsenow and colleagues (2004) evaluated the effectiveness of motivational enhancement therapy and group coping skills treatment in cocaine abusers. The motivational intervention had better substance use outcomes with individuals having a low level of initial motivation to change when compared to those with higher levels of initial motivation.

Proximal Precipitating Factors

The individual will eventually encounter high-risk situations. Marlatt's relapse taxonomy provides a conceptual and methodological framework within which to understand and classify the inter- and intrapersonal factors associated with such situations. Shiffman (1989) has suggested that an exclusive focus on situational determinants in the immediate situation represents an episodic model, which implies that relapse is relatively precipitous and potentially unpredictable.

A cognitive construct that is appropriate to this phase of the relapse process is the level of self-efficacy (Annis & Davis, 1988; Bandura, 1977, 1997; DiClemente, Fairhurst, & Piotrowski, 1995). Self-efficacy has been found fairly consistently to predict treatment outcome; low levels of self-efficacy are predictive of relapse (Drobes et al., 1994; Monti et al., 2001). This construct, which appears to be intimately related to the individual's coping abilities, reflects the degree of confidence the individual has about being confronted with a high-risk relapse situation and successfully avoiding a lapse. For example, Myers and Brown (1990) found that adolescents with the poorest drug use outcome following treatment reported use of significantly fewer problem-solving coping strategies and had less self-efficacy in general high-risk relapse situations. Also, Gwaltney et al. (2002) found that affective and environmental contexts, or situations in which the individual had low levels of abstinence self-efficacy, were associated with lapses among smokers.

Scales of self-efficacy, such as the IDS (Annis et al., 1987) and the Situational Confidence Questionnaire (SCQ; Annis & Graham, 1988), the Alcohol Abstinence Self-Efficacy Questionnaire (DiClemente, Carbonari, Montgomery, & Hughes, 1994), the Drug-Taking Confidence Questionnaire (Sklar, Annis, & Turner, 1997), the Drug Avoidance Self-Efficacy Scale (Martin, Pollock, Cornelius, Lynch, & Martin, 1995), the Smoking Self-Efficacy Questionnaire (Etter, Bergman, Humair, & Perneger, 2000), and others like them, allow self-report and dimensional ratings of the potential temptation or risk associated with a number of situations as well as one's perceived efficacy to deal with them. However, since the situations identified by such measures have only been associated with heavy substance use, one cannot assume a causal link between the types of situations endorsed and the likelihood of relapse (Sobell, Toneatto, & Sobell, 1994). Sobell et al. also indicated that it is important to explore in more depth the unique and personally relevant high-risk situations or areas in which the individual lacks self-confidence or self-efficacy. Gwaltney et al. (2001) found that it is possible to assess the level of self-efficacy for specific situational contexts, thus potentially enabling identification in advance of the situations in which an individual is most likely to lapse. Such context-specific assessments may help to identify not only who will lapse but also the situations in which the lapse will occur (Gwaltney et al., 2001). Given the relationship between self-efficacy and relapse, a number of authors have recommended that self-efficacy should be the appropriate target for interventions (e.g., Vielva & Iraurgi, 2001).

The more immediate and specific aspects of these situations are important to consider, yet are extremely difficult to assess in the moment given their transient and rapidly changing nature. Hodgins and colleagues (Hodgins & el-Guebaly, 2004; Hodgins et al., 1995) have presented a method of assessing mood states in a repeated fashion, so that they will be more contiguous in time to possible lapse, "close call," or relapse "crisis" situations. It is precisely for this type of circumstance that the ecological momentary assessment procedure was developed (Stone et al., 1998). Using this procedure, Shiffman et al. (2000) found that the level of self-efficacy remained relatively high and stable prior to an initial lapse following treatment for smoking; however, it decreased and became more variable after an initial lapse, demonstrating the dynamic nature of efficacy. Similar methods may be usefully employed to assess the nature of the individual's relapse-enhancing or coping-related self-statements preceding or during a potential relapse situation and the degree of craving experienced.

It is likely that the elements of a high-risk situation will elicit a conditioned response to the substance-related cues in the situation, leading to craving and an increased salience of the desired effects of alcohol, drugs, or other addictive behaviors. Heather (Heather & Stallard, 1989; Heather, Stallard, & Tebbutt, 1991) has argued that Marlatt's model pays insufficient attention to the role of craving as a precipitant, in part due to restrictions in the relapse coding guidelines that make assignment of relapses to craving as a precipitant less likely. There has been an increased focus on cue reactivity and craving across a number of addictive behaviors. Heather and Stallard (1989) suggested that craving may serve as the most proximal common pathway through which other interpersonal and intrapersonal factors exert their influence on the probability of relapse.

Monti, Rohsenow, and Hutchison (2000) and Niaura (2000) suggest that it is in the experience and process of craving that the elements of the biopsychosocial model come together. An individual who is genetically more vulnerable due to a family history of addiction and the modeling of parents and peers has an attentional bias that more readily attracts attention to addiction-related cues in situational contexts that threaten his or her perception of control, with a wide range of cues that have been classically conditioned through prior experience to elicit craving, urges, and a strong desire to use in that situation. Such an individual with a deficit in general problem solving, and both general and substance-specific coping skills, and a resultant decrease in self-efficacy, and with an increased focus on the anticipated positive effects of alcohol, drugs, or another addictive behavior, is at extreme risk of a lapse.

Transitional Factors

Marlatt and Gordon (1985) and Saunders and Allsop (1987) suggest that the factors that trigger an initial lapse are different from those that contribute to continued drinking, drug use, or other addictive behavior or a more prolonged relapse. Marlatt's model focuses to a large extent on the tendency to personalize the responsibility for the relapse (an internal attribution) and the negative emotions, such as guilt, remorse, depression, and self-directed anger, that often accompany a relapse, as factors contributing to the transition from lapse to relapse. However, the results of studies investigating the AVE have been mixed (Birke et al., 1990; Curry et al., 1987; Grilo & Shiffman, 1994; Hudson et al., 1992; Mooney et al., 1992; Ross et al., 1988–1989; Shiffman, Hickcox, et al., 1996; Stephens et al., 1994; Ward et al., 1993). Other factors, such as the individual's restorative coping abilities to deal with the negative consequences and emotions, the reaction of family and friends, and the individual's commitment to return to abstinence or moderation/harm reduction, must also be considered. Shiffman, Hickcox, et al. (1996) found that self-efficacy, attributions, and affective reactions to a lapse generally failed to predict progression from an initial lapse to continued use as predicted by the AVE. However, smokers who felt like giving up after an initial lapse progressed more rapidly to a second lapse. Those who attempted restorative coping were less likely to progress to another lapse on the same day.

Dohm et al. (2001) suggest that while their results failed to support the AVE, the most useful variables for differentiating between successful and unsuccessful weight loss maintainers may involve how they respond to a lapse. In addition, the reactions of friends and family members, comprising the individual's social network, are equally important (Beattie & Longabaugh, 1999; Beattie et al., 1993; Longabaugh, 2003). Brown et al. (1995) found that increased coping skills and social networks were related to continued abstinence among drinkers despite their experiencing severe stress. McKay, Merikle, Mulvaney, Weiss, and Koppenhaver (2001) found that support from one's family is an important factor in the outcome of cocaine addicts. It is not just general social support that needs to be taken into account. Support by family and friends for one's treatment goal—to stop drinking, using drugs, or engaging in other addictive behaviors—may be more important (Beattie & Longabaugh, 1999; Beattie et al., 1993; Longabaugh, 2003). While both general and alcohol-specific support were related to reduced drinking behavior among alcoholics over the first 3 months following treatment, only alcohol-specific support helped explain variance over the longer term (15 months posttreatment). Beattie and Longabaugh (1999) concluded that knowing how different types of social support affect drinking behavior at different intervals following treatment may help treatment providers better prepare their clients for the posttreatment social environment.

CONCLUSIONS

Addictive behaviors are complex disorders, with clear contributions of genetic predispositions; psychological vulnerabilities; personality traits and temperaments; cognitive expectations about the anticipated benefits derived from drinking, drug use, or engaging in other addictive behaviors; and lack of adequate coping skills and an attendant low level of self-efficacy. This vulnerability appears to be actuated in a social context in which family and friends serve as models. These factors appear to interact and covary dynamically across time, exerting differential influence at different points along the developmental path in the development, maintenance, and treatment–cessation of the particular addictive behavior.

Relapse is also a complex process. Models that focus exclusively on distal, intermediate, or proximal factors are likely to be inadequate in predicting relapse. Rather, relapse is best understood as having multiple and interactive determinants that vary in temporal proximity and relative influence on relapse. An adequate assessment model must be sufficiently comprehensive to include theoretically relevant variables from each of the multiple domains and different levels of potential predictors. The recently revised model of relapse (Witkiewitz & Marlatt, 2004) has incorporated and elaborated on the dynamic interplay of factors from the biopsychosocial model, from distal to proximal. As such, it will likely provide the field with an updated model in which the determination of relapse precipitants will be more reliable and valid (Donovan, 1996a, 1996b; Marlatt, 1996a, 1996b), and provide better predictive utility in identifying areas of concern, relative to what the individual brings with him or her and in the context of situations perceived as having a high risk of relapse.

The remaining chapters in this volume focus on the application of the heuristic framework that the relapse model provides for the assessment of addictive behaviors. Each chapter provides both a general overview of the assessment issues and process for the particular addictive behavior being covered and information about specific measures that have been developed to assess different aspects of the biopsychosocial model. The goal is to provide a companion volume that interfaces with the application of relapse prevention techniques. Used together, this volume and *Relapse Prevention* (Marlatt & Donovan, 2005) provide information needed to conduct a targeted assessment of relapse risk factors for a given addictive behavior and to develop an appropriate individualized treatment plan to prevent relapse from occurring and to minimize harm, if relapse does occur.

ACKNOWLEDGMENTS

The preparation of this chapter was supported in part by Grant Nos. U10 AA11799 from the National Institute on Alcohol Abuse and Alcoholism and U10 DA13714 from the National Institute on Drug Abuse.

REFERENCES

Allison, D. B., & Heshka, S. (1993). Toward an empirically derived typology of obese persons: Derivation in a nonclinical sample. *International Journal of Eating Disorders, 13*(1), 93–108.

Allsop, S., & Saunders, B. (1989). Relapse and alcohol problems. In M. Gossop (Ed.), *Relapse and addictive behavior* (pp. 11–40). New York: Tavistock/Routledge.

American Psychiatric Association. (1994). *Diagnostic and statistical manual of mental disorders* (4th ed.). Washington, DC: Author.

American Psychiatric Association. (2000). *Diagnostic and statistical manual of mental disorders* (4th ed., text rev.). Washington, DC: Author.

Annis, H., & Davis, C. S. (1988). Self-efficacy and the prevention of alcoholic relapse: Initial findings from a treatment trial. In T. B. Baker & D. S. Cannon (Eds.), *Assessment and treatment of addictive disorders* (pp. 88–112). New York: Praeger.

Annis, H. M. (1991). A cognitive–social learning approach to relapse: Pharmacotherapy and relapse prevention counselling. *Alchohol and Alcoholism Supplement, 1,* 527–530.

Annis, H. M., & Graham, J. M. (1988). *Situational Confidence Questionnaire user's guide.* Toronto: Addiction Research Foundation of Ontario.

Annis, H. M., Graham, J. M., & Davis, C. S. (1987). *Inventory of Drinking Situations (IDS) user's guide.* Toronto: Addiction Research Foundation.

Babor, T. F., Hofmann, M., DelBoca, F. K., Hesselbrock, V., Meyer, R. E., Dolinsky, Z. S., & Rounsaville, B. (1992). Types of alcoholics: I. Evidence for an empirically derived typology based on indicators of vulnerability and severity. *Archives of General Psychiatry, 49*(8), 599–608.

Baer, J. S., Kivlahan, D. R., & Donovan, D. M. (1999). Integrating skills training and motivational therapies: Implications for the treatment of substance dependence. *Journal of Substance Abuse Treatment, 17*(1–2), 15–23.

Ball, S. A., Carroll, K. M., Babor, T. F., & Rounsaville, B. J. (1995). Subtypes of cocaine abusers: Support for a type A–type B distinction. *Journal of Consulting and Clinical Psychology, 63*(1), 115–124.

Bandura, A. (1977). Self-efficacy: Toward a unifying theory of behavioral change. *Psychological Review, 84*(2), 191–215.

Bandura, A. (1997). *Self-efficacy: The exercise of control.* New York: Freeman.

Beattie, M. C., & Longabaugh, R. (1999). General and alcohol-specific social support following treatment. *Addictive Behaviors, 24*(5), 593–606.

Beattie, M. C., Longabaugh, R., Elliott, G., Stout, R. L., Fava, J., & Noel, N. E. (1993). Effect of the social environment on alcohol involvement and subjective well-being prior to alcoholism treatment. *Journal of Studies on Alcohol, 54*(3), 283–296.

Bierut, L. J., Dinwiddie, S. H., Begleiter, H., Crowe, R. R., Hesselbrock, V., Nurnberger, J. I., Jr., Porjesz, B., Schuckit, M. A., & Reich, T. (1998). Familial transmission of substance dependence: Alcohol, marijuana, cocaine, and habitual smoking: A report from the collaborative study on the genetics of alcoholism. *Archives of General Psychiatry, 55,* 982–988.

Birke, S. A., Edelmann, R. J., & Davis, P. E. (1990). An analysis of the abstinence violation effect in a sample of illicit drug users. *British Journal on Addictions, 85*(10), 1299–1397.

Bliss, R. E., Garvey, A. J., Heinold, J. W., & Hitchcock, J. L. (1989). The influence of situation and coping on relapse crisis outcomes after smoking cessation. *Journal of Consulting and Clinical Psychology, 57*(3), 443–449.

Borland, R. (1992). Relationships between mood around slip-up and recovery of abstinence in smoking cessation attempts. *International Journal of Addictions, 27*(9), 1079–1086.

Bradizza, C. M., & Stasiewicz, P. R. (2003). Qualitative analysis of high-risk drug and alcohol use situations among severely mentally ill substance abusers. *Addictive Behaviors, 28*(1), 157–169.

Bradley, B., Field, M., Mogg, K., & De Houwer, J. (2004). Attentional and evaluative biases for smoking cues in nicotine dependence: Component processes of biases in visual orienting. *Behavioral Pharmacology, 15*(1), 29–36.

Bradley, B. P., Mogg, K., Wright, T., & Field, M. (2003). Attentional bias in drug dependence: Vigilance for cigarette-related cues in smokers. *Psychology of Addictive Behaviors, 17*(1), 66–72.

Bradley, B. P. (1990). Behavioural addictions: Common features and treatment implications. *British Journal of Addiction, 85*(11), 1417–1419.

Brady, K. T., & Sonne, S. C. (1999). The role of stress in alcohol use, alcoholism treatment, and relapse. *Alcohol Research and Health, 23*(4), 263–271.

Breslin, C., Sobell, L. C., Sobell, M. B., Buchan, G., & Kwan, E. (1996). Aftercare telephone contacts with problem drinkers can serve a clinical and research function. *Addiction, 91*(9), 1359–1364.

Breslin, C., Sobell, M. B., Sobell, L. C., Sdao-Jarvie, K., & Sagorsky, L. (1996). Relationship between posttreatment drinking and alternative responses to high-risk situations proposed during treatment by problem drinkers. *Journal of Substance Abuse, 8*(4), 479–486.

Brook, D. W., Brook, J. S., Rubenstone, E., Zhang, C., Singer, M., & Duke, M. R. (2003). Alcohol use in adolescents whose fathers abuse drugs. *Journal of Addictive Diseases, 22*(1), 11–34.

Brown, S. A. (1985). Reinforcement expectancies and alcoholism treatment outcome after a one-year follow-up. *Journal of Studies on Alcohol, 46*(4), 304–308.

Brown, S. A. (1993). Drug effect expectancies and addictive behavior change. *Experimental and Clinical Psychopharmacology, 1*(1–4), 55–67.

Brown, S. A., Christiansen, B. A., & Goldman, M. S. (1987). The Alcohol Expectancy Questionnaire: An instrument for the assessment of adolescent and adult alcohol expectancies. *Journal of Studies on Alcohol, 48*(5), 483–491.

Brown, S. A., Tate, S. R., & Goldman, M. S. (1999). Modeling of alcohol use mediates the effect of family history of alcoholism on adolescent alcohol expectancies. *Experimental and Clinical Psychopharmacology, 7*(1), 20–27.

Brown, S. A., Vik, P. W., Patterson, T. L., Grant, I., & Schuckit, M. A. (1995). Stress, vulnerability and adult alcohol relapse. *Journal of Studies on Alcohol, 56*(5), 538–545.

Cannon, D. S., Leeka, J. K., Patterson, E. T., & Baker, T. B. (1990). Principal components analysis of the inventory of drinking situations: Empirical categories of drinking by alcoholics. *Addictive Behaviors, 15*(3), 265–269.

Carels, R. A., Douglass, O. M., Cacciapaglia, H. M., & O'Brien, W. H. (2004). An ecological momentary assessment of relapse crises in dieting. *Journal of Consulting and Clinical Psychology, 72*(2), 341–348.

Carey, K. B. (1997). Challenges in assessing substance use patterns in persons with comorbid mental and addictive disorders. In L. S. Onken, J. Blaine, S. Genser, J. Horton, & A. M. Horton, Jr. (Eds.), *Treatment of drug-dependent individuals with comorbid mental disorders* (pp. 16–32). Rockville, MD: National Institute on Drug Abuse.

Carey, K. B., & Correia, C. J. (1998). Severe mental illness and addictions: Assessment considerations. *Addictive Behaviors, 23*(6), 735–748.

Carpenter, K. M., & Hasin, D. S. (1999). Drinking to cope with negative affect and DSM-IV alcohol use disorders: A test of three alternative explanations. *Journal of Studies on Alcohol, 60*(5), 694–704.

Carpenter, K. M., & Hasin, D. S. (2001). Reliability and discriminant validity of the Type I/II and Type A/B alcoholic subtype classifications in untreated problem drinkers: A test of the Apollonian–Dionysian hypothesis. *Drug and Alcohol Dependence, 63*(1), 51–67.

Carroll, K. M. (1996). Relapse prevention as a psychosocial treatment: A review of controlled clinical trials. *Experimental and Clinical Psychopharmacology, 4*(1), 46–54.

Carroll, K. M., & Rounsaville, B. J. (2002). On beyond urine: Clinically useful assessment instruments in the treatment of drug dependence. *Behaviour Research and Therapy, 40*(11), 1329–1344.

Chassin, L., Pitts, S. C., & Prost, J. (2002). Binge drinking trajectories from adolescence to emerging adulthood in a high-risk sample: Predictors and substance abuse outcomes. *Journal of Consulting and Clinical Psychology, 70*(1), 67–78.

Chiauzzi, E. J. (1991). *Preventing relapse in addictions: A biopsychosocial approach.* New York: Pergamon Press.

Chick, J., Aschauer, H., Hornik, K., & Group, I. (2004). Efficacy of fluvoxamine in preventing relapse in alcohol dependence: A one-year, double-blind, placebo-controlled multicentre study with analysis by typology. *Drug and Alcohol Dependence, 74*(1), 61–70.

Chung, T., Langenbucher, J., Labouvie, E., Pandina, R. J., & Moos, R. H. (2001). Changes in alcoholic patients' coping responses predict 12–month treatment outcomes. *Journal of Consulting and Clinical Psychology, 69*(1), 92–100.

Cloninger, C. R. (1987). Neurogenetic adaptive mechanisms in alcoholism. *Science, 23,* 410–416.

Collins, R. L., Morsheimer, E. T., Shiffman, S., Pat, Y. J. A., Gnys, M., & Papandonatos, G. D. (1998). Ecological momentary assessment in a behavioral drinking moderation training program. *Experimental and Clinical Psychopharmacology, 6*(3), 306–315.

Connors, G. J., Donovan, D. M., & DiClemente, C. C. (2001). *Substance abuse treatment and the stages of change: Selecting and planning interventions.* New York: Guilford Press.

Connors, G. J., Longabaugh, R., & Miller, W. R. (1996). Looking forward and back to relapse: Implications for research and practice. *Addiction, 91*(Suppl. 12), S191–S196.

Connors, G. J., & Maisto, S. A. (1988). The alcohol expectancy construct: Overview and clinical applications. *Cognitive Research and Practice, 12,* 487–504.

Connors, G. J., Maisto, S. A., & Donovan, D. M. (1996). Conceptualizations of relapse: A summary of psychological and psychobiological models. *Addiction, 91*(Suppl. 12), 5–13.

Cooper, M. L., Russell, M., Skinner, J. B., & Windle, M. (1992). Development and validation of a three-dimensional measure of drinking motives. *Psychological Assessment, 4,* 123–132.

Cornelius, J. R., Bukstein, O., Salloum, I., & Clark, D. (2003). Alcohol and psychiatric comorbidity. *Recent Developments in Alcoholism, 16,* 361–374.

Cummings, C., Gordon, J. R., & Marlatt, G. A. (1980). Relapse: Strategies of prevention and prediction. In W. R. Miller (Ed.), *The addictive behaviors* (pp. 291–321). Elmsford, NY: Pergamon Press.

Curry, S., Marlatt, G. A., & Gordon, J. R. (1987). Abstinence violation effect: Validation of an attributional construct with smoking cessation. *Journal of Consulting and Clinical Psychology, 55*(2), 145–149.

Curry, S., Marlatt, G. A., Peterson, A. V., & Lutton, J. (1988). Survival analysis and assessment of relapse. In D. M. Donovan & G. A. Marlatt (Eds.), *Assessment of addictive behaviors* (pp. 454–483). New York: Guilford Press.

De, B., Mattoo, S. K., & Basu, D. (2003). Age at onset typology in opioid-dependent men: An exploratory study from India. *American Journal of Addictions, 12*(4), 336–345.

DiClemente, C. C., Carbonari, J. P., Montgomery, R. P., & Hughes, S. O. (1994). The Alcohol Abstinence Self-Efficacy scale. *Journal of Studies on Alcohol, 55*(2), 141–148.

DiClemente, C. C., Fairhurst, S. K., & Piotrowski, N. A. (1995). Self-efficacy and addictive behaviors. In J. E. Maddux (Ed.), *Self-efficacy, adaptation, and adjustment: Theory, research, and application* (pp. 109–141). New York: Plenum Press.

Dohm, F. A., Beattie, J. A., Aibel, C., & Striegel-Moore, R. H. (2001). Factors differentiating women and men who successfully maintain weight loss from women and men who do not. *Journal of Clinical Psychology, 57*(1), 105–117.

Donovan, D. M. (1988). Assessment of addictive behaviors: Implications of an emerging biopsychosocial model. In D. M. Donovan & G. A. Marlatt (Eds.), *Assessment of addictive behaviors* (pp. 3–48). New York: Guilford Press.

Donovan, D. M. (1996a). Assessment issues and domains in the prediction of relapse. *Addiction, 91*(Suppl. 12), S29–S36.

Donovan, D. M. (1996b). Marlatt's classification of relapse precipitants: Is the Emperor still wearing clothes? *Addiction, 91*(Suppl. 12), S131–S137.

Donovan, D. M. (1998). Assessment and interviewing strategies in addictive behaviors. In B. S. McCrady & E. E. Epstein (Eds.), *Addictions: A comprehensive guidebook for practitioners* (pp. 187–215). New York: Oxford University Press.

Donovan, D. M. (2003a). Assessments to aid in the treatment planning process. In J. P. Allen & V. Wilson (Eds.), *Assessing alcohol problems: A guide for clinicians and researchers* (2nd ed., pp. 125–188). Rockville, MD: National Institute on Alcohol Abuse and Alcoholism, U.S. Department of Health and Human Services, Public Health Service, National Institutes of Health.

Donovan, D. M. (2003b). Relapse prevention in substance abuse treatment. In J. L. Sorensen, R. Rawson, J. R. Guydish, & J. E. Zweben (Eds.), *Drug abuse treatment through collaboration: Practice and research partnerships that work* (pp. 121–137). Washington, DC: American Psychological Association.

Donovan, D. M. (2003c). Self-report assessment instruments. In B. A. Johnson, P. Ruiz, & M. Galanter (Eds.), *Handbook of clinical alcoholism treatment* (pp. 49–61). Baltimore: Lippincott/Williams & Wilkins.

Donovan, D. M., & Chaney, E. F. (1985). Alcoholic relapse prevention and intervention: Models and methods. In G. A. Marlatt & J. R. Gordon (Eds.), *Relapse prevention: Maintenance strategies in the treatment of addictive behaviors* (pp. 351–416). New York: Guilford Press.

Donovan, D. M., & Marlatt, G. A. (Eds.). (1988). *Assessment of addictive behaviors.* New York: Guilford Press.

Donovan, D. M., & Marlatt, G. A. (1993). Behavioral treatment. In M. Galanter & H. Begleiter (Eds.), *Recent developments in alcoholism: Vol. 11. Ten years of progress* (pp. 397–411). New York: Plenum Press.

Donovan, D. M., & Rosengren, D. B. (1999). Motivation for behavior change and treatment among substance abusers. In J. A. Tucker, D. M. Donovan & G. A. Marlatt (Eds.), *Changing addictive behavior: Bridging clinical and public health strategies* (pp. 127–159). New York: Guilford Press.

Dowden, C., Antonowicz, D., & Andrews, D. A. (2003). The effectiveness of relapse prevention with offenders: A meta-analysis. *International Journal of Offender Therapy and Comparative Criminology, 47*(5), 516–528.

Drake, R. E., Mueser, K. T., Brunette, M. F., & McHugo, G. J. (2004). A review of treatments for people with severe mental illnesses and co-occurring substance use disorders. *Psychiatric Rehabilitation Journal, 27*(4), 360–374.

Driessen, M., Veltrup, C., Wetterling, T., John, U., & Dilling, H. (1998). Axis I and Axis II comorbidity in alcohol dependence and the two types of alcoholism. *Alchoholism: Clinical and Experimental Research, 22*(1), 77–86.

Drobes, D. J., Meier, E. A., & Tiffany, S. T. (1994). Assessment of the effects of urges and negative affect on smokers' coping skills. *Behaviour Research and Therapy, 32*(1), 165–174.

Drummond, D. C. (2000). What does cue-reactivity have to offer clinical research? *Addiction, 95*(Suppl.), S129–S144.

Dunn, M. E., & Goldman, M. S. (1998). Age and drinking-related differences in the memory organization of alcohol expectancies in 3rd-, 6th-, 9th-, and 12th-grade children. *Journal of Consulting and Clinical Psychology, 66*(3), 579–585.

Einstein, S. (1994). Relapse revisited: Failure by whom and what? *International Journal of the Addictions, 29*, 409–413.

Eisen, S. A., Lin, N., Lyons, M. J., Scherrer, J. F., Griffith, K., True, W. R., Goldberg, J., & Tsuang, M. T. (1998). Familial influences on gambling behavior: An analysis of 3359 twin pairs. *Addiction, 93*(9), 1375–1384.

Epstein, E. E., Labouvie, E., McCrady, B. S., Jensen, N. K., & Hayaki, J. (2002). A multi-site study of alcohol subtypes: Classification and overlap of unidimensional and multi-dimensional typologies. *Addiction, 97*(8), 1041–1053.

Etter, J. F., Bergman, M. M., Humair, J. P., & Perneger, T. V. (2000). Development and validation of a scale measuring self-efficacy of current and former smokers. *Addiction, 95*(6), 613–625.

Ewing, J. A. (1977). A biopsychosocial look at drinking and alcoholism. *Journal of the American College Health Association, 25*(3), 204–208.

Ewing, J. A. (1980). Alcoholism—Another biopsychosocial disease. *Psychosomatics, 21*(5), 371–372.

Feeney, G. F., Young, R. M., Connor, J. P., Tucker, J., & McPherson, A. (2002). Cognitive behavioural therapy combined with the relapse-prevention medication acamprosate: Are short-term treatment outcomes for alcohol dependence improved? *Australian and New Zealand Journal of Psychiatry, 36*(5), 622–628.

Field, M., Mogg, K., & Bradley, B. P. (2004a). Cognitive bias and drug craving in recreational cannabis users. *Drug and Alcohol Dependence, 74*(1), 105–111.

Field, M., Mogg, K., & Bradley, B. P. (2004b). Eye movements to smoking-related cues: Effects of nicotine deprivation. *Psychopharmacology, 173*(1–2), 116–123.

Field, M., Mogg, K., Zetteler, J., & Bradley, B. P. (2004). Attentional biases for alcohol cues in heavy and light social drinkers: the roles of initial orienting and maintained attention [Electronic version]. *Psychopharmacology, 176*(1), 88–93.

Galizio, M., & Maisto, S. A. (1985). Toward a biopsychosocial theory of substance abuse. In M. Galizio & S. A. Maisto (Eds.), *Determinants of substance abuse: Bi-*

ological, psychological and environmental factors (pp. 425–429). New York: Plenum Press.

Giannetti, V. J. (1993). Brief relapse prevention with substance abusers. In R. A. Wells & V. J. Giannetti (Eds.), *Casebook of the brief psychotherapies: Applied clinical psychology* (pp. 159–178). New York: Plenum Press.

Glautier, S., & Drummond, D. C. (1994a). Alcohol dependence and cue reactivity. *Journal of Studies on Alcohol, 55*(2), 224–229.

Glautier, S., & Drummond, D. C. (1994b). A conditioning approach to the analysis and treatment of drinking problems. *British Medical Bulletin, 50*(1), 186–199.

Goldman, M. S. (1994). The alcohol expectancy concept: Applications to assessment, prevention, and treatment of alcohol abuse. *Applied and Preventive Psychology, 3*(3), 131–144.

Goodman, A. (1990). Addiction: Definition and implications. *British Journal of Addiction, 85*(11), 1403–1408.

Graham, K., Annis, H. M., Brett, P. J., & Venesoen, P. (1996). A controlled field trial of group versus individual cognitive-behavioural training for relapse prevention. *Addiction, 91*(8), 1127–1140.

Grilo, C. M., & Shiffman, S. (1994). Longitudinal investigation of the abstinence violation effect in binge eaters. *Journal of Consulting and Clinical Psychology, 62*(3), 611–619.

Grilo, C. M., Shiffman, S., & Wing, R. R. (1989). Relapse crises and coping among dieters. *Journal of Consulting and Clinical Psychology, 57*(4), 488–495.

Grilo, C. M., Shiffman, S., & Wing, R. R. (1993). Coping with dietary relapse crises and their aftermath. *Addictive Behaviors, 18*(1), 89–102.

Gustafson, R. (1992). The development of alcohol-related expectancies from the age of 12 to the age of 15 for two Swedish adolescent samples. *Alcoholism: Clinical and Experimental Research, 16*(4), 700–704.

Gwaltney, C. J., Shiffman, S., Norman, G. J., Paty, J. A., Kassel, J. D., Gnys, M., Hickcox, M., Waters, A., & Balabanis, M. (2001). Does smoking abstinence self-efficacy vary across situations?: Identifying context-specificity within the Relapse Situation Efficacy Questionnaire. *Journal of Consulting and Clinical Psychology, 69*(3), 516–527.

Gwaltney, C. J., Shiffman, S., Paty, J. A., Liu, K. S., Kassel, J. D., Gnys, M., & Hickcox, M. (2002). Using self-efficacy judgments to predict characteristics of lapses to smoking. *Journal of Consulting and Clinical Psychology, 70*(5), 1140–1149.

Havassy, B. E., Alvidrez, J., & Owen, K. K. (2004). Comparisons of patients with comorbid psychiatric and substance use disorders: Implications for treatment and service delivery. *American Journal of Psychiatry, 161*(1), 139–145.

Hayletta, S. A., Stephenson, G. M., & Lefevera, R. M. H. (2004). Covariation in addictive behaviours: A study of addictive orientations using the Shorter PROMIS Questionnaire. *Addictive Behaviors, 29*, 61–71.

Heather, N., & Stallard, A. (1989). Does the Marlatt model underestimate the importance of conditioned craving in the relapse process? In M. Gossop (Ed.), *Relapse and addictive behaviour* (pp. 180–208). New York: Tavistock/Routledge.

Heather, N., Stallard, A., & Tebbutt, J. (1991). Importance of substance cues in relapse among heroin users: Comparison of two methods of investigation. *Addictive Behaviors, 16*(1–2), 41–49.

Henderson, M. J., & Galen, L. W. (2003). A classification of substance-dependent men on temperament and severity variables. *Addictive Behaviors, 28*(4), 741–760.

Hill, E. M., Stoltenberg, S. F., Bullard, K. H., Li, S., Zucker, R. A., & Burmeister, M. (2002). Antisocial alcoholism and serotonin-related polymorphisms: Association tests. *Psychiatric Genetics, 12*(3), 143–153.

Hill, E. M., Stoltenberg, S. F., Burmeister, M., Closser, M., & Zucker, R. A. (1999). Potential associations among genetic markers in the serotonergic system and the antisocial alcoholism subtype. *Experimental and Clinical Psychopharmacology, 7*(2), 103–121.

Hodgins, D. C., & el-Guebaly, N. (2004). Retrospective and prospective reports of precipitants to relapse in pathological gambling. *Journal of Consulting and Clinical Psychology, 72*(1), 72–80.

Hodgins, D. C., el-Guebaly, N., & Armstrong, S. (1995). Prospective and retrospective reports of mood states before relapse to substance use. *Journal of Consulting and Clinical Psychology, 63*(3), 400–407.

Holahan, C. J., Moos, R. H., Holahan, C. K., Cronkite, R. C., & Randall, P. K. (2001). Drinking to cope, emotional distress and alcohol use and abuse: A ten-year model. *Journal of Studies on Alcohol, 62*(2), 190–198.

Hudson, S. M., Ward, T., & Marshall, W. L. (1992). The abstinence violation effect in sex offenders: A reformulation. *Behaviour Research and Therapy, 30*(5), 435–441.

Hufford, M. R., Witkiewitz, K., Shields, A. L., Kodya, S., & Caruso, J. C. (2003). Relapse as a nonlinear dynamic system: Application to patients with alcohol use disorders. *Journal of Abnormal Psychology, 112*(2), 219–227.

Hunt, W., Barnett, L., & Branch, L. (1971). Relapse rates in addiction programs. *Journal of Clinical Psychology, 27*(4), 455–456.

Irvin, J. E., Bowers, C. A., Dunn, M. E., & Wang, M. C. (1999). Efficacy of relapse prevention: A meta-analytic review. *Journal of Consulting and Clinical Psychology, 67*(4), 563–570.

Isenhart, C. E. (1991). Factor structure of the Inventory of Drinking Situations. *Journal of Substance Abuse, 3*(1), 59–71.

Isenhart, C. E. (1993). Psychometric evaluation of a short form of the inventory of drinking situations. *Journal of Studies on Alcohol, 54*(3), 345–349.

Johnson, B. A., Ait-Daoud, N., Ma, J. Z., & Wang, Y. (2003). Ondansetron reduces mood disturbance among biologically predisposed, alcohol-dependent individuals. *Alcoholism: Clinical and Experimental Research, 27*(11), 1773–1779.

Johnson, B. A., Roache, J. D., Ait-Daoud, N., Zanca, N. A., & Velazquez, M. (2002). Ondansetron reduces the craving of biologically predisposed alcoholics. *Psychopharmacology, 160*(4), 408–413.

Johnson, B. A., Roache, J. D., Javors, M. A., DiClemente, C. C., Cloninger, C. R., Prihoda, T. J., Bordnick, P. S., Ait-Daoud, N., & Hensler, J. (2000). Ondansetron for reduction of drinking among biologically predisposed alcoholic patients: A randomized controlled trial. *Journal of the American Medical Association, 284*(8), 963–971.

Kadden, R. M. (1995). Cognitive-behavioral approaches to alcoholism treatment. *Alcohol Health and Research World, 18*(4), 279–286.

Kadden, R. M. (1999). Cognitive behavior therapy. In P. J. Ott & R. E. Tarter (Eds.), *Sourcebook on substance abuse: Etiology, epidemiology, assessment, and treatment* (pp. 272–283). Boston: Allyn and Bacon.

Kilbey, M. M., Downey, K., & Breslau, N. (1998). Predicting the emergence and persistence of alcohol dependence in young adults: The role of expectancy and other risk factors. *Experimental and Clinical Psychopharmacology, 6*(2), 149–156.

Kranzler, H. R., Burleson, J. A., Brown, J., & Babor, T. F. (1996). Fluoxetine treatment seems to reduce the beneficial effects of cognitive-behavioral therapy in Type B alcoholics. *Alchoholism: Clinical and Experimental Research, 20*(9), 1534–1541.

Kranzler, H. R., & Rosenthal, R. N. (2003). Dual diagnosis: Alcoholism and co-morbid psychiatric disorders. *American Journal of Addictions, 12*(Suppl. 1), S26–S40.

Lamb, S., Greenlick, M. R., & McCarty, D. (Eds.). (1998). *Bridging the gap between practice and research: Forging partnerships with community-based drug and alcohol treatment.* Washington, DC: National Academy Press.

Langbehn, D. R., Cadoret, R. J., Caspers, K., Troughton, E. P., & Yucuis, R. (2003). Genetic and environmental risk factors for the onset of drug use and problems in adoptees. *Drug and Alcohol Dependence, 69*(2), 151–167.

Langenbucher, J., Sulesund, D., Chung, T., & Morgenstern, J. (1996). Illness severity and self-efficacy as course predictors of DSM-IV alcohol dependence in a multisite clinical sample. *Addictive Behaviors, 21*(5), 543–553.

Larimer, M. E., & Marlatt, G. A. (1990). Applications of relapse prevention with moderation goals. *Journal of Psychoactive Drugs, 22*(2), 189–195.

Larimer, M. E., Palmer, R. S., & Marlatt, G. A. (1999). Relapse prevention: An overview of Marlatt's cognitive-behavioral model. *Alcohol Research and Health, 23*(2), 151–160.

Laudet, A., Magura, S., Vogel, H. S., & Knight, E. (2000). Recovery challenges among dually diagnosed individuals. *Journal of Substance Abuse Treatment, 18*(4), 321–329.

Lehman, A. F., Myers, C. P., Thompson, J. W., & Corty, E. (1993). Implications of mental and substance use disorders: A comparison of single and dual diagnosis patients. *Journal of Nervous and Mental Disease, 181*(6), 365–370.

Lesieur, H. R., & Blume, S. B. (1993). Pathological gambling, eating disorders, and the psychoactive substance use disorders. *Journal of Addictive Diseases, 12*(3), 89–102.

Limosin, F., Loze, J. Y., Rouillon, F., Ades, J., & Gorwood, P. (2003). Association between dopamine receptor D1 gene DdeI polymorphism and sensation seeking in alcohol-dependent men. *Alcoholism: Clinical and Experimental Research, 27*(8), 1226–1228.

Litman, G. K. (1986). Alcohol survival: The prevention of relapse. In W. R. Miller & N. Heather (Eds.), *Treating addictive disorders: Processes of change* (pp. 391–405). New York: Plenum Press.

Litman, G. K., Stapleton, J., Oppenheim, A. N., Peleg, M., & Jackson, P. (1983). Situations related to alcoholism relapse. *British Journal of Addiction, 78*(4), 381–389.

Litman, G. K., Stapleton, J., Oppenheim, A. N., Peleg, M., & Jackson, P. (1984). Relationship between coping behaviours, their effectiveness and alcoholism relapse and survival. *British Journal of Addiction, 79*(3), 283–291.

Litt, M. D., Babor, T. F., DelBoca, F. K., Kadden, R. M., & Cooney, N. L. (1992). Types of alcoholics: II. Application of an empirically derived typology to treatment matching. *Archives of General Psychiatry, 49*(8), 609–614.

Litt, M. D., Cooney, N. L., & Morse, P. (2000). Reactivity to alcohol-related stimuli in the laboratory and in the field: Predictors of craving in treated alcoholics. *Addiction, 95*(6), 889–900.

Llorente, J. M., Fernandez, C., & Gutierrez, M. (2000). Prediction of relapse among heroin users treated in Spanish therapeutic communities: A comparison of different models. *Substance Use and Misuse, 35*(11), 1537–1550.

Longabaugh, R. (2003). Involvement of support networks in treatment. *Recent Developments in Alcoholism, 16,* 1332–1147.

Longabaugh, R., Rubin, A., Stout, R. L., Zywiak, W. H., & Lowman, C. (1996). The reliability of Marlatt's taxonomy for classifying relapses. *Addiction, 91*(Suppl. 12), S73–S88.

Lowman, C., Allen, J., & Stout, R. L. (1996). Replication and extension of Marlatt's taxonomy of relapse precipitants: Overview of procedures and results (Relapse Research Group). *Addiction, 91*(Suppl. 12), S51–S71.

Maisto, S. A., Pollock, N. K., Cornelius, J. R., Lynch, K. G., & Martin, C. S. (2003). Alcohol relapse as a function of relapse definition in a clinical sample of adolescents. *Addictive Behaviors, 28*(3), 449–459.

Marks, I. (1990). Behavioural (non-chemical) addictions. *British Journal of Addiction, 85*(11), 1389–1394.

Marlatt, G. A. (1990). Cue exposure and relapse prevention in the treatment of addictive behaviors. *Addictive Behaviors, 15*(4), 395–399.

Marlatt, G. A. (1996a). Lest taxonomy become taxidermy: A comment on the relapse replication and extension project. *Addiction, 91*(Suppl. 12), S147–S153.

Marlatt, G. A. (1996b). Taxonomy of high-risk situations for alcohol relapse: Evolution and development of a cognitive-behavioral model. *Addiction, 91*(Suppl. 12), S37–S49.

Marlatt, G. A., & Donovan, D. M. (1981). Alcoholism and drug dependence: Cognitive social learning factors in addictive behaviors. In E. W. Craighead, A. E. Kazdin, & M. J. Mahoney (Eds.), *Behavior modification: Principles, issues, and applications* (2nd ed., pp. 264–285). Boston: Houghton Mifflin.

Marlatt, G. A., & Donovan, D. M. (Eds.). (2005). *Relapse prevention* (2nd ed.). New York: Guilford Press.

Marlatt, G. A., & George, W. H. (1984). Relapse prevention: Introduction and overview of the model. *British Journal of Addiction, 79*(3), 261–273.

Marlatt, G. A., & Gordon, J. R. (1980). Determinants of relapse: Implications for the maintenance of behavior change. In P. O. Davidson & S. M. Davidson (Eds.), *Behavioral medicine: Changing health lifestyles* (pp. 1410–1452). New York: Brunner/Mazel.

Marlatt, G. A., & Gordon, J. R. (Eds.). (1985). *Relapse prevention: Maintenance strategies in the treatment of addictive behaviors.* New York: Guilford Press.

Marlatt, G. A., & Witkiewitz, K. (2002). Harm reduction approaches to alcohol use: Health promotion, prevention, and treatment. *Addictive Behaviors, 27*(6), 867–886.

Martin, G. W., Pollock, N. K., Cornelius, J. R., Lynch, K. G., & Martin, C. S. (1995). The Drug Avoidance Self-Efficacy Scale. *Journal of Substance Abuse, 7*(2), 151–163.

McCrady, B. S. (1993). Relapse prevention: A couples-therapy perspective. In T. J. O'Farrell (Ed.), *Treating alcohol problems: Marital and family interventions* (pp. 165–182). New York: Guilford Press.

McCrady, B. S. (2000). Alcohol use disorders and the Division 12 Task Force of the American Psychological Association. *Psychology of Addictive Behaviors, 14*(3), 267–276.

McKay, J. R. (1999). Studies of factors in relapse to alcohol, drug and nicotine use: A critical review of methodologies and findings. *Journal of Studies on Alcohol,* 60(4), 566–576.

McKay, J. R., Merikle, E., Mulvaney, F. D., Weiss, R. V., & Koppenhaver, J. M. (2001). Factors accounting for cocaine use two years following initiation of continuing care. *Addiction, 96*(2), 213–225.

McKay, J. R., O'Farrell, T. J., Maisto, S. A., Connors, G. J., & Funder, D. C. (1989). Biases in relapse attributions made by alcoholics and their wives. *Addictive Behaviors, 14*(5), 513–522.

McKay, J. R., Rutherford, M. J., & Alterman, A. I. (1996). An investigation of potential time effects in retrospective reports of cocaine relapses. *Addictive Behaviors, 21*(1), 37–46.

Merikangas, K. R., Stolar, M., Stevens, D. E., Goulet, J., Preisig, M. A., Fenton, B., Zhang, H., O'Malley, S. S., & Rounsaville, B. J. (1998). Familial transmission of substance use disorders. *Archives of General Psychiatry, 55*(11), 973–979.

Meyer, R. E., & Babor, T. F. (1989). Explanatory models of alcoholism. In A. Tasman, R. E. Hales, & A. J. Frances (Eds.), *American Psychiatric Press review of psychiatry* (Vol. 8, pp. 273–292). Washington, DC: American Psychiatric Press.

Miller, P. M., Smith, G. T., & Goldman, M. S. (1990). Emergence of alcohol expectancies in childhood: A possible critical period. *Journal of Studies on Alcohol, 51*(4), 343–349.

Miller, W. R. (1996). What is a relapse?: Fifty ways to leave the wagon. *Addiction, 91*(Suppl. 12), S15–S27.

Miller, W. R., Westerberg, V. S., Harris, R. J., & Tonigan, J. S. (1996). What predicts relapse?: Prospective testing of antecedent models. *Addiction, 91*(Suppl. 12), S155–S172.

Miller, W. R., & Wilbourne, P. L. (2002). Mesa Grande: A methodological analysis of clinical trials of treatments for alcohol use disorders. *Addiction, 97*(3), 265–277.

Moggi, F., Ouimette, P. C., Moos, R. H., & Finney, J. W. (1999). Dual diagnosis patients in substance abuse treatment: Relationship of general coping and substance-specific coping to 1–year outcomes. *Addiction, 94*(12), 1805–1816.

Mokdad, A. H., Marks, J. S., Stroup, D. F., & Gerberding, J. L. (2004). Actual causes of death in the United States, 2000. *Journal of the American Medical Association, 291*(10), 1238–1245.

Monti, P. M., Abrams, D. B., Kadden, R. M., & Cooney, N. L. (1989). *Treating alcohol dependence: A coping skills training guide.* New York: Guilford Press.

Monti, P. M., Gulliver, S. B., & Myers, M. G. (1994). Social skills training for alcoholics: Assessment and treatment. *Alcohol and Alcoholism, 29*(6), 627–637.

Monti, P. M., & O'Leary, T. A. (1999). Coping and social skills training for alcohol and cocaine dependence. *Psychiatric Clinics of North America, 22*(2), 447–470.

Monti, P. M., Rohsenow, D. J., Abrams, D. B., Zwick, W. R., Binkoff, J. A., Munroe, S. M., Fingeret, A. L., Nirenberg, T. D., Liepman, M. R., Pedraza, M., Kadden, R. M., & Cooney, N. L. (1993). Development of a behavior analytically derived alcohol-specific role-play assessment instrument. *Journal of Studies on Alcohol, 54*(6), 710–721.

Monti, P. M., Rohsenow, D. J., Colby, S. M., & Abrams, D. B. (1995). Coping and social skills training. In R. K. Hester & W. R. Miller (Eds.), *Handbook of alcoholism treatment approaches: Effective alternatives* (2nd ed., pp. 221–241). Boston: Ally & Bacon.

Monti, P. M., Rohsenow, D. J., & Hutchison, K. E. (2000). Toward bridging the gap between biological, psychobiological and psychosocial models of alcohol craving. *Addiction, 95*(Suppl.), S229–S236.

Monti, P. M., Rohsenow, D. J., Swift, R. M., Gulliver, S. B., Colby, S. M., Mueller, T. I., Brown, R. A., Gordon, A., Abrams, D. B., Niaura, R. S., & Asher, M. K. (2001). Naltrexone and cue exposure with coping and communication skills training for alcoholics: Treatment process and 1–year outcomes. *Alcoholism: Clinical and Experimental Research, 25*(11), 1634–1647.

Mooney, J. P., Burling, T. A., Hartman, W. M., & Brenner-Liss, D. (1992). The abstinence violation effect and very low calorie diet success. *Addictive Behaviors, 17*(4), 319–324.

Moos, R. H. (2003). Addictive disorders in context: Principles and puzzles of effective treatment and recovery. *Psychology of Addictive Behaviors, 17*(1), 3–12.

Moos, R. H., & Holahan, C. J. (2003). Dispositional and contextual perspectives on coping: Toward an integrative framework. *Journal of Clinical Psychology, 59*(12), 1387–1403.

Moser, A. E., & Annis, H. M. (1996). The role of coping in relapse crisis outcome: A prospective study of treated alcoholics. *Addiction, 91*(8), 1101–1114.

Mulder, R. T. (2002). Alcoholism and personality. *Australian and New Zealand Journal of Psychiatry, 36*(1), 44–52.

Mundt, J. C., Bohn, M. J., King, M., & Hartley, M. T. (2002). Automating standard alcohol use assessment instruments via interactive voice response technology. *Alcohol: Clinical and Experimental Research, 26*(2), 207–211.

Mundt, J. C., Perrine, M. W., & Searles, J. S. (1997). Individual differences in alcohol responsivity: Physiological, psychomotor and subjective response domains. *Journal of Studies on Alcohol, 58*(2), 130–140.

Myers, M. G., & Brown, S. A. (1990). Coping responses and relapse among adolescent substance abusers. *Journal of Substance Abuse, 2*(2), 177–189.

Niaura, R. (2000). Cognitive social learning and related perspectives on drug craving. *Addiction, 95*(Suppl.), S155–S163.

Noble, E. P. (1998). The D2 dopamine receptor gene: A review of association studies in alcoholism and phenotypes. *Alcohol, 16*(1), 33–45.

Noone, M., Dua, J., & Markham, R. (1999). Stress, cognitive factors, and coping resources as predictors of relapse in alcoholics. *Addictive Behaviors, 24*(5), 687–693.

O'Brien, C. P., Childress, A. R., Ehrman, R., & Robbins, S. J. (1998). Conditioning factors in drug abuse: Can they explain compulsion? *Journal of Psychopharmacology, 12*(1), 15–22.

O'Connell, K. A., Gerkovich, M. M., Cook, M. R., Shiffman, S., Hickcox, M., & Kakolewski, K. E. (1998). Coping in real time: Using Ecological Momentary Assessment techniques to assess coping with the urge to smoke. *Research Nursing and Health, 21*(6), 487–497.

Oei, T. P. S., & Baldwin, A. R. (1994). Expectancy theory: A two-process model of alcohol use and abuse. *Journal of Studies on Alcohol, 55*(5), 525–534.

O'Malley, S. S., Jaffe, A. J., Chang, G., Schottenfeld, R. S., Meyer, R. E., & Rounsaville, B. (1992). Naltrexone and coping skills therapy for alcohol dependence: A controlled study. *Archives of General Psychiatry, 49*(11), 881–887.

Palfai, T. P., & Ostafin, B. D. (2003). The influence of alcohol on the activation of outcome expectancies: The role of evaluative expectancy activation in drinking behavior. *Journal of Studies on Alcohol, 64*(1), 111–119.

Patkar, A. A., Thornton, C. C., Mannelli, P., Hill, K. P., Gottheil, E., Vergare, M. J., & Weinstein, S. P. (2004). Comparison of pretreatment characteristics and treatment outcomes for alcohol-, cocaine-, and multisubstance-dependent patients. *Journal of Addictive Diseases, 23*(1), 93–109.

Pattison, E. M. (1980). Bio-psycho-social analysis of alcohol and drug abuse: Implications for social policy. In *Man, drugs, and society—Current perspectives, Proceedings of the First Pan-Pacific Conference on Drugs and Alcohol* (pp. 66–80). Canberra, Australia: Australian Foundation for Alcohol and Drug Dependence.

Pettinati, H. M., Volpicelli, J. R., Kranzler, H. R., Luck, G., Rukstalis, M. R., & Cnaan, A. (2000). Sertraline treatment for alcohol dependence: Interactive effects of medication and alcoholic subtype. *Alcoholism: Clinical and Experimental Research, 24*(10), 1597–1601.

Prochaska, J. O., DiClemente, C. C., & Norcross, J. C. (1992). In search of how people change: Applications to addictive behaviors. *American Psychologist, 47*, 1102–1114.

Rather, B. C., & Goldman, M. S. (1994). Drinking-related differences in the memory organization of alcohol expectancies. *Experimental and Clinical Psychopharmacology, 2*(3), 167–183.

Read, M. R., Penick, E. C., Powell, B. J., Nickel, E. J., Bingham, S. F., & Campbell, J. (1990). Subtyping male alcoholics by family history of alcohol abuse and co-occurring psychiatric disorder: A bi-dimensional model. *British Journal of Addiction, 85*(3), 367–378.

Rohsenow, D. J., Monti, P. M., Martin, R. A., Colby, S. M., Myers, M. G., Gulliver, S. B., Brown, R. A., Mueller, T. I., Gordon, A., & Abrams, D. B. (2004). Motivational enhancement and coping skills training for cocaine abusers: Effects on substance use outcomes. *Addiction, 99*(7), 862–874.

Rohsenow, D. J., Niaura, R. S., Childress, A. R., Abrams, D. B., & Monti, P. M. (1990–1991). Cue reactivity in addictive behaviors: Theoretical and treatment implications. *International Journal of Addictions, 25*(7A–8A), 957–993.

Ross, S. M., Miller, P. J., Emmerson, R. Y., & Todt, E. H. (1988–1989). Self-efficacy, standards, and abstinence violation: A comparison between newly sober and long-term sober alcoholics. *Journal of Substance Abuse, 1*(2), 221–229.

Rotgers, F. (2002). Clinically useful, research validated assessment of persons with alcohol problems. *Behaviour Research and Therapy, 40*(12), 1425–1441.

Sale, E., Sambrano, S., Springer, J. F., & Turner, C. W. (2003). Risk, protection, and substance use in adolescents: A multi-site model. *Journal of Drug Education, 33*(1), 91–105.

Saunders, B., & Allsop, S. (1987). Relapse: A psychological perspective. *British Journal of Addiction, 82*(4), 417–429.

Saunders, B., & Allsop, S. (1989). Relapse: A critique. In M. Gossop (Ed.), *Relapse and addictive behaviour* (pp. 249–277). London: Routledge.

Schmitz, J. M., Rosenfarb, I. S., & Payne, T. J. (1993). Cognitive and affective responses to successful coping during smoking cessation. *Journal of Substance Abuse, 5*(1), 61–72.

Schmitz, J. M., Stotts, A. L., Rhoades, H. M., & Grabowski, J. (2001). Naltrexone and relapse prevention treatment for cocaine-dependent patients. *Addictive Behaviors, 26*(2), 167–180.

Schneider, J. P., & Irons, R. R. (2001). Assessment and treatment of addictive sexual disorders: Relevance for chemical dependency relapse. *Substance Use and Misuse, 36*(13), 1795–1820.

Schuckit, M. A. (1994). Low level of response to alcohol as a predictor of future alcoholism. *American Journal of Psychiatry, 151*(2), 184–189.

Schuckit, M. A. (1998). Biological, psychological and environmental predictors of the alcoholism risk: A longitudinal study. *Journal of Studies on Alcohol, 59*(5), 485–494.

Schuckit, M. A., Edenberg, H. J., Kalmijn, J., Flury, L., Smith, T. L., Reich, T., Bierut, L., Goate, A., & Foroud, T. (2001). A genome-wide search for genes that relate to a low level of response to alcohol. *Alcoholism: Clinical and Experimental Research, 25*(3), 323–329.

Schuckit, M. A., Smith, T. L., Kalmijn, J., Tsuang, J., Hesselbrock, V., & Bucholz, K. (2000). Response to alcohol in daughters of alcoholics: A pilot study and a comparison with sons of alcoholics. *Alchohol and Alcoholism, 35*(3), 242–248.

Schwartz, J. E., Neale, J., Marco, C., Shiffman, S. S., & Stone, A. A. (1999). Does trait coping exist?: A momentary assessment approach to the evaluation of traits. *Journal of Personality and Social Psychology, 77*(2), 360–369.

Shaffer, H. J. (1997). The most important unresolved issue in the addictions: Conceptual chaos. *Substance Use and Misuse, 32*(11), 1573–1580.

Shiffman, S. (1987). Maintenance and relapse: Coping with temptation. In T. D. Nirenberg & S. A. Maisto (Eds.), *Developments in the assessment and treatment of addictive behaviors* (pp. 353–385). Norwood, NJ: Ablex.

Shiffman, S. (1989). Conceptual issues in the study of relapse. In M. Gossop (Ed.), *Relapse and addictive behaviour* (pp. 149–179). London: Tavistock/Routledge.

Shiffman, S., Balabanis, M. H., Paty, J. A., Engberg, J., Gwaltney, C. J., Liu, K. S., Gnys, M., Hickcox, M., & Paton, S. M. (2000). Dynamic effects of self-efficacy on smoking lapse and relapse. *Health Psychology, 19*(4), 315–323.

Shiffman, S., Hickcox, M., Paty, J. A., Gnys, M., Kassel, J. D., & Richards, T. J. (1996). Progression from a smoking lapse to relapse: Prediction from abstinence violation effects, nicotine dependence, and lapse characteristics. *Journal of Consulting and Clinical Psychology, 64*(5), 993–1002.

Shiffman, S., Hufford, M., Hickcox, M., Paty, J. A., Gnys, M., & Kassel, J. D. (1997). Remember that?: A comparison of real-time versus retrospective recall of smoking lapses. *Journal of Consulting and Clinical Psychology, 65*(2), 292–300.

Shiffman, S., Paty, J. A., Gnys, M., Kassel, J. A., & Hickcox, M. (1996). First lapses to smoking: Within-subjects analysis of real-time reports. *Journal of Consulting and Clinical Psychology, 64*, 366–379.

Shiffman, S., & Wills, T. A. (Eds.). (1985). *Coping and substance use.* Orlando, FL: Academic Press.

Siegler, M., Osmond, H., & Newell, S. (1968). Models of alcoholism. *Quarterly Journal of Studies on Alcohol, 29*, 571–591.

Sklar, S. M., Annis, H. M., & Turner, N. E. (1997). Development and validation of the Drug-Taking Confidence Questionnaire: A measure of coping self-efficacy. *Addictive Behaviors, 22*(5), 655–670.

Smith, D. E., & Seymour, R. B. (2004). The nature of addiction. In R. H. Coombs (Ed.), *Handbook of addictive behaviors: A practical guide to diagnosis and treatment* (pp. 3–30). New York: Wiley.

Sobell, L. C., Toneatto, T., & Sobell, M. B. (1994). Behavioral assessment and treat-

ment planning for alcohol, tobacco, and other drug problems: Current status with an emphasis on clinical applications. *Behavior Therapy, 25*(4), 533–580.

Spittle, B. J. (1982). Alcohol use in New Zealand: A review from a biopsychosocial perspective. *New Zealand Medical Journal, 95*(7), 222–225.

Stacy, A. W. (1997). Memory activation and expectancy as prospective predictors of alcohol and marijuana use. *Journal of Abnormal Psychology, 106*(1), 61–73.

Stacy, A. W., Leigh, B. C., & Weingardt, K. R. (1994). Memory accessibility and association of alcohol use and its positive outcomes. *Experimental and Clinical Psychopharmacology, 2*(3), 2690–2282.

Stacy, A. W., Newcomb, M. D., & Bentler, P. M. (1995). Expectancy in mediational models of cocaine use. *Personality and Individual Differences, 19*(5), 655–667.

Stephens, R. S., Curtin, L., Simpson, E. E., & Roffman, R. A. (1994). Testing the abstinence violation effect construct with marijuana cessation. *Addictive Behaviors, 19*(1), 23–32.

Stoffelmayr, B., Wadland, W. C., & Pan, W. (2003). An examination of the process of relapse prevention therapy designed to aid smoking cessation. *Addictive Behaviors, 28*(7), 1351–1358.

Stone, A. A., Schwartz, J. E., Neale, J. M., Shiffman, S., Marco, C. A., Hickcox, M., Paty, J., Porter, L. S., & Cruise, L. J. (1998). A comparison of coping assessed by ecological momentary assessment and retrospective recall. *Journal of Personality and Social Psychology, 74*(6), 1670–1680.

Stout, R. L., Longabaugh, R., & Rubin, A. (1996). Predictive validity of Marlatt's relapse taxonomy versus a more general relapse code. *Addiction, 91*(Suppl. 12), S99–S110.

Stout, R. L., Rubin, A., Zwick, W., Zywiak, W., & Bellino, L. (1999). Optimizing the cost-effectiveness of alcohol treatment: A rationale for extended case monitoring. *Addictive Behaviors, 24*(1), 17–35.

Tapert, S. F., Ozyurt, S. S., Myers, M. G., & Brown, S. .A. (2004). Neurocognitive ability in adults coping with alcohol and drug relapse temptations. *American Journal of Drug and Alcohol and Abuse, 30*(2), 445–460.

Tucker, J. A., Donovan, D. M., & Marlatt, G. A. (Eds.). (1999). *Changing addictive behavior: Bridging clinical and public health strategies.* New York: Guilford Press.

Vielva, I., & Iraurgi, I. (2001). Cognitive and behavioural factors as predictors of abstinence following treatment for alcohol dependence. *Addiction, 96*(2), 297–303.

Wallace, J. (1989). Biopsychosocial model of alcoholism. *Social Casework, 70,* 325–332.

Wallace, J. (1993). Modern disease models of alcoholism and other chemical dependencies: The new biopsychosocial models. *Drugs and Society, 8,* 69–87.

Walton, M. A., Castro, F. G., & Barrington, E. H. (1994). The role of attributions in abstinence, lapse, and relapse following substance abuse treatment. *Addictive Behaviors, 19*(3), 319–331.

Wang, S. J., Winchell, C. J., McCormick, C. G., Nevius, S. E., & O'Neill, R. T. (2002). Short of complete abstinence: An analysis exploration of multiple drinking episodes in alcoholism treatment trials. *Alcohol: Clinical and Experimental Research, 26*(12), 1803–1809.

Ward, T., Hudson, S. M., & Bulik, C. M. (1993). The abstinence violation effect in bulimia nervosa. *Addictive Behaviors, 18*(6), 671–680.

Waters, A. J., Shiffman, S., Bradley, B. P., & Mogg, K. (2003). Attentional shifts to smoking cues in smokers. *Addiction, 98*(10), 1409–1417.

Waters, A. J., Shiffman, S., Sayette, M. A., Paty, J. A., Gwaltney, C. J., & Balabanis, M. H. (2003). Attentional bias predicts outcome in smoking cessation. *Health Psychology, 22*(4), 378–387.

Watkins, K. E., Burnam, A., Kung, F. Y., & Paddock, S. (2001). A national survey of care for persons with co-occurring mental and substance use disorders. *Psychiatric Services, 52*(8), 1062–1068.

Weingardt, K. R., Stacy, A. W., & Leigh, B. C. (1996). Automatic activation of alcohol concepts in response to positive outcomes of alcohol use. *Alcoholism: Clinical and Experimental Research, 20*(1), 25–30.

Weiss, R. D., Najavits, L. M., & Greenfield, S. F. (1999). A relapse prevention group for patients with bipolar and substance use disorders. *Journal of Substance Abuse Treatment, 16*(1), 47–54.

Wilhelmsen, K. C., Schuckit, M., Smith, T. L., Lee, J. V., Segall, S. K., Feiler, H. S., & Kalmijn, J. (2003). The search for genes related to a low-level response to alcohol determined by alcohol challenges. *Alcoholism: Clinical and Experimental Research, 27*(7), 1041–1047.

Wilson, P. H. (1992). Relapse prevention: Conceptual and methodological issues. In P. H. Wilson (Ed.), *Principles and practice of relapse prevention* (pp. 1–22). New York: Guilford Press.

Witkiewitz, K., & Marlatt, G. A. (2004). Relapse prevention for alcohol and drug problems: That was Zen, this is Tao. *American Psychologist, 59*(4), 224–235.

Zucker, R. A., & Gomberg, E. S. (1986). Etiology of alcoholism reconsidered: The case for a biopsychosocial process. *American Psychologist, 41,* 783–793.

Zweben, A., & Cisler, R. A. (2003). Clinical and methodological utility of a composite outcome measure for alcohol treatment research. *Alcohol: Clinical and Experimental Research, 27*(10), 1680–1685.

Zywiak, W. H., Connors, G. J., Maisto, S. A., & Westerberg, V. S. (1996). Relapse research and the Reasons for Drinking Questionnaire: A factor analysis of Marlatt's relapse taxonomy. *Addiction, 91*(Suppl. 12), S121–S130.

Zywiak, W. H., Stout, R. L., Connors, G. J., Maisto, S. A., Longabaugh, R., & Dyck, I. S. (2001). *Factor analysis and predictive validity of the Relapse Questionnaire in Project MATCH.* Paper presented in a symposium, New Perspectives on Relapse and Treatment Outcome, Annual Meeting of the Research Society on Alcoholism, Montreal, Quebec, Canada.

Zywiak, W. H., Westerberg, V. S., Connors, G. J., & Maisto, S. A. (2003). Exploratory findings from the Reasons for Drinking Questionnaire. *Journal of Substance Abuse Treatment, 25*(4), 287–292.

CHAPTER 2

Assessment of Addictive Behaviors in Ethnic-Minority Cultures

ARTHUR W. BLUME
OSVALDO F. MORERA
BERENICE GARCÍA DE LA CRUZ

Addictive behaviors are a serious problem throughout the United States, but ethnic-minority groups may be especially at risk. To begin with, epidemiological data suggests that ethnic-minority abusers of substances may be experiencing disproportionately high numbers of adverse health consequences and may be underserved by treatment services. For example, African Americans have a very high death rate related to the consequences of alcohol when compared to white Americans, even though more African Americans than whites abstain from alcohol (National Institute on Alcohol Abuse and Alcoholism [NIAAA], 2001). Although liver disease (principally substance induced) was absent from the top 10 leading causes of death in the year 2000 for white Americans, it was the sixth leading cause of death for Native Americans and Alaska Natives, and for Hispanics (National Center for Injury Prevention and Control [NCIPC], 2003). Furthermore, ethnic-minority injectable drug users have significantly higher rates of hepatitis and human immunodeficiency virus (HIV) infections related to their drug use behavior than whites (Estrada, 2002). In addition, there is evidence that African American, Hispanic, and Native American adults may experience pathological gambling at rates higher than those for white Americans (Wardman, el-Guebaly, & Hodgins, 2001; Welte, Barnes, Wieczorek, Tidwell, & Parker, 2002).

Finally, there is significant evidence that ethnic-minority abusers of substances are not receiving the treatment services they need, although the cause of this health disparity is not fully understood (NIAAA, 2001; Wells, Klap, Koike, & Sherbourne, 2001). Some have suggested that societal–therapist racism and/or racial bias may be at the core of health disparities (Miranda, Lawson, & Escobar, 2002; Snowden, 2003; Williams & Rucker, 2000). Others have specified factors that may contribute to health disparities, such as basic mistrust of health care providers by ethnic-minority patients (Doescher, Saver, Franks, & Fiscella, 2000; Miranda et al., 2002), language barriers and cultural differences (Fiscella, Franks, Doescher, & Saver, 2002), or lack of financial resources, including health insurance (Miranda et al., 2002; Nazroo, 2003). In some cases, the mistrust of health care providers is the result of real-life aversive experiences (Snowden, 2003; van Ryn & Fu, 2003).

Even though the existence of health disparities for ethnic-minority clients and patients has been well documented among scientists in many domains of health and mental health research (e.g., Institute of Medicine, 2002; U.S. Department of Health and Human Services, 2001, 2003), there has been a recent political effort to downplay these disparities by governmental editing of the reports of some of these scientists (U.S. House of Representatives Committee on Government Reform, 2004). Political efforts like these will likely not decrease the suspicions of people who already feel they have been misled and mistreated by the government in the past.

Health disparity studies suggest that there may be problems in the way ethnic-minority patients are treated when they seek health services. However, treatment or therapy may not be the only avenues that can be improved in order to address the problem of disparities in care. An interesting article in the *Journal of the American Medical Association* (Fiscella, Franks, Gold, & Clancy, 2000) suggests that one important way to address health disparities may be to improve our assessment of ethnic-minority clients. Presumably, making the assessment of addictive behaviors more culturally relevant should improve the quality of care that ethnic-minority patients receive. However, before we embark upon how culturally to enhance addictive behavior assessment of clients, it is important to understand differences between ethnic-minority and majority culture, and the general historical context of testing in ethnic-minority communities.

The worldview of an ethnic-minority group can differ greatly from the majority culture worldview. For example, the worldview of the majority culture in the United States reflects a high sense of individualism. In American majority culture, "self" and "autonomy" commonly define identity and role in society. These majority culture values likely influence assessment. For instance, many Western assessments focus on "self"-assessment constructs that measure individual behavior and cognitions, rather than relational or communal constructs.

However, since many ethnic-minority clients do not necessarily operate with an autonomous worldview, a wealth of information may be missed when majority culture assessment strategies are used exclusively. Collectivism is often more valued than individualism and interdependence more valued than autonomy for many ethnic-minority clients. Actively participating in family and community life is generally a high priority (Gaines et al., 1997; Sue &

Sue, 2003a). Because of these cultural differences, ethnic-minority clients may have significantly different values than those held by majority culture, and vastly different understandings of normative behavior.

ASSESSMENT: ONE SIZE DOES NOT FIT ALL

In addition to cultural differences that may influence assessment, many ethnic-minority communities have a healthy mistrust of being tested, especially if the testing is conducted by people from outside the community. There is a history of testing conducted with little concern for the well-being of the ethnic-minority communities being tested. Because of this history, some ethnic-minority individuals are understandably cautious of being tested. Probably the most notorious examples are from the Barrow alcohol study and the Tuskegee syphilis study; these studies still influence perceptions toward testing, research, and health care within ethnic-minority communities (Freimuth et al., 2001; Gamble, 1993; Guilmet, 1989). In the Barrow study, the drinking behavior of the local indigenous community was portrayed in a highly unfavorable fashion, with little consideration or sensitivity for how the publicity would harm the community. Also, some serious methodological problems with the study made its conclusions suspect. The Tuskegee study is one of the most notorious examples of mistreatment of human subjects in history. African American men unknowingly infected with syphilis were left untreated in some cases for several decades by physicians working with the U.S. Public Health Service in order to study the natural history of this horrible disease.

For many years there has been concern that psychological assessment developed and standardized principally in majority culture populations may be biased, and that the results and interpretations of these assessments may not be accurate for ethnic-minority test takers. The most striking example of test bias has been in the realm of intelligence testing (e.g., Suzuki & Kugler, 1995; Valencia & Suzuki, 2001). In addition, there is evidence that mental health assessment may not accurately measure ethnic-minority mental health. Some researchers have suggested that racial bias in mental health diagnostic assessments has contributed to misdiagnosis and mistreatment of some ethnic-minority clients (Baker & Bell, 1999; Jenkins-Hall & Sacco, 1991; Neighbors et al., 1999; Prieto, McNeill, Walls, & Gomez, 2001; Rosenthal & Berven, 1999; Snowden, 2003; Strakowski et al., 1995; Trierweiler et al., 2000). Although research concerning ethnic–cultural differences on assessment of addictive behaviors is sparse, there is some evidence that ethnic-minority clients may respond differently than white clients on substance use measures, and that such differences can lead to diagnostic misinterpretation (Choca, Shanley, Peterson, & Van Denburg, 1990; Volk, Cantor, Steinbauer, & Cass, 1997; Zager & Megargee, 1981). As an example, the word "craving" in English is not easily translated into Spanish, and we have found that the construct of craving is not generally understood by people of Mexican origin, who have no equivalent construct in their culture.

There are several potential difficulties with using standard assessment measures across cultures. First, the language of the assessment may be difficult for an ethnic-minority client to understand. If English is not the first language, then the assessment may require translation into the client's first language. However, simply translating the measure into the client's preferred language is not adequate. When some measures are translated from English into another language, then back-translated into English, the difference between the original English assessment and the back-translated English assessment can be significant. With regard to addictive behavior assessments, there have been mixed results when items are translated from the original English into another language. Some assessments have been found to be adequate after translation from English to another language (e.g., Leung & Arthur, 2000; Velez-Blasini, 1997), whereas others may become less psychometrically sound (Rodriguez-Martos et al., 2000); in some cases, the questions become incomprehensible (Mason, 1995). There are not always vocabulary equivalents between what is being asked in English and what is ultimately asked in the other language, which can cause problems with simply translating an English instrument into another language. When the assessment is translated, it is being interpreted, and this interpretation may vary widely from the original intent of the English-worded question.

A second difficulty is that many assessments have not been normed on specific ethnic-minority populations. The norms of the majority culture may not be applicable for ethnic-minority group. To use norms developed on another culture to assess an ethnic-minority client is potentially introducing error into the assessment and inviting bias into the interpretation of the assessment.

Third, constructs that may be applicable in one culture may not be applicable in another. One example presented earlier in this chapter concerns how cravings are not necessarily understood among Mexican-origin people. Another example in psychopathology would be assessing for anxiety, which may be considered *nervios* (a physical problem) or even *susto* (a problem with the soul) in Latino cultures. And some constructs in ethnic-minority cultures have no equivalent in majority culture. For example, ghost sickness (an indigenous construct) would not likely be assessed in a majority culture treatment center. Furthermore, assessment instruments that measure specific constructs within one culture may not measure that construct the same way in another culture. Because of these concerns, assessment data for ethnic-minority clients gathered from instruments developed within majority culture should be interpreted with great caution.

As an example, researchers often assume that mean differences on a measure of interest between two populations (e.g., majority vs. ethnic-minority) are indicative of "true" differences between those groups. However, the scores of interest must be invariant across populations for those mean differences to be meaningful. While formal definitions of measurement invariance have been established by psychometricians (Byrne, Shavelson, & Muthen; 1989; Meredith, 1993; Reise, Widaman, & Pugh, 1993; Waller, 1999), this research has not been fully appreciated outside the domain of psychological measurement. According to Meredith (1993), items of any assessment must equally match the latent trait it is intended to measure across groups. In other words, measurement invariance suggests that the item response should be dependent upon the level of the latent trait that is being measured, and not dependent upon group membership.

There are a wide variety of procedures to ensure that measures are commensurable across populations. Means and covariance structure analysis (Chan, 2000; Panter, Swygert, Dahlstrom, & Tanaka, 1997; Widaman & Reise, 1997) proposes to measure the validity of a test's underlying latent ability by explaining covariations between the test items through a limited number of factors. The relationship between the test items and the latent trait is assumed to be linear.

The correlation between an item and a hypothesized factor can be thought of as a factor loading. A weak form of measurement invariance would hold, if the factor loadings were equivalent across groups. Partial measurement invariance (Byrne et al., 1989) states that a majority of items on any scale should have statistically equivalent factor loadings across groups. The testing of stronger forms of measurement invariance via means and covariance structure analysis has been eloquently described by Widaman and Reise (1997).

Another method to evaluate measurement invariance is through item response theory (IRT). For an introduction to IRT, see Hambleton, Swaminathan, and Rogers (1991). Unlike means and covariance structure analysis, IRT posits that the relationship between the latent trait being measured and item responses is nonlinear. This nonlinear relationship between item response and the latent trait is called an item characteristic curve (ICC). Several parameters influence the shape of the ICC. While other parametric item response models have been proposed (McDonald, 1967), three models are the typically estimated. The most popular models that describe this relationship are the one-parameter logistic, the two-parameter logistic, and the three-parameter logistic models.

The one-parameter logistic model, otherwise known as a Rasch model, estimates an item difficulty parameter. Item difficulty represents the amount of latent trait that is necessary in order to have a 50% chance of getting the item correct. The two-parameter model estimates both an item difficulty parameter and an item discrimination parameter. Item discrimination refers to the steepness of the ICC curve. Finally, the three-parameter logistic model estimates item difficulty, item discrimination, and pseudoguessing parameters. The pseudoguessing parameter represents the probability that an examinee with very low ability will correctly answer the test item by guessing. This pseudoguessing parameter is typically evaluated in educational tests. For personality tests and many health-related measures, it is not intuitive to model a pseudoguessing parameter, because examinees do not have a clear incentive to guess at personality items. Suggestions on which IRT model to choose can be found in Suen (1990) or in Camilli and Shepard (1994). For most addictive behavior inventories, we believe a researcher should assess the reasonableness of the assumption that items have equivalent discrimination parameters. If this is not a reasonable assumption, the researcher should estimate the two-parameter logistic model (see Appendix 2.1 at the end of this chapter for more details on these models).

Given concerns about assessment equivalency across cultures and language difficulties, when investigating addictive behaviors among ethnic-minority cultures, researchers must determine whether the assessments being utilized measure the targeted construct accurately. At the minimum, this may require piloting of existing measures among the ethnic-minority study population prior to conducting the research. In some cases, the pilot results may suggest that existing measures are inadequate, and new ones will have to be developed. Finally, both researchers and therapists should be sensitive to the misuse of assessment among ethnic-minority communities and be aware of how this legacy may affect some ethnic-minority clients in assessment situations.

CULTURAL CONSIDERATIONS IN ASSESSING ADDICTIVE BEHAVIORS

Considering Cultural Differences in Behavioral Assessment

In collectivistic cultures, where there may be highly proscribed expectations about social roles and obligations (Gushue & Sciarra, 1995; McGoldrick, Pearce, & Giordano, 1982; Sue & Sue, 2003b, 2003c), behavior is best understood in the context of social interactions. A comprehensive behavioral analysis of an ethnic-minority client should include how that person's behavior fits into a larger social context. The social context may include family life and larger community life, including important social institutions within the community.

For example, a thorough behavioral analysis for addictive behaviors should include not only a determination of how the addiction is affecting the client, but also how the addiction may have affected the client's roles in and obligations to family and community. Assessment should include important interpersonal consequences related to addictive behaviors, especially with regard to how the addictive behaviors have affected relationships with family members. Finally, the therapist would want to know the exact community views and norms concerning the addictive behavior in question, since those norms will likely exert strong influences on the behavior of the client.

One example of the differences in behavioral analysis of ethnic-minority clients can be illustrated in self-monitoring of addictive behaviors. For clients who have a collectivistic worldview, self-monitoring may be culturally enhanced by assigning the client the task to observe and record how the addictive behavior affects social interactions. So in addition to asking the client about linking the addictive behavior with personal consequences, thoughts, and feelings, it also may be important to link the substance use behavior to the consequences for, and the thoughts and feelings of the extended family and the greater community. Some ethnic-minority clients may have difficulty understanding self-monitoring as a written task, so it may be helpful to include an oral component. For instance, it might be more useful for an ethnic-minority client to complete self-monitoring in narrative form (relational) rather than in chart form.

Another important part of behavioral assessment is to ascertain whether a client has a repertoire of coping skills and is able to generate those skills at the appropriate times. To begin with, it is important to remember to assess whether the client has effective interpersonal skills to negotiate both majority and minority culture. Specifically, the therapist would want to determine social expectations placed upon the ethnic-minority client by both cultures, and then assess how well the client is meeting those expectations. This is discussed later in greater detail. In addition, it is important to determine whether the client is meeting expectations for his or her roles within the family and the community, and if not, whether the client has the requisite skills to do so.

Specific contexts for the addictive behavior pattern are important to identify, just as would be the case for a client from the majority culture, but assessing context should be conducted in a way that reflects an understanding of how the culture may be different than majority culture. For example, in assessing potentially risky relapse situations in ethnic-minority clients, the therapist may want to assess community or family social demands that may place the person at risk. Extended family members may exercise a great deal of influence on the ethnic-minority client, and it will be very important to conduct a risk assessment related to relapse associated with family interactions. Substance refusal skills should be assessed to determine whether the client can negotiate high-risk community and family activities in a socially respectful way.

In assessing problem-solving skills, it is important to understand the normative ways to solve problems within the ethnic-minority community. In the same way, goal setting is different for many ethnic-minority clients than what is expected among clients from majority culture. Some cultures find it disrespectful and rude to focus on individual goals, so it would be helpful to understand the cultural views about personal goals before emphasizing them in treatment. Alternatively, it may be quite helpful to establish client goals that are congruent with community goals, and to illustrate to the client how meeting those personal goals also would be helpful for both family and community.

Assessing Skills Sets for Multiple Cultures

Since ethnic-minority clients often live in two (or more) cultures, it has been hypothesized that they have to develop competence in the skills of each culture. This particular model has been referred to as "bicultural competence" (LaFromboise & Rowe, 1983). As a consequence of conceptualizing coping in this fashion, many intervention programs in ethnic communities have incorporated culturally enhanced skills training in order to promote bicultural competence. Successful programs have developed these bicultural skills training components in close consultation with community members in order to determine which skills are important and relevant for community well-being.

Conceptualizing that coping skills should be developed within a cultural context has led to assessment for ethnic identity becoming a more common practice. Assessing ethnic identity may be a way to ascertain what culturally enhanced skills may be important to a client, which can provide a road map for the type of skills training program (ethnic-minority or/and majority skills programs) to use with a client. Two ways to conceptualize ethnic identity may be helpful for understanding and treating addictive behaviors among ethnic-minority clients. First, ethnic identity can be conceptualized as the level of acculturation into majority society by the client. An assessment of acculturation can provide useful information concerning the level of comfort that a person may have with majority culture constructs, skills, and language. Many acculturation measures have been developed, and a few of the more commonly known measures are mentioned below.

For example, several acculturation measures have been developed and tested among Latino/Hispanic samples. First, the Bidimensional Acculturation Scale for Hispanics (BAS; Marín & Gamba, 1997), a 24-item measure, assesses acculturation into non-Hispanic majority culture and enculturation into Hispanic/Latino culture. Second, the Multidimensional 97 Acculturative Stress Inventory (MASI; Rodriguez, Myers, Mira, Flores, & Garcia-Hernandez, 2000), a 36-item instrument, measures acculturation stress among Mexican Americans. Third, the Acculturation, Habits, and Interests Multicultural Scale for Adolescents (AHIMSA; Unger et al., 2000) has four different scales that measure different levels of acculturation into American culture and of enculturation into Mexican American culture. As the name implies, the AHIMSA was developed specifically for use with Hispanic youth. Finally, the Bicultural Involvement Questionnaire (BIQ; Szapocznik, Kurtines, & Fernandez, 1980) was developed to assess enculturation into Hispanic culture and acculturation into majority culture, and the Cultural Lifestyle Inventory (CLSI; Mendoza, 1990) was developed to measure acculturation on five different dimensions among Mexican Americans.

Variations of the BIQ and CLSI have been developed and used among many other groups. The BIQ has been used to measure acculturation and enculturation among Dominican Americans (Rodriguez, 1999), Asian Americans (Borek, 1998), and Native Americans (Byington, 2001). The CLSI has been used to measure acculturation among Puerto Rican college students (De Leon & Mendez, 1996), Vietnamese American women (Nguyen, 1999), Armenian Americans (Khanjian, 2002), Iranian Americans (Ghaffarian, 1998; Ostovar, 1997; Rouhparvar, 2001), and Chinese Americans (Fu, 2002; Lau, 1998).

Assessing acculturation and enculturation may be potentially helpful for determining risk for addictive behaviors among specific ethnic-minority populations. For example, among Mexican American men, increased risky drinking behavior has been linked to increased acculturation into mainstream society (e.g., Caetano, 1987a, 1987b), and a study conducted with Native American youth found evidence that increased enculturation may protect against drug problems (Zimmerman, Ramirez, Washienko, Walter, & Dyer, 1998). However, not enough research has been conducted to fully understand the relationship between acculturation–enculturation and addictive behaviors. Some have speculated that a balance between acculturation and enculturation may be ideal for preventing and treating addictive behaviors (e.g., LaFromboise & Rowe, 1983), but research studies testing this assumption are minimal.

Second, ethnic identity also can be conceptualized as multifaceted, so that the level of identity with one culture is independent of the level of identity with another culture. An assessment of ethnic identity in this fashion can help to determine how engaged–disengaged a person may be in all the cultures in which he or she identifies or participates. This may provide information about the relevance of teaching bicultural or multicultural skills. The prevailing model for understanding ethnic identity is called the orthogonal cultural identification theory (OCIT; Oetting & Beauvais, 1991). Instruments to assess orthogonal cultural identification have been developed for African American youth (Strunin & Demissie, 2002), Native American youth (Oetting, Swaim, & Chiarella, 1998), and Korean Americans (Lee, 1995).

In addition, there is the Acculturation Rating Scale for Mexican Americans–II (ARSMA-II; Cuellar, Arnold, & Maldonado, 1995) which is a second-generation instrument that measures identification with Mexican American and majority white cultures. Similarly, the Asian Self-Identity Acculturation Scale (Suinn, Rickard-Figueroa, Lew, & Vigil, 1987) has been used to assess cultural identification among a wide range of Asian American groups, and the Multigroup Ethnic Identity Measure has been successfully among youth from many different ethnicities (Phinney, 1992).

Obviously, many different instruments are available to aid therapists in identifying acculturation, enculturation, and ethnic identity among ethnic-minority clients of many populations (see Table 2.1). A recommended resource for therapists is the book *Acculturation: Advances in Theory, Measurement, and Applied Research*, edited by Chun, Organista, and Marín (2002), which has a wealth of additional information that cannot be adequately covered in this particular forum.

TABLE 2.1. Measures of Ethnic Identity

Purpose	Domain/construct	Instrument(s)	Author(s)
Measure ethnic identity	Assessing skill sets for multiple cultures	BAS	Marín & Gamba (1997)
		MASI	Rodriguez, Myers, Mira, Flores, & Garcia-Hernandez (2000)
		AHIMSA	Unger et al. (2002)
		BIQ	Szapocznik, Kurtines, & Fernandez (1980)
		CLSI	Mendoza (1990)
		OCIT	Oetting & Beauvais (1991)
		ARSMA-II	Cuellar, Arnold, & Maldonado (1995)
		Asian Self-Identity Acculturation Scale	Suinn, Rickard-Figueroa, Lew, & Vigil (1987)
		Multigroup Ethnic Identity Measure	Phinney (1992)

Assessing the Experience of Racism

Finally, behavioral assessments of ethnic-minority clients are incomplete without assessing for racial or ethnic bias. Prejudice and racism are commonly reported experiences for people from ethnic-minority groups. Epidemiological research has suggested that racism can be a contributing factor to increased psychopathology, including substance abuse (Carter, 1994; Wingo, 2001). Unfortunately, assessing racial and ethnic bias as part of a more comprehensive behavioral analysis is frequently absent. By not conducting such an analysis, important information that links addictive behaviors with incidents of bias and pressure may be missed (Rhodes & Johnson, 1997).

Considering Cultural Differences in Assessing Cognitive Factors

Several cognitive factors have been found to be important determinants of the course of addictive behaviors after they have been initiated, including motivation and self efficacy to change the behaviors, and outcome expectancies about engaging in the addictive behaviors. In addition, self-efficacy related to addictive behaviors is predictive of relapse. However, little research has been conducted on how to assess these cognitive constructs among ethnic-minority clients. Furthermore, it is not clear whether the constructs are equivalent across cultures.

For example, key constructs within the transtheoretical stages-of-change model (TTM; Prochaska, DiClemente, & Norcross, 1992), including motivation to change, have not been investigated among ethnic-minority clients. Although the model itself was developed by using meta-analytical research from many outcome studies, those studies were principally conducted among samples drawn largely from the majority culture. With the limited research available, there is some reason to suspect that there may be differences in how motivation to change may be expressed across cultures.

The TTM posits that ambivalence about change is typical, and that people often use a decisional balance to weigh the benefits of change, as well as the benefits of not changing behavior. If the decisional balance tips in favor of change (i.e., if the pros for change outweigh the cons for change), then ambivalence toward change may be resolved in favor of motivation to change, which may result in commitment to a plan of action (e.g., Prochaska et al., 1992).

However, several studies have found slight group differences in results that have investigated the use of decisional balance among white and nonwhite smokers. One study that examined decisional balance differences between white and African American smokers found that white smokers had higher "pros" for smoking than did African Americans (Audrain et al., 1997), and another study that focused upon the decisional balance differences solely among women smokers found significantly greater numbers of "cons" for African Americans than for whites (Ahijevych & Parsley, 1999). In one other study, the investigators found decisional balance response among Southeast Asian American smokers that differed from more general population samples in the literature (Lafferty, Heaney, & Chen, 1999). Although the research is sparse in this area of inquiry, these findings suggest the possibility that the decisional balance could have a slightly different presentation in nonmajority clients.

It cannot be taken for granted that the construct of motivation is the same across all cultures. What little research has been conducted suggests that care must be taken when assessing ethnic-minority clients for motivation to change addictive behaviors, or when using a decisional balance method, because the results may suggest a level of motivation that is not necessarily accurate.

Cultural Differences and Self-Efficacy

Self-efficacy has been associated with changes in addictive behaviors in the general population, and there is some evidence that this may be true for ethnic-minority clients as well (e.g., Kercher, 2000). Interestingly, one smoking study found an inverse relationship between level of acculturation and reported self-efficacy among Hispanic study participants (Sabogal, Otero-Sabogal, Perez-Stable, Marín, & Marín, 1989), suggesting that cultural identity may influence self-efficacy.

Other research suggests that the construct of self-efficacy may be different among people from ethnic-minority populations than it is for whites. For instance, in studies concerning organizational behavior, participants from a collectivistic culture were more likely to develop efficacy in tasks from collective feedback and success rather than from individual feedback or success (Earley, 1994; Earley, Gibson, & Chen, 1999). These studies did not specifically examine the relationship between self-efficacy and addictive behaviors, but they do suggest the possibility that self-efficacy may develop differently among people from collectivistic cultures.

In fact, assessing collective efficacy may be as critical as assessment of self-efficacy among people from collectivistic societies. Collective efficacy is the shared belief by a group of people in their ability to organize successfully and complete particular tasks in order to achieve specified goals (Bandura, 1997). Since collective institutions such as the family or the community are the principle reference groups for normative behavior in many minority cultures, it would follow that efficacy would occur in the context of these social groups. As an example, a study examined the relationship of self-efficacy and collective efficacy with mental health and job satisfaction across both United States (individualistic) and Chinese (collectivistic) cultures. The researchers found that for workers in the United States, increased self-efficacy predicted better mental health and job satisfaction, but for Chinese workers, increased collective efficacy predicted better mental health and job satisfaction (Schaubroeck, Lam, & Xie, 2000).

With attention to the research, it is recommended that both self-efficacy and collective efficacy related to addictive behaviors be assessed. Although it is unclear whether either construct can be adequately measured across cultures, there is evidence that efficacy may be better understood in the context of social relations in some cultures, and that assessing self-efficacy alone may not provide the total picture of a person's competence and confidence in mastering particular situations.

Cultural Differences and Expectancies

Another important cognitive construct to assess relative to addictive behaviors is outcome expectancies, but like other constructs, there may cultural differences. For example, several studies have found significant cross-cultural differences in alcohol expectancies; one group studied expectancies among Japanese and American college students (Nagoshi, Nakata, Sasano, & Wood, 1994) and another studied expectancies among Irish and American adolescents (Christiansen & Teahan, 1987). Yet another study found cultural differences in the level of alcohol expectancies for aggressive behavior among college students across eight countries (Lindman & Lang, 1994).

Even within the United States, cultural differences have been found for alcohol expectancies. Researchers have found significant ethnic group differences in alcohol expectancies among college students (Daisy, 1989), between native Puerto Ricans and college students in the United States (Velez-Blasini, 1997), in alcohol expectancies between Puerto Ricans and Irish Americans

that mirrored cultural norms concerning the appropriateness for loss of control (Johnson & Glassman, 1999), and in smoking expectancies between Hispanic and non-Hispanic whites. Interestingly, the last study mentioned also found that acculturation level for Hispanics moderated differences in expectancies; the smoking expectancies of highly acculturated Hispanics tended to be very similar to smoking expectancies of non-Hispanic whites (Marín, Marín, Perez-Stable, Sabogal, & Otero-Sabogal, 1989). And just to complicate things further, in one intergenerational epidemiological study, the investigators found that expectancies varied across generations within ethnic-minority groups, and that those changes could reflect increased acculturation within groups over time (Caetano & Clark, 2002).

Although the assessment of expectancies may be important across cultures, there may be cultural differences that complicate such assessment. Research about expectancies in different cultures needs to be expanded, so that new, culturally relevant assessment tools for ethnic-minority cultures can be developed. However, the Caetano and Clark study (2002) also reminds researchers and therapists that expectancies may be subject to cohort effects, which could mean that assessments developed for use with one generation may not necessarily be applicable to the next.

Considering Cultural Differences in Neuropsychological Assessment

Much has been written about the deleterious effects of alcohol and other substances upon the brain (e.g., Bates, Bowden, & Barry, 2002; Brown, Tapert, Granholm, & Delis, 2000). Because of the considerable evidence that substance abuse can be associated with cognitive difficulties, conducting a neuropsychological screen or full assessment has become a standard of care for those clinics that have the resources. Generally speaking, it seems appropriate to administer some form of neuropsychological assessment as part of a larger behavioral and cognitive assessment.

For ethnic-minority clients, conducting such an assessment is complicated. Several studies using a variety of neuropsychological assessments, some very well known, have found patterns of response that suggest potential cultural biases that may affect performance (Ardila & Moreno, 2001; Barker-Collo, 2001; Loewenstein, Argueelles, Argueelles, & Linn-Fuentes, 1994; Teresi, Holmes, Ramirez, Gurland, & Lantigua, 2001). Some of the difficulties may be a result of the neuropsychological tests being administered in English (e.g., Lu & Bigler, 2000). However, administration of tests in a second language cannot account for all potential biases. There had been some thought that potential cultural biases might be circumvented through the use of nonverbal testing, but even nonverbal tests have the potential for bias (Mahurin, Espino, & Holifield, 1992). Because of concerns about cultural bias, a neuropsychological assessment conducted with an ethnic-minority client should be interpreted with caution, especially if the person has limited English-language skills or is not highly acculturated into majority culture.

Considering Cultural Differences in Objective Assessment

Objective assessment, such as using laboratory tests, can be quite helpful when working with an ethnic-minority client, but suggesting that these tests be conducted may be greeted by suspicion. Western medicine and medical tests may not be sought out by patients who are less acculturated into majority society (Doescher et al., 2000; Miranda et al., 2002), and often those patients will prefer to participate in traditional folk medicine and healing practices. The risk with the use of objective tests is that a client may not show for the testing when it is requested, even if he or she appeared to be committed to doing so. Furthermore, the client may not disclose symptoms, so it would be unlikely that laboratory tests would be ordered.

Even if a client discloses symptoms, there is no guarantee that the symptoms will be understood by the treating professional. Recalling the previous discussion concerning language differences, vocabulary means different things across cultures, which complicates communication between client and provider. An example from an area of research outside of addictions illustrates this concern. In a study investigating how people with asthma described their airway obstruction symptoms, researchers found that African Americans described their symptoms differently than did white patients, and that those differences could prompt misunderstandings by physicians of the symptoms being reported (Hardie, Janson, Gold, Carrieri-Kohlman, & Boushey, 2000). Although similar research has not been conducted in the area of addictions, the implications are obvious. It is possible that ethnic-minority clients may not describe their addictive symptoms in ways that would be readily understood by health care professionals. Furthermore, the results of substance use may be misinterpreted. For example, some Native Americans and Alaska Natives use substances to seek visions. "Visions" could be mistaken for psychotic behavior as "a consequence" of substance use, when in fact the substance use was "a means" to have a religious or spiritual experience. Understanding cultural functions for substance use will help to avoid potential misunderstandings by professionals.

In spite of the potential difficulties, laboratory tests would be quite helpful to identify undetected addiction cases among ethnic-minority clients. Between the staggering figures concerning health problems subsequent to addictive behaviors among some ethnic minority groups (Estrada, 2002; NCIPC, 2003) and the reports of disparities in treatment services (NIAAA, 2001; Wells et al., 2001), any effort to expose undetected cases would be useful. The most likely place of contact with an undetected case would probably be a primary medical care clinic or an emergency department of a hospital—clinical settings that would have the staff and resources to administer objective assessment if it was determined to be warranted.

CONCLUSIONS

Assessment is extremely important in the diagnosis and treatment of addictive behaviors. However, there may be cultural differences that present challenges to accurately assessing addictive behavior. Many psychological assessments were developed within the majority culture, and some have been used in minority culture settings, with little regard for whether they validly assess behavior within those cultures. Because of these difficulties, some clients from ethnic-minority communities may not have sought or received the care they needed.

One of the great challenges ahead for addiction researchers is to develop and validate assessment tools suitable for use across very diverse cultures. The demographics of the United States are changing rapidly, and ethnic minorities are likely to become the ethnic majority in the next century or so (U.S. Bureau of the Census, 2003). Because of these changes, the cultural norms of the minority may well become the cultural norms for the majority. These monumental societal changes will likely have a broad impact on the treatment of addictive behaviors in American society. In order to meet the treatment needs of this rapidly changing society, the assessment of addictive behaviors will need to be conducted accurately and with sensitivity across a broad range of ethnic and cultural backgrounds.

APPENDIX 2.1. DETAILS ON
ITEM RESPONSE THEORY (IRT) MODELS

Expressed mathematically, the one-parameter logistic model is $P_i(\theta) = 1 / \{1 + \exp[-1.7(\theta - b)]\}$. The one-parameter model estimates an item difficulty parameter and is also known as the Rasch model. This model assumes that all of the items have equal item discriminations and pseudoguessing parameters equal to zero. The two-parameter logistic model is expressed mathematically as $P_i(\theta) = 1 / \{1 + \exp[-1.7 a(\theta - b)]\}$. The two-parameter model estimates both the difficulty parameter and the item difficulty. In other words, the two-parameter model assumes that the c parameter equals 0. Although the a and b parameters constitute the two-parameter model, they are measured on different metric systems and are not comparable. Finally, the three-parameter logistic model is expressed mathematically as

$$P(\theta) = c + \frac{1-c}{1 + \exp[-1.7\,a(\theta - b)]}$$

The three-parameter model estimates the a, b, and c parameters. The c parameter represents the probability that an examinee with very low ability will correctly answer the test item by guessing. The a parameter represents the discrimination of a test item and is related to the slope of the ICC (Waller, 1999). A steep slope indicates the ability of the item to discriminate within a small range of ability continuum. The b parameter, which represents the difficulty of each test item, is typically measured in the same metric as the ability (θ) parameter. The b parameter can represent the level of ability that an individual must possess to have a 50% probability of endorsing the item.

REFERENCES

Ahijevych, K., & Parsley, L. A. (1999). Smoke constituent exposure and stage of change in black and white women cigarette smokers. *Addictive Behaviors, 24,* 115–120.

Ardila, A., & Moreno, S. (2001). Neuropsychological test performance on Aruaco Indians: An exploratory study. *Journal of the International Neuropsychological Society, 7,* 510–515.

Audrain, J., Gomez-Caminero, A., Robertson, A. R., Boyd, R., Orleans, C. T., & Lerman, C. (1997). Gender and ethnic differences in readiness to change smoking behavior. *Women's Health, 3,* 139–150.

Baker, F. M., & Bell, C. C. (1999). Issues in the psychiatric treatment of African Americans. *Psychiatric Services, 50,* 362–368.

Bandura, A. (1997). Collective efficacy. In *Self-efficacy: The exercise of control* (pp. 477–525). New York: Freeman.

Barker-Collo, S. L. (2001). The 60–item Boston Naming Test: Cultural bias and possible adaptations for New Zealand. *Aphasiology, 15,* 85–92.

Bates, M. E., Bowden, S. C., & Barry, D. (2002). Neurocognitive impairment associated with alcohol use disorders: Implications for treatment. *Experimental and Clinical Psychopharmacology, 10,* 193–212.

Borek, N. T. (1998). *Collective self-esteem as related to acculturation and commitment to school in Latino and southeast Asian immigrant and refugee adolescents.* Unpublished doctoral dissertation, George Washington University, Washington, DC.

Brown, S. A., Tapert, S. F., Granholm, E., & Delis, D. C. (2000). Neurocognitive functioning of adolescents: Effects of protracted alcohol use. *Alcoholism: Clinical and Experimental Research, 24,* 164–171.

Byington, M. L. (2001). *Bicultural involvement, psychological differentiation, and time perspective as mediators for depression and anxiety in Native Americans living on and off-reservation.* Unpublished doctoral dissertation, Columbia University, New York.

Byrne, B. M., Shavelson, R. J., & Muthen, B. (1989). Testing for the equivalence of factor covariance and mean structures: The issue of partial measurement invariance. *Psychological Bulletin, 105,* 456–466.

Caetano, R. (1987a). Acculturation and drinking patterns among U.S. Hispanics. *British Journal of Addictions, 82,* 789–799.

Caetano, R. (1987b). Acculturation, drinking and social settings among U.S. Hispanics. *Drug and Alcohol Dependence, 19,* 215–226.

Caetano, R., & Clark, C. L. (2002). Acculturation, alcohol consumption, smoking, and drug use among Hispanics. In K. M. Chun, P. B. Organista, & G. Marín (Eds.), *Acculturation: Advances in theory, measurement, and applied research* (pp. 223–239). Washington, DC: American Psychological Association.

Camilli, G., & Shepard, L. A. (1994). *Methods for identifying biased test items.* Thousand Oaks, CA: Sage.

Carter, J. H. (1994). Racism's impact on mental health. *Journal of the American Medical Association, 86,* 543–547.

Chan, D. (2000). Detection of differential item functioning on the Kirton Adaption–Innovation Inventory using multi-group mean and covariance structure analyses. *Multivariate Behavioral Research, 35,* 169–199.

Choca, J. P., Shanley, L. A., Peterson, C. A., & Van Denburg, E. (1990). Racial bias and the MCMI. *Journal of Personality Assessment, 54,* 479–490.

Christiansen, B. A., & Teahan, J. E. (1987). Cross-cultural comparisons of Irish and American adolescent drinking practices and beliefs. *Journal of Studies on Alcohol, 48,* 558–562.

Chun, K. M., Organista, P. B., & Marín, G. (Eds.). (2002). *Acculturation: Advances in theory, measurement, and applied research.* Washington, DC: American Psychological Association.

Cuellar, I., Arnold, B., & Maldonado, R. (1995). Acculturation Rating Scale for Mexican Americans–II: A revision of the original ARMSA scale. *Hispanic Journal of Behavioral Sciences, 17,* 275–304.

Daisy, F. (1989). *Ethnic differences in alcohol outcome expectancies and drinking patterns.* Unpublished doctoral dissertation, University of Washington, Seattle.

De Leon, B., & Mendez, S. (1996). Factorial structure of a measure of acculturation in a Puerto Rican population. *Educational and Psychological Measurement, 56,* 155–165.

Doescher, M. P., Saver, B. G., Franks, P., & Fiscella, K. (2000). Racial and ethnic disparities in perceptions of physician style and trust. *Archives of Family Medicine, 9,* 1156–1163.

Earley, P. C. (1994). Self or group?: Cultural effects of training on self-efficacy and performance. *Administrative Science Quarterly, 39,* 89–117.

Earley, P. C., Gibson, C. B., & Chen, C. C. (1999). "How did I do?" versus "how did we do?": Cultural contrasts of performance feedback use and self-efficacy. *Journal of Cross-Cultural Psychology, 30,* 594–619.

Estrada, A. L. (2002). Epidemiology of HIV/AIDS, hepatitis B, hepatitis C, and tuberculosis among minority injection drug users. *Public Health Reports, 117,* S126–S134.

Fiscella, K., Franks, P., Doescher, M. P., & Saver, B. G. (2002). Disparities in health care by race, ethnicity, and language among the insured: Findings from a national sample. *Medical Care, 40,* 52–59.

Fiscella, K., Franks, P., Gold, M. R., & Clancy, C. M. (2000). Inequality in quality: Addressing socioeconomic, racial, and ethnic disparities in health care. *Journal of the American Medical Association, 283,* 2579–2584.

Freimuth, V. S., Quinn, S. C., Thomas, S. B., Cole, G., Zook, E., & Duncan, T. (2001). African American's views on research and the Tuskegee syphilis study. *Social Science and Medicine, 52,* 797–808.

Fu, M. (2002). *Acculturation, ethnic identity, and family conflict among first- and second-generation Chinese Americans.* Unpublished doctoral dissertation, Alliant International University, San Francisco, CA.

Gaines, S. O., Jr., Marelich, W. D., Bledsoe, K. L., Steers, W. N., Henderson, M. C., Granrose, C. S., Barajas, L., Hicks, D., Lyde, M., Takahashi, Y., Yum, N., Rios, D. I., Garcia, B. F., Farris, K. R., & Page, M. S. (1997). Links between race/ethnicity and cultural values as mediated by racial/ethnic identity and moderated by gender. *Journal of Personality and Social Psychology, 72,* 1460–1476.

Gamble, V. N. (1993). A legacy of distrust: African Americans and medical research. *American Journal of Preventive Medicine, 9,* S35–S38.

Ghaffarian, S. (1998). The acculturation of Iranian immigrants in the United States and the implications for mental health. *Journal of Social Psychology, 138,* 645–654.

Guilmet, G. M. (1989). Miscontinence and the Barrow alcohol study. *American Indian and Alaska Native Mental Health Research, 2,* 29–34.

Gushue, G. V., & Sciarra, D. T. (1995). Culture and families: A multidimensional approach. In J. G. Ponterotto, J. M. Casas, L. A. Suzuki, & C. M. Alexander (Eds.), *Handbook of multicultural counseling* (pp. 586–606). Thousand Oaks, CA: Sage.

Hambleton, R. K., Swaminathan, H., & Rogers, H. J. (1991). *Fundamentals of item response theory* (Measurement Methods for the Social Sciences, Series Vol. 2). Thousand Oaks, CA: Sage.

Hardie, G. E., Janson, S., Gold, W. M., Carrieri-Kohlman, V., & Boushey, H. A. (2000). Ethnic differences: Word descriptors used by African-Americans and white patients during induced bronchoconstriction. *Chest, 117,* 935–943.

Institute of Medicine. (2002). *Unequal treatment: What healthcare providers need to know about racial and ethnic disparities in health-care.* Washington, DC: National Academies Press.

Jenkins-Hall, K., & Sacco, W. P. (1991). Effects of client race and depression on evaluations by white therapists. *Journal of Social and Clinical Psychology, 10,* 322–333.

Johnson, P. B., & Glassman, M. (1999). The moderating effects of gender and ethnicity on the relationship between effect expectancies and alcohol problems. *Journal of Studies on Alcohol, 60,* 64–69.

Kercher, L. S. (2000). *Alcohol expectancies, coping responses, and self-efficacy judgments: Predictors of alcohol use and alcohol-related problems for Anglo-American and Mexican-American college students.* Unpublished doctoral dissertation, California School of Professional Psychology, San Diego.

Khanjian, E. (2002). *Gender role ideology and its relationship with acculturation, gender, age, education, and wife employment among married Armenian Americans.* Unpublished doctoral dissertation, Alliant International University, San Francisco, CA.

Lafferty, C. K., Heaney, C. A., & Chen, M. S., Jr. (1999). Assessing decisional balance from smoking cessation among Southeast Asian males in the U.S. *Health Education Research, 14,* 139–146.

LaFromboise, T. D., & Rowe, W. (1983). Skills training for bicultural competence: Rationale and application. *Journal of Counseling Psychology, 30,* 589–595.

Lau, A. (1998). *Acculturation, intergenerational conflict, and level of self-esteem in Chinese immigrant women.* Unpublished doctoral dissertation, California School of Professional Psychology, San Diego.

Lee, K. S. (1995). *Korean American cultural identifications: Effects on mental stress and self-esteem.* Unpublished doctoral dissertation, Arizona State University, Tempe.

Leung, S. F., & Arthur, D. (2000). The Alcohol Use Disorders Identification Test (AUDIT): Validation of an instrument for enhancing nursing practice in Hong Kong. *International Journal of Nursing Studies, 37,* 57–64.

Lindman, R. E., & Lang, A. R. (1994). The alcohol–aggression stereotype: A cross-cultural comparison of beliefs. *International Journal of the Addictions, 29,* 1–13.

Loewenstein, D. A., Argueelles, T., Argueelles, S., & Linn-Fuentes, P. (1994). Potential cultural bias in the neuropsychological assessment of the older adult. *Journal of Clinical and Experimental Neuropsychology, 16,* 623–629.

Lu, L., & Bigler, E. D. (2000). Performance on original and a Chinese version of Trail

Making Test Part B: A normative bilingual sample. *Applied Neuropsychology, 7,* 243–246.

Mahurin, R. K., Espino, D. V., & Holifield, E. B. (1992). Mental status testing in elderly Hispanic populations: Special concerns. *Psychopharmacology Bulletin, 28,* 391–399.

Marín, G., & Gamba, R. J. (1997). A new measurement of acculturation for Hispanics: The Bidimensional Acculturation Scale for Hispanics (BAS). *Hispanic Journal of Behavioral Sciences, 18,* 297–316.

Marín, G., Marín, B. V., Perez-Stable, E. J., Sabogal, F., & Otero-Sabogal, R. (1990). Cultural differences in attitudes and expectancies between Hispanic and non-Hispanic white smokers. *Hispanic Journal of Behavioral Sciences, 12,* 422–436.

Mason, M. J. (1995). A preliminary language validity analysis of the Problem Oriented Screening Instrument for Teenagers (POSIT). *Journal of Child and Adolescent Substance Abuse, 4,* 61–68.

McDonald, R. P. (1967). *Nonlinear factor analysis* (Psychometric Monograph, No. 15). Iowa City, IA: Psychometric Society.

McGoldrick, M., Pearce, J. K., & Giordano, J. (Eds.). (1982). *Ethnicity and family therapy.* New York: Guilford Press.

Mendoza, R. H. (1990). An empirical scale to measure type and degree of acculturation in Mexican-American adolescents and adults. *Journal of Cross-Cultural Psychology, 20,* 372–385.

Meredith, W. (1993). Measurement invariance, factor analysis and factorial invariance. *Psychometrika, 58,* 525–543.

Miranda, J., Lawson, W., & Escobar, J. (2002). Ethnic minorities. *Mental Health Services Research, 4,* 231–237.

Nagoshi, C. T., Nakata, T., Sasano, K., & Wood, M. D. (1994). Alcohol norms, expectancies and reasons for drinking and alcohol use in a U. S. versus a Japanese college sample. *Alcoholism: Clinical and Experimental Research, 18,* 671–678.

National Center for Injury Prevention and Control. (2003). *Leading causes of death reports.* Retrieved February 3, 2004, from webapp.cdc.gov/sasweb/ncipc/leadcaus10.html.

National Institute on Alcohol Abuse and Alcoholism. (2001). *Forecast for the future: Strategic plan to address health disparities.* Bethesda, MD: Author.

Nazroo, J. Y. (2003). The structuring of ethnic inequalities in health: Economic position, racial discrimination, and racism. *American Journal of Public Health, 93,* 277–284.

Neighbors, H. W., Trierweiler, S. J., Munday, C., Thompson, E. E., Jackson, J. S., Binion, V. J., & Gomez, J. (1999). Psychiatric diagnosis of African Americans: Diagnostic divergence in clinician-structured and semistructured interviewing conditions. *Journal of the National Medical Association, 91,* 601–612.

Nguyen, K. O. T. (1999). *Acculturation and gender role attitudes as related to caregiving for elderly family members among Vietnamese women.* Unpublished doctoral dissertation, California School of Professional Psychology, Los Angeles.

Oetting, G. R., & Beauvais, F. (1991). Orthogonal cultural identification theory: The cultural identification of minority adolescents. *International Journal of the Addictions, 25,* 655–685.

Oetting, E. R., Swaim, R. C., & Chiarella, M. C. (1998). Factor structure and invariance of the Orthogonal Cultural Identification Scale among American Indian and Mexican American youth. *Hispanic Journal of Behavioral Sciences, 20,* 131–154.

Ostovar, R. (1997). *Predictors of acculturation among Iranian immigrant adults living in the United States.* Unpublished doctoral dissertation, California School of Professional Psychology, Los Angeles.

Panter, A. T., Swygert, K. A., Dahlstrom, W. G., & Tanaka, J. S. (1997). Factor analytic approaches to personality item-level data. *Journal of Personality Assessment, 68,* 561–589.

Phinney, J. S. (1992). The Multigroup Ethnic Identity Measure: A new scale for use with diverse groups. *Journal of Adolescent Research, 7,* 156–176.

Prieto, L. R., McNeill, B. W., Walls, R. G., & Gomez, S. P. (2001). Chicanas/os and mental health services: An overview of utilization, counselor preference, and assessment issues. *Counseling Psychologist, 29,* 18–54.

Prochaska, J. O., DiClemente, C. C., & Norcross, J. C. (1992). In search of how people change: Applications to addictive behaviors. *American Psychologist, 47,* 1102–1114.

Reise, S. P., Widaman, K. F., & Pugh, R. H. (1993). Confirmatory factor analysis and item response theory: Two approaches for exploring measurement invariance. *Psychological Bulletin, 114,* 552–566.

Rhodes, R., & Johnson, A. (1997). A feminist approach to treating alcohol and drug addicted African-American women. *Women and Therapy, 20,* 23–37.

Rodriguez, M. M. (1999). *The relationships among acculturation style, family functioning, and adolescent psychopathology and competence in non-immigrant and immigrant Dominicans.* Unpublished doctoral dissertation, Columbia University, New York.

Rodriguez, N., Myers, H. F., Mira, C. B., Flores, T., & García-Hernandez, L. (2000). Development of the Multidimensional Stress Inventory for adults of Mexican origin. *Psychological Assessment, 14,* 451–461.

Rodriguez-Martos, A., Rubio, G., Auba, J., Santo-Domingo, J., Torralba, L. I., & Campillo, M. (2000). Readiness to Change Questionnaire: Reliability study of its Spanish version. *Alcohol and Alcoholism, 35,* 270–275.

Rosenthal, D. A., & Berven, N. L. (1999). Effects of client race on clinical judgment. *Rehabilitation Counseling Bulletin, 42,* 243–264.

Rouhparvar, A. (2001). *Acculturation, gender, and age as related to somatization in Iranians.* Unpublished doctoral dissertation, California School of Professional Psychology, Los Angeles.

Sabogal, F., Otero-Sabogal, R., Perez-Stable, E. J., Marín, B. V., & Marín, G. (1990). Perceived self-efficacy to avoid cigarette smoking and addiction: Differences between Hispanics and non-Hispanic whites. *Hispanic Journal of Behavioral Sciences, 11,* 136–147.

Schaubroeck, J., Lam, S. S. K., & Xie, J. L. (2000). Collective efficacy versus self-efficacy in coping responses to stressors and control: A cross-cultural study. *Journal of Applied Psychology, 85,* 512–525.

Snowden, L. R. (2003). Bias in mental health assessment and intervention: Theory and evidence. *American Journal of Public Health, 93,* 239–243.

Strakowski, S. M., Lonczak, H. S., Sax, K. W., West, S. A., Crist, A., Mehta, R., & Thienhaus, O. J. (1995). The effects of race on diagnosis and disposition from a psychiatric emergency service. *Journal of Clinical Psychiatry, 56,* 101–107.

Strunin, L., & Demissie, S. (2002). Cultural identification and alcohol use among "black" adolescents. *Substance Use and Misuse, 36,* 2025–2041.

Sue, D. W., & Sue, D. (2003a). Barriers to effective multicultural counseling/therapy. In *Counseling the culturally diverse: Theory and practice* (pp. 95–121). New York: Wiley.

Sue, D. W., & Sue, D. (2003b). Counseling and therapy with racial/ethnic minority populations. In *Counseling the culturally diverse: Theory and practice* (pp. 291–376). New York: Wiley.

Sue, D. W., & Sue, D. (2003c). Multicultural family counseling and therapy. In *Counseling the culturally diverse: Theory and practice* (pp. 151–176). New York: Wiley.

Suen, H. K. (1990). *Principles of test theories.* Mahwah, NJ: Erlbaum.

Suinn, R. M., Rickard-Figueroa, K., Lew, S., & Vigil, P. (1987). The Suinn–Lew Asian Self-Identity Acculturation Scale: An initial report. *Educational and Psychological Measurement, 47,* 401–407.

Suzuki, L. A., & Kugler, J. F. (1995). Intelligence and personality assessment: Multicultural perspectives. In J. G. Ponterotto, J. M. Casas, L. A. Suzuki, & C. M. Alexander (Eds.), *Handbook of multicultural counseling* (pp. 493–515). Thousand Oaks, CA: Sage.

Szapocznik, J., Kurtines, W. M., & Fernandez, T. (1980). Bicultural involvement and adjustment in Hispanic-American youths. *International Journal of Intercultural Relations, 4,* 353–365.

Teresi, J. A., Holmes, D., Ramirez, M., Gurland, B. J., & Lantigua, R. (2001). Performance of cognitive tests among different racial/ethnic and education groups: Findings of differential item functioning and possible item bias. *Journal of Mental Health and Aging, 7,* 79–89.

Trierweiler, S. J., Neighbors, H. W., Munday, C., Thompson, E. E., Binion, V. J., & Gomez, J. P. (2000). Clinician attributions associated with the diagnosis of schizophrenia in African American and non-African American patients. *Journal of Consulting and Clinical Psychology, 68,* 171–175.

Unger, J. B., Gallaher, P., Shakib, S., Ritt-Olson, A., Palmer, P. H., & Johnson, C. A. (2002). The AHIMSA Acculturation Scale: A new measure of acculturation for adolescents in a multicultural society. *Journal of Early Adolescence, 22,* 225–251.

U.S. Bureau of the Census. (2003). *Population projections.* Retrieved February 3, 2004, www.census.gov/population/www/projections/popproj.html.

U.S. Department of Health and Human Services. (2001). *Mental health: Culture, race, and ethnicity. A supplement to mental health: A report of the surgeon general.* Rockville, MD: Author.

U.S. Department of Health and Human Services. (2003). *National healthcare disparities report* (July draft). Rockville, MD: Author.

U.S. House of Representatives Committee on Government Reform. (2004). *A case study in politics and science: Changes to the national healthcare disparities report.* Retrieved February 12, 2004, www.reform.house.gov/min.

Valencia, R. R., & Suzuki, L. A. (2001). *Intelligence testing and minority students: Foundations, performance factors, and assessment issues* (Racial and Ethnic Minority Series, Vol. 3). Thousand Oaks, CA: Sage.

Van Ryn, M., & Fu, S. S. (2003). Paved with good intentions: Do public health and human service providers contribute to racial/ethnic disparities in health? *American Journal of Public Health, 93,* 248–255.

Velez-Blasini, C. J. (1997). A cross-cultural comparison of alcohol expectancies in Puerto Rico and the United States. *Psychology of Addictive Behaviors, 11,* 124–141.

Volk, R. J., Cantor, S. B., Steinbauer, J. R., & Cass, A. R. (1997). Item bias in the CAGE screening test for alcohol use disorders. *Journal of General Internal Medicine, 12,* 763–769.

Waller, N. G. (1999). Searching for structure in the MMPI. In S. E. Embretson & S. L. Hershberger (Eds.), *The new rules of measurement: What every psychologist and educator should know* (pp. 185–217). Mahwah, NJ: Erlbaum.

Wardman, D., el-Guebaly, N., & Hodgins, D. (2001). Problem and pathological gambling in North American Aboriginal populations: A review of the empirical literature. *Journal of Gambling Studies, 17,* 81–100.

Wells, K., Klap, R., Koike, A., & Sherbourne, C. (2001). Ethnic disparities in unmet need for alcoholism, drug abuse, and mental health care. *American Journal of Psychiatry, 158,* 2027–2032.

Welte, J. W., Barnes, G. M., Wieczorek, W. F., Tidwell, M. C., & Parker, J. (2002). Gambling participation in the U. S.: Results from a national survey. *Journal of Gambling Studies, 17,* 81–100.

Widaman, K. F., & Reise, S. P. (1997). Exploring the measurement invariance of psychological instruments: Applications in the substance use domain. In K. J. Bryant, M. Windle, & S. G. West (Eds.), *The science of prevention: Methodological advances from alcohol and substance abuse research* (pp. 281–324). Washington, DC: American Psychological Association.

Williams, D. R., & Rucker, T. D. (2000). Understanding and addressing racial disparities in health care. *Health Care Financial Review, 21,* 75–90.

Wingo, L. K. (2001). Substance abuse in African American women. *Journal of Cultural Diversity, 20,* 23–37.

Zager, L. D., & Megargee, E. I. (1981). Seven MMPI alcohol and drug abuse scales: An empirical investigation of their interrelationships, convergent and discriminant validity, and degree of racial bias. *Journal of Personality and Social Psychology, 40,* 532–544.

Zimmerman, M. A., Ramirez, J., Washienko, K. M., Walter, B., & Dyer, S. (1998). Enculturation hypothesis: Exploring direct and protective effects among Native American youth. In H. I. McCubbin, E. A. Thompson, A. I. Thompson, & J. E. Fromer (Eds.), *Resiliency in Native American and immigrant families* (pp. 199–220). Thousand Oaks, CA: Sage.

CHAPTER 3

Assessment of Alcohol Problems

NED L. COONEY
RONALD M. KADDEN
HOWARD R. STEINBERG

Forty-four percent of the adult U.S. population report that they are current drinkers and have consumed at least 12 drinks in the preceding year (Dawson, Grant, Chou, & Pickering, 1995). Although most current drinkers do not experience problems, those who drink heavily have a significant impact on themselves and their friends, families, and communities. As described in the *10th Special Report to Congress on Alcohol and Health* (U.S. Department of Health and Human Services, 2000), 14 million Americans (7.4% of the population) meet diagnostic criteria for alcohol abuse or dependence; traffic crashes involving alcohol killed more than 16,000 people in 1997 alone; approximately one in four victims of violent crime (2.7 million victims per year) reports that the offender had been drinking alcohol prior to committing the crime; and the estimated economic costs of heavy alcohol consumption in the United States was $185 billion for 1998 alone.

The assessment of alcohol problems involves a number of related dimensions, including the fourth edition of the *Diagnostic and Statistical Manual of Mental Disorders* (DSM-IV; American Psychiatric Association, 1994) disorders of alcohol abuse and alcohol dependence, the continuous dimension of severity of alcohol dependence, alcohol-related negative consequences, and hazardous or at-risk drinking. This chapter reviews the major screening and assessment instruments, and describes their characteristics. This review is not exhaustive, but it attempts to cover the most widely used or promising measures. The following domains of assessment of alcohol problems are reviewed: screening tests, diagnostic instruments, measures of severity of alcohol dependence and alcohol consumption, alcohol consumption biomarkers, severity of alcohol withdrawal, and alcohol-related consequences. Also reviewed

71

are the following domains of assessments of personal factors associated with alcohol problems: readiness to change, antecedents to drinking, self-efficacy, coping skills, drinking outcome expectations, spirituality and religiosity, 12-step affiliation, alcohol craving, comorbid psychopathology, and neuropsychological deficits. Finally, multidimensional assessments and patient placement criteria are reviewed. It is difficult to recommend a single instrument in each assessment domain, because the instruments have various strengths and weaknesses depending on the measurement context. The reader is encouraged to use this review as a starting point in evaluating and selecting appropriate alcohol assessment tools.

SCREENING STAGE

"Alcohol screening" is defined as the use of specific procedures to identify individuals with alcohol problems or those who are at risk for developing such problems. Alcohol screening programs are justified, because alcohol problems are common; they are associated with serious health and social consequences; they are often undetected; effective treatment is available; and simple, valid, cost-effective screening methods are also available (Institute of Medicine, 1990). The Institute of Medicine strongly recommended that health care and community agencies identify individuals with alcohol problems and provide intervention or referrals.

There are two conceptual models for screening (Safer, 1986). Screening for disease detection seeks to identify individuals who have clear evidence of alcohol abuse or dependence. Screening for risk reduction, on the other hand, seeks to identify those who are not experiencing problems but who have behavioral risk factors that can be modified with counseling. Early alcohol screening instruments were developed primarily for disease detection. However, the development of brief intervention methods has led to increased development of screening tools designed to detect hazardous drinking, for the purpose of risk reduction. Although there is no firm consensus regarding the criterion for safe versus hazardous drinking (Bradley, Donovan, & Larson, 1993), the National Institute on Alcohol Abuse and Alcoholism (NIAAA) guidelines define "moderate drinking" as no more than an average of two drinks per day (no more than four drinks on any one occasion) for men, and no more than an average of one drink per day (no more than three drinks per occasion) for women or anyone over age 65 (National Institute on Alcohol Abuse and Alcoholism, 1995). Drinking more than 14 (men) or 7 (women and over 65) drinks per week would indicate at least hazardous drinking.

It is important to understand the difference between screening and assessment. The goal of screening is to detect individuals with possible alcohol problems or those at risk of developing such problems. Screening procedures should be brief and capable of being administered by individuals with limited clinical experience. The goal of assessment is to gather more detailed information in order to develop a diagnosis, guide treatment planning, or evaluate treatment process.

Alcohol Screening Tests

A recent review identified 17 alcohol screening measures (Connors & Volk, 2003). This review focuses on simple screening tests that can be administered in 1–2 minutes. Longer measures could more accurately be called assessment measures rather than screening tools.

The *CAGE* (Ewing, 1984) is a four-question test:

1. "Have you ever felt the need to *Cut* down on your drinking?"
2. "Have you ever felt *Annoyed* by someone criticizing your drinking?"
3. "Have you ever felt bad or *Guilty* about your drinking?"
4. "Have you ever had a drink the first thing in the morning to steady your nerves and get rid of a hangover [*Eye-opener*]?"

Two positive responses is the cutoff for a positive test. Although the CAGE is popular in primary care settings, it does not assess current problems, levels of alcohol consumption, or binge drinking. It is better at detecting dependence. Consequently, it is not recommended when screening to identify hazardous drinkers for risk reduction.

The *Alcohol Use Disorders Identification Test* (AUDIT) was developed as a cross-cultural screening tool for the early identification of problem drinkers (Saunders, Aasland, Babor, de la Fuente, & Grant, 1993). It consists of 10 questions that include 3 questions on alcohol consumption, 4 questions on dependence symptoms, and 3 questions about alcohol-related problems. It can be administered by an interviewer or self-administered using pencil-and-paper or computer. An Internet-based version of the AUDIT has been evaluated, with good reliability for the AUDIT total score, but lower reliability for the Dependence subscale (E. T. Miller et al., 2002).

Quantity–Frequency Questions

A shorter version of the AUDIT may be useful to physicians in a busy primary care practice. Gordon and colleagues (2001) compared the full AUDIT with a test consisting of only the first three quantity–frequency questions (AUDIT-C), and with a test consisting of only the third binge-drinking question (AUDIT-3). The AUDIT and AUDIT-C were better at identifying hazardous drinkers than the AUDIT-3. This study suggests that the three quantity, frequency, and binge-drinking items may be as useful for screening as the full 10-question AUDIT.

Another example of a rapid, simple alcohol screening test is the single question suggested by Williams and Vinson (2001). Responses to the question "When was the last time you had more than four drinks (women) or five drinks (men) in one day?" were compared with a calendar measure of hazard-ous drinking and with a structured diagnostic interview measure of past-year alcohol use disorder. A positive answer within the past 3 months detected 86% of individuals with recent hazardous drinking or current alcohol use dis-order. Fleming (2001) recommended the use of quantity–frequency and binge-drinking questions as a first-line alcohol screening test, with the CAGE recom-mended as a second-line test for patients who test positive on the basis of quantity–frequency questions.

Russell (1994) developed the *TWEAK*, based on the CAGE, substituting a question on tolerance for the question on guilt, modifying the question about annoyance, and adding a question about blackouts. Cherpitel (1997) reported that the TWEAK (and the full AUDIT) correctly identified more indi-viduals with alcohol problems (i.e., it was more sensitive) than the CAGE. Al-though the TWEAK was originally developed for use with women, Cherpitel found that it was more sensitive for men than for women.

The *Rapid Alcohol Problems Screen* (RAPS), a five-item alcohol screen-ing test, was empirically derived from an item pool consisting of the CAGE, brief Michigan Alcoholism Screening Test (MAST), AUDIT, and TWEAK. The RAPS outperformed the standard screening instruments in identifying emergency room patients meeting criteria for alcohol dependence or harmful drinking (Cherpitel, 1995). A four-item version, called the RAPS4 (Cherpitel, 2000), had a sensitivity of 93% for alcohol dependence, and sensitivity was consistently high across gender and ethnic subgroups. Sensitivity for hazard-ous drinking was lower, at 55%. The RAPS4 items are as follows:

1. "During the last year, have you had a feeling of guilt or remorse after drinking? (Remorse)."
2. "During the last year, has a friend or family member ever told you about things you said or did while you were drinking that you could not remember?" (Amnesia, also called Blackout).
3. "During the last year, have you failed to do what was normally ex-pected of you because of drinking?" (Perform).
4. "Do you sometimes take a drink in the morning when you first get up?" (Starter, also called Eye-Opener).

Improving Referral Compliance

An important step in the screening process is making a referral for further as-sessment and possibly intervention. Many individuals identified as having al-cohol problems or hazardous drinking do not accept or follow through with referrals. Referral compliance ranges from 14% (Babor, Ritson, & Hodgson, 1986) to 30% (Soderstrom & Cowley, 1987). Cooney, Zweben, and Fleming (1995) describe a referral compliance intervention process drawn from the work on brief intervention and motivational interviewing (Miller & Rollnick, 2002). The overall goal of the referral compliance intervention is to increase the client's motivation for change and to initiate client action, either through self-change or participation in further assessment and intervention. The model attends to discrepancies between the client's present drinking behavior and important personal goals or values. Alcohol use is discussed in the language of health promotion rather than disease detection. Labels such as "alcoholism" are avoided, and further assessment is described as a Drinker's Check-Up (Miller, Sovereign, & Krege, 1989). Referral options will depend on local resources, but screening programs will need to contend with the fact that most individuals who drink in a harmful or hazardous way are not dependent on alcohol (Kreitman, 1986), and many may be best served by brief intervention rather than traditional abstinence-oriented, intensive programs. The ASAM Patient Placement Criteria (American Society of Addiction Medicine, 2001), described later in this chapter, are useful for determining the appropriate level of care.

PROBLEM ASSESSMENT STAGE

The conceptual basis of alcohol problem assessment has been strongly influenced over the past 25 years by the dependence syndrome concept described by Griffith Edwards and colleagues (1976). The essential postulates of the dependence syndrome include (1) the clustering of specified cognitive, behavioral, and physiological elements that are related to a common process; (2) the distribution of these elements along a continuum of severity; and (3) the independence of dependence elements from negative consequences of substance use. The following section reviews categorical measures of alcohol diagnosis and continuous measures of severity of alcohol dependence, alcohol consumption, and alcohol-related negative consequences.

Diagnostic Assessment

Diagnostic criteria provide a common language for identifying alcohol problems and serve as a consistent means of communication in both research and clinical settings. In the United States, the DSM categorical system is most influential. The criteria for alcohol dependence and alcohol abuse in the DSM-IV (American Psychiatric Association, 1994), are similar to the *International Classification of Diseases and Related Health Problems* (ICD-10) published by the World Health Organization (1992).

Alcohol Dependence

A maladaptive pattern of substance use leading to clinically significant impairment or distress as manifested by three or more of the following occurring within a 12-month period: tolerance, withdrawal, impaired control over amount or duration of drinking, desire or unsuccessful efforts to control or stop drinking, excessive time spent obtaining alcohol, drinking, or recovering from drinking, neglect of activities because of drinking, and continued drinking despite problems.

Alcohol Abuse

A maladaptive pattern of alcohol use leading to clinically significant impairment or distress as manifested by one or more of the following occurring within a 12-month period: failure to fulfill major role obligations due to drinking, drinking in hazardous situations, alcohol-related legal problems, and continued drinking despite social or interpersonal problems.

Six assessment instruments designed to provide an alcohol problem diagnosis are described below. These instruments provide not only an alcohol diagnosis but also offer a full range of other DSM Axis I or Axis II diagnoses. This is potentially useful given the high rate of comorbidity of alcohol and other psychiatric disorders.

The *Diagnostic Interview Schedule–IV* (DIS-IV) was designed for epidemiological research (Robins et al., 2000). It is highly structured and can be administered by interviewers without clinical training. An available computer-administered version, known as the CDIS-IV, provides only lifetime diagnostic information (epi.wustl.edu/dis/discdis.htm). The CDIS-IV can be interviewer-administered or computer-administered. Advantages of the CDIS-IV over the paper-and-pen version include added specification for each question on the screen, reduced cost of interviewer training, elimination of missing data due to incorrect skips, and elimination of data entry and cleaning. Although published psychometric data are not available on the CDIS-IV, an earlier version of the C-DIS was found to overdiagnose individuals when compared with the Structured Clinical Interview for DSM-III-R and a consensus clinical diagnosis (Ross, Swinson, Larkin, & Doumani, 1994). A DIS version for children and adolescents is available, known as the DISC-IV. The DISC has demonstrated reliability and validity comparable with that of other diagnostic measures (Shaffer, Fisher, Lucas, Dulcan, & Shwab-Stone, 2000). A computer-assisted version, known as the C-DISC-4.0, is also available. Described by Schaffer et al., the C-DISC-4.0 is owned and distributed by the Division of Child and Adolescent Psychiatry at Columbia University (www.c-disc.com/index.htm). This program is available in both English and Spanish, and can be run in DOS or Windows. Given the complex branching and skipping instructions in the interview, the computer-administered versions rather than the interviewer-administered version it is recommended when more than one diagnostic module is needed. To our knowledge, published psychometric data on the computer-administered version are not available.

The *Structured Clinical Interview for DSM-IV* Axis I Disorders, Patient edition, version 2.0 (SCID-I/P; First, Spitzer, Gibbon, & Williams, 1996) is semistructured, allowing the interviewer the opportunity to probe for information. The SCID is systematic and comprehensive. It facilitates definitive diagnoses of DSM-IV mood, anxiety, psychotic, and substance use disorders. Since it is modular, it can be shortened to focus only on diagnoses of interest. The interview has shown good interrater reliability, especially for substance use disorders, and is widely used, but it requires a skilled interviewer and clinical judgment, and takes an hour or more to administer in its entirety. A computer-assisted interview version and a self-administered computer screening version of the SCID are also available (First, Gibbon, Williams, Spitzer, & MHS Staff, 2001).

The *Psychiatric Research Interview for Substance and Mental Disorders* (PRISM) was designed to improve the reliability of psychiatric diagnosis in individuals with alcohol and drug problems. It is similar to the SCID, with a semistructured format and flexible probes, and designed for administration by clinically experienced interviewers. Scoring guidelines explicitly address comorbidity issues. A computer program is available to score the interview. A study of patients from substance abuse and dual-diagnosis treatment settings suggests that the PRISM has very good reliability for diagnosis of current and past major depressive disorder (Hasin et al., 1996). The DSM-IV PRISM is described by Hasin, Traitman, and Endicott (1998).

The *WHO/NIH Composite International Diagnostic Interview—Substance Abuse Module* (CIDI-SAM; Robbins, Cottler, & Babor, 1995), a highly structured interview designed for epidemiological research, obtains information on current and lifetime symptoms of substance abuse and dependence needed to determine DSM-IV and WHO ICD-10 diagnoses. The Substance Abuse Module provides a greater focus on substance use disorders than the CIDI Core interview. Past-year quantity and frequency of drinking is also obtained. Nonclinicians can conduct the CIDI interview after completing a rigorous 1-week course. The CIDI has benefited from extensive cross-cultural feedback (Ustun et al., 1997).

The *Semi-Structured Assessment for the Genetics of Alcoholism* (SSAGA) was developed by the Collaborative Study on the Genetics of Alcoholism (COGA) for use in its large scale, multisite study. Reliability and validity data are available (Bucholz et al., 1994, 1995; Hesselbrock, Easton, Bucholz, Schuckit, & Hesselbrock, 1999). It is a highly structured interview designed for use by well-trained nonclinicians using prescribed probes to assess current and past psychiatric problems in clinical and general population samples. The latest version, the SSAGA-II, provides DSM-IV and ICD-10 diagnoses. It is being used in over 50 studies in the United States and has been translated into seven foreign languages. It also provides a detailed assessment of alcohol and drug use, an assessment of their consequences, and an assessment of comorbid psychiatric disorders. There is also a set of diagnostic instruments, using the SSAGA format, to assess children ages 7–12 years (C-SSAGA-C) and adolescents ages 13–17 years (C-SSAGA-A), and a parent interview to assess the psychiatric history of their individual children (C-SSAGA-P). At this time, copies of the SSAGA-II and associated documentation are available via the NIAAA website at zork.wustl.edu/niaaa/form.htm.

The *Schedule for Clinical Assessment in Neuropsychiatry* (SCAN; Wing et al., 1990) is a semistructured diagnostic interview designed for use by mental health professionals already trained in diagnosis. The interview allows for flexibility in probing responses and clinical judgment in rating symptom severity. Current and lifetime psychiatric diagnoses are obtained according to the DSM-III-R, DSM-IV, and ICD-10 systems. Reliability and validity of judgments of diagnoses of alcohol abuse and dependence derived from assessments with the SCAN have been documented (Compton, Cottler, Dorsey, Spitznagel, & Mager, 1996; Cottler et al., 1997).

Severity of Alcohol Dependence

While a psychiatric diagnosis indicates the presence or absence of alcohol problems, these problems vary across a continuum of severity, from relatively mild to severe, life-threatening disorders. Although some researchers recommended that substance dependence severity ratings be incorporated into the DSM-IV (Woody & Cacciola, 1994), such severity specifiers were not included in the system. A number of measures of severity of alcohol dependence, however, have been developed based on the alcohol dependence syndrome originally described by Edwards and Gross (1976). The assessment of dependence severity is relevant to treatment planning and selecting drinking goals. Individuals with greater dependence severity tend to be poor candidates for moderate drinking outcomes (Rosenberg, 1993). Measurement time frame of symptoms and length of administration are important considerations when deciding upon which alcohol dependence measure to choose.

The *Alcohol Dependence Scale* (ADS; Skinner & Allen, 1982) is a 25-item scale, with a 12-month time frame covering alcohol withdrawal symptoms, impaired control over drinking, awareness of compulsion to drink, tolerance to alcohol, and salience of drink-seeking behavior. It is administered by pencil and paper or computer, and is widely used as a research and clinical tool. Normative data are available (Skinner & Horn, 1984). An Internet-based version of the ADS was found to be reliable (E. T. Miller et al., 2002).

The *Ethanol Dependence Syndrome Scale* (EDSS; Babor, 1996) consists of 16 items, with balanced coverage of five dependence syndrome elements: salience of drink seeking, impaired control, tolerance, withdrawal, and withdrawal relief drinking. The time frame is the past 3 months or a recent period of heavy drinking.

The *Severity of Alcohol Dependence Questionnaire* (SADQ; Stockwell, Murphy, & Hodgson, 1983) is a 20-item scale focused on alcohol withdrawal symptoms, alcohol craving, and heavy alcohol consumption. Time frame is a recent 30-day period of heavy drinking.

The *Substance Dependence Severity Scale* (SDSS; Miele et al., 2000) was designed to assess the severity and frequency of substance dependence and abuse symptoms based on DSM-IV and ICD-10 criteria. The symptoms are assessed with a 30-day time frame across a range of substances, including alcohol, cocaine, heroin, stimulants, licit opiates, sedatives, methadone, cannabis, and hallucinogens. The SDSS differs from other severity measures in that it is a semistructured interview, designed to be administered by an interviewer with a Master's degree and clinical experience.

Alcohol Consumption

This section provides a selective review of alcohol consumption measures. A more thorough review of such instruments can be found in Sobell and Sobell (2003). As with most other assessment domains, assessment of alcohol consumption is largely based on self-report. Although the accuracy of self-reported drinking is often questioned, the literature suggests that self-reports of alcohol use from clinical and nonclinical samples are relatively accurate when people are interviewed under the proper conditions. The following procedures are recommended to enhance validity of reported alcohol consumption (Babor, Brown, & Del Boca, 1990; Room, 2000; Sobell & Sobell, 2003): (1) Ensure that the respondent is completely alcohol-free when interviewed; (2) provide assurance of confidentiality; (3) interview in a setting that does not punish reported drinking; (4) use clearly worded, objective questions; (5) carefully determine alcohol content and serving size of the respondent's preferred beverages; (6) use memory aids such as calendars; (7) load questions by assuming the presence of heavy drinking; (8) provide nonjudgmental feedback about discrepancies between self-report data and other sources of information; and (9) include questions not only about typical or usual drinking pattern, but also about heavy or atypical drinking occasions. Alcohol consumption measures can be classified into three general methods: estimates of average quantity–frequency of consumption, daily drinking estimation procedures, and daily diaries.

There are numerous *quantity–frequency* (QF) estimates of alcohol consumption (Room, 1990; Sobell & Sobell, 2003). Simple QF measures ask about the average frequency of drinking (days/week or days/month) and average quantity per occasion within a specific time period, often with separate questions for wine, beer, and distilled spirits. Such simple QF items are often part of alcohol screening tests. As with any alcohol consumption measure, it is important to determine serving size when asking about quantity consumed. Simple QF measures can provide quick, reliable information about total consumption and number of drinking days. However, QF measures have some major limitations. Many fail to measure heavy-drinking occasions along with more typical, lighter drinking days, so that days of sporadic heavier drinking go unreported. Because QF methods typically inquire separately about each beverage type, they may fail to correct for days when more than one type of alcoholic beverage was consumed. The net result is that simple QF measures may seriously underestimate heavy consumption.

The *graduated frequency* (GF) measure (Midanik, 1994) was designed to address the criticism of QF measures. The GF measure asks respondents to report the frequency of different levels of drinking (i.e., 1–2 drinks, 3–4 drinks, 5–7 drinks, 8–11 drinks, 12 or more drinks) for all alcoholic beverages combined. This measure takes longer to administer than simple QF measures; however, it does not require as much averaging by the respondent, and it captures more information on atypical heavy-drinking occasions than other QF instruments. In a comparative evaluation of alcohol consumption measures, the GF measure yielded prevalence estimates of harmful drinking that were almost three times higher than a QF measure and almost five times higher than a weekly drinking measure that asked for the number of drinks consumed on each of the 7 days preceding the survey (Rehm et al., 1999).

The *Lifetime Drinking History* (LDH) method (Skinner & Sheu, 1982) is used to obtain information about alcohol consumption over an entire drinking career, or very long time periods. Distinct phases and changes in a person's lifetime drinking patterns are identified, then QF information is obtained for average and maximum drinking days within each phase. Although the LDH provides an overall picture of alcohol consumption, it lacks precision for the most recent drinking period.

The *Cognitive Lifetime Drinking History* (CLDH; Russell et al., 1997) is a computer-administered assessment based on Skinner's LDH, incorporating some of the memory aids from the Sobells' Timeline Followback technique. The CLDH can be administered with floating assessment intervals based on the respondent's report of when drinking patterns changed, or with fixed assessment intervals defined in terms of decades. To date it has only been evaluated in nonclinical populations.

The *Alcohol Timeline Followback* (TLFB) is an extensively evaluated daily drinking estimation procedure (Sobell & Sobell, 1992, 2000). The procedure can also be employed to obtain information about illicit drug use and cigarette smoking. A calendar is used to obtain retrospective estimation of daily drinking and abstinent days across a specified time period up to 12 months. The TLFB is recommended when relatively precise estimates of drinking are needed, and when the pattern and/or variability in alcohol consumption are of interest. The amount of time necessary to administer the TLFB varies as a function of the assessment interval (e.g., 90 days = 10–15 minutes; 12 months = 30 minutes), although the time needed grows considerably if use of other substances is included, and if other behaviors such as Alcoholics Anonymous (AA) meeting attendance are assessed. It is available in interview, paper-and-pencil format, or computerized versions (Sobell & Sobell, 1996). It has been translated and is available in seven languages.

The *Form 90* (Miller, 1996; Miller & Del Boca, 1994) is a family of instruments developed by the Project MATCH Research Group (1993). Daily drinking information across a 90-day period is gathered using a combination of a calendar method (like the TLFB) and a grid-averaging method (Miller & Marlatt, 1984). The Form 90 also collects data on other aspects of functioning, including use of drugs, experience with medical and substance abuse treatments, and attendance at 12-step meetings. The following Form 90 interview formats have been developed: (1) intake (in person); (2) follow-up (in person); (3) telephone follow-up; (4) a quick form to collect minimal essential data; and (5) a telephone collateral interview for intake or follow-up.

The *daily diary* or self-monitoring method involves recording alcohol consumption either once a day or at the time of each drink. One concern about self-monitoring is that it may be reactive, leading to changes in drinking (Sobell, Bogardis, Schuller, Leo, & Sobell, 1989). However, studies conducted with problem drinkers did not demonstrate significant enduring reactive effects of self-monitoring (Harris & Miller, 1990; Kavanagh, Sitharthan, Spilsbury, & Vignaendra, 1999). There is also concern about poor self-monitoring compliance or faked compliance, in which participants complete missed recordings hours or days later (Litt, Cooney, & Morse, 1998).

Compliance concerns have been addressed by the use of *interactive voice response* (IVR) systems (Searles, Perrine, Mundt, & Helzer, 1995). Daily self-reports of drinking and other relevant variables are obtained by asking participants to dial in to a computer-automated interviewing system, and to key in responses to queries on a touch-tone telephone. Advantages of this methodology include the accurate attribution of the date and time of responses, the ability to monitor compliance with data collection on a daily basis, and the potential greater willingness of participants to disclose sensitive information to a computer that might be withheld from another person (Greist, 1998). Comparisons of drinking data obtained by an IVR system and by TLFB interviews show that less drinking is reported on the TLFB, especially among individuals with diagnosed alcohol problems (Searles, Helzer, & Walter, 2000).

Ecological momentary assessment (EMA) methodology is another recent advance in the technology of self-monitoring (Shiffman & Stone, 1998). Participants self-monitor on a handheld computer in the natural environment, completing both event-contingent recordings (e.g., at the start of each drinking episode) and randomly timed, signal-contingent recordings. A comparison of event-contingent recordings and randomly sampled recordings allows one to determine whether specific processes (e.g., negative mood states) are simply occurring at a high base rate or are uniquely associated with drinking episodes. Compliance with EMA recordings of alcohol consumption has been good in moderate drinkers (Carney, Tennen, Affleck, Del Boca, & Kranzler, 1998). Alcohol-dependent clients also showed good compliance with EMA recordings of cravings and other variables when they were abstinent, but their compliance deteriorated during periods of alcohol relapse (Litt, Cooney, & Morse, 1998). Recently, Collins, Kashdan, and Gollnisch (2003) tested a new system for collecting EMA data using cellular telephones linked to an IVR system. This system combines the advantages of both IVR and EMA technology: the ability to collect real-time event contingent and randomly prompted *in vivo* recordings, and the ability to immediately examine data collected, allowing an investigator to identify and address compliance problems right away. Preliminary results suggest that cellular telephones are a viable alternative to handheld computers for collecting EMA data.

Alcohol Biomarkers

Biological assessment of alcohol consumption can be an important adjunct to self-report assessments. Most importantly, they are not vulnerable to problems of inaccurate recall or reluctance of individuals to give candid reports of their drinking. They can thus add credibility to self-reported outcomes in studies of alcohol treatment efficacy, and can provide clinicians a source of objective information on patients' drinking. This section provides recommended alcohol biomarkers, based on the thorough review by Allen, Sillanaukee, Strid, and Litten (2003).

Ethanol can be easily detected in breath, serum, urine, or saliva. Ethanol tests are often used in clinical and law enforcement settings, and there are virtually no false positive results. Unfortunately, the rapid elimination of ethanol from the blood usually makes it impossible to assess alcohol consumption beyond the most recent 6–8 hours. False-negative results are likely if a drinker avoids alcohol on the day of the ethanol test.

Serum *gamma-glutamyl transpeptidase* (GGT), an indicator of liver function, is the most widely used marker of alcohol abuse. Levels typically rise after several weeks of continuous heavy alcohol intake (Allen, Litten, Anton, & Cross, 1994) and decrease to normal with 4–6 weeks of abstinence. The half-life of GGT is 14–26 days. GGT levels can also be elevated by hepatobiliary disorders, obesity, diabetes, hypertension, and hypertriglyceridemia, resulting in many false-positive findings. Laboratory tests for evaluating GGT are inexpensive and readily available.

Carbohydrate-deficient transferrin (CDT) levels are also indicative of liver dysfunction. They usually rise after 2–3 weeks of heavy drinking, and normalize with a half-life of 12–17 days of abstinence. False-positive CDT results can be found in patients with an inborn error of glycoprotein metabolism; genetic D-variant of transferrin; severe nonalcoholic liver diseases, such as primary biliary cirrhosis; diseases characterized by high total transferrin; and in patients who have received combined kidney and pancreas transplants. Although the sensitivities of CDT and GGT appear approximately equal, CDT is far more specific than GGT and other liver function tests (Litten, Allen, & Fertig, 1995). The cost of a CDT test in a clinical laboratory is two to five times higher than the cost of a GGT test.

Allen and colleagues (2003) suggest the use of a combination of biomarkers in alcohol treatment research, because individuals vary regarding which biomarker will respond to heavy drinking. CDT and GGT are recommended at the present time. Several emerging biomarkers are promising, although further research is needed before they can be recommended for treatment research. These include the ratio 5-hydroxytryptophol (5HTOL)/5-hydroxyindoleacetic acid (5HIAA) in urine, acetaldehyde adducts in blood and urine, and transdermal devices.

Allen and colleagues (2003) also suggest using combinations of biomarkers in clinical settings. The combination of GGT, CDT, and MCV (mean corpuscular volume) is suggested for alcohol screening purposes, and the combination of CDT and GGT is recommended for monitoring drinking status of patients in treatment. Biomarker assessment can be used to provide feedback to clients as part of a strategy to motivate reductions in drinking (e.g., Kristenson, Ohlin, Hulten-Nosslin, Trell, & Hood, 1983; Miller, Zweben, DiClemente, & Rychtarik, 1994).

Severity of Alcohol Withdrawal

The *Clinical Institute Withdrawal Assessment for Alcohol revised* (CIWA-Ar; Sullivan, Sykora, Schneiderman, Naranjo, & Sellers, 1989) is an instrument based on assessment of vital signs and 10 items that measure severity of the alcohol withdrawal syndrome (nausea and vomiting, paroxysmal sweats, agitation, headache, anxiety, tremor, disorientation and clouding of sensorium, and visual, tactile, and auditory disturbances). The CIWA-Ar can be used as part of a symptom-triggered alcohol detoxification protocol (e.g., Reoux & Miller, 2000) and can assist with treatment decisions. Additionally, the measure may be administered by a range of medical and clinical research staff trained in its use.

The *Alcohol Withdrawal Syndrome* scale (AWS; Wetterling et al., 1997) was developed by item analysis of the CIWA-A scale. It consists of a six-item Somatic subscale and a five-item Mental subscale. The authors of the AWS suggest differential medication strategies based on subscale scores.

Alcohol-Related Consequences

An adequate assessment must extend beyond determination of a diagnosis and assaying severity of dependence to ascertain the impact of problem drinking on the full range of drinkers' life functioning and activities. In addition to depicting the full scope of alcohol's impact on a person's life, information about alcohol-related problems can also be used to assess treatment-related change and outcome. Such information collected at treatment intake is an important part of motivational interventions, to show clients the connections between their alcohol consumption and the consequences they experience (Miller & Rollnick, 2002).

The *Drinker Inventory of Consequences* (DrInC; Miller, Tonigan, & Longabaugh, 1995) is a family of measures of adverse consequences of drinking. There are forms assessing lifetime and recent (past 3 months) consequences of drinking, assessing the consequences of both drinking and drug use, and for obtaining information from collaterals. The items ask the respondent to make a causal connection between drinking and problems; thus, responses are influenced by perceptions of the extent to which drinking is inflicting harm. The DrInC is subdivided according to the following subscales: Physical Consequences, Social Responsibility Consequences, Intrapersonal Consequences, Interpersonal Consequences, and Impulse Control Consequences. The DrInC can be combined with alcohol consumption measures to generate a composite outcome measure (Zweben & Cisler, 1996). A 15-item short form (Short Inventory of Problems; SIP) was developed and has been found to be a reliable and valid measure in a sample of problem drinkers (Feinn, Tennen, & Kranzler, 2003).

The *Rutgers Alcohol Problem Index* (RAPI; White & Labouvie, 1989) is a 23-item measure of alcohol problems designed for adolescents, and the *Drinking Problem Index* (DPI; Finney, Moos, & Brennan, 1991) is a 17-item measure specifically designed to assess alcohol problems in older adults.

Alcohol consequences are also measured on several of the multidimensional assessment tools, such as the Comprehensive Drinker Profile (Miller & Marlatt, 1984), the Alcohol Use Inventory (Horn, Wanberg, & Foster, 1987), the Personal Experience Inventory for Adults (Winters, 1999), and the Addiction Severity Index (McLellan, Kushner, et al., 1992). These measures are described later in this chapter.

PERSONAL ASSESSMENT STAGE

A comprehensive assessment must include measurement of an array of factors that have been found to be associated with the initiation and maintenance of alcohol problems, the likelihood of relapse, and the achievement of long-term sobriety. In addition, each individual's life experiences, beliefs, psychopathology, and level of functioning should be assessed to broaden the context within which the individual is perceived. An inclusive approach such as this is consistent with a biopsychosocial model of addiction (Donovan, 1988).

Assessing Cognitive and Behavioral Dimensions

Alcohol researchers have identified a number of psychological factors related to problematic drinking patterns and treatment outcome that should be considered when developing treatment plans. This section provides a brief review of a number of instruments that have been found to be useful in the assessment of the following areas: readiness to change, antecedents to drinking, coping skills, self-efficacy, outcome expectations, spirituality, 12-step affiliation, craving, and cue reactivity.

Readiness to Change

It is not safe to assume that everyone presenting for treatment is equally motivated to make changes in his or her alcohol use behavior. It may be apparent to the clinician that an individual ought to engage in treatment and initiate a change process. However, it is often the case that individuals vary in their readiness to make life changes (Carey, Maisto, Carey, & Purnine, 2001), even if they offer statements professing agreement with diagnoses and the need for treatment (Miller & Rollnick, 2002).

Prochaska and DiClemente (1986) provided a conceptual framework within which motivation to change substance use behavior may be placed. They proposed that individuals progress through a series of stages (precontemplation, contemplation, determination, action, maintenance, and relapse) that characterize the dynamic state of readiness to change behavior that individuals experience. As one moves through the stages, commitment to change is increased and ambivalence is resolved. Self-report measures based on this model have been used to assess various stages of change-readiness with regard to alcohol use.

The *University of Rhode Island Change Assessment* (URICA—alcohol version; DiClemente & Hughes, 1990) was developed to measure four of the stages of change (precontemplation, contemplation, action, and maintenance), as described by the Transtheoretical Model (Prochaska & DiClemente, 1986). The 28-item scale has been used in many investigations in order to classify treatment-seeking individuals according to the stages of readiness for change. In Project MATCH, the URICA was scored to yield a single continuous Readiness score, which was calculated by adding the means of the Contemplation, Action, and Maintenance subscales together and then subtracting the Precontemplation subscale mean (DiClemente, Carbonari, Zweben, Morrel, & Lee, 2001). This URICA Readiness score was a strong predictor of drinking outcome in the Project MATCH outpatient sample (Project MATCH Research Group, 1997). An internet-based version of the URICA has been evaluated, with good reliability reported for the Readiness score and lower reliabilities for the URICA subscale scores (E. T. Miller et al., 2002).

The *Stages of Change Readiness and Treatment Eagerness Scale* (SOCRATES; Miller & Tonigan, 1996) is a 39-item (or 19-item) self-report scale intended to measure each of the five stages of change (precontemplation, contemplation, determination, action, and maintenance). The authors identified an empirically derived three-factor solution characterized by (1) recognition of the severity of the drinking problem, (2) ambivalence or thinking about making changes, and (3) taking active steps for change.

The *Readiness to Change Questionnaire* (RTCQ; Rollnick, Heather, Gold, & Hall, 1992) is composed of 12 items that measure three of the stages of change (precontemplation, contemplation, and action), with four items per stage. The scale was initially developed for use in medical settings with hazardous drinkers who were not seeking alcohol treatment, and it can serve to assess change readiness quickly. A 15-item treatment version (RTCQ-TV; Heather, Luce, Peck, Dunbar, & James, 1999) was developed for use with individuals seeking treatment.

A thorough review of these and other instruments that may be used to assess readiness to change (Carey, Purnine, Maisto, & Carey, 1999) has identified the strengths and limitations of each method.

Antecedents to Drinking

Drinking contexts vary, as does an individual's risk for relapse in specific circumstances. The model of relapse proposed by Marlatt (Marlatt & Gordon, 1985) includes an identification of eight high-risk contexts for drinking. This taxonomy of drinking situations comprises negative emotional states, interpersonal conflict, physical discomfort, testing personal control, urges and temptations, social pressure to drink, pleasant social situations, and pleasant emotions. Ideally, accurate detection of an individual's high-risk situations should form the basis for teaching coping skills targeted at these specific situations.

The *Inventory of Drinking Situations* (IDS; Annis, Graham, & Davis, 1987) is likely the most widely used method to assess triggers for drinking. The 100-item instrument was developed to reflect each of Marlatt's eight drinking contexts described earlier. Responses on the IDS may be calculated to form a problem index, which provides an indication of the individual's frequency of heavy drinking in each of the eight types of situations. A 42-item version of the IDS (IDS-42; Annis et al., 1987; Isenhart, 1993) was developed in an effort to address item redundancy on the 100-item version and to provide for shorter administration time. The two versions have been found to be psychometrically similar (Cannon, Leeka, Patterson, & Baker, 1990; Carrigan, Samoluk, & Stewart, 1998), though decisions regarding which version to use should take into account the benefits of capturing all eight relapse situations with the larger scale at twice the cost of administration time compared to the shorter version.

The *Reasons for Drinking Questionnaire* (RFDQ; Zywiak, Connors, Maisto, & Westerberg, 1996) is a 16-item self-report measure derived from a scale designed to assess relapse risk in heroin abusers (Heather, Stallard, & Tebbutt, 1991). The RFDQ asks respondents to rate the importance of 16 situations (reasons) in their return to drinking alcohol. Each item of the questionnaire is designed to represent a category or subcategory from Marlatt's relapse taxonomy. The psychometric properties of the RFDQ were tested in the multisite Relapse Replication and Extension Project, and a factor analysis revealed that this brief measure adequately represents Marlatt's taxonomic system. Evidence for the predictive validity of the RFDQ was also provided: factor scores were correlated with drinking data, alcohol dependence, and other outcome factors (Zywiak et al., 1996).

The *Relapse Precipitants Inventory* (RPI; Litman, Stapleton, Oppenheim, Peleg, & Jackson, 1983), a 25-item questionnaire developed from responses that individuals with alcohol problems provided to sentence completion and interview questions, presents to the respondent a variety of situations and asks for a rating on a 4-point scale as to how "dangerous" each situation is in terms of risk for relapse.

Miller and Harris (2000) developed the 37-item *Assessment of Warning Signs of Relapse* (AWARE) scale based on Gorski's model of relapse (Gorski

& Miller, 1982). Each item of the scale presents a different situation that could possibly trigger a drinking episode. Based upon their analysis, the authors suggest using 28 of the items for the final scale, because these appear to represent a single coherent factor.

Self-Efficacy

Self-efficacy theory (Bandura, 1977) provides an integration of cognitive and behavioral processes that affect behavioral performance. The theory states that individuals vary regarding their belief in their ability to cope effectively with various situations. Self-efficacy theory provides a heuristic for understanding clients' confidence in their ability to cope effectively with high risk drinking situations (Annis & Graham, 1988). This conceptualization has direct implications for the evaluation of risk for relapse: Individuals with greater confidence in their ability to cope with high-risk drinking contexts are inclined to engage in more coping behaviors and are thus less likely to relapse (Annis & Graham, 1988; Greenfield et al., 2000). The following instruments have been used to measure self-efficacy expectations in individuals with alcohol problems.

The *Situational Confidence Questionnaire* (SCQ-39; Annis & Graham, 1988) was created to measure respondents' beliefs that they could refrain from drinking alcohol in a variety of potentially high-risk situations. These situations were taken from the eight contexts assessed by the IDS described earlier. The 39-item questionnaire asks individuals to rate on a 6-point scale their level of confidence that they would be able to resist drinking heavily in each of the situations presented. Greater self-efficacy for not drinking, as measured by the SCQ-39, has been associated with decreased drinking at follow-up (Solomon & Annis, 1990), as well as higher abstinence rates at 6 months (Burling, Reilly, Moltzen, & Ziff, 1989), and 12 months (Greenfield et al., 2000).

The *Alcohol Abstinence Self-Efficacy Scale* (AASE; DiClemente, Carbonari, Montgomery, & Hughes, 1994) is actually two scales in one. Twenty situations are presented, and individuals rate how "tempted" they would be to drink in each of the situations, and how confident they are that they would not drink in each. The 20 items have been separated into four subscales; Negative Affect, Social/Positive, Physical and Other Concerns, and Withdrawal and Urges.

The *Drinking Refusal Self-Efficacy Questionnaire* (DRSEQ; Young, Oei, & Crook, 1991) is a 31-item self-report measure of an individual's perceived ability to resist drinking alcohol in a variety of situations. A number of possible drinking contexts are presented, representing three content areas: social pressure, opportunistic drinking, and emotional relief.

In an effort to obtain a more individualized assessment of one's ability to resist drinking, which could then be incorporated into treatment, a few semistructured methods have been developed. For example, the *Substance Abuse Relapse Assessment* (SARA; Schonfeld, Peters, & Dolente, 1993) is a multidimensional measure of the elements that may lead to an eventual relapse, and the *Individualized Self-Efficacy Survey* (ISS; Miller, McCrady, Abrams, & Labouvie, 1994) was developed to gain a more personalized set of efficacy expectations.

Coping Skills

Cognitive-behavioral approaches to treating alcohol problems rely heavily upon teaching individuals a range of skills that may be utilized to help manage potential relapse situations. Appraisal of clients' coping skills is an essential component of treatment planning and treatment outcome assessment. Some self-report and behavioral methods of assessing coping skills are reviewed here.

The *Coping Behaviours Inventory* (CBI; Litman, Stapleton, Oppenheim, & Peleg, 1983) is a 36-item self-report measure of how individuals attempt to avoid relapse. The items yield four factors: Positive Thinking, Negative Thinking, Avoidance/Distraction, and Seeking Social Support. The *Effectiveness of Coping Behaviours Inventory* (ECBI; Litman, 1984) contains the same items as the CBI, but instructs the individual to provide a rating of the usefulness of the strategies.

The *Coping Response Inventory* (CRI; Moos, 1992), a 48-item measure of coping skills, focuses upon a recent drinking trigger situation as defined by the individual. The CRI is scored to yield eight dimensions, with four subscales reflecting approach coping (Logical Analysis, Positive Reappraisal, Seeking Guidance and Support, and Taking Problem-Solving Action), and four subscales reflecting avoidance coping (Cognitive Avoidance, Acceptance/ Resignation, Seeking Alternative Rewards, and Emotional Discharge).

Role-play measures of coping skills have been developed to assess individuals' responses to potential drinking situations. These measures typically involve an audiotaped presentation of a variety of scenarios. Individuals are asked either to act out their response to the situation or to provide a verbal response describing what they might do or say when such a situation arises. Some of these measures include the *Situational Competency Test* (SCT; Chaney, O'Leary, & Marlatt, 1978), the *Adaptive Skills Battery* (ASB; Jones & Lanyon, 1981), and the *Problem Situation Inventory* (PSI; Hawkins, Catalano, & Wells, 1986). The *Alcohol-Specific Role-Play Test* (ASRPT; Monti et al., 1993) involves interactive role play of situations with a confederate.

Drinking Outcome Expectations

Expectations concerning the anticipated reinforcing and punishing consequences of drinking, based on prior experience with alcohol, may influence decisions whether or not to drink (Goldman, Darkes, & Del Boca, 1999). Information about expectancies may be useful clinical data concerning one's reason for drinking in certain environments. Additionally, modifying alcohol expectancies shows promise as an intervention for the disruption of drinking patterns (Darkes & Goldman, 1993, 1998).

There is no shortage of alcohol expectancy scales in the literature. A review of these instruments has revealed that the most reliable measures, and those covering the broadest range of content, demonstrated the largest effect sizes (McCarthy & Smith, 1996). Some of the most commonly used alcohol expectancy scales are listed below.

The *Alcohol Expectancy Questionnaire* (AEQ; Brown, Goldman, Inn, & Anderson, 1980), a 90-item measure, comprises six empirically derived factors that characterize the positive effects of drinking alcohol. These factors identify alcohol as (1) being a global, positive transforming agent; (2) enhancing sexual performance; (3) enhancing social and physical pleasure; (4) increasing social assertiveness; (5) providing relaxation/tension reduction; and (6) increasing power and aggression. Higher scores on the AEQ were related to higher levels of drinking (Brown, Goldman, & Christiansen, 1985), predicted college drinking styles (Brown, 1985a), and were related to treatment outcome at 1-year follow-up (Brown, 1985b).

Modifications to the items, length, and response structure of the AEQ have led to the development of other alcohol expectancy measures including the *Alcohol Effects Questionnaire* (AEQ; Rohsenow, 1983) and the *AEQ-3* (George et al., 1995).

The *Drinking Expectancy Questionnaire* (DEQ; Young & Knight, 1989) is a 43-item scale measuring both positive and negative alcohol expectancies across five scales, while a sixth scale measures a general level of alcohol involvement. A recent investigation of the factor structure of the scale found a five-factor solution to be a more robust measure of expectancies, and a new scoring method has been devised, appropriate to the new structure (Lee, Oei, Greeley, & Baglioni, 2003).

The *Comprehensive Effects of Alcohol* scale (CEOA; Fromme, Stroot, & Kaplan, 1993) measures both positive and negative expected effects of drinking across seven empirically derived domains. The 41-items of the scale are administered one time to measure an individual's agreement with each expectancy statement, and again to determine one's subjective evaluation (good–bad) of the anticipated effects of drinking.

The *Negative Alcohol Expectancy Questionnaire* (NAEQ; Jones & McMahon, 1994) was developed to measure anticipated negative consequences of drinking that may occur over three periods of time (same day, next day, and long term). The 60-item questionnaire consists of statements regarding possible negative effects of drinking alcohol, and respondents are asked to rate each item based on the likelihood that they believe the negative outcome would occur.

The *Alcohol Expectancy Questionnaire—Adolescent Version* (AEQ-A; Christiansen, Goldman, & Inn, 1982), a 100-item instrument developed for use with adolescents, measures expectancies in seven different domains: global positive changes, improved cognitive and motor functioning, sexual enhancement, increased arousal, relaxation, social enhancement or impairment, and deteriorated cognitive and motor functioning. Assessment of seventh- and eighth-grade students' alcohol expectancies using the AEQ-A discriminated non-problem drinkers from those who went on to become problem drinkers over a 1-year period (Christansen, Smith, Roehling, & Goldman, 1989).

Spirituality and Religiosity

An individual's sense of spirituality and religiosity may be viewed as an additional coping resource against relapse (Miller, Westerberg, Harris, & Tonigan, 1996). Research investigations have provided support for a relationship between spiritual/religious involvement and prevention of relapse (Miller, 1998). More specific attention has been paid to this area as it relates to referrals to, affiliation with, and maintenance of abstinence through 12-step self-help programs. However, evidence has indicated that benefits of such programs are likely independent of prior levels of spirituality or religious affiliation (Connors, Tonigan, & Miller, 2001; Winzelberg & Humphreys, 1999). Few measures have been designed specifically for individuals with alcohol problems, but the scales that follow have demonstrated utility in this area.

The *Religious Background and Behavior* questionnaire (RBB; Connors, Tonigan, & Miller, 1996) was designed for use in Project MATCH as a brief measure of religious practices. The 13-item scale assesses an individual's religious affiliation and frequency of engagement in various religious practices during the past year and throughout his or her lifetime. Analysis of the RBB has yielded two factors labeled God Consciousness and Formal Practices.

The *Purpose in Life Test* (PIL; Crumbaugh, 1969) and the *Seeking of Noetic Goals* scale (SONG; Crumbaugh, 1977) are complementary measures that have been used in substance abuse research (Black, 1991; Miller et al., 1996; Tonigan, Miller, & Connors, 2001) to determine one's current sense of meaning in life (PIL) and the extent of one's desire for and seeking of greater meaning in life (SONG). In Project MATCH, a difference score (SONG—PIL) was utilized to operationalize the degree to which one had "hit bottom," as described in AA literature.

Many additional measures developed to assess spirituality and religiosity have not been extensively tested. Some of these measures include the Mathew Materialism–Spiritualism Scale (MMSS; Mathew, Mathew, Wilson, & Georgi, 1995), which has been used with individuals recovering from substance use problems; the Spiritual Well-Being Scale (SWBS; Ellison & Paloutzian, 1982); and the Spiritual Involvement and Beliefs Scale (SIBS; Hatch, Burg, Naberhaus, & Hellmich, 1998), which is a 26-item self-report measure designed to assess an individual's spiritual beliefs and participation in activities of a spiritual nature.

Twelve-Step Affiliation

Twelve-step-oriented treatment encourages attendance and involvement in AA meetings. Assessment instruments have been developed to measure engagement in AA. The *Alcoholics Anonymous Involvement (AAI) Scale* (Tonigan, Miller, & Connors, 1996) is a 13-item, self-administered questionnaire that measures lifetime and recent attendance and involvement in AA. The *Steps Questionnaire* (Gilbert, 1991), a 21-item scale, measures attitudes and beliefs related to the first three of AA's 12 steps. The *Brown–Peterson Recovery Progress Inventory* (B-PRPI; H. P. Brown & Peterson, 1991) is a 53-item assessment of behaviors, beliefs, and attitudes that measures progress in a 12-step program. The 8-item *Self-Help Group Participation Scale* and the 4-item *Adoption of Self-Help Group Beliefs Scale* measure self-help group involvement (McKay Alterman, McLellan, & Snider, 1994). The *Alcoholics Anonymous Affiliation Scale* (AAAS; Humphreys, Kaskutas, & Weisner, 1998), a 9-item scale, measures attendance at AA meetings, having a sponsor, and reading AA literature. A review and critique of these instruments can be found in Allen (2000) and Finney (2003).

Craving and Cue Reactivity

Definition and measurement of craving for alcohol are controversial topics in the alcohol literature (Anton, 1999; Potgieter, Deckers, & Geerlings, 1999; Sayette et al., 2000). In general, craving has been described as the subjective desire to use alcohol (Sayette et al., 2000), or as intense thoughts about drinking, or a powerful urge to drink (National Institute on Alcohol Abuse and Alcoholism, 2001). While the term is widely used among patients, clinicians, and researchers alike, there is great debate as to its role in the development and maintenance of alcohol problems as well as relapse after treatment. Additionally, craving measurement has ranged from simple, single-item instruments (e.g., "How strong is your craving for alcohol?") to more elaborate behavioral and psychophysiological measures. Due to the growing interest in the use of nonaversive medications aimed at reducing alcohol craving, assessment of craving experiences has become increasingly important (Potgieter et al., 1999).

Craving for alcohol can be assessed in a variety of ways. Research on craving may employ a methodology involving the induction of craving in controlled laboratory settings. Techniques for inducing craving have included exposure to actual alcoholic beverages (with or without consumption of a priming dose), exposure to visual representations of alcoholic beverages, and induction of negative mood states through the use of guided imagery (Litt & Cooney, 1999). Although there is evidence that laboratory assessments of alcohol cue reactivity are predictive of alcohol relapse (Cooney, Litt, Morse, Bauer, & Gaupp, 1997; Rohsenow et al., 1994), this methodology has been criticized because of the artificial nature of the laboratory environment. Recent investigations have assessed alcohol craving in the natural environment using EMA methodology described earlier in this chapter in the section on measures of alcohol consumption.

The following is a description of alcohol craving assessment scales. For a more extensive review of craving assessment issues, see Sayette et al. (2000).

The *Yale–Brown Obsessive Compulsive Scale—Heavy Drinkers* (YBOCS-hd; Modell, Glaser, Mountz, Schmaltz, & Cyr, 1992), a 10-item measure, consists of two subscales reflecting obsessional thought patterns and compulsive behaviors that may be related to problematic alcohol use. The scale is adapted from the Yale–Brown Obsessive Compulsive Scale (YBOCS; Goodman et al., 1989) and can be administered either as a structured interview or as a questionnaire.

The *Obsessive Compulsive Drinking Scale* (OCDS; Anton, Moak, & Latham, 1995) was developed as a modification of the YBOCS-hd (Modell et al., 1992). This widely used measure comprises Obsessive and Compulsive subscales, each measured by 14 self-report items. Respondents are asked to complete the measure based upon their experiences of craving over a 1- to 2-week period. A recent investigation found the predictive capacity of the Obsessive subscale of the OCDS to be more robust than two other measures of alcohol craving for the prediction of drinking during alcohol treatment (Flannery et al., 2001).

The *Alcohol Urge Questionnaire* (AUQ; Bohn, Krahn, & Staehler, 1995) is an 8-item measure of one's current urge to drink alcohol. This brief self-report instrument consists of questions regarding one's desire for alcohol, expected positive effects from drinking, and the inability to resist drinking in the presence of alcohol. The AUQ has been demonstrated to be an easily administered, reliable, state measure of craving for use in laboratory settings (Sinha & O'Malley, 1999).

The *Alcohol Craving Questionnaire* (ACQ-Now; Singleton, 1996) is a 47-item self-report measure adapted from the Cocaine Craving Questionnaire (Tiffany, Singleton, Haertzen, & Henningfield, 1993). The scale was designed to assess current craving for alcohol. Factor analysis of the items indicated the presence of four factors labeled Emotionality, Purposefulness, Compulsivity, and Expectancy (Singleton & Gorelick, 1998).

The *Penn Alcohol Craving Scale* (PACS; Flannery, Volpicelli, & Pettinati, 1999) is a brief scale of five self-report items measuring the intensity, frequency, and duration of craving, as well as the ability to resist alcohol, if it were available. Additionally, average level of craving during the past week is assessed. Weekly PACS scores were found to clearly differentiate between individuals who had relapsed to alcohol use during treatment and those who remained abstinent or drank less than five drinks per week (Flannery et al., 2001).

Assessing Co-Occurring Clinical Problems

There is consistent evidence that individuals with alcohol use disorders are often troubled by a number of other psychological and behavioral problems (e.g., Kessler et al., 1997). Some of the most common co-occurring difficulties include the use of other substances, affective disturbance, anxiety disorders, and neuropsychological deficits. Many of these problems are severe enough to warrant a clinical diagnosis and should likely be an additional focus of intervention at some point in the treatment process. However, the dynamic interaction between alcohol use, psychiatric symptoms, and personality factors often adds complexity to treatment decisions (Modesto-Lowe & Kranzler, 1999). An initial screening allows for identification of these issues in affected individuals. More extensive assessment, determination of level of care, and selection of interventions may follow this initial step. The following section provides a limited overview of measures that may be used to identify difficulties frequently seen in individuals with alcohol use disorders. The assessment of other addictive disorders, including other substance use, tobacco use, gambling problems, and eating disorders, is not covered in this section, because each is a significant issue reviewed in detail elsewhere in this volume.

Comorbid Psychopathology

As was stated earlier, the coexistence of alcohol use disorders with other psychological problems is common. Epidemiological investigations have found lifetime co-occurrence rates for both men and women with alcohol dependence to exceed 75% (Kessler et al., 1997). Similar comorbidity rates have been found for current diagnoses in clinical settings (Driessen, Veltrup, Wetterling, John, & Dilling, 1998). Mood, anxiety, psychotic, and personality disorders (e.g., antisocial personality disorder), when comorbid with alcohol dependence, frequently involve substantial clinical complexity. In addition, it is often difficult to differentiate exacerbations of previously existing syndromes, development of new pathology, and symptoms that are tied to alcohol use. Therefore, evaluation of these symptoms is necessary, because they can affect treatment process and outcome, as well as significantly heighten the risk of relapse.

The *Beck Depression Inventory* (BDI-II; Beck, Steer, & Brown, 1996), and the *Center for Epidemiologic Studies—Depression Questionnaire* (CES-D; Radloff, 1977) are frequently utilized self-report questionnaires designed to assess depressive symptoms in a short amount of time. Brief measures of anxiety used often in the literature include the *State–Trait Anxiety Inventory* (STAI; Spielberger, Gorsuch, Lushene, Vagg, & Jacobs, 1983) and the *Beck Anxiety Inventory* (BAI; Beck, Epstein, Brown, & Steer, 1988). Multidimensional measures of psychological symptoms can be useful in screening for the presence of a wide variety of psychological complaints, and such instruments can be administered multiple times to evaluate changes in symptoms over time. The *Brief Symptom Inventory* (BSI; Derogatis & Melisaratos, 1983), derived from the highly utilized *Symptom Checklist 90—Revised* (SCL-90-R; Derogatis, 1983) is a good example of such a measure; it is a widely used self-report scale assessing nine primary symptom dimensions, while also providing a Global Severity Index.

Neuropsychological Deficits

Chronic alcohol abuse typically leads to some form of cognitive impairment, ranging from mild functional deficits to the severe damage seen in Korsakoff's disease. Though there is some dispute as to the chronicity of drinking necessary for deficits to emerge (Beatty, Tivis, Stott, Nixon, & Parsons, 2000; Eckardt et al., 1998), studies of detoxified alcoholics have typically found impairments in the areas of abstract thinking and problem-solving skills, verbal and/or memory skills, visuospatial skills, and perceptual–motor skills (Nixon, 1995). Significant individual differences have been found in the nature of these impairments (Parsons, 1998), and the extent and speed of recovery of functioning (Goldman, 1995; Mann, Guenther, Stetter, & Ackermann, 1999).

Evaluation of neuropsychological deficits in individuals with alcohol use problems can provide useful information regarding their cognitive capacity for treatment and domains of functioning that may affect their likelihood of relapse. Although a comprehensive neuropsychological assessment takes a good deal of time and expertise to conduct, a number of instruments have become popular due to their sensitivity to alcohol-related impairments, ease of administration, and brevity. Some of these are listed below; however, it is important to note that while cognitive deficits may be observed by such instruments, questions have been raised regarding the clinical or functional significance of what are often subtle impairments (Nixon, 1995).

The *Wisconsin Card Sorting Test* (WCST; Heaton, 1981) and the Abstraction Test from the *Shipley Institute of Living Scale* (Zachary, 1986) are frequently used measures of abstract thinking and problem-solving deficits. A computer administration and scoring program for the WCST is available. Although measures of verbal performance generally appear to be less affected by chronic alcohol use, measures of memory often provide significant evidence of alcohol-related impairment. Elements of the *Wechsler Memory Scale—Revised* (WMS-R; Wechsler, 1987) have often been used for this purpose, as well as the *California Verbal Learning Test* (CVLT; Delis, Kramer, Kaplan, & Ober, 1987). In addition to memory, visuospatial and perceptual–motor tasks are typically sensitive to the effects of drinking. Some of the instruments frequently used to assess these impairments include the *Trail Making Test* from the Halstead–Reitan Battery (HRB; Halstead, 1947) and the *Digit Symbol Substitution Test* from the Wechsler Adult Intelligence Scale—Revised (WAIS-R; Wechsler, 1981).

Multidimensional Assessment Measures

Choosing from the many possible domains of assessment and the multiple measures available can be a daunting task. If the battery of instruments used to measure alcohol use and related problems is too large, time for other aspects of the treatment process may be sacrificed, and clients may feel overwhelmed by the initial assessment. On the other hand, if the evaluation is too brief, important information concerning factors that may influence treatment outcome may be missed. Multidimensional assessment measures have been developed in an attempt to provide a comprehensive picture of an individual's alcohol use and other, associated issues in a single instrument. Some widely used and promising measures are reviewed below.

The *Addiction Severity Index* (ASI; McLellan et al., 1992; McLellan, Luborsky, O'Brien, & Woody, 1980) is a widely-used, semistructured interview designed to obtain information about seven possible problem areas, including medical status, employment/support status, drug use, alcohol use, legal status, family/social relationships, and psychiatric status. While the focus of the ASI is not specific to alcohol use, it does cover a broad range of problems that are often seen in individuals suffering from alcohol use problems. In approximately 1 hour or less, an interviewer can obtain lifetime and recent (past 30 days) problem information, patient and interviewer severity ratings for each area evaluated, and interviewer confidence ratings of the patient's responses. Computerized scoring of the ASI is available, and composite scores for each problem area can be derived. Additionally, a computer-administered version of the ASI has been developed, and shows promising reliability compared with the original version (Butler et al., 2001). A self-administered paper-and-pencil version of the ASI has also been developed (Rosen, Henson, Finney, & Moos, 2000). The *Comprehensive Addiction Severity Index for Adolescents* (CASI-A; Meyers, McLellan, Jaeger, & Pettinati, 1995) similarly covers seven broad areas of functioning in a semistructured interview format, which the authors suggest may be used for the assessment of adolescents with a variety of presenting problems.

In an effort to evaluate treatment process, McLellan and his colleagues developed the *Treatment Services Review* (TSR; McLellan, Alterman, Cacciola, & Metzger, 1992). This brief interview is designed to measure the number and type of treatment and services received by individuals during the course of substance treatment. The seven areas covered by the TSR correspond to those of the ASI, as described earlier. This facilitates a direct evaluation of whether problems identified at intake by the ASI have been addressed during treatment. A similar instrument has been developed to assess treatment process in adolescents, the *Teen-Treatment Services Review* (T-TSR; Kaminer, Blitz, Burleson, & Sussman, 1998).

The *Comprehensive Drinker Profile* (CDP; Miller & Marlatt, 1984) is an extensive interview intended to gather information concerning multiple areas related to alcohol use. CDP items assess drinking history, including drinking

patterns, usual settings, related problems, reasons for drinking, alcohol expectancies, and self-efficacy. Approximately 2 hours are required for administration of all 88 items, though an abbreviated version has been developed (*Brief
Drinker Profile*). Corresponding follow-up (*Follow-up Drinker Profile*) and
collateral interviews (*Collateral Interview Form*) are also available (Miller &
Marlatt, 1987).

Self-report, multidimensional assessment measures have also been widely
used in the alcohol field. The *Alcohol Use Inventory* (AUI; Horn et al., 1987)
has been extensively utilized in both clinical and research settings. The 228-
item measure yields 17 primary scales, 6 second-order scales, and 1 general
alcohol involvement third-order factor. Broad domains measured by the primary scales include the perceived benefits of drinking (e.g., improved sociability, mood management), styles of drinking (e.g., gregarious vs. solo, compulsive), drinking consequences (e.g., loss of behavioral control, dependence
symptoms), and concerns and acknowledgment of problems (e.g., awareness,
guilt and worry, readiness for change). Computerized administration and
scoring, including interpretive reports and profiles, are available.

The *Personal Experience Inventory for Adults* (PEI-A; Winters, 1996,
1999) is a self-report, multiscale measure of adult substance abuse problems.
The design of the PEI-A was influenced by the development of the *Personal
Experiences Inventory* (PEI; Winters & Henly, 1989), which is an adolescent
substance abuse inventory. The PEI-A consists of two parts: the Problem Severity section comprises 120 items that make up 10 problem severity scales,
three validity indices, alcohol and drug use consumption characteristics, and a
scale measuring receptiveness to treatment. The Psychosocial section comprises 150 items broken down into eight personal risk adjustment scales, three
environmental scales, 10 problem screens, and two indicators of validity.
Computerized administration and scoring, including the production of a narrative clinical report, along with standardized scores, are available.

American Society of Addiction
Medicine Patient Placement Criteria

The American Society of Addiction Medicine Patient Placement Criteria
(ASAM PPC) were designed to help clinicians and third-party payers match
patients to levels of care in a rational manner based on an individualized multidimensional assessment. The PPC have been endorsed by a broad consensus
process (Center for Substance Abuse Treatment, 1995), and concurrent validity studies suggest that the ASAM PPC is clinically meaningful (Turner,
Turner, Reif, Gutowski, & Gastfriend, 1999; Staines et al., 2003). The latest
version, the ASAM PPC-2R (Mee-Lee, Shulman, Fishman, Gastfriend, & Griffith, 2001), identifies and describes six biopsychosocial assessment dimensions
that are used to differentiate patient needs for services across levels of care.
These dimensions include Acute Intoxication and/or Withdrawal Potential;
Biomedical Conditions and Complications; Emotional, Behavioral or Cogni-

tive Conditions and Complications; Readiness to Change; Relapse, Continued Use or Continued Problem Potential; and Recovery Environment. The PPC contain five basic levels of care: Early Intervention; Outpatient Services; Intensive Outpatient/Partial Hospitalization; Residential/Inpatient Services; and Medically Managed Intensive Inpatient Services.

The complexity of the PPC makes it difficult for even experienced clinicians to apply consistently the patient placement rules, so an automated approach to facilitate the interviewing and scoring required for the PPC was proposed and developed (Turner et al., 1999). It consists of a computer-guided sequence of questions and scoring options for use by a counselor or research assistant. Items were drawn from standardized assessment instruments including the CIWA, ASI, Global Assessment of Function, and the Recovery Attitude and Treatment Evaluator (RAATE; Najavits et al., 1997). Duration of administration is less than 60 minutes per patient (Turner et al., 1999).

A new version of the PPC assessment software has been released (Gastfriend & Mee-Lee, 2004). This software guides the interviewer in a multidimensional evaluation, and provides comprehensive narrative reports for use at intake, continuing review, or discharge/transfer. In addition, the software allows assessment data to be uploaded via the Web to a central data repository that produces periodic reports of case mix, utilization, and (with repeat administration to patients) outcomes. The assessment data are also available for use by the treatment program for custom analyses and research purposes.

CONCLUSIONS

The alcohol field is blessed with a wide array of screening and assessment instruments (see Table 3.1). We have tried to identify and describe the more established and promising instruments. Probably the reason there are so many assessment instruments is because there are so many varied assessment needs. Alcohol assessment settings range from primary care to emergency departments, specialized substance abuse clinics, and funded clinical research projects. Assessment needs range from identification of individuals with possible alcohol problems to determination of alcohol and comorbid problems for treatment planning, to obtaining information for use in motivational feedback, to validating self-reported alcohol consumption, and measuring change and treatment outcome. Practical limitations of resources (i.e., staff time and training) and client time also influence assessment decisions.

Given the lack of consensus regarding which variables are most significant, or which measures are the best for assessing them, we cannot make recommendations as to which is the best instrument in each assessment domain. Such a designation would likely be premature at this stage of development of this field. Although it requires considerably greater effort, clinicians and researchers alike must review the available instruments to determine which ones are most appropriate to the particular needs in their setting.

TABLE 3.1. Summary of Alcohol Assessment Measures

Purpose	Domain/construct	Instrument(s)	Author(s)
Screening	Screening for alcohol problems	CAGE	Ewing (1984)
		AUDIT	Saunders et al. (1993)
		AUDIT-C	Gordon et al. (2001)
		TWEAK	Russell (1994)
		RAPS/RAPS4	Cherpitel (1995, 2000)
Problem assessment	Diagnosis of alcohol problems	DIS-IV	Robins et al. (2000)
		SCID-I/P	First et al. (1996)
		PRISM	Hasin et al. (1996, 1998)
		CIDI-SAM	Robins et al. (1995)
		SSAGA	Bucholz et al. (1994)
		SCAN	Wing et al. (1990)
	Severity of alcohol dependence	ADS	Skinner & Allen (1982)
		EDSS	Babor (1996)
		SADQ	Stockwell et al. (1983)
		SDSS	Miele et al. (2000)
	Alcohol consumption	QF measures	
		GF	Midanik (1994)
		LDH	Skinner & Sheu (1982)
		CLDH	Russell et al. (1997)
		TLFB	Sobell & Sobell (1992, 2000)
		Form 90	Miller (1996)
		Daily diary	
		IVR/EMA	
	Alcohol biomarkers	Ethanol tests	
		GGT	
		CDT	
	Severity of alcohol withdrawal	CIWA-Ar	Sullivan et al. (1989)
		AWS	Wetterling et al. (1997)
	Alcohol-related consequences	DrInC	Miller et al. (1995)
		RAPI	White & Labouvie (1989)
Personal assessment	Readiness to change	URICA	DiClemente & Hughes (1990)
		SOCRATES	Miller & Tonigan (1996)
		RTCQ-TV	Heather et al. (1999)
	Antecedents to drinking	IDS	Annis et al. (1987)
		RFDQ	Zywiak et al. (1996)
		RPI	Litman et al. (1983)
		AWARE	Miller & Harris (2000)
	Self-efficacy	SCQ-39	Annis & Graham (1988)
		AASE	DiClemente et al. (1994)

(continued)

TABLE 3.1. *(continued)*

Purpose	Domain/construct	Instrument(s)	Author(s)
Personal assessment *(cont.)*	Self-efficacy *(cont.)*	DRSEQ	Young & Knight (1991)
		SARA	Schonfeld et al. (1993)
		ISS	Miller et al. (1994)
	Coping skills	CBI	Litman et al. (1983)
		CRI	Moos (1992)
		ASRPT	Monti et al. (1993)
	Drinking outcome expectations	AEQ	Brown et al. (1980)
		DEQ	Young & Knight (1989)
		CEOA	Fromme et al. (1993)
		NAEQ	Jones & McMahon (1994)
		AEQ-A	Christiansen et al. (1982)
	Spirituality and religiosity	RBB	Connors et al. (1996)
		PIL/SONG	Crumbaugh (1969, 1977)
	Twelve-step affiliation	AAI	Tonigan et al. (1996)
		Steps	Gilbert (1991)
		B-PRPI	Brown & Peterson (1994)
		AAAS	Humphreys et al. (1998)
	Craving	YBOCS-hd	Modell et al. (1992)
		OCDS	Anton et al. (1995)
		AUQ	Bohn et al. (1995)
		ACQ-Now	Singleton (1996)
		PACS	Flannery et al. (1999)
	Comorbid psychopathology	BDI-II	Beck et al. (1996)
		CES-D	Radloff (1977)
		STAI	Spielberger et al. (1983)
		BAI	Beck et al. (1988)
		BSI	Derogatis & Melisaratos (1983)
	Neuropsychological deficits	WCST	Heaton (1981)
		Shipley	Zachary (1986)
		WMS	Wechsler (1987)
		CVLT	Delis et al. (1987)
		Trail Making	Halstead (1947)
		Digit Symbol	Wechsler (1981)
	Multidimensional measures	ASI	McLellan et al. (1992)
		CASI-A	Meyers et al. (1995)
		CDP	Miller & Marlatt (1984)
		AUI	Horn et al. (1987)
		PEI-A	Winters (1996, 1999)
	Patient placement	ASAM criteria	Mee-Lee et al. (2001)

REFERENCES

Allen, J. P. (2000). Measuring treatment process variables in Alcoholics Anonymous. *Journal of Substance Abuse Treatment, 18,* 227–230.

Allen, J. P., Litten, R. Z., Anton, R. F., & Cross, G. M. (1994). Carbohydrate-deficient transferrin as a measure of immoderate drinking: Remaining issues. *Alcoholism: Clinical and Experimental Research, 18,* 799–812.

Allen, J. P., Sillanaukee, P., Strid, N., & Litten, R. Z. (2003). Biomarkers of heavy drinking. In J. P. Allen & V. B. Wilson (Eds.), *Assessing alcohol problems: A guide for clinicians and researchers* (2nd ed., pp. 37–53). Rockville, MD: U.S. Department of Health and Human Services, National Institute on Alcohol Abuse and Alcoholism.

American Psychiatric Association. (1994). *Diagnostic and statistical manual of mental disorders* (4th ed.). Washington, DC: Author.

American Society of Addiction Medicine. (2001). *ASAM Patient Placement Criteria for the treatment of substance-related disorders* (2nd ed., rev.). Chevy Chase, MD: Author.

Annis, H. M., & Graham, J. M. (1988). *Situational Confidence Questionnaire (SCQ-39) user's guide.* Toronto: Addiction Research Foundation.

Annis, H. M., Graham, J. M., & Davis, C. S. (1987). *Inventory of Drinking Situations (IDS) user's guide.* Toronto: Addiction Research Foundation.

Anton, R. F. (1999). What is craving?: Models and implications for treatment. *Alcohol Research and Health, 23,* 165–173.

Anton, R. F., Moak, D. H., & Latham, P. K. (1995). The Obsessive Compulsive Drinking Scale: A self-rated instrument for the quantification of thoughts about alcohol and drinking behavior. *Alcoholism: Clinical and Experimental Research, 19,* 92–99.

Babor, T. F. (1996). Reliability of the ethanol dependence syndrome scale. *Psychology of Addictive Behaviors, 10,* 97–103.

Babor, T. F., Brown, J., & Del Boca, F. K. (1990). Validity of self-reports in applied research on addictive behaviors: Fact or fiction? *Addictive Behaviors, 12,* 5–32.

Babor, T. F., Ritson, E. B., & Hodgson, R. J. (1986). Alcohol-related problems in the primary health care setting: A review of early intervention strategies. *British Journal of Addiction, 81,* 23–46.

Bandura, A. (1977). Self-efficacy: Toward a unifying theory of behavior change. *Psychological Review, 84,* 191–215.

Beatty, W. W., Tivis, R., Stott, H. D., Nixon, S. J., & Parsons, O. A. (2000). Neuropsychological deficits in sober alcoholics: Influences of chronicity and recent alcohol consumption. *Alcoholism: Clinical and Experimental Research, 24,* 149–154.

Beck, A. T., Epstein, N., Brown, G., & Steer, R. (1988). An inventory for measuring clinical anxiety: Psychometric properties. *Journal of Consulting and Clinical Psychology, 56,* 893–897.

Beck, A. T., Steer, R. A., & Brown, G. K. (1996). *Beck Depression Inventory–II.* San Antonio, TX: Psychological Corporation.

Black, W. A. M. (1991). An existential approach to self-control in the addictive behaviours. In N. Heather, W. R. Miller, & J. Greeley (Eds.), *Self control and the addictive behaviours* (pp. 262–279). Sydney: Maxwell Macmillan.

Bohn, M. J., Krahn, D. D., & Staehler, R. A. (1995). Development and initial validation of a measure of drinking urges in abstinent alcoholics. *Alcoholism: Clinical and Experimental Research, 19,* 600–606.

Bradley, K. A., Donovan, D. M., & Larson, E. B. (1993). How much is too much?: Advising patients about safe levels of alcohol consumption. *Archives of Internal Medicine, 153,* 2734–2740.

Brown, H. P., & Peterson, J. H. (1991). Assessing spirituality in addiction treatment and follow-up: Development of the Brown–Peterson Recovery Process Inventory (B-PRPI). *Alcoholism Treatment Quarterly, 8,* 21–50.

Brown, S. A. (1985a). Expectancies versus background in the prediction of college drinking patterns. *Journal of Consulting and Clinical Psychology, 53,* 123–130.

Brown, S. A. (1985b). Reinforcement expectancies and alcoholism treatment outcome after a one-year follow-up. *Journal of Studies on Alcohol, 46,* 304–308.

Brown, S. A., Goldman, M. S., & Christiansen, B. A. (1985). Do alcohol expectancies mediate drinking patterns of adults? *Journal of Consulting and Clinical Psychology, 53,* 512–519.

Brown, S. A., Goldman, M. S., Inn, A., & Anderson, L. (1980). Expectations of reinforcement from alcohol: Their domain and relation to drinking pattern. *Journal of Consulting and Clinical Psychology, 48,* 419–426.

Bucholz, K., Cadoret, R., Cloninger, C. R., Dinwiddie, S., Hesselbrock, V., Nurnberger, J., Reich, T., Schmidt, I., & Schuckit, M. (1994). A new, semistructured psychiatric interview for use in genetic linkage studies: A report of the reliability of the SSAGA. *Journal of Studies on Alcohol, 55,* 149–158.

Bucholz, K. K., Hesselbrock, V. M., Shayka, J. J., Nurnberger, J. I., Schuckit, M. A., & Reich, T. R. (1995). Reliability of individual diagnostic criterion items for psychoactive substance dependence and impact on diagnosis. *Journal of Studies on Alcohol, 56,* 500–505.

Burling, T. A., Reilly, P. M., Moltzen, J. O., & Ziff, D. C. (1989). Self-efficacy and relapse among inpatient drug and alcohol users: A predictor of outcome. *Journal of Studies on Alcohol, 50,* 354–360.

Butler, S. F., Budman, S. H., Goldman, R. J., Newman, F. L., Beckley, K. E., Trottier, D., & Cacciola, J. S. (2001). Initial validation of a computer-administered Addiction Severity Index: The ASI-MV. *Psychology of Addictive Behaviors, 15,* 4–12.

Cannon, D. S., Leeka, J. K., Patterson, E. T., & Baker, T. B. (1990). Principal components analysis of the Inventory of Drinking Situations: Empirical categories of drinking by alcoholics. *Addictive Behaviors, 15,* 265–269.

Carey, K. B., Maisto, S. A., Carey, M. P., & Purnine, D. M. (2001). Measuring readiness-to-change substance misuse among psychiatric outpatients: I. Reliability and validity of self-report measures. *Journal of Studies on Alcohol, 66,* 79–88.

Carey, K. B., Purnine, D. M., Maisto, S. A., & Carey, M. P. (1999). Assessing readiness to change substance abuse: Critical review of instruments. *Clinical Psychology, 6,* 245–266.

Carney, M. A., Tennen, H., Affleck, G., Del Boca, F., & Kranzler, H. R. (1998). Levels and patterns of alcohol consumption using timeline follow-back, daily diaries and real-time "electronic interviews." *Journal of Studies on Alcohol, 59,* 447–454.

Carrigan, G., Samoluk, S. B., & Stewart, S. H. (1998). Examination of the short form of the Inventory of Drinking Situations (IDS-42) in a young adult university student sample. *Behaviour Research and Therapy, 36,* 789–807.

Center for Substance Abuse Treatment. (1995). *The role and current status of patient placement criteria in the treatment of substance use disorders.* Treatment Improvement Protocol (TIP) Series No. 13 (DHHS Publication No. (SMA) 953021). Rockville, MD: U.S. Department of Health and Human Services.

Chaney, E. F., O'Leary, M. R., & Marlatt, G. A. (1978). Skill training with alcoholics. *Journal of Consulting and Clinical Psychology, 46,* 1092–1104.

Cherpitel, C. J. (1995). Screening for alcohol problems in the emergency room: A rapid alcohol problems screen. *Drug and Alcohol Dependence, 40,* 133–137.

Cherpitel, C. J. (1997). Brief screening for alcohol problems. *Alcohol Health and Research World, 21,* 348–351.

Cherpitel, C. J. (2000). A brief screening instrument for problem drinking in the emergency room: The RAPS4. *Journal of Studies on Alcohol, 61,* 447–449.

Christiansen, B. A., Goldman, M. S., & Inn, A. (1982). Development of alcohol related expectancies in adolescents: Separating pharmacological from social-learning influences. *Journal of Consulting and Clinical Psychology, 50,* 336–344.

Christiansen, B. A., Smith, G. T., Roehling, P. V., & Goldman, M. S. (1989). Using alcohol expectancies to predict adolescent drinking behavior at one year. *Journal of Consulting and Clinical Psychology, 57,* 93–99.

Collins, R. L., Kashdan, T. B., & Gollnisch, G. (2003). The feasibility of using cellular phones to collect ecological momentary assessment data: Application to alcohol consumption. *Experimental and Clinical Psychopharmacology, 11,* 73–78.

Compton, W. M., Cottler, L. B., Dorsey, K. B., Spitznagel, E. L., & Mager, D. E. (1996). Comparing assessments of DSM-IV substance dependence disorders using CIDI-SAM and SCAN. *Drug and Alcohol Dependence, 41,* 179–187.

Connors, G. J., Tonigan, J. S., & Miller, W. R. (1996). Measure of religious background and behavior for use in behavior change research. *Psychology of Addictive Behaviors, 10,* 90–96.

Connors, G. J., Tonigan, J. S., & Miller, W. R. (2001). Religiosity and responsiveness to alcoholism treatments. In R. H. Longabaugh & P. W. Wirtz (Eds.), *Project MATCH hypotheses: Results and causal chain analyses* (NIAAA Project MATCH Monograph Series, Vol. 8, pp. 166–175, NIH Publication No. 01-4238). Rockville, MD: National Institute on Alcohol Abuse and Alcoholism.

Connors, G. J., & Volk, R. J. (2003). Self-report screening for alcohol problems among adults. In J. P. Allen & V. Wilson (Eds.), *Assessing alcohol problems: A guide for clinicians and researchers* (2nd ed.). Rockville, MD: U.S. Department of Health and Human Services, National Institute on Alcohol Abuse and Alcoholism.

Cooney, N. L., Babor, T. F., & Litt, M. D. (2001). Matching clients to alcoholism treatment based on severity of alcohol dependence. In R. H. Longabaugh & P. W. Wirtz (Eds.), *Project MATCH hypotheses: Results and causal chain analyses* (NIAAA Project MATCH Monograph Series, Vol. 8, pp. 30–43, NIH Publication No. 01-4238). Rockville, MD: National Institute on Alcohol Abuse and Alcoholism.

Cooney, N. L., Litt, M. D., Morse, P. M., Bauer, L. O., & Gaupp, L. (1997). Alcohol cue reactivity, negative mood reactivity, and relapse in treated alcoholics. *Journal of Abnormal Psychology, 106,* 243–250.

Cooney, N. L., Zweben, A., & Fleming, M. F. (1995). Screening for alcohol problems and at-risk drinking in health care settings. In R. K. Hester & W. R. Miller (Eds.), *Handbook of alcoholism treatment approaches: Effective alternatives* (2nd ed., pp. 45–60). New York: Allyn & Bacon.

Cottler, L. B., Grant, B. F., Blaine, J., Mavreas, V., Pull, C., Hasin, D., Compton, W. M., Rubio-Stipec, M., & Mager, D. (1997). Concordance of DSM-IV alcohol and drug use disorder criteria and diagnoses as measured by AUDADIS-ADR, CIDI and SCAN. *Drug and Alcohol Dependence, 47,* 195–205.

Crumbaugh, J. C. (1969). *Purpose in Life test.* Murfreesboro, TN: Psychometric Affiliates.

Crumbaugh, J. C. (1977). The Seeking of Noetic Goals test (SONG): A complementary scale to the Purpose in Life test (PIL). *Journal of Clinical Psychology, 33,* 900–907.

Darkes, J., & Goldman, M. S. (1993). Expectancy challenge and drinking reduction: Experimental evidence for a mediational process. *Journal of Consulting and Clinical Psychology, 61,* 344–353.

Darkes, J., & Goldman, M. S. (1998). Expectancy challenge and drinking reduction: Structure and process in expectancy challenge. *Experimental and Clinical Psychopharmacology, 6,* 64–76.

Dawson, D. A., Grant, B. F., Chou, S. P., & Pickering, R. P. (1995). Subgroup variation in U. S. drinking patterns: Results of the 1992 National Longitudinal Alcohol Epidemiologic Survey. *Journal of Substance Abuse, 7,* 331–344.

Delis, D. C., Kramer, J. H., Kaplan, E., & Ober, B. A. (1987). *The California Verbal Learning Test.* New York: Psychological Corporation.

Derogatis, L. R. (1983). *SCL-90-R: Administration, scoring and procedures manual II* (rev.). Towson, MD: Clinical Psychometric Research.

Derogatis, L. R., & Melisaratos, N. (1983). The Brief Symptom Inventory: An introductory report. *Psychological Medicine, 13,* 595–605.

DiClemente, C. C., Carbonari, J. P., Montgomery, R. P. G., & Hughes, S. O. (1994). The Alcohol Abstinence Self-Efficacy Scale. *Journal of Studies on Alcohol, 55,* 141–148.

DiClemente, C. C., Carbonari, J. P., Zweben, A., Morrel, T., & Lee, R. E. (2001). Motivation hypothesis causal chain analysis. In R. H. Longabaugh & P. W. Wirtz (Eds.), *Project MATCH hypotheses: Results and causal chain analyses* (NIAAA Project MATCH Monograph Series, Vol. 8, pp. 206–222, NIH Publication No. 01-4238). Rockville, MD: National Institute on Alcohol Abuse and Alcoholism.

DiClemente, C. C., & Hughes, S. O. (1990). Stages of change profiles in outpatient alcoholism treatment. *Journal of Substance Abuse, 2,* 217–235.

Donovan, D. M. (1988). Assessment of addictive behaviors: Implications of an emerging biopsychosocial model. In D. M. Donovan & G. A. Marlatt (Eds.), *Assessment of addictive behaviors* (pp. 3–48). New York: Guilford Press.

Driessen, M., Veltrup, C., Wetterling, T., John, U., & Dilling, H. (1998). Axis I and Axis II comorbidity in alcohol dependence and the two types of alcoholism. *Alcoholism: Clinical and Experimental Research, 22,* 77–86.

Eckardt, M. J., File, S. E., Gessa, G. L., Grant, K. A., Guerri, C., Hoffman, P. L., Kalant, H., Koob, G. F., Li, T. K., & Tabakoff, B. (1998). Effects of moderate alcohol consumption on the central nervous system. *Alcoholism: Clinical and Experimental Research, 22,* 998–1040.

Edwards, G., & Gross, M. M. (1976). Alcohol dependence: Provisional description of a clinical syndrome. *British Medical Journal, 1,* 1058–1061.

Ellison, C. W., & Paloutzian, R. F. (1982). *The Spiritual Well-Being Scale.* Nyack, NY: Life Advance.

Ewing, J. (1984). Detecting alcoholism: The CAGE questions. *Journal of the American Medical Association, 252,* 1905–1907.

Feinn, R., Tennen, H., & Kranzler, H. R. (2003). Psychometric properties of the short index of problems as a measure of recent alcohol-related problems. *Alcoholism: Clinical and Experimental Research, 27,* 1436–1441.

Finney, J. W. (2003). Assessing treatment and treatment processes. In J. P. Allen & V. Wilson (Eds.), *Assessing alcohol problems: A guide for clinicians and researchers* (2nd ed., pp. 189–217). Rockville, MD: U.S. Department of Health and Human Services, National Institute on Alcohol Abuse and Alcoholism.

Finney, J. W., Moos, R. H., & Brennan, P. L. (1991). The Drinking Problems Index: A measure to assess alcohol-related problems among older adults. *Journal of Substance Abuse, 3,* 395–404.

First, M. B., Gibbon, M., Williams, J. B. W., Spitzer, R. L., & the MHS Staff. (2001). *SCID Screen Patient Questionnaire (SSPQ) and SCID Screen Patient Questionnaire—Extended (SSPQ-X): Computer programs for Windows software manual.* Canada: Multi-Health Systems/American Psychiatric Press.

First, M. B., Spitzer, R. L., Gibbon, M., & Williams, J. B. W. (1996). *Structured Clinical Interview for DSM-IV Axis I Disorders—Patient Edition (SCID-I/P, Version 2.0).* Biometrics Research Department, New York City, New York State Psychiatric Institute.

Flannery, B. A., Roberts, A. J., Cooney, N., Swift, R. M., Anton, R. F., & Rohsenow, D. J. (2001). The role of craving in alcohol use, dependence, and treatment. *Alcoholism: Clinical and Experimental Research, 25,* 299–308.

Flannery, B. A., Volpicelli, J. R., & Pettinati, H. M. (1999). Psychometric properties of the Penn Alcohol Craving Scale. *Alcoholism: Clinical and Experimental Research, 25,* 1289–1295.

Fleming, M. F. (2001). In search of the Holy Grail for the detection of hazardous drinking. *Journal of Family Practice, 504,* 321–322.

Fromme, K., Stroot, E., & Kaplan, D. (1993). Comprehensive effects of alcohol: Development and psychometric assessment of a new expectancy questionnaire. *Psychological Assessment, 5,* 19–26.

Gastfriend, D. R., & Mee-Lee, D. (2004). The ASAM Patient Placement Criteria: Context, concepts and continuing development. In D. R. Gastfriend (Ed.), *Addiction treatment matching: Research foundations of the American Society of Addiction Medicine (ASAM) criteria* (pp. 1–8). Binghamton, NY: Haworth Press.

George, W. H., Frone, M. R., Cooper, M. L., Russell, M., Skinner, J. B., & Windle, M. (1995). A revised Alcohol Expectancy Questionnaire: Factor structure confirmation and invariance in a general population sample. *Journal of Studies on Alcohol, 56,* 177–185.

Gilbert, F. S. (1991). The development of a "Steps Questionnaire." *Journal of Studies on Alcohol, 52,* 353–360.

Goldman, M. S. (1995). Recovery of cognitive functioning in alcoholics: The relationship to treatment. *Alcohol Health and Research World, 19,* 148–154.

Goldman, M. S., Darkes, J., & Del Boca, F. K. (1999). Expectancy mediation of biopsychosocial risk for alcohol use and alcoholism. In I. Kirsch (Ed.), *How expectancies shape experience* (pp. 233–262). Washington, DC: American Psychological Association Books.

Goodman, W. K., Price, L. H., Rasmussen, S. A., Mazure, C., Fleischmann, R. L., Hill, C. L., Heninger, G. R., & Charney, D. S. (1989). The Yale–Brown Obsessive Compulsive Scale: I. Development, use, and reliability. *Archives of General Psychiatry, 46,* 1006–1011.

Gordon, A. J., Maisto, S. A., McNeil, M., Kraemer, K. L., Conigliaro, R. L., Kelley, M. E., & Conigliaro, J. (2001). Three questions can detect hazardous drinkers. *Journal of Family Practice, 504,* 313–320.

Gorski, T. T., & Miller, M. (1982). *Counseling for relapse prevention.* Independence, MO: Herald House–Independence Press.

Greenfield, S. F., Hufford, M. R., Vagge, L. M., Muenz, L. R., Costello, M. E., & Weiss, R. D. (2000). The relationship of self-efficacy expectancies to relapse among alcohol dependent men and women: A prospective study. *Journal of Studies on Alcohol, 61,* 345–351.

Greist, J. H. (1998). Computer-based assessment of patients. *Journal of Clinical Psychopharmacology, 18,* 359–361.

Halstead, W. C. (1947). *Brain and Intelligence: A quantitative study of the frontal lobes.* Chicago: University of Chicago Press.

Harris, K. B., & Miller, W. R. (1990). Behavioral self-control training for problem drinkers: Components of efficacy. *Psychology of Addictive Behavior, 4,* 82–90.

Hasin, D., Trautman, K., & Endicott, J. (1998). Psychiatric Research Interview for Substance and Mental Disorders: Phenomenologically based diagnosis in patients who abuse alcohol or drugs. *Psychopharmacology Bulletin, 34,* 3–8.

Hasin, D. S., Trautman, K. D., Miele, G. M., Samet, S., Smith, M., & Endicott, J. (1996). Psychiatric Research Interview for Substance and Mental Disorders (PRISM): Reliability for substance abusers. *American Journal of Psychiatry, 153,* 1195–1201.

Hatch, R. L., Burg, M. A., Naberhaus, D. S., & Hellmich, L. K. (1998). The Spiritual Involvement and Beliefs Scale: Development and testing of a new instrument. *Journal of Family Practice, 46,* 476–486.

Hawkins, J. D., Catalano, R. F., & Wells, E. A. (1986). Measuring effects of a skills training intervention for drug abusers. *Journal of Consulting and Clinical Psychology, 54,* 661–664.

Heather, N., Luce, A., Peck, D., Dunbar, B., & James, I. (1999). The development of a treatment version of the Readiness to Change Questionnaire. *Addiction Research, 7,* 63–68.

Heather, N., Stallard, A., & Tebbutt, J. (1991). Importance of substance cues in relapse among heroin users: Comparison of two methods of investigation. *Addictive Behaviors, 16,* 41–49.

Heaton, R. K. (1981). *Wisconsin Card Sorting Test manual.* Odessa, FL: Psychological Assessment Resources.

Hesselbrock, M., Easton, C., Bucholz, K. K., Schuckit, M., & Hesselbrock, V. (1999). A validity study of the SSAGA-A comparison with the SCAN. *Addiction, 94,* 1361–1370.

Horn, J. L., Wanberg, K. W., & Foster, F. M. (1987). *Guide to the Alcohol Use Inventory.* Minneapolis: National Computer Systems.

Humphreys, K., Kaskutas, L. A., & Weisner, C. (1998). The Alcoholics Anonymous Affiliation Scale: Development, reliability, and norms for diverse treated and untreated populations. *Alcoholism: Clinical and Experimental Research, 22,* 974–978.

Institute of Medicine. (1990). *Broadening the base of treatment for alcohol problems.* Washington, DC: National Academy Press.

Isenhart, C. E. (1993). Psychometric evaluation of a short form of the Inventory of Drinking Situations. *Journal of Studies on Alcohol, 54,* 345–349.

Jones, B. T., & McMahon, J. (1994). Negative and positive alcohol expectancies and predictors of abstinence after discharge from a residential treatment program: A one-month and three-month follow-up study in men. *Journal of Studies on Alcohol, 55,* 543–548.

Jones, S. L., & Lanyon, R. I. (1981). Relationship between adaptive skills and outcome of alcoholism treatment. *Journal of Studies on Alcohol, 42,* 521–525.

Kaminer, Y., Blitz, C., Burleson, J. A., & Sussman, J. (1998). The Teen Treatment Services Review (T-TSR). *Journal of Substance Abuse Treatment, 15,* 291–300.

Kavanagh, D. J., Sitharthan, T., Spilsbury, G., & Vignaendra, S. (1999). An evaluation of brief correspondence programs for problem drinkers. *Behavior Therapy, 30,* 641–656.

Kessler, R. C., Crum, R. M., Warner, L. A., Nelson, C. B., Schulenberg, J., & Anthony, J. C. (1997). Lifetime co-occurrence of DSM-III-R alcohol abuse and dependence with other psychiatric disorders in the National Comorbidity Survey. *Archives of General Psychiatry, 54,* 313–321.

Kreitman, N. (1986). Alcohol consumption and the preventative paradox. *British Journal of Addiction, 81,* 353–363.

Kristenson, H., Ohlin, H., Hulten-Nosslin, M. B., Trell, E., & Hood, B. (1983). Identification and intervention of heavy drinking in middle-aged men: Results and follow-up of 24–60 months of long-term study with randomized controls. *Alcoholism: Clinical and Experimental Research, 7,* 203–209.

Lee, N. K., Oei, T. P. S., Greeley, J. D., & Baglioni, A. J., Jr. (2003). Psychometric properties of the drinking expectancy questionnaire: A review of the factor structure and a proposed new scoring method. *Journal of Studies on Alcohol, 64,* 432–436.

Litman, G. K. (1984). The relationship between coping behaviours, their effectiveness and alcoholism relapse and survival. *British Journal of Addiction, 79,* 283–291.

Litman, G. K., Stapleton, J., Oppenheim, A. N., & Peleg, M. (1983). An instrument for measuring coping behaviours in hospitalized alcoholics: Implications for relapse prevention treatment. *British Journal of Addictions, 78,* 269–276.

Litman, G. K., Stapleton, J., Oppenheim, A. N., Peleg, M., & Jackson, P. (1983). Situations related to alcoholism relapse. *British Journal of Addiction, 78,* 381–389.

Litt, M. D., & Cooney, N. L. (1999). Inducing craving for alcohol in the laboratory. *Alcohol Research and Health, 23,* 174–178.

Litt, M. D., Cooney, N. L., & Morse, P. (1998). Ecological momentary assessment (EMA) with treated alcoholics: Methodological problems and potential solutions. *Health Psychology, 17,* 48–52.

Litten, R. Z., Allen, J. P., & Fertig, J. B. (1995). Gamma-glutamyltranspeptidase and carbohydrate deficient transferrin: Alternative measures of excessive alcohol consumption. *Alcoholism: Clinical and Experimental Research, 19,* 1541–1546.

Mann, K., Guenther, A., Stetter, F., & Ackermann, K. (1999). Rapid recovery from cognitive deficits in abstinent alcoholics: A controlled test–retest study. *Alcohol and Alcoholism, 34,* 567–574.

Marlatt, G. A., & Gordon, J. R. (Eds.). (1985). *Relapse prevention: Maintenance strategies in the treatment of addictive behaviors.* New York: Guilford Press.

Mathew, R. J., Mathew, V. G., Wilson, W. H., & Georgi, J. M. (1995). Measurement of materialism and spiritualism in substance abuse research. *Journal of Studies on Alcohol, 56,* 470–475.

McCarthy, D. M., & Smith, G. T. (1996, June). *Meta-analysis of alcohol expectancy.* Paper presented at the annual meeting of the Research Society on Alcoholism, Washington, DC.

McKay, J. R., Alterman, A. I., McLellan, A. T., & Snider, E. C. (1994). Treatment goals, continuity of care, and outcome in a day hospital substance abuse rehabilitation program. *American Journal of Psychiatry, 151,* 254–259.

McLellan, A. T., Alterman, A. I., Cacciola, J., & Metzger, D. (1992). A new measure of substance abuse treatment: Initial studies of the Treatment Services Review. *Journal of Nervous and Mental Disease, 180,* 101–110.

McLellan, A. T., Kushner, H., Metzger, D., Peters, R., Smith, I., Grisson, G., Pettinati, H., & Argeriou, M. (1992). The fifth edition of the Addiction Severity Index. *Journal of Substance Abuse Treatment, 9,* 199–213.

McLellan, A. T., Luborsky, L., O'Brien, C. P., & Woody, G. E. (1980). An improved diagnostic evaluation instrument for substance abuse patients: The Addiction Severity Index. *Journal of Nervous and Mental Disease, 168,* 26–33.

Mee-Lee, D., Shulman, G. D., Fishman, M., Gastfriend, D. R., & Griffith, J. H. (Eds.). (2001). *ASAM Patient Placement Criteria for the treatment of substance-related disorders, second edition—Revised (ASAM PPC-2R).* Chevy Chase, MD: American Society of Addiction Medicine.

Meyers, K., McLellan, A. T., Jaeger, J. L., & Pettinati, H. M. (1995). The development of the comprehensive addiction severity index for adolescents (CASI-A): An interview for assessing multiple problems of adolescents. *Journal of Substance Abuse Treatment, 12,* 181–193.

Midanik, L. T. (1994). Comparing usual quantity/frequency and graduated frequency scales to assess yearly alcohol consumption: Results from the 1990 United States National Alcohol Survey. *Addiction, 89,* 407–412.

Miele, G. M., Carpenter, K. M., Cockerham, M. S., Trautman, K. D., Blaine, J., & Hasin, D. S. (2000). Substance Dependence Severity Scale (SDSS): Reliability and validity of a clinician-administered interview for DSM-IV substance use disorders. *Drug and Alcohol Dependence, 59,* 63–75.

Miller, E. T., Neal, D. J., Roberts, L. J., Baer, J. S., Cressler, S. O., Metrik, J., & Marlatt, G. A. (2002). Test–retest reliability of alcohol measures: Is there a difference between internet-based assessment and traditional methods? *Psychology of Addictive Behaviors, 16,* 56–63.

Miller, K. J., McCrady, B. S., Abrams, D. B., & Labouvie, E. W. (1994). Taking an individualized approach to the assessment of self-efficacy and the prediction of alcoholic relapse. *Journal of Psychopathology and Behavioral Assessment, 16,* 111–120.

Miller, W. R. (1996). *Form 90: A structured assessment interview for drinking and related behaviors* (NIAAA Project MATCH Monograph Series, Vol. 5, NIH Publication No. 96-4004). Rockville, MD: National Institute on Alcohol Abuse and Alcoholism.

Miller, W. R. (1998). Researching the spiritual dimensions of alcohol and other drug problems. *Addiction, 93,* 979–990.

Miller, W. R., & Del Boca, F. K. (1994). Measurement of drinking behavior using the Form 90 family of instruments. *Journal of Studies on Alcohol, 12*(Suppl.), 112–118.

Miller, W. R., & Harris, R. J. (2000). A simple scale of Gorski's warning signs for relapse. *Journal of Studies on Alcohol, 61,* 759–765.

Miller, W. R., & Marlatt, G. A. (1984). *Manual for the Comprehensive Drinker Profile*. Odessa, FL: Psychological Assessment Resources.

Miller, W. R., & Marlatt, G. A. (1987). *Comprehensive Drinker Profile manual supplement for use with Brief Drinker Profile, Followup Drinker Profile, Collateral Interview Form*. Odessa, FL: Psychological Assessment Resources.

Miller, W. R., & Rollnick, S. (2002). *Motivational interviewing: Preparing people for change* (2nd ed.). New York: Guilford Press.

Miller, W. R., & Tonigan, J. S. (1996). Assessing drinkers' motivations for change: The Stages of Change Readiness and Treatment Eagerness Scale (SOCRATES). *Psychology of Addictive Behaviors, 10,* 81–89.

Miller, W. R., Tonigan, J. S., & Longabaugh, R. (1995). *The Drinker Inventory of Consequences (DrInC): An instrument for assessing adverse consequences of alcohol abuse* (Project MATCH Monograph Series Vol. 4., NIH Publication No. 95-3911). Rockville, MD: National Institute on Alcohol Abuse and Alcoholism.

Miller, W. R., Sovereign, R. G., & Krege, B. (1989). Motivational interviewing with problem drinkers: II. The Drinkers Check-up as a preventive intervention. *Behavioral Psychotherapy, 16,* 251–268.

Miller, W. R., Westerberg, V. S., Harris, R. J., & Tonigan, J. S. (1996). What predicts relapse?: Prospective testing of antecedent models. *Addiction, 91*(Suppl.), S155–S171.

Miller, W. R., Zweben, A., DiClemente, C. C., & Richtarik, R. G. (1992). *Motivational enhancement therapy manual: A clinical research guide for therapists treating individuals with alcohol abuse and dependence* (Project MATCH Monograph Series Vol. 2., NIH Publication No. 94-3723). Rockville, MD: National Institute on Alcohol Abuse and Alcoholism.

Modell, J. G., Glaser, F. B., Mountz, J. M., Schmaltz, S., & Cyr, L. (1992). Obsessive and compulsive characteristics of alcohol abuse and dependence: Quantification by a newly developed questionnaire. *Alcoholism: Clinical and Experimental Research, 16,* 266–271.

Modesto-Lowe, V., & Kranzler, H. R. (1999). Diagnosis and treatment of alcohol-dependent patients with comorbid psychiatric disorders. *Alcohol Research and Health, 23,* 144–150.

Monti, P. M., Rohsenow, D. J., Abrams, D. B., Zwick, W. R., Binkoff, J. A., Munroe, S. M., et al. (1993). Development of a behavior analytically derived alcohol specific role play assessment instrument. *Journal of Studies on Alcohol, 54,* 710–721.

Moos, R. H. (1992). *Coping Response Inventory: Adult form manual*. Palo Alto, CA: Center for Health Care Evaluation, Stanford University and Department of Veterans Affairs Medical Centers.

Najavits, L. M., Gastfriend, D. R., Nakayama, E. Y., Barber, J. P., Blaine, J., Frank, A., Muenz, L. R., & Thase, M. (1997). A measure of readiness for substance abuse treatment: Psychometric properties of the RAATE-R interview. *American Journal on Addictions, 6,* 74–82.

National Institute on Alcohol Abuse and Alcoholism. (1995). *The physician's guide to helping patients with alcohol problems* (NIH Publication No. 95-3769). United States Public Health Service. Retrieved March 17th, 2005, from www. niaaa. nih. gov/publications/physicn. htm.

National Institute on Alcohol Abuse and Alcoholism. (2001). Craving research: Implications for treatment. *Alcohol Alert, 54,* 1–4.

Nixon, S. J. (1995). Assessing cognitive impairment. *Alcohol Health and Research World, 19,* 97–103.

Parsons, O. A. (1998). Neurocognitive deficits in alcoholics and social drinkers: A continuum? *Alcoholism: Clinical and Experimental Research, 22,* 954–961.

Potgieter, A. S., Deckers, F., & Geerlings, P. (1999). Craving and relapse measurement in alcoholism. *Alcohol and Alcoholism, 34,* 254–260.

Prochaska, J. O., & DiClemente, C. C. (1986). Toward a comprehensive model of change. In W. R. Miller & N. Heather (Eds.), *Treating addictive behaviors: Processes of change* (pp. 3–27). New York: Plenum Press.

Project MATCH Research Group. (1993). Project MATCH (Matching Alcoholism Treatment to Client Heterogeneity): Rationale and methods for a multisite clinical trial matching patients to alcoholism treatment. *Alcoholism: Clinical and Experimental Research, 17,* 1130–1145.

Project MATCH Research Group. (1997). Matching alcoholism treatments to client heterogeneity: Project MATCH posttreatment drinking outcomes. *Journal of Studies on Alcohol, 58,* 7–29.

Radloff, L. S. (1977). The CES-D scale: A self-report depression scale for research in the general population. *Applied Psychological Measurement, 1,* 385–401.

Rehm, J., Greenfield, T. K., Walsh, G., Xie, X., Robson, L., & Single, E. (1999). Assessment methods for alcohol consumption, prevalence of high risk drinking and harm: A sensitivity analysis. *International Journal of Epidemiology, 28,* 219–224.

Reoux, J. P., & Miller, K. (2000). Routine hospital alcohol detoxification practice compared to symptom triggered management with an objective withdrawal scale (CIWA-Ar). *American Journal on Addictions, 9,* 135–144.

Robins, L. N., Cottler, L. B., & Babor, T. (1995). *CIDI substance abuse module.* St. Louis, MO: Washington University School of Medicine.

Robins, L. N., Cottler, L. B., Bucholz, K. K., Compton, W. M., North, C. S., & Rourke, K. M. (2000). *Diagnostic Interview Schedule for the DSM-IV (DIS-IV).* St Louis, MO: Washington University School of Medicine.

Rohsenow, D. J. (1983). Drinking habits and expectancies about alcohol's effect for self versus others. *Journal of Consulting and Clinical Psychology, 51,* 752–756.

Rohsenow, D. J., Monti, P. M., Rubonis, A. V., Sirota, A. D., Nuaura, R. S., Colby, S. M., Wunschel, S. M., & Abrams, D. B. (1994). Cue reactivity as a predictor of drinking among male alcoholics. *Journal of Consulting and Clinical Psychology, 62,* 620–626.

Rollnick, S., Heather, N., Gold, R., & Hall, W. (1992). Development of a short "Readiness to Change Questionnaire" for use in brief, opportunistic interventions among excessive drinkers. *British Journal of Addiction, 87,* 743–754.

Room, R. (1990). Measuring alcohol consumption in the United States: Methods and rationales. In L. T. Kozlowski, H. M. Annis, H. D. Cappell, F. B. Glaser, M. S. Goodstadt, Y. Israel, H. Kalant, E. M. Sellers, & E. R. Vingilis (Eds.), *Research advances in alcohol and drug problems* (Vol. 10, pp. 39–80). New York: Plenum Press.

Room, R. (2000). Measuring drinking patterns: The experience of the last half century. *Journal of Substance Abuse, 12,* 23–31.

Rosen, C. S., Henson, B. R., Finney, J. W., & Moos, R. H. (2000). Consistency of self-administered and interview-based Addiction Severity Index composite scores. *Addiction, 95,* 419–425.

Rosenberg, H. (1993). Prediction of controlled drinking by alcoholics and problem drinkers. *Psychological Bulletin, 113,* 129–139.

Ross, H. E., Swinson, R., Larkin, E. J., & Doumani, S. (1994). Diagnosing co-morbidity in substance abusers: Computer assessment and clinical validation. *Journal of Nervous and Mental Disease, 182,* 556–563.

Russell, M. (1994). New assessment tools for drinking in pregnancy: T-ACE, TWEAK, and others. *Alcohol Health and Research World, 18,* 55–61.

Russell, M., Marshall, J. R., Trevisan, M., Freudenheim, J. L., Chan, A. W., Markovic, N., Vana, J. E., & Priore, R. L. (1997). Test–retest reliability of the Cognitive Lifetime Drinking History. *American Journal of Epidemiology, 146,* 975–981.

Safer, M. A. (1986). A comparison of screening for disease detection and screening for risk factors. *Health Education Research: Theory and Practice, 1,* 131–138.

Saunders, J. B., Aasland, O. G., Babor, T. F., de la Fuente, J. R., & Grant, M. (1993). Development of the alcohol use disorders identification test (AUDIT): WHO col-laborative project on early detection of persons with harmful alcohol consump-tion-II. *Addiction, 88,* 791–804.

Sayette, M. A., Shiffman, S., Tiffany, S. T., Niaura, R. S., Martin, C. S., & Shadel, W. G. (2000). The measurement of drug craving. *Addiction, 95*(Suppl.), 189–210.

Schonfeld, L., Peters, R., & Dolente, A. (1993). *SARA: Substance Abuse Relapse As-sessment: Professional manual.* Odessa, FL: Psychological Assessment Resources.

Searles, J. S., Helzer, J. E., & Walter, D. E. (2000). Comparison of drinking patterns measured by daily reports and timeline followback. *Psychology of Addictive Be-haviors, 14,* 277–286.

Searles, J. S., Perrine, M. W., Mundt, J. C., & Helzer, J. E. (1995). Self-report of drink-ing using touch-tone telephone: Extending the limits of reliable daily contact. *Journal of Studies on Alcohol, 56,* 375–382.

Shaffer, D., Fisher, P., Lucas, C. P., Dulcan, M. K., & Schwab-Stone, M. E. (2000). NIMH Diagnostic Interview Schedule for Children Version IV (NIMH DISC-IV): Description, differences from previous versions, and reliability of some common diagnoses. *Journal of the American Academy of Child and Adolescent Psychiatry, 39,* 28–38.

Shiffman, S., & Stone, A. A. (1998). Introduction to the special section: Ecological mo-mentary assessment in health psychology. *Health Psychology, 17,* 3–5.

Singleton, E. G. (1996). Alcohol Craving Questionnaire (ACQ-NOW) [Abstract]. *Al-cohol and Alcoholism, 32,* 344.

Singleton, E. G., & Gorelick, D. A. (1998). Mechanisms of alcohol craving and their clinical implications. In M. Galanter (Ed.), *Recent developments in alcoholism: Volume 14. The consequences of alcoholism* (pp. 177–195). New York: Plenum Press.

Sinha, R., & O'Malley, S. S. (1999). Craving for alcohol: Findings from the clinic and the laboratory. *Alcohol and Alcoholism, 34,* 223–230.

Skinner, H. A., & Allen, B. A. (1982). Alcohol dependence syndrome: Measurement and validation. *Journal of Abnormal Psychology, 91,* 199–209.

Skinner, H. A., & Horn, J. L. (1984). *Alcohol Dependence Scale (ADS) users guide.* Toronto: Addiction Research Foundation.

Skinner, H. A., & Sheu, W. J. (1982). Reliability of alcohol use indices: The Lifetime Drinking History and the MAST. *Journal of Studies on Alcohol, 43,* 1157–1170.

Sobell, L. C., & Sobell, M. B. (1992). Timeline Follow-back: A technique for assessing self-reported alcohol consumption. In R. Z. Litten & J. Allen (Eds.), *Measuring alcohol consumption: Psychosocial and biological methods* (pp. 41–72). Towota, NJ: Humana Press.

Sobell, L. C., & Sobell, M. B. (1996). *Timeline Followback (TLFB) for alcohol (Version 4. 0b)* (computer software). Toronto: Addiction Research Foundation.

Sobell, L. C., & Sobell, M. B. (2000). Alcohol Timeline Followback (TLFB). In American Psychiatric Association (Ed.), *Handbook of psychiatric measures* (pp. 477–479). Washington, DC: American Psychiatric Association.

Sobell, L. C., & Sobell, M. B. (2003). Alcohol consumption measures. In J. P. Allen & V. Wilson (Eds.), *Assessing alcohol problems: A guide for clinicians and researchers* (rev. ed.). Rockville, MD: U.S. Department of Health and Human Services, National Institute on Alcohol Abuse and Alcoholism.

Sobell, M. B., Bogardis, J., Schuller, R., Leo, G. I., & Sobell, L. C. (1989). Is self-monitoring of alcohol consumption reactive? *Behavioral Assessment, 11,* 447–458.

Soderstrom, C. A., & Cowley, R. A. (1987). A National Alcohol and Trauma Center survey. *Archives of Surgery, 122,* 1067–1071.

Solomon, K. E., & Annis, H. M. (1990). Outcome and efficacy expectancy in the prediction of post-treatment drinking behaviour. *British Journal of Addiction, 85,* 659–665.

Spielberger, C., Gorsuch, R., Lushene, R., Vagg, P., & Jacobs, G. (1983). *Manual for the State–Trait Anxiety Inventory.* Palo Alto, CA: Consulting Psychologists Press.

Staines, G., Kosanke, N., Magura, S., Bali, P., Foote, J., & Deluca, A. (2003). Convergent validity of the ASAM Patient Placement Criteria using a standardized computer algorithm. *Journal of Addictive Diseases, 22,* 61–77.

Stockwell, T., Murphy, D., & Hodgson, R. (1983). The Severity Alcohol Dependence Questionnaire. *British Journal of Addiction, 78,* 145–156.

Sullivan, J. T., Sykora, K., Schneiderman, J., Naranjo, C. A., & Sellers, E. M. (1989). Assessment of alcohol withdrawal: The revised Clinical Institute Withdrawal Assessment for Alcohol scale (CIWA-Ar). *British Journal of Addiction, 84,* 1353–1357.

Tiffany, S. T., Singleton, E., Haertzen, C. A., & Henningfield, J. E. (1993). The development of a cocaine craving questionnaire. *Drug and Alcohol Dependence, 34,* 19–28.

Tonigan, J. S., Miller, W. R., & Connors, G. J. (1996). Alcoholics Anonymous Involvement (AAI) scale: Reliability and norms. *Psychology of Addictive Behaviors, 10,* 75–80.

Tonigan, J. S., Miller, W. R., & Connors, G. J. (2001). The search for meaning in life as a predictor of alcoholism treatment outcome. In R. H. Longabaugh & P. W. Wirtz (Eds.), *Project MATCH hypotheses: Results and causal chain analyses* (NIAAA Project MATCH Monograph Series, Vol. 8, pp. 154–165, NIH Publication No. 01-4238). Rockville, MD: National Institute on Alcohol Abuse and Alcoholism.

Turner, W. M., Turner, K. H., Reif, S., Gutowski, W. E., & Gastfriend, D. R. (1999). Feasibility of multidimensional substance abuse treatment matching: Automating the ASAM Patient Placement Criteria. *Drug and Alcohol Dependence, 55,* 35–43.

U.S. Department of Health and Human Services. (2000). *10th Special Report to Congress on Alcohol and Health.* Rockville, MD: Author.

Ustun, B., Compton, W., Mager, D., Babor, T., Baiyewu, O., Chatterji, S., et al. (1997). WHO study on the reliability and validity of the alcohol and drug use disorder instruments: Overview of methods and results. *Drug and Alcohol Dependence, 47,* 161–169.

Wechsler, D. (1981). *WAIS-R manual.* New York: Harcourt Brace Jovanovich.

Wechsler, D. (1987). *Wechsler Memory Scale—Revised.* New York: Psychological Corporation.

Wetterling, T., Kanitz, R. D., Bestiers, B., Fischer, D., Zerfass, B., John, U., Spranger, H., & Driessen, M. (1997). A new rating scale for the assessment of the alcohol-withdrawal syndrome (AWS scale). *Alcohol and Alcoholism, 32,* 753–760.

White, H. R., & Labouvie, E. W. (1989). Toward the assessment of adolescent problem drinking. *Journal of Studies on Alcohol, 50,* 30–37.

Williams, R., & Vinson, R. C. (2001). Validation of a single screening question for problem drinking. *Journal of Family Practice, 50,* 307–312.

Wing, J. K., Babor, T., Brugha, T., Burke, J., Cooper, J. E., Giel, R., Jablenski, A., Regier, D., & Sartorius, N. (1990). SCAN, Schedule for Clinical Assessment in Neuropsychiatry. *Archives of General Psychiatry, 47,* 589–593.

Winters, K. C. (1996). *Personal Experience Inventory—Adults user's manual.* Los Angeles: Western Psychological Services.

Winters, K. C. (1999). A new multiscale measure of adult substance abuse. *Journal of Substance Abuse Treatment, 16,* 237–246.

Winters, K. C., & Henly, G. A. (1989). *Personal Experience Inventory.* Los Angeles: Western Psychological Services.

Winzelberg, A., & Humphreys, K. (1999). Should patients' religiosity influence clinicians' referral to 12–step self-help groups?: Evidence from a study of 3,018 male substance abuse patients. *Journal of Consulting and Clinical Psychology, 67,* 790–794.

Woody, G. E., & Cacciola, J. (1994). Severity of dependence. In T. A. Widger, A. J. Frances, H. A. Pincus, R. Ross, M. B. First, & W. W. Davis (Eds.), *DSM-IV sourcebook* (Vol. 1, pp. 81–92). Washington, DC: American Psychiatric Association Press.

World Health Organization. (1992). *The ICD-10 classification of mental and behavioural disorders: Clinical descriptions and diagnostic guidelines.* Geneva: Author.

Young, R. M., & Knight, R. G. (1989). The Drinking Expectancy Questionnaire: A revised measure of alcohol related beliefs. *Journal of Psychopathology and Behavioral Assessment, 11,* 99–112.

Young, R. M., Oei, T. P. S., & Crook, C. M. (1991). Development of a drinking self-efficacy scale. *Journal of Psychopathology and Behavioral Assessment, 13,* 1–15.

Zachary, R. A. (1986). *Shipley Institute of Living Scale: Revised manual.* Los Angeles: Western Psychological Services.

Zweben, A., & Cisler, R. (1996). Composite outcome measures in alcoholism treatment research: Problems and potentialities. *Substance Use and Misuse, 31,* 1783–1805.

Zywiak, W. H., Connors, G. J., Maisto, S. A., & Westerberg, V. S. (1996). Relapse research and the Reasons for Drinking Questionnaire: A factor analysis of Marlatt's relapse taxonomy. *Addiction, 91*(Suppl.), 121–130.

CHAPTER 4

Assessment of Smoking Behavior

WILLIAM G. SHADEL
SAUL SHIFFMAN

THE PURPOSE OF ASSESSMENT IN SMOKING

Cigarette smoking contributes to half a million deaths annually in the United States (U.S. Department of Health and Human Services, 1989), and quitting clearly reduces the mortality associated with smoking (National Cancer Institute, 1997). Any level of formal smoking cessation treatment may confer some incremental benefit on a given smokers' ability to quit (Fiore et al., 2000). Brief (less than 3 minutes) advice to quit delivered in an office setting by a primary care provider yields 1-year quit rates of nearly 10%; increasing numbers of treatment sessions and time spent in those sessions increases smokers' odds of quitting in a dose–response fashion; and multisession, multicomponent cognitive-behavioral cessation interventions with a pharmacological adjunct— the most intensive and efficacious interventions currently available—yield relatively high long-term quit rates (about 35%).

These abstinence rates, while very encouraging on the one hand, very clearly indicate that the vast majority of smokers relapse or fail in their efforts to quit, even with the best programs. Indeed, as with most addictive behaviors, relapse is the most common outcome of any given cessation attempt (Piasecki, Fiore, McCarthy, & Baker, 2002). One context for understanding these findings is that individual smokers or groups of smokers can vary in their responses to the same smoking treatment, in their overt smoking behavior, and/or in key psychological (e.g., self-efficacy) and behavioral parameters (e.g., coping) associated with successful smoking cessation (Abrams et al., 1996; Shadel & Mermelstein, 1996; Shadel, Niaura, & Abrams., 2000; Shadel, Cervone, Niauria, & Abrams, 2004). Because of these differences, the same standardized treatments would not be expected to work uniformly well with all smokers. As such, it would seem to be important for assessment to measure *individual differences* that are important to smoking, smoking cessation, and relapse (Abrams et al., 2003; Fiore et al., 2000; Shadel & Mermelstein, 1996; Shadel et al., 2000, 2004; Shiffman, 1993b; see also Shadel, 2004). Once key individual differences are assessed and identified, smokers could—in theory—be assigned to specific treatments that are matched to those individual difference characteristics, under the assumption that matching ultimately will improve treatment outcome (Abrams, Borrelli, Shadel, King, Bock, & Niaura, 1998; Kassel & Yates, 2002; Shadel et al., 2004; Shiffman, 1993b).

Our goal in this chapter is to review types and methods of assessments that we feel should probably take center stage when researching and treating smokers. Certainly, myriad assessments are used in both research and clinical contexts with smokers, and it would be a nearly impossible task within the bounds of this chapter to cover in detail every single assessment that has been developed in this domain. Indeed, we periodically direct the reader to other resources for more in-depth coverage of topics and assessments that are clearly beyond the scope of this chapter. Our specific aims, then, are to cover the most widely researched and traditional topics and strategies for assessment, and also to introduce several exciting recent developments in the assessment of smoking behavior (i.e., those that may have significant potential for identifying individual differences that are relevant for treatment planning and intervention design). In doing so, we provide guidance as to when (in preparing for cessation or in relapse prevention training after cessation) particular assessments are potentially most useful (recognizing, though, given the state of the science, that most assessments can probably be given at any time). Finally, we provide, in tables throughout the chapter, key examples of several of the assessments we discuss; in cases in which more than one established assessment exists in a given domain, we offer, wherever possible, data-driven pros and cons to using each assessment device and leave choice of assessment to the reader's discretion.

DOES ASSESSMENT MATTER?

Although the idea that treatment should be guided by individual assessment is a core tenet of treatment planning, particularly of cognitive-behavioral treatment, we must admit at the outset to some skepticism that this kind of matching paradigm itself has much value with smokers at present. While many of the assessments we discuss have some degree of demonstrated validity, their ability to improve treatment outcomes has typically not been demonstrated (Fiore et al., 2000; Kassel & Yates, 2002; Niaura & Abrams, 2002; Shiffman, 1993b), primarily because the field *lacks* different treatment options that can be administered to individuals who differ on some validly assessed dimension.

Assessment by treatment interactions—that is, finding that one treatment works best for one group of smokers, while another works best for a different group of smokers—has almost never been demonstrated (cf. Niaura, Goldstein, & Abrams, 1994). In addition, and as we emphasized earlier in this chapter, treatment efficacy is overall quite limited. As such, at present, it seldom makes sense to administer a particular intervention only to those whose assessment results indicate that they "need" it. In fact, current consensus recommendations (Fiore et al., 2000) are to treat every smoker with some form of both cognitive-behavioral intervention pharmacotherapy: All smokers should be offered evidence-based treatments, regardless of what the results of assessment show.

In the absence of more convincing and better supported models of assessment guiding treatment, our view is that clinicians need to soldier on using primarily theory and conceptual rationale to integrate assessment with treatment. The current state of affairs cries out for more empirical work that meaningfully links assessment to treatment. We hope that this review will stimulate additional clinical research that more fully integrates assessment with treatment.

INITIAL ASSESSMENTS

Demographics

Demographics and cultural variables should be assessed. Age, gender, ethnicity, education, and income all have been associated with cessation success (Centers for Disease Control and Prevention, 1994; Ockene et al., 2000). Smokers of minority and low socioeconomic status may be particularly vulnerable to unsuccessful quit attempts (King, Borrelli, Black, Pinto, & Marcus, 1997). This information is also important, for example, because providers of smoking cessation services must be culturally sensitive, and intervention materials should be written in the appropriate languages and at the appropriate education level (King et al., 1997).

Smoking and Quitting History

Certain historical variables are relevant to treatment outcome. For example, early initiation of smoking predicts cessation failure (Pomerleau, Adkins, & Pertschuk, 1978) and may indicate a later higher level of nicotine dependence (Lando, Haddock, Robinson, Klesges, & Talcott, 2000). Assessment of the timing and length of past smoking quit attempts (Figure 4.1) is important: The longest past quit attempt and length of most recent quit attempt have been shown to predict cessation success (Farkas et al., 1996). The critical time period seems to be a longest lifetime past quit attempt of a year or more and length of most recent quit of over 5 days (Farkas et al., 1996). The total number of past quit attempts does not seem to be as important for predicting later

1. How old were you when you had your first cigarette?_____

2. How many years have you been smoking every day?   _____

3. How long ago was your most recent attempt (greater than 12 hours) to quit smoking (date)?

    __/__/__

    3a. How long were you able to quit for during this most recent attempt? ____ days

4. In the past year, how many times have you quit smoking for at least 24 hours?

    ____ times   0   *If never quit, circle "0"*

5. How many times in the past year have you made what you would consider a "serious" attempt to quit smoking?

    ____ times   0   *If never quit, circle "0"*

6. How many times in your life have you quit smoking for at least 24 hours?

    ____ times   0   *If never quit, circle "0"*

7. How many times in your life have you made what you would consider a "serious" attempt to quit smoking?

    ____ times   0   *If never quit, circle "0"*

FIGURE 4.1. Smoking and quitting history.

cessation success (Cohen et al., 1989). Though its value has not been supported empirically, from a clinical standpoint, it may useful to ask about prior treatment approaches that the smoker may have tried (and presumably failed with) and what treatment components from these past attempts the smoker found to be especially helpful (or not). Review of past treatment efforts may also uncover problems with treatment compliance (e.g., trouble with adhering to self-monitoring), and suggest the need, in treatment, to boost commitment and compliance.

Amount of Smoking and Nature of Smoking Habit

Some of the most critical areas that need to be assessed initially have to do with the amount of smoking (or daily smoking rate), where smoking occurs and does not occur, and what situations or contexts seem to trigger smoking. Smoking rate is important to assess, because the amount smoked can be a crude index of nicotine dependence (Radzius, Moolchan, Henningfield, Heishman, & Gallo, 2001) and can predict smoking cessation outcomes (Farkas et al., 1996). Tracking daily smoking rate prior to, during, and (if not successful) after a cessation attempt can be a useful index of progress and compliance with treatment recommendations.

Cigarette smoking may occur in response to specific triggers. Exposure to various smoking triggers can lead to increased physiological (e.g., heart rate), cognitive–affective (e.g., mood, expectancies for use), and craving responses in smokers (Abrams et al., 1988; Niaura et al., 1998), and these responses may predict smoking lapse and/or relapse (Abrams et al., 1987, 1988). Thus, knowing about factors related to smoking serves to establish baseline data and to increase knowledge about the factors that trigger and maintain the smoking habit. Those triggers can become the targets for cognitive-behavioral self-management and relapse prevention training.

Several formats and methods are available to assess both smoking rate and smoking patterns, and each has implications for the validity of those assessments. As such, we discuss each variable that can be assessed and the implications for each assessment method in turn.

Global Self-Report

SMOKING RATE

One of the most common, face valid (but see below), and easiest ways to measure smoking rate or amount of smoking is via a self-report assessment that requires smokers to reflect on their smoking behavior. Typical questions assess the number of cigarettes smoked per day in a given interval (i.e., "How many cigarettes per day have you smoked in the last 7 days?"; see Ossip-Klein et al., 1986), and the results of such assessments have been used as the "gold standard" outcome in many controlled smoking cessation studies (Hughes et al., 2003; Ockene et al., 2000).

Smoking researchers have also used timeline followback methods for assessing smoking rates and patterns over longer periods of time (Brandon, Copeland, & Saper, 1995; Brown et al., 1998; Shiffman, Paty, Kassel, Gnys, & Zettler-Segal, 1994). This procedure requires trained interviewers to record, in detail, daily smoking rates and/or other variables (e.g., craving, mood, other substance use), by providing smokers with calendars and specifically prompting them with key dates and events that occurred during the assessment interval (e.g., a holiday or a birthday). This procedure has demonstrated both test-retest reliability and validity with collateral reports of smoking behavior and biochemical measures (Brown et al., 1998).

SMOKING PATTERNS

One method of measuring smoking patterns is to assess reasons for smoking. The most commonly cited motive is stress reduction (see Kassel, Stroud, & Paronis, 2003), but other motives include facilitation of social encounters, the perceived stimulant or sedative properties of nicotine, addiction, habit, and the sensorimotor aspects of smoking. These smoking "motives" are thought to be important for understanding the etiology of nicotine dependence and maintenance of smoking (McKennel, 1970). Assessment of a given patient's smoking motives is seen as potentially important for identifying potential high-risk situations for relapse. For example, if a patient clearly attributes his or her smoking to social facilitations motives, then times of social contact and interaction following cessation may prove to be of an especially high risk. There are numerous smoking motive (e.g., Ikard, Green, & Horn, 1969; McKennel, 1970) questionnaires available to the clinician who seeks to assess such constructs, most of which are relatively short and easy to administer and score. However, considerable evidence suggests that these scales are not valid as measures of actual smoking patterns, and may be especially influenced by smokers' prevailing levels of nicotine dependence (Shiffman, 1993a).

Self-Monitoring Diaries

Self-monitoring, or recording (most typically via paper-and-pencil methods) number of cigarettes smoked, situations under which the cigarette was smoked, and consequences of smoking seemingly confer an added benefit over retrospective daily logs of smoking in that self-monitoring is (or should be) completed concurrently with the actual smoking event (see Figure 4.2). Self-monitoring also may confer some incremental treatment benefit, in that it has been shown to reduce the total number of cigarettes smoked per day (Abrams & Wilson, 1979). Self-monitoring with smokers typically involves attaching a preprinted card or sheet to the cigarette pack (e.g., "wrap sheets"), which is then (in concept, at least) completed with a pen or pencil prior to or concur-

Name: _____

Day of week: _____   Date: _____

Cigarette #	Time of day	A.M. or P.M.?	**Craving** 1 = None 10 = A lot	**Mood** 1 = Very sad 10 = Very happy	**Activity** (describe)	**Need rating** 1 = Least 10 = Most
1	:					
2	:					
3	:					
4	:					
5	:					
6	:					
7	:					
8	:					
9	:					
10	:					

FIGURE 4.2. Sample "wrap-sheet" to assess smoking patterns.

rent with a smoking episode. Variables assessed during self-monitoring can include time of day each cigarette is smoked, the situation or context in which the cigarette is smoked, and mood and craving prior to smoking. The situational notations are often interpreted to reveal the environmental and emotional influences that trigger smoking (or at least that the smoker perceives as related to his or her smoking), as well as provide a tally of the number of cigarettes that are smoked during particular intervals of interest (i.e., daily, weekly).

Despite the fact that self-monitoring is a cornerstone of the majority of cognitive-behavioral treatment approaches, it has limitations as an assessment method per se. Perhaps foremost, monitoring of smoking contexts does not in itself reveal what contexts are associated with smoking, because the self-monitoring data are heavily influenced by base rates (Paty, Kassell, & Shiffman, 1992). Thus, a smoker who reports being depressed on most smoking occasions may simply be depressed much of the time, whether smoking or not (see Shiffman et al., 2002). Another conceptual problem is that the linkage between situations where ad lib smoking occurs at baseline and situations that promote relapse, even though conceptually and clinically compelling, has not been established. Finally, a significant practical problem is that written diaries are often filled out en masse after the fact or immediately prior to a meeting with a clinician (Stone & Shiffman, 2002), negating the rationale for field monitoring as a more accurate representation of behavior *in vivo*.

Ecological Momentary Assessment

Researchers have increasingly recognized the limits of global self-reports and even self-monitoring for analyses of behavioral processes. An additional major flaw of most self-reports is their almost total reliance on retrospective recall. In addition to simple forgetting, such recall is subject to a host of cognitive biases that are built into the process of autobiographical memory. Research on autobiographical memory suggests that long-term recall of events often amounts to a narrative reconstruction of events (Hammersley, 1994), which is influenced by the need to make the narrative coherent and to provide what appears to be an adequate explanation for the event. For example, respondents tend to "recall" things in a way that is consistent with their own theories of human behavior (Ross, 1989), or that explains or justifies their behavior (see Brown, 1978). Such retrospective reconstructions are particularly likely to be biased when intervening events have modified the meaning of the initial event (e.g., subjects who are currently ill are more likely to recall stress). With respect to smoking, Shiffman and colleagues (1997) demonstrated that retrospective recall of past events (in this case, a smoking relapse episode) was both inaccurate and biased: The correlation of recall with real-time data was only .30. These biases are not deliberate distortions, but are inherent in the normal operation of autobiographical memory (Hammersley, 1994). This finding suggests that both researchers and clinicians should exercise considerable skepticism in interpreting such self-reports, even when they are the only data practically available.

Concerns about retrospective report have caused researchers in many areas to adopt what has been labeled the ecological momentary assessment (EMA; Stone & Shiffman, 1994) approach, which involves collecting data in real time about momentary events as they occur in the subject's natural environment. This is particularly important when one is interested in studying how subjects react to environmental stimuli, which are often difficult to model adequately in the laboratory, or when one is interested in dynamic or transient phenomena, such as the situational contexts that may provoke craving, smoking, lapse, or relapse. Momentary measures are particularly important when the phenomena of interest are subject to rapid change. Studying fleeting effects such as these requires real-time data collection. Using the computerized methods described below, Shiffman, Paty, et al. (1996; Shiffman et al., 1997) have demonstrated the ability of these methods to capture momentary emotional responses to small-scale daily events. They found that real-time diary data could discriminate the mood and activity correlates of quite minor daily events, such as having a nice dinner with friends or being in a traffic jam. Thus, real-time EMA monitoring is ideally suited to studying processes that may be affected by transient mood swings.

To facilitate collection of valid EMA data, Shiffman, Paty, et al. (1996; Shiffman et al., 1997) developed a method for using small, palm-top computers to collect data from subjects in the field. The electronic diary (ED) functions both to prompt subjects for data (e.g., beeping them at random to collect self-report data) and to arrange for collection of clean data. The computer presents questions and response alternatives on-screen, and accepts the user's response. It prevents entry of formally invalid responses (one cannot respond "6" on a 1–5 response scale), prevents missing data (items cannot be skipped), handles all skip patterns (i.e., making presentation of some items contingent on responses to others), and does online data-quality checks (i.e., rejecting logically inconsistent responses or clearly flawed response patterns). Thus, the computer not only ensures that data are entered in real time but also can enhance the quality of the data themselves.

The use of palm-top computers to collect real-time data in real-world environments also provides an opportunity to truly study the linkages between smoking end environmental contexts. One design (see Shiffman et al., 2002) uses palm-top-based self-monitoring of smoking situations (i.e., the smoker notifies the computer when he or she is about to smoke, and is administered an assessment of mood, craving, etc.), supplemented by also assessing randomly selected nonsmoking situations, which serve as a comparison. The approach logically resembles a case–control design in epidemiology, where characteristics of cases (smoking episodes) are compared to those of controls (nonsmoking situations). Analyses of such data have yielded surprising conclusions: For example, there appears to be little association, on average, between mood and ad lib smoking (Shiffman et al., 2002). However, this finding about average associations does not preclude the possibility that there are meaningful individual differences that may prove useful for guiding treatment. Similar EMA approaches have been used to assess lapse episodes (Shiffman, Paty, et al., 1996; O'Connell et al., 1998) and progression to relapse (Shiffman, Hickcox, et al., 1996).

Palm-top, computer-based EMA methods are just beginning to be applied to research studies of smoking and cessation (Shiffman, Paty, et al., 1996; O'Connell et al., 1998; Jamner, Shapiro, & Jarvik, 1999; Cooney, Litt, & Cooney, 2002). As the technology and methodology matures, EMA methods have the potential to become mainstays of clinical assessment as well, and may provide new and useful insights to guide treatment. As of this writing, however, those applications are not well developed or well supported.

Biochemical Measures

Biological and biochemical indices, such as expired air carbon monoxide (CO) and cotinine, can be used to measure strength of smoking habit and/or to serve as an index of level of nicotine in the smoker's body. These more objective measures can serve two related purposes. First, the measures can be used to verify self-reports. Abstinence self-reports, especially reports of abstinence in clinical trials, are subject to distortions or outright fabrications by smokers (Velicer, Prochaska, Rossi, & Snow, 1992). Having the ability to objectively verify whether smokers' self-reports are truthful is of substantial value on both clinical and research grounds. Second, biochemical indices can be used as a quantitative assessment of amount of smoking and, as such, be utilized to provide feedback to smokers about their progress in reducing their smoking. Clinically, smokers may come to rely on reductions in weekly CO levels as "evidence" that they are making progress in the face of potentially substantial difficulties with quitting. For this reason, such biochemical feedback has been used in clinical trials as part of interventions (e.g., Risser & Belcher, 1990).

CO is a very approximate index of recent smoking and/or exposure to cigarette smoke (Kozlowski & Herling, 1988). It is modestly associated with actual levels of nicotine in the blood (Kozlowski & Herling, 1988) and self-report measures of nicotine dependence (Fagerstrom & Schneider, 1989). Measuring CO levels requires the use of automated equipment (e.g., over $1,200 for some units) and is only accurate up to about 12 hours (Kozlowski & Herling, 1988). CO is cleared from the body overnight and rises through the smoking day, so measures must be obtained in the afternoon, if they are to indicate overall exposure. CO is particularly sensitive to recent smoking, so the interval since the last cigarette should ideally be controlled.

Plasma or blood levels of nicotine, and the active nicotinic metabolite cotinine, are more stable indices of recent tobacco smoking and may be obtained trough the peripheral veins of the arms (Kozlowski & Herling, 1988), and cotinine may be obtained via analysis of saliva samples. Cotinine is a far better indicator of nicotine intake, because its long half-life results in an integrated assessment of exposure, whereas nicotine varies depending on recent smoking. However, it is expensive to obtain the proper assays of nicotine and cotinine (up to $50 per assay).

On balance, then, the choice to utilize a biochemical index requires one to weigh the real (dollar) costs involved (i.e., purchasing and maintaining equipment, assay analysis) with the stated use of those indices (verification of abstinence in clinical settings vs. clinical feedback on progress).

Nicotine Dependence

Nicotine is an addicting or dependence-producing drug (Shadel et al., 2000). Formally, dependence can be diagnosed by DSM-IV (American Psychiatric Association, 1994) if the smoker exhibits three or more of the following symptoms and/or behaviors: tolerance, withdrawal upon cessation, smoking in greater amounts over time to achieve the same effect, unsuccessful efforts to quit despite a desire to do so, a great deal of time spent on activities to procure cigarettes, giving up important life activities as a result of smoking, and continuing to smoke despite knowledge of adverse consequences. However, diagnosing nicotine dependence according to DSM-IV criteria is often not particularly helpful in a clinical sense, because most smokers can be diagnosed as nicotine-dependent (Breslau, Kilbey, & Andreski, 1994), especially among smokers seeking treatment. This limits the utility of DSM-IV diagnoses in treatment and motivates the search for alternative assessments of dependence that can be utilized in clinical contexts.

There is a consensus that individuals differ in *degree* of dependence, with a continuum of dependence from mild to severe (Shiffman, 1991). Although a precise assessment of nicotine dependence is still being refined (Fagerstrom & Schneider, 1989; Shadel et al., 2000; Shiffman, 2004; Etter, Le-Houezec, & Perneger, 2003), several scales have been developed to measure degree of nicotine dependence. The Fagerstrom Tolerance Questionnaire (FTQ; Fagerstrom, 1978) emerged as one of earliest assessments. The FTQ is a brief (8-item) questionnaire to which the smoker can respond about their smoking habit, and the resulting score serves as an index of degree of dependence. FTQ scores taken at the beginning of treatment have been shown in numerous studies to predict treatment outcome (Fagerstrom & Schneider, 1989) and recent studies have suggested that high scorers on the FTQ are more likely than low scorers to benefit from nicotine replacement therapy (Fagerstrom & Schneider, 1989; Niaura et al., 1994) (although even low-dependent smokers have been shown to benefit). A more psychometrically sound revision of the FTQ, the Fagerstrom Test for Nicotine Dependence (FTND; Heatherton, Kozlowski, Frecker, & Fagerstrom, 1991) has demonstrated good reliability and validity (Figure 4.3). If the time constraints preclude administration of the FTQ and

1. How soon after waking do you smoke your first cigarette? 0. After 60 minutes
    1. 31–60 minutes
    2. 6–30 minutes
    3. Within 5 minutes

2. Do you find it difficult to refrain from smoking in places where it is forbidden (e.g., in a church, at the library, at the movies, etc.)?

    Yes (1)   No (0)

3. Which cigarette would you hate to give up most?

    The first one in the morning (1)
    Any other (0)

4. How many cigarettes per day do you smoke? 0. 10 or less
    1. 11–20
    2. 21–30
    3. 31 or more

5. Do you smoke more frequently during the first hours after waking than during the rest of the day?

    Yes (1)   No (0)

6. Do you smoke even when you are so ill that you are in bed most of the day?

    Yes (1)   No (0)

FIGURE 4.3. Fagerstrom Test for Nicotine Dependence. From Heatherton, Kozlowski, Frecker, and Fagerstrom (1991). Copyright 1991 by Blackwell Publishing. Reprinted by permission.

FTND, the History of Smoking Index (HSI; Heatherton et al., 1989) can be administered. The HSI, which consists of an item that assesses time to first morning cigarette and the individual's daily smoking rate, can be a valid assessment of the smoker's current dependence level. The FTQ, FTND, and HSI are all highly interrelated (Kozlowski et al., 1994).

Other recently developed scales assess severity of nicotine dependence as well. The Cigarette Dependence Scale (CDS; Etter et al., 2003), a self-report measure that draws its items from DSM-IV and ICD-10 criteria, underwent psychometric development to yield two versions: CDS-12 and CDS-5. Both versions cover, to greater and lesser degrees, the content of the DSM and ICD and were shown to have adequate construct validity, internal consistency, and retest reliability. Both versions also proved to be better at differentiating between daily and occasional smokers than the FTND, though neither version predicted success with smoking cessation in an uncontrolled assessment of smoking behavior over time.

The Nicotine Dependence Syndrome Scale (NDSS; Shiffman, Waters, & Hickox, 2004) addresses a different facet of dependence compared to these other scales (Figure 4.4). It explicitly views dependence as a *multidimensional*

INSTRUCTIONS: Using the scale below, fill in the circle corresponding to the number that indicates how well each of the following statements describes you.

		Not at all true	Somewhat true	Moderately true	Very true	Extremely true
1	My smoking pattern is very irregular throughout the day. It is not unusual for me to go smoke many cigarettes in an hour, then not have another one until hours later.	1 O	2 O	3 O	4 O	5 O
2	My smoking is not much affected by other things. I smoke about the same amount whether I'm relaxing or working, happy or sad, alone or with others, etc.	1 O	2 O	3 O	4 O	5 O
3	Even if traveling a long distance, I'd rather not travel by airplane because I wouldn't be allowed to smoke.	1 O	2 O	3 O	4 O	5 O
4	Sometimes I decline offers to visit with my nonsmoking friends because I know they'll feel uncomfortable if I smoke.	1 O	2 O	3 O	4 O	5 O
5	I tend to avoid restaurants that don't allow smoking, even if I would otherwise enjoy the food.	1 O	2 O	3 O	4 O	5 O
6	I smoke consistently and regularly throughout the day.	1 O	2 O	3 O	4 O	5 O
7	I smoke at different rates in different situations.	1 O	2 O	3 O	4 O	5 O
8	Compared to when I first started smoking, I need to smoke a lot more now in order to really get what I want out of it.	1 O	2 O	3 O	4 O	5 O
9	Compared to when I first started smoking, I can smoke much, much more now before I start to feel nauseated or ill.	1 O	2 O	3 O	4 O	5 O
10	After not smoking for a while, I need to smoke in order to keep myself from experiencing any discomfort.	1 O	2 O	3 O	4 O	5 O

(continued)

FIGURE 4.4. Nicotine Dependence Syndrome Scale. From Shiffman, Waters, and Hickcox (in press). Copyright by Taylor & Francis. Reprinted by permission.

		Not at all true	Somewhat true	Moderately true	Very true	Extremely true
11	It's hard to estimate how many cigarettes I smoke per day because the number often changes.	1 ○	2 ○	3 ○	4 ○	5 ○
12	I feel a sense of control over my smoking. I can "take it or leave it" at any time.	1 ○	2 ○	3 ○	4 ○	5 ○
13	The number of cigarettes I smoke per day is often influenced by other factors—how I'm feeling, what I'm doing, etc.	1 ○	2 ○	3 ○	4 ○	5 ○
14	When I'm really craving a cigarette, it feels like I'm in the grip of some unknown force that I cannot control.	1 ○	2 ○	3 ○	4 ○	5 ○
15	Since the time when I became a regular smoker, the amount I smoke has either stayed the same or has decreased somewhat.	1 ○	2 ○	3 ○	4 ○	5 ○
16	Whenever I go without a smoke for a few hours, I experience craving.	1 ○	2 ○	3 ○	4 ○	5 ○
17	My cigarette smoking is fairly regular throughout the day.	1 ○	2 ○	3 ○	4 ○	5 ○
18	After not smoking for a while, I need to smoke to relieve feelings of restlessness and irritability.	1 ○	2 ○	3 ○	4 ○	5 ○
19	I smoke about the same amount on weekends as on weekdays.	1 ○	2 ○	3 ○	4 ○	5 ○

FIGURE 4.4. *(continued)*

syndrome composed of several dimensions (Shiffman, Waters, et al., 2004; Edwards & Gross, 1976; Shadel et al., 2000) and yields subscale scores for different aspects of dependence: Drive (craving, withdrawal, compulsion to smoke), Priority (giving priority to smoking over other reinforcers), Tolerance (diminishing effects of smoking or the need to smoke more for effects), Stereotypy (fixed, inflexible patterns of smoking), and Continuity (smoking continuously). The NDSS can also be scored for a single, omnibus dependence score. It has been shown to capture variance that is not captured by the Fagerstrom scales, and the five subscales have demonstrated discriminant validity. Further research is required to assess the implications of various subscale profiles of the NDSS, especially in relation to treatment.

Withdrawal Symptoms

The nicotine withdrawal syndrome has been well described and can be a hallmark sign of dependence (Hughes & Hatsukami, 1986; Hughes, Higgins, & Hatsukami, 1990). Symptoms of the nicotine withdrawal syndrome include irritability, frustration, or anger; anxiety; difficulty concentrating; restlessness; decreased heart rate; and increased appetite or weight gain (see DSM-IV; American Psychiatric Association, 1994). Symptoms of nicotine withdrawal typically appear within 2 hours after the last cigarette, peak between 24 and 48 hours after cessation, and last up to a few weeks on average (Hughes et al., 1990; Piasecki, Fiore, & Baker, 1997). However, recent studies have demonstrated that there can be substantial variability in both the trajectory of symptoms and time course of withdrawal (Piasecki et al., 1997). In any case, withdrawal symptoms can predict lapse and relapse after a cessation attempt (Killen & Fortman, 1997; Shiffman et al., 1997). Relief of withdrawal, then, is thought to mediate the clinical effect of treatment on abstinence. For example, nicotine replacement therapy is thought to work largely by reducing craving and withdrawal symptoms (Hughes, 1993). Withdrawal measures can also be used as markers for treatment efficacy in the absence of complete abstinence.

Of the several scales developed to assess nicotine withdrawal, two have been most studied. The Shiffman–Jarvik scale (1976), a 23-item scale, assesses facets of nicotine withdrawal (i.e., craving, psychological symptoms, physical symptoms, arousal disturbance, and appetite disturbance). Although the Shiffman–Jarvik scale has demonstrated good reliability, it was one of the first scales developed (i.e., prior to the refinement of the withdrawal construct) and as such includes a number of items that are no longer considered a core part of the withdrawal syndrome (Figure 4.5). A shorter clinical checklist was later developed by Hughes and Hatsukami (1986) to assess severity of individual symptoms corresponding to the DSM-III-R criteria for withdrawal. Hughes, Gust, Skoog, Kennan, and Fenwick (1991) reported that factor analysis suggests three factors: mood, appetite, and sleep disturbance. These results suggest that it may not be prudent to aggregate the entire list of withdrawal symptoms into a total scale score. On the other hand, with one item per symptom, reliability of each symptom is hard to assess and is likely to be limited.

The newer Wisconsin Smoking Withdrawal Scale (Welsch et al., 1999), which was developed via factor analysis from items designed to tap DSM-IV criteria, was tested in two studies of nicotine replacement therapy. The scales contain 28 items and assess seven constructs or symptoms. The subscales correlate with each other, and confirmatory factor analysis suggests that they can also be summarized as a single underlying factor (Welsch et al., 1999). The subscales were shown to be reliable and were validated by demonstrating changes with abstinence and effects of nicotine patches. Thus, the scale appears reliable and valid in at least some conditions. Further experience with

Shiffman–Jarvik (1976) Withdrawal Scale

In response to each of the following items, please mark the appropriate box. We are interested in how you feel *at the time you are filling out the questionnaire.* You will be filling out a number of questionnaires and your responses on each one should reflect your state *at the time you fill out.*

____ Very Definitely

____ Definitely

____ Probably

____ Possibly

____ Probably Not

____ Definitely Not

____ Very Definitely Not

1. If you could smoke freely, would you like a cigarette this minute?
2. Is your heart beating faster than usual?
3. Do you feel more calm than usual?
4. Are you able to concentrate as well as usual?
5. Do you feel wide awake?
6. Do you feel content?
7. If you had just eaten, would you want a cigarette?
8. Do you feel more restless than usual?
9. Are you thinking of cigarettes more than usual?
10. Are you unusually sleepy for this time of day?
11. Do you have fluttery feelings in your chest right now?
12. Do you feel hungrier than usual for this time of day?
13. If you were permitted to smoke would you refuse a cigarette right now?
14. Do you feel unusually tired?
15. Do you feel more tense than usual?
16. Do you miss a cigarette?
17. Do you feel alert?
18. Do you feel anxious?
19. Do you have an urge to smoke a cigarette right now?
20. Are you feeling irritable?
21. Would you find a cigarette unpleasant right now?
22. Are your hands shaky?
23. Is your appetite smaller than normal?

Hughes and Hatsukami (1986) Withdrawal Assessment

Please check any items on the following list which may apply to how you feel right now.

____ restless	____ healthy
____ irritated	____ headachy
____ anxious, nervous	____ tired
____ angry	____ confused
____ hungry	____ bored
____ aggressive	____ other (please specify)
____ sweaty	_____

FIGURE 4.5. Withdrawal scales. From Shiffman and Jarvik (1976) and Hughes and Hatsukami. Copyright 1976 by the American Medical Association. Copyright 1986 by the American Medical Association. Reprinted by permission.

the scale in a variety of contexts may be needed before it is adopted as a matter of routine in those contexts. For an extensive review of withdrawal scales, see Shiffman, West, et al. (2004).

Cravings and Urges

Craving is a subjectively "felt" desire to smoke and an important part of the nicotine dependence syndrome (American Psychiatric Association, 1994; Shadel et al., 2000). However, there is continuing debate over how best to define and assess cravings (Sayette et al., 2000; Kassell & Shiffman, 1992), and also over the most appropriate technique to measure cravings (Sayette et al., 2000). Sayette and colleagues review the issues that surround craving assessment and the reader is directed here for a complete discussion of craving assessment. Shiffman, West, et al. (2004) also review measures of craving for use in clinical trials.

Self-report measures of craving have the benefit of immediate clinical utility. Like withdrawal, craving can be used as one rough marker for treatment efficacy and can additionally be used to help identify the cigarettes that will be most difficult to "give up" during treatment (i.e., the stronger the craving associated with a cigarette, the harder that cigarette may be to quit). Two prominent measures of cravings and urges are available for assessing this construct among smokers. First, the Questionnaire of Smoking Urges (QSU) is a multi-item, self-report scale (Tiffany & Drobes, 1991) that purports to measure multiple aspects of craving (e.g., desires for smoking, expectancies about cravings). The scale is available in both a long form (Tiffany & Drobes, 1991) and a short form (Cox, Tiffany, & Christen, 2001), though there are concerns with the content validity of the QSU scales, in that they tap constructs, such as smoking expectancies and intentions, that may not be part of craving per se (Kozlowski, Pillitteri, Sweeney, Whitfield, & Graham, 1996). Shiffman and colleagues (2003) have used a more homogeneous, 5-item scale to assess craving that has been shown to have strong internal consistency in prior studies (> .95; see Figure 4.6). Finally, single-item assessments of craving (e.g., "On a scale from 1 to 10, how strong are your cravings to smoke right now?") have been shown to be as reliable and as valid as longer scales, and demonstrate ability to predict smoking behaviors (Niaura et al., 1998).

Motivation to Quit

In the population of adult smokers, 70% say they want to quit, but a significant majority (up to 80 %) are not ready to quit within 30 days, and 30–45% do not intend to quit within 6 months (Centers for Disease Control and Prevention, 1994). Motivation to quit appears to be important in predicting whether a given cessation attempt will be successful (Miller & Rollnick,

Shiffman et al. (2003)

1. I have a desire for a cigarette right now.
2. If it were possible, I would smoke right now.
3. All I want right now is a cigarette.
4. I have an urge for a cigarette.
5. I crave a cigarette right now.

Questionnaire of Smoking Urges (Short Form) (Cox et al., 2001)

Indicate how much you agree or disagree with each of the following statements by placing a checkmark (like this: √) along each line between STRONGLY DISAGREE and STRONGLY AGREE. The closer you place your checkmark to one end or the other indicates the strength of your disagreement or agreement. Please complete every item. We are interested in how you are thinking or feeling *right now* as you are filling out the questionnaire.

1. I have a strong urge for a cigarette right now.
   STRONGLY DISAGREE: : : : : : : STRONGLY AGREE
2. Nothing would be better than smoking a cigarette right now.
   STRONGLY DISAGREE: : : : : : : STRONGLY AGREE
3. If it were possible, I would probably smoke now.
   STRONGLY DISAGREE: : : : : : : STRONGLY AGREE
4. I could control things better right now if I could smoke.
   STRONGLY DISAGREE: : : : : : : STRONGLY AGREE
5. All I want right now is a cigarette.
   STRONGLY DISAGREE: : : : : : : STRONGLY AGREE
6. I have an urge for a cigarette.
   STRONGLY DISAGREE: : : : : : : STRONGLY AGREE
7. A cigarette would taste good now.
   STRONGLY DISAGREE: : : : : : : STRONGLY AGREE
8. I would do almost anything for a cigarette right now.
   STRONGLY DISAGREE: : : : : : : STRONGLY AGREE
9. Smoking would make me less depressed.
   STRONGLY DISAGREE: : : : : : : STRONGLY AGREE
10. I am going to smoke as soon as possible.
    STRONGLY DISAGREE: : : : : : : STRONGLY AGREE

FIGURE 4.6. Craving scales. From Shiffman et al. (2003) and Cox, Tiffany, and Christen (2001). Copyright 2003 by Springer. Copyright 2001 by Taylor & Francis. Reprinted by permission.

1991), and evidence has suggested that initial levels of motivation to quit smoking can predict success with smoking cessation (e.g., Biener & Abrams, 1991; Curry, Grothaus, & McBride, 1997). However, there are many different ways to define and assess motivation; each of these methods has its own set of associated costs and benefits and in fact, any assessment of motivation may be limited in a clinical context (where motivation is likely to be uniformly "high"). We review and evaluate some of the more popular methods of assessing motivation below.

The *stages-of-change* algorithm, part of the broader *transtheoretical model of behavioral change* (Prochaska, DiClemente, & Norcross, 1992), is a widely adopted measure of motivation or readiness to change smoking behavior or quit smoking. Staging smokers involves categorizing smokers and ex-smokers into five discrete classes (precontemplation, contemplation, preparation, action, maintenance) based on their current smoking (or nonsmoking) behavior, quit attempts in the last year, and intention to quit during the next 6 months. Progression through the stages (i.e., from preparation to action) is thought to be driven by various behavioral change strategies that a provider may deliver (e.g., education through consciousness raising), termed the "processes of change" (Prochaska et al., 1988).

Despite prominence in the field of behavior change and its application to numerous health risk behaviors (Prochaska et al., 1994), stages-of-change measures may not be very useful in treatment settings, since all the smokers presenting for treatment will typically fall into the Preparation phase. Additionally, the appropriateness and adequacy of discrete assessments of motivation, like stages, and the use of the results of these assessments to match smokers to treatments have been extensively questioned (Bandura, 1997; Farkas et al., 1996). Moreover, there is no consistent evidence that the processes of change actually predict movement through the stages (e.g., Herzog, Abrams, Emmons, Linnan, & Shadel, 1999). These factors may make staging smokers a less desirable option for measuring motivation, especially in cessation-oriented treatment contexts.

An alternative measure of readiness, the readiness-to-change ladder, is a measure with 11 response options designed to assess motivation along a continuum from "not at all considering quitting smoking in the near future" to "already having quit smoking" (Abrams & Beiner, 1992; Beiner & Abrams, 1991). The readiness-to-change ladder has been shown to be associated with objective measures of readiness to quit smoking (e.g., intention to quit; nicotine dependence, number of prior quit attempts; Abrams & Beiner, 1992; Beiner & Abrams, 1991) and with making quit attempts. Thus, the ladder has the advantage of being a short, efficient, and face-valid measure that is generalizable for use with many diverse populations (e.g., it can be easily understood by both blue- and white-collar workers alike; Abrams & Beiner, 1992). As with stages of change, though, its utility in an active cessation treatment context is probably limited.

Social Support

Although evidence suggests that social support influences smoking cessation outcomes (e.g., Murray et al., 1995), interventions to increase patients' social support during treatment for nicotine dependence have met with mixed results (Carlson, Goodey, Bennett, Taenzer, & Koopmans, 2002; McMahon & Jason, 2000). Nevertheless, there are methods to assess social support available to the smoker. The Partner Interaction Questionnaire (PIQ; Mermelstein, Cohen, Lichtenstein, Baer, & Karmack, 1983), a 61-item questionnaire, was designed to assess the level of support the smoker perceives that a significant other is contributing to his or her efforts to quit smoking. Pretreatment scores on the PIQ have been found to predict smoking cessation and relapse: High levels of perceived support of a significant other were associated with greater success at quitting smoking (Mermelstein et al., 1986).

Assessment of Mood and Other Psychiatric Disorders

Mood and psychiatric disorders are becoming increasingly important to understanding smoking and smoking cessation. However, myriad self-report and interviewer-administered assessments can be used in this context, and it is beyond the scope of this chapter to review these assessments. Thus, we focus our brief discussion below on the rationale for assessing additional mood and psychiatric disorders among smokers, and direct the reader to other resources for more explicit information on assessment (Bauer, 2003). Assessment of other substance use among smokers is also becoming increasingly important; the reader is directed to other chapters in this volume for in-depth coverage.

Depressed Mood

Some studies have demonstrated significant relations between self-reported depression and the frequency of smoking; recent theory has suggested that avoidance of negative affect should be considered among the most important motivators of substance use (Baker, Piper, McCarthy, Majeskie, & Fiore, 2004). For example, among the general population of adults in the United States, smokers with major depressive disorder (Glassman et al., 1990) or depressive symptoms (Anda et al., 1990) are less likely to quit smoking than nondepressed smokers, and smokers report higher levels of depression than nonsmokers (Frederick, Frerichs, & Clark, 1988). The presence of a mood disorder or even low levels of dysphoria may play a role in precipitating a relapse to smoking after attempted abstinence. Among smokers undergoing cessation treatment, depressed mood at pretreatment predicts failure to achieve abstinence during treatment (Niaura, Britt, Shadel, Goldstein, & Abrams, 2001), and depressive symptoms following initial cessation predict subsequent relapse to smoking (West, Hajek, & Belcher, 1989). However, recent data have called into question whether a lifetime history of major depressive disorder (Hitsman, Borrelli, McChargue, Spring, & Niaura, 2003) predict smoking cessation outcomes and whether transient changes in mood are associated with smoking (Shiffman et al., 2002).

Stress and Anxiety

Smokers report that they smoke or relapse most frequently under stressful conditions (e.g., Shiffman, 1982, 1986), smokers report greater levels of stress compared to nonsmokers (e.g., Breslau et al., 1994), and experimental studies that have manipulated negative affect suggest a causal association with smoking intensity (via topography assessment; e.g., Dobbs, Strickler, & Maxwell, 1981). Stress has also been found, in experimental studies, to predict urge or craving to smoke (Perkins & Grobe, 1992). Real-time analysis of smokers' relapse situations found that lapses and relapses were very significantly related to acute stress and negative affect, even when more stable levels of mood were controlled (Shiffman, Paty, Kassel, & Hickox, 1996). In fact, a recent comprehensive review of the complex and extensive database of research on stress and smoking has indicated that stress has a clear, most probably causal relationship to both lapse and relapse (Kassel et al., 2003).

Substance Use

Smoking rates over 85% have been noted in alcoholics (Battjes, 1988), opiate addicts (Rounsaville et al., 1985), and polydrug users (Burling & Ziff, 1988). Even persons who are taking methadone for help with opiate dependence have smoking rates well over 90% (Clarke, Stein, McGarry, & Gogineni, 2001). Alcohol use and abuse, and possibly abuse of other drugs, are also associated with difficulty giving up smoking. Drinking alcohol is reported to be a significant precipitant of smoking relapse in the general population (Shiffman, 1986). Moreover, alcoholics are considerably less likely to be successful than nonalcoholics in their attempts to quit smoking (DiFranza & Guerrera, 1990).

Other Psychiatric Disorders

A number of studies have established that psychiatric patients, especially those with psychoses, are much more likely to smoke than the general population or even nonpsychiatric patients (Hughes, Hatsukami, Mitchell, & Dahlgren, 1986). Given the multiple complex issues that need to be addressed with psychiatric patients who smoke (i.e., due to the interactions between smoking and psychotropic drug levels; see Glassman, 1993) and the likelihood that patients with more severe psychiatric disorders may have more difficulty with quitting smoking (Hall et al., 1995), an assessment of comorbid psychiatric involvement seems prudent.

ASSESSMENTS RELEVANT
FOR UNDERSTANDING RELAPSE

Self-Efficacy

Self-efficacy, the belief in one's ability to perform a particular action or behavior within a given domain (Bandura, 1997), is typically measured by asking about an individual's confidence to perform that behavior or activity. Smoking research has used self-efficacy to great benefit in predicting response to treatment. Indeed, in the two decades following the initial studies (e.g., Condiotte & Lichtenstein, 1981), self-efficacy appraisals of one's ability to quit smoking assessed at the end of treatment remain the most consistently strong predictor of later lapse and relapse (reviewed by Ockene et al., 2000). Naturalistic studies of self-efficacy over time demonstrate that efficacy can vary across time and situations (Shiffman et al., 1997; Shiffman, Balabanis, et al., 2000), and that self-efficacy to refrain from smoking commonly varies across different contexts (Gwaltney et al., 2001). Despite these findings, the vast majority of studies of self-efficacy among smokers treat the construct as a global trait (i.e., averaged across situations), assessing it globally on one occasion (e.g., at baseline or at the end of treatment). As such, self-efficacy to quit smoking (averaged across situations) measured at the end of treatment typically predicts later lapse and relapse (Ockene et al., 2000).

The *Confidence Questionnaire* (Condiotte & Lichtenstein, 1981) is a 46-item questionnaire designed to assess levels of confidence to resist smoking in a number of common situations (e.g., "when you feel anxious"; "when you see others smoking"). This assessment of self-efficacy has the advantage of demonstrating strong psychometric properties covering many situations and domains, and predicting smoking relapse (Baer & Lichtenstein, 1988). However, in a clinical context, this scale tends to be cumbersome and time-consuming to complete. A short form (14 items) of the Confidence Questionnaire (Form S) was developed to address this concern; it also predicts smoking relapse (Baer & Lichtenstein, 1988). In either case, the items of the questionnaires are summed to produce a final score that may be taken to refer to a general sense of self-efficacy to quit smoking.

The *Confidence Inventory* (Velicer, DiClemente, Rossi & Prochaska, 1990), an alternative measure of self-efficacy, consists of items similar in structure and content to the items represented in the Confidence Questionnaire, in that smokers respond according to their level of confidence to resist smoking in the situations represented by the items. However, the Confidence Inventory differs from the Confidence Questionnaire in that it may be divided into subscales that assess self-efficacy in three broad situational domains: Positive/Social; Negative/Affective; and Habit/Addictive. The authors of the Confidence Inventory suggest that it is best to use the subscales to target problem areas for relapse after a cessation attempt, whereas the total scale score should be used to index general level of confidence to quit smoking.

The newer *Relapse Situation Efficacy Questionnaire* (RSEQ; Gwaltney et al., 2001) similarly assesses context-specific vulnerability across the following domains: Negative Affect, Positive Affect, Restrictive Situations (to smoking), Idle Time, Social–Food Situations, Low Arousal, and Craving (Figure 4.7). Uniquely, the RSEQ context subscores have been shown to predict the situation in which smokers may lapse, making this a useful tool for identifying situational challenges that need to be addressed in treatment (Shiffman, Read, & Jarvik, 1985). One approach is to target the smoker's "Achilles' heel"—the situation associated with the lowest confidence. This proved to be the best predictor of outcome (Gwaltney et al., 2001). Whatever scale is used, situation-specific efficacy measures appear more promising for treatment, because they help the smoker and the clinician think about and address the smoker's vulnerabilities.

Outcome Expectancies

Myriad theories focus on the regulatory role that outcome expectancies play in motivating action and performance (e.g., Ajzen & Fishbein, 1980). In smoking research, outcome expectancies are thought of as beliefs about the consequences that result from smoking (e.g., "How much does smoking help you to relax?"; "How much does smoking help you to control your weight?"). Most research on outcome expectancies among smokers has focused on developing assessments that tap the multidimensional nature of the consequences of smoking (e.g., *Smoking Consequences Questionnaire* [SCQ]; Brandon & Baker, 1991) and on using this measure to predict outcomes or show associations with important smoking variables (Figure 4.8). The SCQ is associated with measures of nicotine dependence (Copeland, Brandon, & Quinn, 1995), severity of withdrawal, and experienced negative affect and stress during a cessation attempt (Wetter et al., 1994), and cessation outcomes (Copeland et al., 1995; Wetter et al., 1994). Outcome expectancies for positive smoking effects have been shown to decrease more among abstinent individuals in treatment compared to smoking individuals in treatment (Copeland et al., 1995). However, several studies of outcome expectancies among smokers have found contradictory or no relations to treatment outcome (e.g., Shadel & Mermelstein, 1993; see also Brandon, Juliano, & Copeland, 1999). Outcome expectancies have been manipulated to test for their effects on withdrawal relief from pharmacological treatment (Gottleib, Killen, Marlatt, & Taylor, 1987) and from smoking a cigarette (Juliano & Brandon, 2002). Assessment of outcome expectancies maybe most useful in treatment as a way of drawing out smokers' often unrealistic beliefs about the effects of smoking, so that they can be addressed and debunked. For example, many smokers believe smoking relaxes them and reduces stress, even though evidence suggests otherwise (Kassel et al., 2003); it is important to debunk these unrealistic beliefs.

Instructions: Some situations may tempt you to smoke during the process of quitting smoking. Use the scale below to rate your confidence in staying abstinent under a variety of conditions. Indicate on the line to the right of each item the number that best describes your confidence level. (1 = Not at all confident, 2 = Somewhat confident, 3 = Very confident, 4 = Extremely confident.)

How confident are you that you can resist the temptation to smoke when you are—
1. Restless? _____
2. Tired? _____
3. Happy? _____
4. Irritable? _____
5. Spacey? _____
6. Miserable? _____
7. Sleepy? _____
8. Tense? _____
9. Contented? _____
10. Frustrated or angry? _____
11. Energetic? _____
12. Sad? _____
13. Finding it hard to concentrate? _____
14. Hungry? _____

How confident are you that you can resist the temptation to smoke when you are feeling—
15. Very bad? _____
16. Bad? _____
17. Neutral? _____
18. Good? _____
19. Very good? _____

How confident are you that you can resist the temptation to smoke when your arousal or energy level is—
20. Very low? _____
21. Low? _____
22. Moderate? _____
23. High? _____
24. Very high? _____

How confident are you that you can resist the temptation to smoke when—
Eating and Drinking
25. You have had food or drink in the last 15 minutes? _____
26. You have had a meal? _____
27. You have had a snack? _____
28. You have had coffee or tea? _____
29. You have had alcohol? (missing if subject is nondrinker) _____

(continued)

FIGURE 4.7. Relapse Situation Efficacy Questionnaire. From Gwaltney et al. (2001). Copyright 2001 by the American Psychological Association. Reprinted by permission.

Situations and Activities

30. You are home?   ____
31. You are at your workplace?   ____
32. You are at another's home?   ____
33. You are in a bar or restaurant?   ____
34. You are in a vehicle?   ____
35. You are outside?   ____
36. You are alone?   ____
37. You must change locations to be able to smoke?   ____
38. You are with others?   ____
39. You are socializing?   ____
40. You are interacting with others for business?   ____
41. You are interacting with others on household issues?   ____
42. You are arguing with others?   ____
43. You are engaged in job-related work or chores?   ____
44. You are engaged in home or personal work or chores?   ____
45. You are engaged in leisure?   ____
46. You are inactive while you are waiting?   ____
47. You are inactive while you are between activities?   ____
48. You are inactive while you are doing nothing?   ____
49. You are on the telephone?   ____
50. You are lost in thought?   ____
51. You are doing something you want to do?   ____
52. You are doing something you should do?   ____
53. You are doing something you both want and should do?   ____
54. You are where smoking is forbidden?   ____
55. You are where smoking is discouraged?   ____
56. You are where smoking is allowed?   ____
57. You are where people are smoking in your group?   ____
58. You are where people are smoking in view?   ____

How confident are you that you can resist the temptation to smoke when—

59. Your urge to smoke is low?   ____
60. Your urge to smoke is moderate?   ____
61. Your urge to smoke is high?   ____
62. Your craving is low?   ____
63. Your craving is moderate?   ____
64. Your craving is high?   ____
65. You are in a bad mood?   ____
66. You are experiencing stress?   ____
67. You are in a good mood?   ____
68. You are around others' smoking, and ashtrays, etc.?   ____
69. You are eating or drinking?   ____
70. You are relaxing?   ____
71. You are bored?   ____
72. You are in transition, between activities?   ____
73. Cigarettes are easily available?   ____
74. Cigarettes are available with difficulty?   ____

FIGURE 4.7. *(continued)*

INSTRUCTIONS: Below is a list of statements about smoking. Each statement contains a possible consequence of smoking. For each of the statements listed below, please rate how LIKELY or UNLIKELY you believe each consequence is for you when you smoke. If the consequences seem unlikely to you, mark a number 5–9. That is, if you believe that a consequence would never happen, make the number 0; if you believe that a consequence would happen every time you smoke, make the number 9. Use the guide below to aid you further.

0	1	2	3	4	5	6	7	8	9
Completely	Extremely	Very little	Somewhat	A little	A little	Somewhat	Very	Extremely	Completely
UNLIKELY					LIKELY				

	UNLIKELY					LIKELY			
1. Cigarettes taste good.	0	1	2	3	4	5	6	7	8	9
2. Smoking controls my appetite.	0	1	2	3	4	5	6	7	8	9
3. My throat burns after smoking.	0	1	2	3	4	5	6	7	8	9
4. Cigarettes help me deal with anxiety or worry.	0	1	2	3	4	5	6	7	8	9
5. Nicotine "fits" can be controlled by smoking.	0	1	2	3	4	5	6	7	8	9
6. When I'm angry, a cigarette can calm me down.	0	1	2	3	4	5	6	7	8	9
7. When I'm alone, a cigarette can help me pass the time.	0	1	2	3	4	5	6	7	8	9
8. I become more addicted the more I smoke.	0	1	2	3	4	5	6	7	8	9
9. If I'm tense, a cigarette can help me to relax	0	1	2	3	4	5	6	7	8	9
10. Cigarettes keep me from overeating.	0	1	2	3	4	5	6	7	8	9
11. Smoking a cigarette energizes me.	0	1	2	3	4	5	6	7	8	9
12. Cigarettes help me deal with anger.	0	1	2	3	4	5	6	7	8	9
13. Smoking calms me down when I feel nervous.	0	1	2	3	4	5	6	7	8	9
14. Cigarettes make my lungs hurt.	0	1	2	3	4	5	6	7	8	9
15. I feel like I do a better job when I am smoking.	0	1	2	3	4	5	6	7	8	9
16. A cigarette can give me energy when I'm bored and tired.	0	1	2	3	4	5	6	7	8	9
17. Cigarettes can really make me feel good.	0	1	2	3	4	5	6	7	8	9
18. When I'm feeling happy, smoking helps keep that feeling.	0	1	2	3	4	5	6	7	8	9
19. I will enjoy the flavor of a cigarette.	0	1	2	3	4	5	6	7	8	9
20. If I have nothing to do, a smoke can help kill time.	0	1	2	3	4	5	6	7	8	9
21. I will enjoy feeling a cigarette on my tongue and lips.	0	1	2	3	4	5	6	7	8	9
22. Smoking will satisfy my nicotine craving.	0	1	2	3	4	5	6	7	8	9
23. I feel like part of a group when I'm around other smokers.	0	1	2	3	4	5	6	7	8	9
24. Smoking makes me seem less attractive.	0	1	2	3	4	5	6	7	8	9
25. By smoking I risk heart disease and lung cancer.	0	1	2	3	4	5	6	7	8	9
26. Smoking helps me enjoy people more.	0	1	2	3	4	5	6	7	8	9

(continued)

FIGURE 4.8. Smoking Consequences Questionnaire. From Brandon and Baker (1991). Copyright 1991 by the American Psychological Association. Reprinted by permission.

	UNLIKELY					LIKELY				
27. Cigarettes help me reduce tension.	0	1	2	3	4	5	6	7	8	9
28. I feel better physically after having a smoke.	0	1	2	3	4	5	6	7	8	9
29. I enjoy parties more when I am smoking.	0	1	2	3	4	5	6	7	8	9
30. People think less of me if they see me smoking.	0	1	2	3	4	5	6	7	8	9
31. A cigarette can satisfy my urge to smoke	0	1	2	3	4	5	6	7	8	9
32. Just handling a cigarette is pleasurable.	0	1	2	3	4	5	6	7	8	9
33. If I'm feeling irritable, a smoke will help me relax.	0	1	2	3	4	5	6	7	8	9
34. Smoking irritates my mouth and throat.	0	1	2	3	4	5	6	7	8	9
35. When I feel bored and tired a cigarette can really help.	0	1	2	3	4	5	6	7	8	9
36. I will become more dependent on nicotine if I continue smoking.	0	1	2	3	4	5	6	7	8	9
37. Smoking helps me control my weight.	0	1	2	3	4	5	6	7	8	9
38. When I'm upset with someone, a cigarette helps me cope.	0	1	2	3	4	5	6	7	8	9
39. The more I smoke, the more I risk my health.	0	1	2	3	4	5	6	7	8	9
40. Cigarettes keep me from eating more than I should.	0	1	2	3	4	5	6	7	8	9
41. I enjoy the steps I take to light up.	0	1	2	3	4	5	6	7	8	9
42. Conversations seem more special if we are smoking.	0	1	2	3	4	5	6	7	8	9
43. I look ridiculous while smoking.	0	1	2	3	4	5	6	7	8	9
44. Smoking keeps my weight down.	0	1	2	3	4	5	6	7	8	9
45. I like the way a cigarette makes me feel physically.	0	1	2	3	4	5	6	7	8	9
46. Smoking is hazardous to my health.	0	1	2	3	4	5	6	7	8	9
47. I enjoy feeling the smoke hit my mouth and back of my throat.	0	1	2	3	4	5	6	7	8	9
48. When I smoke, the taste is pleasant.	0	1	2	3	4	5	6	7	8	9
49. I like to watch the smoke from my cigarette.	0	1	2	3	4	5	6	7	8	9
50. When I am worrying about something, a cigarette is helpful.	0	1	2	3	4	5	6	7	8	9
51. Smoking temporarily reduces those repeated urges for cigarettes.	0	1	2	3	4	5	6	7	8	9
52. I enjoy the taste sensations while smoking.	0	1	2	3	4	5	6	7	8	9
53. I feel more at ease with other people if I have a cigarette.	0	1	2	3	4	5	6	7	8	9
54. Cigarettes are good for dealing with boredom.	0	1	2	3	4	5	6	7	8	9
55. Smoking is taking years off my life.	0	1	2	3	4	5	6	7	8	9

FIGURE 4.8. *(continued)*

Attributions

Theory has suggested that internal (located within the actor), stable (unchanging), and global (applicable across a range of contexts and situations) attributions are associated more with relapse (Marlatt & Gordon, 1985); that is, smoking lapse episodes that are perceived by the recently abstinent smoker to have resulted from internal factors (e.g., personal weakness), that are both stable (e.g., person weakness as an enduring characteristic of themselves) and global (e.g., personal weakness as a characteristic that can be applied in the smoking setting, as well as in countless other settings) are more likely to lead to relapse. However, empirical work has found either the opposite effect (Curry et al., 1987) or no support for the importance of attributions in the relapse process (Shiffman et al., 1997). Thus, while these variables are interesting, they clearly are in need of further study before they can be incorporated into a comprehensive, treatment-oriented assessment of smoking behavior.

Coping Resources

Relapse prevention theory (Marlatt & Gordon, 1985) proposes that the ability to cope with "high-risk" situations determines an individual's probability of maintaining abstinence. Successful coping in high-risk situations is thought to lead to an increased sense of self-efficacy, but failure to cope initiates a chain of events in which diminished self-efficacy may lead to a slip and perhaps to a full-blown relapse. Coping after a lapse episode may prevent relapse (Shiffman, Hickox, et al., 1996), though it is not clear that negative emotional reactions following a lapse can lead to a full blown relapse.

It is worth distinguishing different types of coping that smokers must field in order to maintain abstinence and forestall relapse: (1) *anticipatory coping*, which is designed to help the smoker avoid high-risk situations and is enacted prior to facing an acute crisis; (2) *immediate coping*, synonymous with temptation coping, in which the smoker copes with an immediate craving or temptation to smoke in order to avoid a lapse; and (3) *restorative coping*, in which the smoker copes with the aftermath of a lapse in order to try and prevent progression to relapse. All of these coping responses can be assessed by open-ended questioning of past and/or present quit experiences.

More formally, the Coping with Temptation Inventory (Shiffman, 1988) provides a questionnaire method with which to assess anticipatory, immediate, and restorative coping (Figure 4.9). It lists both cognitive coping strategies (e.g., willpower, delay thoughts) and behavioral coping strategies (e.g., physical activity, distraction) in each of these domains. Alternatively, self-monitoring of coping responses "as they occur" may be achieved by having smokers keep a written record (via self-monitoring or EMA, as reviewed earlier). In any case, increased use of both cognitive and behavioral forms of coping predicts increased chances of abstinence, although it is not clear whether

INSTRUCTIONS: For each of the items below, please indicate whether you have used this strategy to manage cravings or urges to smoke when you are trying not to smoke.

Behavioral coping responses	Yes	No

Used alternative consumption
- Food and drink (e.g., allowed yourself to eat more to avoid smoking, chewed gum, drank water/ juice)
- Nicotine (e.g., chewed nicotine gum or used snuff)

Used alternative activities
- Exercise (e.g., lifted weights, took walks)
- Distraction (e.g., kept busy, doodles when talking on the phone)
- Relaxation (e.g., practiced deep breathing exercises, took hot shower to relax)

Engaged in self-care activities
- Stress reduction (e.g., isolated yourself for a relaxing weekend, kept out of stressful situations)
- Other self-care activities (e.g., ate better, took more time for yourself)

Practiced stimulus control
- Cigarettes and smoking paraphernalia (e.g., bought cigarettes by the pack rather than the carton, got rid of ashtrays, refused to keep cigarettes in the house)
- Other substances (e.g., avoided alcohol and coffee, drank fruit juice)
- People (e.g., avoided friends who smoke, did not visit with smokers)
- Situations (e.g., sat in nonsmoking section of restaurants, avoided situations in which you typically smoke, change places of relaxation at home)

Asked for help from others
- Social support (e.g., asked your children to throw away your cigarettes, called a "buddy" for support, talked with an ex-smoker for support)
- Wagers, dares (e.g., made a bet or wager with a friend as a motivator for quitting)
- Treatment (e.g., attended a stop smoking clinic, enrolled in a clinic)

Practiced direct control of smoking
- Cut down (e.g., bought low tar cigarettes, cut back, stopped smoking in the car)
- Satiation (e.g., smoked a cigar or chain smoked to make yourself sick)

Used other techniques
- Self-reward (e.g., put $1 in jar for each day quit, rewarded yourself for 3-hour periods of abstinence)
- Cognitive cueing (e.g., reread your list of reasons for quitting, hung list on refrigerator)
- Other behavioral responses? (list here):

Cognitive coping responses	Yes	No

Thought about the positive health consequences for yourself
- Future (e.g., living longer, being alive for grandchildren, improved health with quitting)
- Immediate (e.g., being able to breathe deeply, no longer waking up coughing, feeling better physically if you quit)

Thought about the negative health consequences for yourself
- Future (e.g., getting cancer, dying, leaving your children and spouse)
- Immediate (e.g., getting frequent colds or chest pains from smoking, feeling sick often)

(continued)

FIGURE 4.9. Coping with Temptation Inventory. From Shiffman (1988). Copyright 1988 by The Guilford Press. Reprinted by permission.

Cognitive coping responses *(continued)*	Yes	No

Thought about the health consequences of smoking on others
- Realized that the health problems of children are due to your smoking, decided that it would be nice for them to have fresh air in the house and car)

Thought about the social consequences
- Positive (e.g., setting a good example for pregnant daughter, making family members happy/proud)
- Negative (e.g., getting nagged by friends, disappointing family members)

Thought about financial consequences
- Thought about having additional money for other purposes, saving more money each month

Thought about other consequences
- Realized that food would taste better, house would smell cleaner if you quit
- Decided you wanted to improve your complexion, feel less nervous/jittery by quitting
- Decided smoking smells bad and is offensive to others
- Thought about yellow teeth and discolored fingers from smoking
- Thought about having bad breath and not being "kissable"

Downplayed the value of smoking
- General devaluation (e.g., told yourself "It's not worth it; smoking is gross; I'm sick of cigarettes")
- Disappointment in smoking habit (e.g., realized that cigarettes are not a solution to daily hassles, smoking doesn't make you feel better, smoking doesn't improve anything)
- Sensory devaluation (e.g., reminded yourself that smoking tasted bad)

Used self-talk
- Self-motivation (e.g., kept telling yourself that you don't want cigarettes and don't need them, reviewed your reasons for quitting)
- Willpower (e.g., gave yourself orders not to smoke, told yourself "no" when you were tempted)
- Self-redefinition (e.g., told yourself "I'm a nonsmoker" and visualized yourself as a nonsmoker)
- Positive thoughts (e.g., told yourself "I can do it," gave yourself pats on the back for each period of abstinence, reminded yourself that quitting smoking would get easier each day)
- General positive attitudes (e.g., kept a positive attitude toward the process of quitting)

Used orienting thoughts
- Planning (e.g., made specific plans for coping with temptations, set a quit date, practiced self-monitoring of smoking)
- Temporal orientation (e.g., thought about quitting smoking 1 hour at a time, reminded yourself about getting through day by day, remembered that there would be ups and downs)

Used alternative cognitions
- Distraction (e.g., pushed thoughts about smoking out of your head, kept your mind busy)
- Relaxation (e.g., took "mental vacations" to manage stress, thought about peaceful memories)

Experienced other cognitions
- Remorse (e.g., accused yourself of being weak or lacking willpower, told yourself "I'm an idiot")
- Guilt (e.g., felt guilty about slipping or relapsing, told yourself "I haven't really tried hard enough")
- Consequences of the slips (e.g., said to yourself "If I have one cigarette, I will relapse; it must be all or nothing"; told yourself "I've gotten this far; it's not worth blowing it now")
- Minimizing slips (e.g., told yourself "One cigarette doesn't mean complete relapse; I don't have to go back to being a smoker")

FIGURE 4.9. *(continued)*

one form of coping is better suited to preventing relapses than the other (Shiffman, Paty, et al., 1996; Shiffman, Hickox, et al., 1996).

Lapse and Relapse Crises

Assuming that a given smoker is initially successful at quitting, there is a high probability that he or she will lapse within the first 2 weeks of this attempt. As such, it is important to be able to conduct an assessment as soon as possible after the lapse or relapse to determine three factors: (1) circumstances surrounding the event (e.g., trigger situation, craving, withdrawal experienced, affect, presence–absence of others); (2) attempts at immediate coping (as reviewed earlier); and (3) attempts at restorative coping (Figure 4.10). This information provides a framework within which additional interventions may be directed.

The following questions deal with the circumstances in which you were recently tempted to smoke or did not smoke. Please answer each one:

Where were you?

____ Home ___ Work ___ Someone else's home   ___ A restaurant or bar
____ A vehicle   ___ Other (please identify) _____

What were you doing?

____ Working   ___ Eating or drinking ___ Socializing ___ Relaxing
____ Other (please identify)_____

Had you been consuming: ____ coffee ___ alcohol

Were other people with you? ____ Yes ___ No
   If Yes: How many of them were smoking? ____

Were cigarettes available?   ____ Yes ___ No
   If Yes: From what source? _____

If you smoked, how did you get the cigarette? _____

How were you feeling? ____ Happy___ Depressed   ___ Relaxed
____ Anxious   ___ Neutral   ___ Angry

How did you feel after the episode was over?

_____

If you did not smoke, what did you do to keep yourself from smoking?

_____

FIGURE 4.10. Relapse Debriefing Form.

SPECIAL ISSUES IN ASSESSMENT

Assessment for Harm Reduction

The goal of smoking cessation treatment is ultimately to reduce death and disease due to tobacco use. Thus, for smokers who cannot quit smoking completely, behavior changes that reduce the harm of smoking may have some benefit. The promotion of harm reduction strategies raises a host of policy issues too complex to review or address here. Suffice it to say the benefits of various harm reduction strategies and the potential risks of promoting them are difficult to assess at this time. This is in contrast to complete abstinence, whose benefits are well-documented. Broadly, then, harm reduction strategies make the most sense when two conditions are met: (1) when complete cessation is not a realistic option, and (2) when the pattern of alternative behavior has a realistic prospect of reducing the harm due to smoking.

This suggests the assessment strategy needed to consider harm-reduction strategies. The clinician must first evaluate whether complete cessation is a realistic option using the measures of motivation described earlier. Cessation might be considered an unrealistic near-term option under two circumstances:

1. When a smoker expresses willingness to attempt smoking reduction but rejects cessation as a goal. To establish this, it is important to assess interest in cessation and confirm rejection of abstinence in the near or middle term. In this situation, it may be fruitful to engage the smoker in a program of reduction.
2. When a smoker who has attempted cessation is relapsing, and rejects the possibility of recycling into another cessation attempt.

Second, the clinician must ensure that the behavior adopted under the guide of harm reduction in fact has some realistic prospect of reducing harm. When the harm reduction strategy involves adoption of some new product (e.g., oral tobacco or novel cigarettes claiming reduced harm), this involves assessing whether the product itself is less toxic. The clinician will rarely be in a position to judge this directly, but must rely on credible scientific sources. The absence of a science-based regulatory authority, such as the Food and Drug Administration, with authority over tobacco products, vastly complicates this assessment. The clinician will have more opportunity to assess the individual smoker's behavior, to ensure that it is consistent with harm reduction. If reduced smoking is adopted as a goal, it is essential to ensure that there are real reductions in exposure to tobacco-related toxins. Because smokers seek to maintain nicotine levels and because cigarettes are very flexible dosing forms, even smokers who truly reduce the number of cigarettes smoked may inadvertently maintain their original exposure to tobacco toxins. This makes it essential to monitor biochemical exposure, using biochemical markers. Carbon monoxide (CO), while far from an adequate marker of toxic exposures, is probably the most practical marker for clinical use. If CO levels are not dropping sharply, it is unlikely that exposure to tobacco toxins is being reduced. (The converse is not true: There could be substantial reductions in CO without meaningful reductions in toxicity, because other toxins in smoke may not be reduced.)

If a smoker adopts use of an alternative tobacco product, it is also essential to ensure that it is adopted in place of smoking and not in addition to it. For example, a smoker who starts using oral tobacco in addition to smoking (a common pattern) may well increase rather than decrease risk. In general, adoption of harm reduction strategies for tobacco use is fraught with complexity and risk, and should be undertaken cautiously.

Assessment for Medication

As we noted at the outset, efficacy of cognitive-behavioral treatments can be improved with the addition of a pharmacological adjunct (Fiore et al., 2000). Several different pharmacotherapies are currently available as adjuncts to cognitive-behavioral treatment. Nicotine gum and transdermal nicotine replacement are currently available over the counter. The nicotine inhaler and nicotine nasal spray are also relatively recent (by prescription) additions to this market. Zyban is also available by prescription as the only approved non-nicotine replacement product for use with smoking cessation. Some data have indicated that ad lib use of nicotine gum is effective at combating acute, breakthrough craving (Shiffman et al., 2003) and that 24-hour nicotine patches may effectively blunt early morning craving, making people who experience more craving in the morning less susceptible to smoking (Shiffman, Elash, et al., 2000). This suggests that smokers with morning craving should be steered toward 24-hour patch treatment. Although more highly dependent smokers derive greater benefit from pharmacotherapy (because they do more poorly in the absence of treatment), the research clearly indicates that all smokers benefit from pharmacological treatment, and clinical guidelines (Fiore et al., 2000) dictate that all smokers be offered pharmacological treatment. There is not yet an adequate evidence base for treatment matching between smoker types and particular forms of treatment (e.g., patch vs. gum). In the absence of specific guidelines recommending one form of treatment over another, though, a useful clinical approach is to interview the smoker about prior experiences (relative successes and failures) with pharmacological treatments and any specific problems (i.e., side effects) experienced during a last attempt. Personal preference is also a useful indicator of which pharmacological intervention is best suited to a particular smoker.

Assessment of Genetic Risk

Genetic testing has become an important component for primary prevention of a number of a number of diseases and disorders (Harper, 1997). Genetic susceptibility to lung cancer has been identified (Law, Hetzel, & Idel, 1989). Given that smoking is a major risk factor for developing lung cancer (U.S. Department of Health and Human Services, 1989), genetic testing has been implemented as part of an intervention to boost personal motivation for smoking cessation: Studies have shown that giving feedback about genetic susceptibility to lung cancer to smokers as part of a brief smoking cessation treatment can predict some smoking outcomes (Lerman et al., 1997). The testing itself can be expensive and is not normally considered a routine part of assessment, however. Future research is needed to understand more fully the role that genetic testing may or may not have in smoking cessation assessment. More germane to treatment itself, some research is beginning to demonstrate gene × treatment interactions for particular forms of pharmacotherapy (Niaura & Abrams, 2002), suggesting that the future may allow tailoring of pharmacological strategy to genetic patterns.

CONCLUSIONS

Substantial progress has been made in developing and validating smoking-related measures covering a broad array of domains, including behavior, biological attributes, attitudes, and beliefs. Thus, a clinician has a large corpus of mostly reliable and valid assessments available for use, many of which have been reviewed here (see Table 4.1 for an abbreviated summary of all theory-driven assessments reviewed in this chapter). Concomitant progress has not been made, though, in establishing empirically validated algorithms that the assessment to treatment, and in demonstrating that such assessments can constructively influence and guide treatment to enhance clinical outcomes. As a result, the clinical application of assessment in smoking cessation remains more art or intuition than science.

AUTHOR NOTES

Saul Shiffman consults to GlaxoSmithKline exclusively on matters related to smoking cessation. He also has an interest in a new smoking cessation product, and is a cofounder of and stakeholder in invivodata, inc., which markets electronic diaries for clinical trials.

ACKNOWLEDGMENTS

Preparation of this chapter was supported, in part, by Grant No. R01 CA081291. Both authors have acted as consultants to companies marketing pharmaceutical products for smoking cessation.

TABLE 4.1. Summary of Smoking Assessment Measures

Purpose	Domain/ construct	Instrument(s)/method(s)	Author(s)
Assessment of severity, habit	Smoking rate	—	—
	Smoking patterns	Global self-report	Ossip-Klein et al. (1986)
	Smoking motives	Ikard et al. (1969) McKennel (1970)	
		Time-line follow-back	Brown et al. (1998)
		Self-monitoring	Abrams & Wilson (1979)
		EMA	Stone & Shiffman (1994) Shiffman, Gwaltney, et al. (2002)
		CO, cotinine	Kozlowski & Herling (1988)
	Nicotine dependence	DSM-IV	American Psychiatric Association (1994)
		FTND	Heatherton et al. (1991)
		Cigarette Dependence Scale	Etter et al. (2003)
		Nicotine Dependence Syndrome Scale	Shiffman, Waters, et al. (2004)
	Withdrawal	DSM IV	American Psychiatric Association (1994)
		Shiffman–Jarvik Scale	Shiffman & Jarvik (1976)
		Withdrawal Checklist	Hughes & Hatsukami (1986)
		Wisconsin Smoking Withdrawal Scale	Welsch et al. (1999)
	Craving	Questionnaire of Smoking Urges	Tiffany & Drobes (1990) Cox et al. (2001)
		Shiffman–Jarvik Scale	Shiffman & Jarvik (1976)
		Craving scale	Shiffman et al. (2003)
Quitting related	Motivation to quit	Stages of change	Prochaska et al. (1992)
		Readiness to quit ladder	Abrams & Beiner (1992)
	Social support	Partner Interaction Questionnaire	Mermelstein et al. (1983)
	Self-efficacy	Confidence Questionnaire	Condiotte & Lichtenstein (1981)
		Confidence Inventory	Velicer et al. (1990)
		Relapse Situation Efficacy Questionnaire	Gwaltney et al. (2001)
	Outcome expectancies	Smoking Consequences Questionnaire	Brandon & Baker (1991)
	Coping	Coping with Temptation Inventory	Shiffman (1988)

REFERENCES

Abrams, D. B., & Biener, L. (1992). Motivational characteristics of smokers at the worksite: A public health challenge. *International Journal of Preventive Medicine, 21*, 679–687.

Abrams, D. B., Borrelli, B., Shadel, W. G., King, T., Bock, B., & Niaura, R. (1998). Adherence to treatment for nicotine dependence. In S. A. Shumaker, E. Schron, J. Ockene, & W. McBee (Eds.), *Handbook of health behavior change* (pp. 137–165). New York: Springer.

Abrams, D. B., Monti, P. M., Carey, K., Pinto, R., & Jacobus, S. I. (1988). Reactivity to smoking cues and relapse: Two studies of discriminant validity. *Behaviour Research and Therapy, 26*(3), 225–233.

Abrams, D. B., Monti, P. M., Pinto, R., Elder, J. P., Brown, R. A., & Jacobus, S. I. (1987). Psychosocial stress and coping in smokers who relapse or quit. *Health Psychology, 6*(4), 289–303.

Abrams, D. B., Niaura, R., Brown, R. A., Emmons, K. M., Goldstein, M. G., & Monti, P. M. (Eds.). (2003). *The tobacco dependence treatment handbook.* New York: Guilford Press.

Abrams, D. B., & Wilson, G. T. (1979). Self-monitoring and reactivity in the modification of cigarette smoking. *Journal of Consulting and Clinical Psychology, 47*(2), 243–251.

Ajzen, I., & Fishbein, M. (1980). *Understanding attitudes and predicting social behavior.* Angle Cliffs, NJ: Prentice-Hall.

American Psychiatric Association (1994). *Diagnostic and statistical manual of mental disorders* (4th ed.). Washington, DC: Author.

Anda, R. F., Williamson, D. F., Escobedo, L. G., Mast, E. E., Giovino, G. A., & Remington, P. L. (1990). Depression and the dynamics of smoking. *Journal of the American Medical Association, 264*(12), 1541–1545.

Baer, J., & Lichtenstein, E. (1988). Cognitive assessment. In D. M. Donovan & G. A. Marlatt (Eds.), *Assessment of addictive behaviors* (pp. 189–213). New York: Guilford Press.

Baker, T., Piper, M., McCarthy, D., Majeskie, M., & Fiore, M. (2004). Addiction motivation reformulated: An affective processing model of negative reinforcement. *Psychological Review, 111*, 33–51.

Bandura, A. (1997). *Self-efficacy: The exercise of control.* New York: Freeman.

Battjes, R. J. (1988). Smoking as an issue in alcohol and drug abuse treatment. *Addictive Behaviors, 13*, 225–230.

Bauer, M. S. (2003). *Field guide to psychiatric assessment and treatment.* Philadelphia: Lippincott Williams & Wilkins.

Biener, L., & Abrams, D. B. (1991). The contemplation ladder: Validation of a meaure of readiness to consider smoking cessation. *Health Psychology, 10*, 360–365.

Brandon, T., & Baker, T. (1991). The smoking consequences questionnaire: The subjective expected utility of smoking in college students. *Psychological Assessment, 3*, 484–491.

Brandon, T., Juliano, L., & Copeland, A. (1999). Expectancies for tobacco smoking. In I. Kirsch (Ed.), *How expectancies shape experience* (pp. 263–299). Washington, DC: American Psychological Association.

Brandon, T. H., Copeland, A. L., & Saper, Z. L. (1995). Programmed therapeutic messages as a smoking treatment adjunct: Reducing the impact of negative affect. *Health Psychology, 14*, 41–47.

Breslau, N., Kilbey, M., & Andreski, P. (1994). DSM-III-R nicotine dependence in young adults: Prevalence, correlates and associated psychiatric disorders. *Addiction, 89,* 743–754

Brown, L. (1978). Nonanalytic concept formation and memory for instances. In E. Rosch & B. Lloyd (Eds.), *Cognition and categorization* (pp. 169–211). Hillsdale, NJ: Erlbaum.

Brown, R. A., Burgess, E. S., Sales, S. D., Whiteley, J. A., Evans, D., & Miller, I. W. (1998). Reliability and validity of a smoking timeline follow-back interview. *Psychology of Addictive Behaviors, 12*, 101–112.

Burling, T. A., & Ziff, D. C. (1988). Tobacco smoking: A comparison between alcohol and drug abuse inpatients. *Addictive Behaviors, 13,* 185–190.

Carlson, L., Goodey, E., Bennett, M. H., Taenzer, P., & Koopmans, J. (2000). The addition of social support to a community-based large-group behavioral smoking cessation intervention: Improved cessation rates and gender differences. *Addictive Behaviors, 27*, 547–559.

Centers for Disease Control and Prevention. (1994). Cigarette smoking among adults—United States 1993. *Morbidity and Mortality Weekly Report, 43*, 925–930.

Clarke, J. G., Stein, M. D., McGarry, K. A., & Gogineni, A. (2001). Interest in smoking cessation among injection drug users. *American Journal on Addictions, 10*, 159–166.

Cohen, S., Lichtenstein, E., Prochaska, J. O., Rossi, J. S., Gritz, E. R., Carr, C. R., et al. (1989). Debunking myths about self-quitting: Evidence from 10 prospective studies of persons who attempt to quit smoking by themselves. *American Psychologist, 44*, 1355–1365.

Condiotte, M. M., & Lichtenstein, E. (1981). Self-efficacy and relapse in smoking cessation programs. *Journal of Consulting and Clinical Psychology, 49*, 648–658.

Cooney, N., Litt, M., & Cooney, J. (2002). *In vivo* assessment of the effects of smoking cessation in alcoholic smokers. *Alcoholism: Clinical and Experimental Research, 26*, 1952–1953.

Copeland, A., Brandon, T., & Quinn, E. (1995). The Smoking Consequences Questionnaire—Adult: Measurement of smoking outcome expectancies of experienced smokers. *Psychological Assessment, 7*, 484–494.

Cox, L. S., Tiffany, S. T., & Christen, A. G. (2001). Evaluation of the brief questionnaire of smoking urges (QSU—Brief) in laboratory and clinical settings. *Nicotine and Tobacco Research, 3*, 7–16.

Curry, S. J., Grothaus, L., & McBride, C. M. (1997). Reasons for quitting: Intrinsic and extrinsic motivation for smoking cessation in a population-based sample of smokers. *Addictive Behaviors, 22*, 727–739.

DiFranza, J. R., & Guerrera, M. P. (1990). Alcoholism and smoking. *Journal of Studies on Alcohol, 51,* 130–135.

Dobbs, S. D., Strickler, D. P., & Maxwell, W. A. (1981). The effects of stress and relaxation in the presence of stress on urinary pH and smoking behaviors. *Addictive Behaviors, 6*, 345–353.

Edwards, G., & Gross, M. (1976). Alcohol dependence: Provisional description of a clinical syndrome. *British Medical Journal, 1*, 1058–1061.

Etter, J. F., Le-Houezec, J., & Perneger, T. (2003). A self-administered questionnaire to measure dependence on cigarettes: The Cigarette Dependence Scale. *Neuropsychopharmacology, 28,* 359–370.

Fagerstrom, K. O. (1978). Measuring degree of physical dependence to tobacco smoking with reference to individuation of treatment. *Addictive Behaviors, 3,* 235–241.

Fagerstrom, K., & Schneider, N. (1989). Measuring nicotine dependence: A review of the Fagerstrom Tolerance Questionnaire. *Journal of Behavioral Medicine, 12*(2), 159–182.

Farkas, A. J., Pierce, J. P., Zhu, S., Rosbrook, B., Gilpin, E. A., Berry, C., & Kaplan, R. M. (1996). Addiction versus stage of change models in predicting smoking cessation. *Addiction, 91*(9), 1271–1280.

Fiore, M., Baily, W. C., Cohen, S. J., et al. (2000). *Treating tobacco use and dependence: Clinical practice guideline.* Rockville, MD: U.S. Department of Health and Human Services.

Frederick, T., Frerichs, R. R., & Clark, V. A. (1988). Personal health habits and symptoms of depression at the community level. *Preventive Medicine, 17,* 173–182.

Glassman, A. H. (1993). Cigarette smoking: Implications for psychiatric illness. *American Journal of Psychiatry, 150,* 546–553.

Glassman, A. H., Helzer, J. E., Covey, L. S., Cottler, L. B., Stetner, F., Tipp, J. E., & Johnson, J. (1990). Smoking, smoking cessation, and major depression. *Journal of the American Medical Association, 264,* 1546–1549.

Gottlieb, A. M., Killen, J. D., Marlatt, G. A., & Taylor, C. B. (1987). Psychological and pharmacological influences in cigarette smoking withdrawal: Effects of nicotine gum and expectancy on smoking withdrawal symptoms and relapse. *Journal of Consulting and Clinical Psychology, 55*(4), 606–608.

Gwaltney, C. J., Shiffman, S., Norman, G. J., Paty, J. A., Kassel, D., Gnys, M., et al. (2001). Does smoking abstinence self-efficacy vary across situations?: Identifying context-specificity within the Relapse Situation Efficacy Questionnaire. *Journal of Consulting and Clinical Psychology, 69,* 516–527.

Hall, R., Duhamel, M., McClanahan, R., Miles, G., Nason, C., Rosen, S., Schiller, P., Tao-Yonenaga, L., & Hall, S. M. (1995). Level of functioning, severity of illness, and smoking status among chronic psychiatric patients. *Journal of Nervous and Mental Disease, 183*(7), 468–471.

Hammersley, R. (1994). A digest of memory phenomena for addiction research. *Addiction, 89,* 283–293.

Harper, P. S. (1997). What do we mean by genetic testing? *Journal of Medical Genetics, 34,* 749–752.

Heatherton, T. F., Kozlowski, L. T., Frecker, R. C., & Fagerstrom, K. O. (1991). The Fagerstrom Test for Nicotine Dependence: A revision of the Fagerstrom Tolerance Questionnaire. *British Journal of Addiction, 86,* 1119–1127.

Heatherton, T. F., Kozlowski, L. T., Frecker, R. C., Rickert, W., & Robinson, T. E. (1989). Measuring the heaviness of smoking: Using self-reported time to the first cigarette of the day and number of cigarettes smoked per day. *British Journal of Addiction, 84,* 791–799.

Herzog, T. H., Abrams, D. B., Emmons, K. M., Linnan, L., & Shadel, W. G. (1999). Do processes of change predict smoking stage movements?: A prospective analysis of the transtheoretical model. *Health Psychology, 18,* 369–375.

Hitsman, B., Borrelli, B., McChargue, D., Spring, B., & Niaura, R. (2003). History of depression and smoking cessation outcome: A meta-analysis. *Journal of Consulting and Clinical Psychology, 71,* 657–663.

Hughes, J. R. (1993). Pharmacotherapy for smoking cessation: Unvalidated assumptions, anomalies, and suggestions for future research. *Journal of Consulting and Clinical Psychology, 61,* 751–760.

Hughes, J. R., Gust, S. W., Skoog, K. P., Keenan, R. M., & Fenwick, J. W. (1991). Symptoms of tobacco withdrawal: A replication and extension. *Archives of General Psychiatry, 48,* 52–59.

Hughes, J. R., & Hatsukami, D. (1986). Signs and symptoms of tobacco withdrawal. *Archives of General Psychiatry, 43,* 289–294.

Hughes, J. R., Hatsukami, D. K., Mitchell, J. E., & Dahlgren, L. A. (1986). Prevalence of smoking among psychiatric outpatients. *American Journal of Psychiatry, 143*(8), 993–997.

Hughes, J. R., Higgins, S. T., & Hatsukami, D. K. (1990). Effects of abstinence from tobacco. In L. T. Kozlowski, H. M. Annis, & H. D. Cappell (Eds.), *Recent advances in alcohol and drug problems* (pp. 317–398). New York: Plenum Press.

Hughes, J. R., Keeley, J. P., Niaura, R., Ossip-Klein, D., Richmond, R., & Swan, G. (2003). Measures of abstinence in clinical trials: Issues and recommendations. *Nicotine and Tobacco Research, 5,* 13–26.

Ikard, F., Green, P., & Horn, D. (1969). A scale to differentiate between types of smoking as related to the management of affect. *International Journal of the Addictions, 4,* 649–659.

Jamner, L., Shapiro, D., & Jarvik, M. (1999). Nicotine reduces the frequency of anger reports in smokers and nonsmokers with high but not low hostility: An ambulatory study. *Experimental and Clinical Psychopharmacology, 7,* 454–463.

Juliano, L., & Brandon, T. (2002). Effect of nicotine dose, instructional set, and outcome expectancies on the subjective effects of smoking in the presence of a stressor. *Journal of Abnormal Psychology, 111,* 88–97.

Kassel, J., & Shiffman, S. (1992). What can hunger teach us about drug craving?: A comparative analysis of the two constructs. *Advances in Behaviour Research and Therapy, 14,* 141–167.

Kassel, J., Stroud, L., & Paronis, C. (2003). Smoking, stress, and negative affect: Correlation, causation, and context across stages of smoking. *Psychological Bulletin, 129,* 270–304.

Kassel, J., & Yates, M. (2002). Is there a role for assessment in smoking cessation treatment? *Behaviour Research and Therapy, 40,* 1457–1470.

Killen, J., & Fortman, S. (1997). Craving is associated with smoking relapse: Evidence from three prospective studies. *Experimental and Clinical Psychopharmacology, 5*(2), 137–142.

King, T. K., Borrelli, B., Black, C., Pinto, B. M., & Marcus, B. H. (1997). Minority women and tobacco: Implications for smoking cessation interventions. *Annals of Behavioral Medicine, 19,* 301–313.

Kozlowski, L., & Herling, S. (1988). Objective measures. In D. M. Donovan & G. A. Marlatt (Eds.), *Assessment of addictive behaviors* (pp. 214–238). New York: Guilford Press.

Kozlowski, L., Pillitteri, J., Sweeney, C., Whitfield, K., & Graham, J. (1996). Asking about urges or cravings for cigarettes. *Psychology of Addictive Behaviors, 10,* 248–260.

Kozlowski, L. T., Porter, C. Q., Orleans, C. T., Pope, M. A., & Heatherton, T. (1994). Predicting smoking cessation with self-reported measures of nicotine dependence: FTQ, FTND, and HSI. *Drug and Alcohol Dependence, 34*, 211–216.

Lando, H., Haddock, C. K., Robinson, L. A., Klesges, R. C., & Talcott, GW. (2000). Ethnic differences in patterns and correlates of age of initiation in a population of Air Force recruits. *Nicotine and Tobacco Research, 2*, 337–344.

Law, M. R., Hetzel, M. R., & Idel, J. R. (1989). Debrisoquine metabolism and genetic predisposition to lung cancer. *British Journal of Cancer, 59*, 686–687.

Lerman, C., Gold, K., Audrain, J., et al. (1997). Incorporating biomarkers of exposure and genetic susceptibility into smoking cessation treatment: Effects on smoking-related cognitions, emotions, and behavior change. *Health Psychology, 16*, 87–99.

Marlatt, G. A., & Gordon, J. (1985). *Relapse prevention*. New York: Guilford Press.

McKennel, Z. (1970). Smoking motivation factors. *British Journal of Social and Clinical Psychology, 9*, 8–22.

McMahon, S., & Jason, L. A. (2000). Social support in a worksite smoking intervention: A test of theoretical models. *Behavior Modification, 24*, 184–201.

Mermelstein, R., Cohen, S., Lichtenstein, E., Baer, J., & Kamarck, T. (1986). Social support and smoking cessation and maintenance. *Journal of Consulting and Clinical Psychology, 54*, 447–453.

Mermelstein, R., Lichtenstein, E., & McIntyre, K. (1983). Partner support and relapse in smoking cessation programs. *Journal of Consulting and Clinical Psychology, 51*, 465–466.

Miller, W., & Rollnick, S. (1991). *Motivational interviewing*. New York: Guilford Press.

Murray, R., Johnston, J., Dolce, J., Lee, W., & O'Hara, P. (1995). Social support for smoking cessation and abstinence: The Lung Health Study. *Addictive Behaviors, 20*(2), 159–170.

National Cancer Institute. (1997). *Changes in cigarette-related disease risks and their implication for prevention and control* (NIH Publication No. 97-4213). Washington, DC: U.S. Government Printing Office.

Niaura, R., & Abrams, D. (2002). Smoking cessation: Progress, priorities, and prospectus. *Journal of Consulting and Clinical Psychology, 70*, 494–509.

Niaura, R., Britt, D., Shadel, W. G., Goldstein, M. G., & Abrams, D. B. (2001). Symptoms of depression and survival experience in three samples of smokers. *Psychology of Addictive Behaviors, 15*, 13–17.

Niaura, R., Goldstein, M., & Abrams, D. (1994). Matching high- and low-dependence smokers to self-help treatment with or without nicotine replacement. *Preventive Medicine, 23*, 70–77.

Niaura, R., Shadel, W. G., Abrams, D., Monti, P., Rohsenow, D., & Sirota, A. (1998). Individual differences in cue reactivity among smokers trying to quit: Effects of gender and cue type. *Addictive Behaviors, 23*, 209–224.

Ockene, J., Emmons, K., Mermelstein, R., Perkins, K., Bonollo, D., Voorhees, C., & Hollis, J. (2000). Relapse and maintenance issues for smoking cessation. *Health Psychology, 19*(Suppl.), 17–31.

O'Connell, K. A., Gerkovich, M. M., Cook, M. R., Shiffman, S., Hickcox, M., & Kakolewski, K. E. (1998). Coping in real time: Using Ecological Momentary Assessment techniques to assess coping with the urge to smoke. *Research in Nursing and Health, 21*(6), 487–497.

Ossip-Klein, D. J., Bigelow, G., Parker, S. R., Curry, S., Hall, S., & Kirkland, S. (1986) Task Force 1: Classification and assessment of smoking behavior. *Health Psychology, 5,* 3–11.

Paty, J., Kassel, J., & Shiffman, S. (1992). The importance of assessing base rates for clinical studies: An example of stimulus control of smoking. In M. W. deVries (Ed.), *The experience of psychopathology: Investigating mental disorders in their natural settings* (pp. 347–352). New York: Cambridge University Press.

Perkins, K. A., & Grobe, J. E. (1992). Increased desire to smoke during acute stress. *British Journal of Addiction, 87,* 1037–1040.

Piasecki, T., Fiore, M., & Baker, T. (1997). Profiles in discouragement: Two studies of variability in the timecourse of smoking withdrawal symptoms. *Journal of Abnormal Psychology, 107,* 238–251.

Piasecki, T. M., Fiore, M. C., McCarthy, D. E., & Baker, T. B. (2002). Have we lost our way? The need for dynamic formulations of smoking relapse proneness. *Addiction, 97,* 1093–1108.

Pomerleau, O., Adkins, D., & Pertschuk, M. (1978). Predictors of outcome and recidivism in smoking cessation treatment. *Addictive Behaviors, 3*(2), 65–70.

Prochaska, J. O., DiClemente, C. C., & Norcross, J. C. (1992). In search of how people change: Applications to addictive behaviors. *American Psychologist, 47,* 1102–1114.

Prochaska, J. O., Velicer, W. F., Rossi, J. S., Goldstein, M. G., Marcus, B. H., Rakowski, W., Fiore, C., Harlow, L. L., Redding, C. A., Rosenbloom, D., & Rossi, S. R. (1994). Stages of change and decisional balance for 12 problem behaviors. *Health Psychology, 13,* 39–46.

Razdius, A., Moolchan, E., Henningfield, J., Heishman, S. J., & Gallo, J. (2001). A factor analysis of the Fagerstrom Tolerance Questionnaire. *Addictive Behaviors, 26,* 303–310.

Risser, N. L., & Belcher, D. W. (1990). Adding spirometry, carbon monoxide, and pulmonary symptom results to smoking cessation counseling: A randomized trial. *Journal of General Internal Medicine, 5,* 16–22.

Ross, L. (1989). The relation of implicit theories to the construction of personal histories. *Psychological Review, 96,* 341–357.

Rounsaville, B. J., Kosten, T. R., Weissman, M. M., & Kleber, H. D. (Eds.). (1985). *Evaluating and treating depressive disorders in opiate addicts* (DHHS Publication No. [ADM] 85-1406]. Washington, DC: U.S. Government Printing Office.

Sayette, M., Shiffman, S., Tiffany, S., Niaura, R., Carter, C., & Shadel, W. G. (2000). The measurement of drug craving. *Addiction, 95,* 189–210.

Shadel, W. G. (2004). Introduction to the special series: What can personality science offer cognitive-behavioral therapy and research? *Behavior Therapy, 35*(1), 101–111.

Shadel, W. G., Cervone, D., Niaura, R., & Abrams, D. B. (2004). Developing an integrative social-cognitive strategy for personality assessment at the level of the individual: An illustration with regular cigarette smokers. *Journal of Research in Personality, 38*(4), 394–419.

Shadel, W. G., & Mermelstein, R. J. (1993). Cigarette smoking under stress: The role of coping expectancies among smokers in a clinic-based smoking cessation program. *Health Psychology, 12,* 443–450.

Shadel, W. G., & Mermelstein, R. (1996). Individual differences in self-concept among smokers attempting to quit: Validation and predictive utility of measures of the

Smoker Self-Concept and Abstainer Self-Concept. *Annals of Behavioral Medicine, 18,* 151–156.

Shadel, W. G., Niaura, R., & Abrams, D. (2000). An idiographic approach to understanding personality structure and individual differences among smokers. *Cognitive Therapy and Research, 24,* 345–359.

Shadel, W. G., Shiffman, S., Niaura, R., Nichter, M., & Abrams, D. B. (2000). Current models of nicotine dependence: What is known and what is needed to advance understanding of tobacco etiology among youth. *Drug and Alcohol Dependence, 59,* 9–22.

Shiffman, S. (1982). Relapse following smoking cessation: A situational analysis. *Journal of Consulting and Clinical Psychology, 50,* 71–86.

Shiffman, S. (1986). A cluster-analytic classification of smoking relapse episodes. *Addictive Behaviors, 11,* 295–307.

Shiffman, S. (1988). Behavioral assessment. In D. M. Donovan & G. A. Marlatt (Eds.), *Assessment of addictive behavior* (pp. 139–199). New York: Guilford Press.

Shiffman, S. (1991). Refining models of dependence: Variations across persons and situations. *British Journal of Addiction, 86,* 611–615.

Shiffman, S. (1993a). Assessing smoking patterns and motives. *Journal of Consulting and Clinical Psychology, 61,* 732–742.

Shiffman, S. (1993b). Smoking cessation treatment: Any progress? *Journal of Consulting and Clinical Psychology, 61,* 718–722.

Shiffman, S., Balabanis, M., Paty, J., Engberg, J., Gwaltney, C., Liu, K., Hickcox, M., Gnys, M., & Paton, S. (2000). Dynamic effects of self-efficacy on smoking lapse and relapse. *Health Psychology, 19,* 315–323.

Shiffman, S., Elash, C. A., Paton, S. M., Gwaltney, C. J., Paty, J. A., & Clark, D. B. (2000). Comparative efficacy of 24–hour and 16–hour transdermal nicotine patches for relief of morning craving. *Addiction, 95,* 1185–1195.

Shiffman, S., Engberg, J., Paty, J. A., Perz, W., Gnys, M., Kassel, J. D., & Hickcox, M. (1997). A day at a time: Predicting smoking lapse from daily urge. *Journal of Abnormal Psychology, 106,* 104–116.

Shiffman, S., Gwaltney, C., Balabanis, M. H., Liu, K. S., Paty, J. A., Kassel, J. D., Hickcox, M., & Gnys, M. (2002). Immediate antecedents of cigarette smoking: An analysis from ecological momentary assessment. *Journal of Abnormal Psychology, 111*(4), 531–545.

Shiffman, S., Hickcox, M., Paty, J., Gnys, M., Kassel, J., & Richards, T. (1996). Progression from a smoking lapse to relapse: Prediction from abstinence violation effects, nicotine dependence, and lapse characteristics. *Journal of Consulting and Clinical Psychology, 64,* 993–1002.

Shiffman, S., & Jarvik, M. (1976). Trends in withdrawal symptoms in abstinence from cigarette smoking. *Psychopharmacologia, 50,* 35–39.

Shiffman, S., Paty, J. A., Kassel, J. D., Gnys, M., & Zettler-Segal, M. (1994). Smoking behavior and smoking history of tobacco chippers. *Experimental and Clinical Psychopharmacology, 2,* 126–142.

Shiffman, S., Paty, J., Kassel, J., & Hickcox, M. (1996). First lapses to smoking: Within-subjects analysis of real-time reports. *Journal of Consulting and Clinical Psychology, 62,* 366–379.

Shiffman, S., Read, L., & Jarvik, M. (1985). Smoking relapse situations: A preliminary typology. *International Journal of the Addictions, 20,* 311–318.

Shiffman, S., Shadel, W. G., Niaura, R., Khayrallah, M., Jorenby, D., Ryan, C., & Ferguson, C. (2003). Efficacy of acute administration of nicotine gum in relief of cue-provoked cigarette craving. *Psychopharmacology, 166,* 343–350.

Shiffman, S., Waters, A., & Hickcox, M. (2004). The Nicotine Dependence Syndrome Scale: A multidimensional measure of nicotine dependence. *Nicotine and Tobacco Research, 6,* 327–348.

Shiffman, S., West, R., & Gilbert, D. (2004). Recommendation for the assessment of tobacco craving and withdrawal in smoking cessation trials. *Nicotine and Tobacco Research, 6,* 599–614.

Stone, A. A., & Shiffman, S. (1994). Ecological momentary assessment (EMA) in behavioral medicine. *Annals of Behavioral Medicine, 16,* 199–202.

Stone, A. A., & Shiffman, S. (2002). Capturing momentary, self-report data: A proposal for reporting guidelines. *Annals of Behavioral Medicine, 24,* 236–243.

Tiffany, S., & Drobes, D. (1990). The development and initial validation of a questionnaire on smoking urges. *British Journal of Addiction, 86,* 1467–1476.

U.S. Department of Health and Human Services. (1989). *Reducing the health consequences of smoking: A report of the Surgeon General* (DHHS Publication No. CDC-89-8411). Washington, DC: U.S. Government Printing Office.

Velicer, W., DiClemente, C., Rossi, J., & Prochaska, J. (1990). Relapse situations and self-efficacy: An integrative model. *Addictive Behaviors, 15,* 271–283.

Velicer, W. F., Prochaska, J. O., Rossi, J. S., & Snow, M. G. (1992). Assessing outcome in smoking cessation studies. *Psychological Bulletin, 111,* 23–41.

Welsch, S. K., Smith, S. S., Jorenby, D. E., Wetter, D. W., Fiore, M. C., & Baker, T. B. (1999). Development and validation of the Wisconsin Smoking Withdrawal Scale. *Experimental and Clinical Psychopharmacology, 7,* 354–361.

West, R. J., Hajek, P., & Belcher, M. (1989). Severity of withdrawal symptoms as a predictor of outcome of an attempt to quit smoking. *Psychological Medicine, 19,* 981–985.

Wetter, D., Smith, S., et al. (1994). Smoking outcome expectancies: Factor structure, predictive validity, and discriminant validity. *Journal of Abnormal Psychology, 103,* 801–811.

CHAPTER 5

Assessment of Cocaine Abuse and Dependence

KATHLEEN M. CARROLL
SAMUEL A. BALL

Cocaine dependence remains a serious public health problem in the United States. The 2002 National Survey on Drug Use and Health estimated that in 2002, there were 2 million current cocaine users in the United States (approximately 0.9% of the population) (Substance Abuse and Mental Health Services Administration [SAMHSA], 2003). Although there are some indications that the number of individuals seeking treatment for a primary cocaine use disorder is decreasing (Community Epidemiology Work Group, 2003), the percentage of young adults ages 18–25 who had ever used cocaine increased slightly from 14.9% in 2001 to 15.4% in 2002 (SAMHSA, 2003).

Assessment plays a critical role in understanding, preventing use, and treating individuals with cocaine use disorders. As noted in the landmark first edition of this book (Donovan & Marlatt, 1988), the trend in assessment of addictive behaviors has been to focus on commonalities rather than differences among types of substance abuse. Although there are important differences across drugs of abuse in terms of use patterns, abuse liability, tolerance and withdrawal syndromes, half-life, nature of the clinical population, and so on, in recent years, both research and clinical conceptions of substance use have moved toward recognizing broad similarities in pathological patterns of use across various psychoactive substances (Donovan, 1999; Donovan & Marlatt, 1988; Edwards, Arif, & Hodgson, 1981; Kosten, Rounsaville, & Kleber, 1987). This broader conception of substance use disorders, stressing commonalities across addictive behaviors and substances of abuse, has been codified by the adoption of a uniform set of dependence criteria across substances beginning with the *Diagnostic and Statistical Manual of Mental Disor-*

ders (DSM-III-R) (Rounsaville, Spitzer, & Williams, 1986) and extending through DSM-IV (Cottler et al., 1997; Nathan, 1989). A broader conception of substance use has also been reinforced by research that has pointed to consistencies in factors associated with the development of substance use disorders (Kandel, 1985; Kandel & Logan, 1984; Kandel, Yamaguchi, & Chen, 1992), comorbid disorders and co-occurring problems (McLellan, Luborsky, Woody, & O'Brien, 1980; Rounsaville et al., 1991; Rounsaville, Weissman, Kleber, & Wilber, 1982), predictors of outcome (McLellan et al., 1994), the nature of relapse (Brownell, Marlatt, Lichtenstein, & Wilson, 1986; Hunt, Barnet, & Branch, 1971; Marlatt & Gordon, 1985), and processes of change (Miller & Heather, 1998; Prochaska, DiClemente, & Norcross, 1992) across substance use disorders (Carroll, 1995).

While this chapter focuses specifically on the assessment of cocaine use and dependence and therefore highlights issues that may be specific to or deserving of special focus when working with cocaine-using populations, we also emphasize those assessment strategies and instruments that can be used across a diverse range of populations (see Table 5.1). Using the organizing framework articulated by Peterson and Sobell (1994), we review issues relevant to clinical assessment of cocaine users in four general domains that cut across addictive behaviors: (1) issues related to the diagnosis of cocaine dependence and assessing severity of cocaine dependence, (2) evaluating problems and disorders that co-occur with cocaine dependence, (3) assessment of issues important for treatment planning, and (4) indicators of treatment outcome (Carroll & Rounsaville, 2002). Finally, we explore a small number of issues that are of special consideration among cocaine-using populations.

DIAGNOSIS AND SEVERITY OF DEPENDENCE

There are a wealth of strategies and well-validated instruments for establishing a formal diagnosis of a cocaine use disorder according to DSM or International Classification of Diseases (ICD) criteria (see Babor, 1993, for a detailed summary). These include the Structured Clinical Interview for DSM-IV (SCID; First, Spitzer, Gibbon, & Williams, 1995), the Diagnostic Interview Schedule (DIS; Robins, Helzer, Croughan, & Ratcliff, 1981), and the Composite International Diagnostic Interview (CIDI; Robins, Wing, & Helzer, 1983), all of which apply a similar set of criteria across the various types of substance use disorders (e.g., marijuana, alcohol, cocaine, heroin, and hallucinogen abuse and dependence).

Large-scale epidemiological surveys using these instruments have enhanced our understanding of the nature of cocaine dependence relative to other drug use disorders. For example, compared with marijuana or alcohol use, cocaine dependence tends to develop most quickly after initial use. Using data from the National Comorbidity Survey (NCS; Kessler et al., 1994), Wagner and Anthony (2002) reported that 15–16% of cocaine users developed de-

TABLE 5.1. Major Domains and Selected Assessments for Cocaine-Using Populations

Purpose	Domain/construct	Instrument(s)	Authors
Diagnosis, assessment of severity	Diagnosis of substance use and psychiatric disorders	CIDI	Robins et al. (1983)
		SCID	First et al. (1995)
		DIS	Robins et al. (1981)
	Withdrawal severity	Cocaine Selective Severity Assessment	Kampman et al. (1998)
	Severity of dependence	Substance Dependence Severity Scale (SDSS)	Miele et al. (2000)
		Severity of Dependence Scale (SDS)	Gossop et al. (1995)
	Cocaine craving	Cocaine Craving Questionnaire	Tiffany et al. (1993)
Comorbid disorders and problems	Psychosocial functioning	Addiction Severity Index (ASI)	McLellan et al. (1992)
	HIV risk behaviors	Risk Assessment Battery	Navaline et al. (1994)
		HIV Risk-Taking Behavior Scale	Darke et al. (1991)
	Consequences of use	SIP-R	Miller et al. (1995)
	Neuropsychological functioning	Neuropsychological Screening Battery	Heaton et al. (1990)
Treatment planning	Areas to target	ASI	
	Motivation	URICA	DiClemente & Hughes (1990)
		SOCRATES	Miller & Tonigan (1996)
		Contemplation Ladder	Biener & Abrams (1991)
		Alcohol and Drug Consequences	Cunningham et al. (1997)
		Readiness to Change Questionnaire	Rollnick et al. (1992)
	Commitment to abstinence	Commitment to Abstinence Questionnaire	Hall et al. (1991)
	High-risk situations	Inventory of Drug-Taking Situations	Turner et al. (1997)
	Patterns of drug use, frequency, and intensity of use	Timeline Followback	Sobell & Sobell (1992)

(continued)

TABLE 5.1. *(continued)*

Purpose	Domain/construct	Instrument(s)	Authors
Treatment planning *(cont.)*	Self-efficacy	Situational Confidence Questionnaire	Breslin et al. (2000)
		Drug-Taking Confidence Questionnaire	Sklar et al. (1997)
	Coping skills	Situational Competency Test	Chaney et al. (1978)
		Cocaine Risk Response Test	Carroll et al. (1999)
Treatment outcome	Urine toxicology screening		
	Frequency, quantity of use	Timeline Followback	Sobell & Sobell (1992)
	Concurrent problems	ASI	McLellan et al. (1992)

pendence within 10 years of first cocaine use. In contrast, progression to marijuana or alcohol dependence after initial use tends to occur more slowly, with 8% of first-time marijuana users and 13% of alcohol users becoming dependent within 10 years (Wagner & Anthony, 2002). Furthermore, 5–6% of cocaine users develop dependence within the first year of use, and the peak risk period for cocaine dependence occurs around the ages of 23–25.

Epidemiological research has also confirmed a strong relationship between frequency–quantity of cocaine use and the development of cocaine dependence, with more frequent users and those that use larger amounts per episode more likely to meet dependence criteria (Chen & Kandel, 2002), and between particular routes of administration and cocaine dependence (with intravenous use and smoking associated with higher rates of dependence than intranasal use) (Chen & Kandel, 2002). There has also been considerable controversy regarding differences between crack (smoked) cocaine and cocaine in its powdered form (cocaine hydrochloride), fueled in part by the U.S. judicial system, which imposes much more severe penalties for possessing crack versus cocaine powder. In a thoughtful and highly influential review, Hatsukami and Fischman (1996) noted that the physiological and subjective effects of cocaine are similar regardless of the form used. However, the immediacy of effect, as well as the frequency and amount of use, tend to be much higher when cocaine is smoked or used intravenously. Thus, the greater abuse liability, risk of dependence, and severe consequences associated with using cocaine via smoking or intravenous use appears to be driven more by the efficiency of the delivery systems (e.g., route of administration) than by the specific form of cocaine used.

An important development regarding the DSM diagnosis of cocaine dependence since the first edition of this book is that a more nuanced understanding of the significance of individual dependence criteria is emerging. For example, the specific constellation of dependence criteria met by an individual and the relative sequence with which they develop over time may be important markers of cocaine use severity and progression; that is, among cocaine users, particular temporal patterns of dependence symptoms have been linked to greater risk of progression to cocaine dependence. Shaffer and Eber (2002), using data from the NCS (Anthony, Warner, & Kessler, 1994; Kessler et al., 1994), found that cocaine users whose first symptom is tolerance or withdrawal were several times more likely to develop cocaine dependence than individuals whose early symptoms reflected social consequences only.

As one of its criteria for cocaine dependence, DSM-IV includes withdrawal, defined as a syndrome characterized by depression plus at least two of the following five symptoms: fatigue; vivid, unpleasant dreams; insomnia or hypersomnia; increased appetite; and psychomotor retardation or agitation (American Psychiatric Association, 1994). However, the significance, consistency, and nature of cocaine withdrawal remains controversial (Cottler, Shillington, Compton, Mager, & Spitznagel, 1993; Satel, Kosten, Schuckit, & Fischman, 1993; Satel et al., 1991; Sofuoglu, Dudish-Poulsen, Brown, & Hatsukami, 2003). Several researchers have identified a cocaine withdrawal syndrome that, while not uniformly present during early abstinence in all cocaine abusers, occurs in a significant proportion and is characterized by craving for cocaine, sleep disturbance, fatigue, depression and anxiety, increased appetite, and poor concentration (Cottler et al., 1993). To assess cocaine withdrawal symptoms, Kampman and colleagues (1998) developed the Cocaine Selective Severity Assessment (CSSA), an 18-item measure of cocaine withdrawal severity that has been shown to predict treatment retention among cocaine users without comorbid psychiatric disorders, particularly when used in conjunction with urine toxicology testing (Kampman et al., 2001).

In addition to determining whether a given individual meets criteria for cocaine abuse or dependence, it is also important to determine severity of dependence, which has been shown to be associated with treatment outcome in several studies (McLellan et al., 1994). There are several strategies for assessing severity of dependence, including the newly developed Substance Dependence Severity Scale (Miele et al., 2000), a clinician-rated interview that has been shown to have good psychometric properties and to predict treatment outcome. The Severity of Dependence Scale (SDS; Gossop, Best, Marsden, & Strang, 1997) is a short (5-item) scale that can be used to measure severity of dependence across different classes of drug use (Gossop et al., 1995; Topp & Mattick, 1997). Finally, age of onset of cocaine use or dependence, which is associated with severity of cocaine dependence (as it is for other drug use disorders and alcohol dependence) (Babor et al., 1992; Ball, Carroll, Rounsaville,

& Babor, 1995), may provide a "rough marker" of severity and is comparatively easy to evaluate.

COMORBID DISORDERS AND PROBLEMS

It is rare that treatment-seeking cocaine users have problems solely with cocaine use itself. Like other forms of drug dependence, cocaine dependence is
associated with a host of medical, psychiatric, legal, employment, and social
problems that complicate treatment and confer poorer prognosis if left untreated (Appleby, Dyson, Altman, & Luchins, 1997; Carroll, Powers, Bryant,
& Rounsaville, 1993; McLellan et al., 1994; McLellan, Luborsky, Woody,
O'Brien, & Druley, 1983; McLellan, Luborsky, Woody, O'Brien, & Kron,
1981; Rounsaville, Tierney, Crits-Christoph, Weissman, & Kleber, 1982;
Rounsaville, Weissman, et al., 1982). Moreover, it is often not the drug use itself, but the medical, legal, social, and financial complications of drug use that
lead most cocaine users to seek treatment (Downey, Rosengren, & Donovan,
2001). It is also comparatively well established that treatments that assess and
address comorbid problems among drug users are typically more effective
than those that target cocaine use alone (Alterman, McLellan, & Shifman,
1993; Leshner, 1999; McLellan, Arndt, Metzger, Woody, & O'Brien, 1993;
McLellan, Grissom, Zanis, & Randall, 1997; McLellan et al., 1999; Simpson,
Joe, Fletcher, Hubbard, & Anglin, 1999).

Given the multidimensional nature of cocaine users' comorbid problems,
one of the most useful assessment tools in planning and assessing treatment
outcome for drug-abusing populations, including cocaine users, is the Addiction Severity Index (ASI; McLellan et al., 1980, 1992). It is a semistructured
interview that assesses history, frequency, and consequences of alcohol and
drug use, as well as five additional domains that are commonly associated
with drug use: medical, legal, employment, social/family, and psychological
functioning. Higher scores on the ASI indicate greater severity and need for
treatment in each of these areas. Thus, ASI scores on the six major domains
may be used to profile the individual's major problem areas and thus to plan
effective treatment. Elevations in the psychological section indicate need for
attention to psychological symptoms; elevations in the medical section indicate need for medical intervention, and so on. Although there is some evidence
that reduction of cocaine use is associated with improved functioning in other
domains (Carroll, Powers, et al., 1993), several studies have demonstrated
that patients who receive treatment services that target their problem areas
have better outcome than those who do not (McLellan et al., 1997).

The ASI has been used for over 20 years in a wide number of substance-
using populations and has strong support for its reliability and validity in a
number of formats and settings (Alterman, Brown, Zaballero, & McKay,
1994; Alterman et al., 2000; Butler et al., 1998; Kosten, Rounsaville, &
Kleber, 1983; Rosen, Henson, Finney, & Moos, 2000; Zanis, McLellan, &

Corse, 1997), including predictive validity (Alterman, Bovasso, Cacciola, & McDermott, 2001; Bovasso, Alterman, Cacciola, & Cook, 2001). The ASI is available free of charge and takes roughly 45–60 minutes to administer at baseline. Computerized versions of the ASI with computerized scoring and clinically useful summaries are available (McDermott, Alterman, Brown, & Zaballero, 1996).

There are, however, a number of domains not covered by the ASI that have clinical relevance in working with cocaine-using populations. In particular, comorbid psychopathology is common among cocaine users, with roughly 60–80% meeting criteria for another lifetime Axis I psychiatric disorder (Kessler et al., 1997; Levin, Evans, & Kleber, 1998; Regier et al., 1990; Rounsaville et al., 1991, 1998). Moreover, the presence of an unrecognized or untreated psychiatric disorder generally confers poor prognosis among drug users (Carroll, Powers, et al., 1993; McLellan & McKay, 1998; Rounsaville, Kosten, Weissman, & Kleber, 1986). The most commonly diagnosed co-occurring psychiatric disorders among treatment-seeking cocaine users include affective disorders, anxiety disorders, antisocial personality disorder, and history of childhood attention-deficit/hyperactivity disorder (Kessler et al., 1997; Rounsaville et al., 1991). Accurate and timely diagnosis of comorbid psychiatric disorders is crucial, because many of the psychiatric disorders that frequently co-occur with substance use are treatable, particularly affective disorders (McDowell, Levin, Seracini, & Nunes, 2000; O'Brien, 1997). Although the ASI provides a clinically useful continuous measure of psychological symptoms and history, it does not provide a specific psychiatric diagnosis. Thus, standardized diagnostic instruments such as the SCID, DIS, CIDI, or Psychiatric Research Interview for Substance and Mental Disorders (PRISM; Hasin et al., 1996) can be used to make diagnoses of concurrent psychiatric disorder.

Assessing Personality Disorders in Cocaine Users

Personality disorders appear to be especially prevalent in cocaine abusers (J. P. Barber, Frank, Weiss, & Blaine, 1996; Marlowe, Husband, Lamb, & Kirby, 1995; Rounsaville et al., 1998; Sonne & Brady, 1998; Weiss, Mirin, Griffin, Gunderson, & Hufford, 1993), with median rates of 70% having at least one personality disorder (see summary in Verheul, Ball, & van den Brink, 1998a). Of these, antisocial disorder is the most prevalent (median 24%), followed by borderline personality disorder (median 18%) in cocaine abusers with the paranoia seen in a significant minority of patients. However, there is wide variability noted across studies, depending on the method (self-report vs. structured interview), setting (residential, inpatient, methadone, outpatient), diagnostic system, and assessment procedure (timing of assessment, separating acute symptoms of intoxication or withdrawal) (Verheul et al., 1998).

Effective treatment depends in part on first obtaining an accurate and meaningful assessment of the problem. The difficulties associated with the reliable and valid diagnosis of DSM Axis II personality disorders have been summarized by several excellent reviews (e.g., Perry, 1992; Zimmerman, 1994). The reliability or diagnostic stability of personality disorders may be even more problematic in cocaine abusers, especially when patients are assessed at the beginning of treatment, when they are intoxicated or experiencing acute or protracted withdrawal. Cocaine intoxication and withdrawal are characterized by marked changes in cognitive, emotional, and social functioning that mimic many symptoms of personality disorders. As such, if assessment occurs during this time, it may lead to inflated estimates of personality disorders. However, this is also the time of greatest clinical relevance from the standpoint of treatment planning. Although this problem can be overcome in inpatient settings by waiting for 2 weeks of abstinence, decreased lengths of inpatient stay greatly limit the clinical usefulness of this assessment. Among cocaine-abusing outpatients, it is more difficult to ensure that a completely drug-free state has been achieved and maintained throughout the assessment period.

Part of the reliability and validity issue for personality disorder diagnosis in cocaine and other substance abusers centers on whether to include or exclude Axis II symptoms that seem to be substance related (i.e., intoxication, withdrawal, or other behaviors required to maintain an addiction). Weiss et al. (1993) found a negligible effect for substance-related symptoms in an inpatient sample of cocaine abusers, except for decreased rates of antisocial and borderline personality disorder (see also (Carroll, Ball, & Rounsaville, 1993; Rounsaville et al., 1991). Others have not found such a change in rates even for antisocial or borderline personality disorder (Hasin & Grant, 1987; Ross, Glaser, & Germanson, 1988). As Verheul et al. (1998) suggest, these inconsistencies seem partly attributable to the strategy used for exclusion. Measures with more stringent criteria exclude any symptoms that have ever been linked to substance abuse and yield significant rate changes. Measures that exclude symptoms only if they were completely absent before substance abuse or during periods of extended abstinence show minimal rate changes.

Intuitively, one might predict that excluding cocaine-related symptoms would make other psychiatric diagnoses more reliable (although not necessarily more valid). However, the task of differentiating between substance-related symptoms and personality traits is not an easy task for patients or clinical interviewers, and may not be reliable. Although many cocaine abusers can distinguish between behaviors that are only related to intoxication or withdrawal, they often have greater difficulty making the same distinction for other activities, such as lying or breaking the law, which may be related to obtaining cocaine. Such a distinction requires a high level of introspection and cognitive competence in making the motivational judgments necessary to differentiate between a trait and a situation or state (i.e., cocaine-seeking) behavior. It also requires an empathic awareness of the impact of one's behavior on self and others, and a willingness to accept responsibility for one's actions (Zimmerman, 1994). Substance abusers may be particularly impaired in the skills necessary to make these discriminations. Depending on their stage of recovery and motivation, they may be more prone to make dispositional attribution for their behaviors or, in contrast, project responsibility for their negative traits onto others, the situation, or the effects of the substance.

Diagnosing personality disorders independent of substance use disorders is consistent with guidelines suggested by DSM-IV. However, the evidence is inconclusive whether it is more valid to include or exclude substance-related symptoms from the diagnosis of personality disorders. If one does choose to exclude substance-related symptoms, several suggestions can be made. First, interviewers should determine whether a symptom should be eliminated as substance-related on an item-by-item basis. It is probably less reliable and less valid to wait until the end of each disorder to ask whether the diagnosis is substance related. Second, criteria in which substance dependence is an inherent part should be scored as being due to substance abuse unless non-substance-related behavioral indicators of the trait (e.g., impulsivity, unlawful behaviors) are also present. Finally, when another Axis I disorder is suspected or present, the interviewer should periodically remind patients that questions refer to the way they are even when they are not symptomatic with either substance abuse or another Axis I disorder.

Multidimensional Assessment for Addiction Typologies

There have been several attempts to subtype substance abusers based on single dimensions such as comorbid psychopathology, age of onset, family history, gender, and personality. Addicted individuals are likely to have coexisting psychopathology (Rounsaville et al., 1991; Rounsaville, Dolinsky, Babor, & Meyer, 1987; Rounsaville, Kosten, et al., 1986). Age of onset is another important alcoholism subtyping variable, with earlier onset predicting more severe substance-related social problems, coexistent psychopathology, criminality, psychopathy, and familial or genetic risk (Irwin, Schuckit, & Smith, 1990; McGue, Pickens, & Svikis, 1992; Roy, DeJong, Lamparksi, & Adinoff, 1991; Turnbull, George, Landerman, Swartz, & Blazer, 1990). There is an extensive literature (particularly using the Minnesota Multiphasic Personality Inventory [MMPI]) of subtyping substance abusers on the basis of abnormal personality dimensions (e.g., neurotic, psychopathic, psychotic) (Anglin, Weisman, & Fisher, 1989; Graham & Strenger, 1988).

Although single-dimension subtyping systems have greater clinical appeal from the standpoint of parsimony, they tend to predict a narrower range of outcomes than a more comprehensive, multidimensional typology (Babor et al., 1992). Such a broader theoretical framework helps organize diverse variables into meaningful constructs that may play a role in the etiology, patterning, and course of the disorder. Babor et al.'s Type A and Type B alcoholism systems categorize individuals into one of two broader types. Type A is characterized by lower heritability, fewer childhood risk factors, later age of onset, less severe dependence, and lower novelty seeking. Type B is characterized by higher heritability, more childhood risk factors, earlier onset, more severe dependence and psychiatric comorbidity, impulsivity, high novelty seeking, and antisocial behavior.

Ball et al. (1995) and Feingold, Ball, Kranzler, and Rounsaville (1996) have found that the Type A–Type B distinction is also reliable and valid for cocaine, opiate, and marijuana users. In addition, this typology has predicted outcome and response to specific treatment. Type B cocaine-dependent patients exhibit more severe substance use severity, associated psychosocial problems, and psychiatric symptoms, and may relapse faster than Type A's (Ball et al., 1995).

Other Specific Comorbid Problems

Because of the significance of negative affect, particularly depression, among cocaine users (McDowell et al., 2000; Nunes et al., 1998), evaluating depression via instruments such as the Beck Depression Inventory (Beck, Ward, Mendelson, Mock, & Erbaugh, 1961) or the Brief Symptom Inventory (Derogatis & Melisaratos, 1983) is usually helpful. However, depression should be reassessed following stabilization or prolonged abstinence (see Husband et al., 1996; Strain, Stitzer, & Bigelow, 1991), because self-reports may overestimate depressive disorders and symptoms, particularly early in treatment, when patients may be experiencing withdrawal.

HIV remains a major problem among cocaine-using populations and its assessment in clinical populations is important, because effective treatment often results in substantially lowered levels of risk behaviors (Sorenson & Copeland, 2000). There are a number of reliable instruments for evaluating HIV risk behaviors, including the Risk Assessment Battery (RAB; Navaline et al., 1994) and the HIV Risk-Taking Behavior Scale (HRBS; Darke, 1998; Darke, Hall, Heather, Ward, & Wodak, 1991) among the instruments that are suitable for general populations of cocaine users.

To assess negative consequences of cocaine use across multiple domains (e.g., medical, legal, family/social, psychological, employment), the ASI can be used. In addition, several measures of negative consequences of substance use that are appropriate for use with cocaine users have been derived from instruments first developed to assess negative consequences of alcohol use, such as the Short Inventory of Problems (SIP), which was derived from the Drinker Inventory of Consequences (DrInC) (Miller, Tonigan, & Longabaugh, 1995).

TREATMENT PLANNING

Since the initial edition of this volume (Donovan & Marlatt, 1988), assessment and treatment planning have been increasingly closely and explicitly linked for several reasons. First, behavioral therapies that have strong empirical support as treatment for cocaine-using populations often require the integration of specific assessments in order to be delivered effectively. For example, contingency management approaches (Budney & Higgins, 1998; Higgins, Budney, Bickel, & Hughes, 1993; Petry et al., 2002) require repeated assessment of urine specimens, timed to detect new episodes of use, for verification of abstinence or close assessment of other target goals (Petry, 2000). Motivational interviewing (Miller & Rollnick, 1991) uses delivery of objective feedback based on a pretreatment assessment of substance use and consequences, including results of neuropsychological tests, reasons for quitting, and consequences of use (Miller & Heather, 1998; Miller, Zweben, DiClemente, & Rychtarik, 1992). Second, there has been growing recognition of the strong relationship between the provision of services directly linked to specific needs of individual drug users and improved outcomes (McLellan et al., 1993, 1997, 1983); thus, assessment is an important strategy for assessing the individual's need for specific interventions and services.

Another major advance in the treatment of addictive behaviors was the transtheoretical model, which suggests that individuals attempting to change problem behavior go through a predictable series of stages of change, from precontemplation to contemplation, to action and maintenance (Prochaska & DiClemente, 1982; Prochaska et al., 1992). A wide range of instruments has been developed to measure stages of change, motivation, and related constructs that have been used with cocaine users, with minor adaptations. These include the University of Rhode Island Change Assessment (URICA; DiClemente & Hughes, 1990), the Stages of Change Readiness and Treatment Eagerness Scale (SOCRATES; Miller & Tonigan, 1996), the Contemplation Ladder (Biener & Abrams, 1991), the Alcohol and Drug Consequences Questionnaire (ADCQ; Cunningham, Sobell, Gavin, Sobell, & Breslin, 1997), the Recovery Attitude and Treatment Evaluator (RAATE; Gastfriend, Filstead, Reif, & Najavits, 1995; Mee-Lee, 1988), and the Readiness to Change Questionnaire (Rollnick, Heather, Gold, & Hall, 1992). However, it should be noted that psychometric support for some of these instruments and, in particular, for their predictive validity among samples of cocaine and other drug users, has been mixed (Carey, Purnine, Maisto, & Carey, 1999; Pantalon, Nich, Frankforter, & Carroll, 2002). A related but more narrowly defined construct, commitment to abstinence, has been shown to predict treatment outcome in cocaine users (Carroll & Rounsaville, 2002; Hall, Havassy, & Wasserman, 1991; McKay, Merikle, Mulvaney, Weiss, & Koppenhaver, 2001; Milligan, Nich, & Carroll, 2004).

Since the first edition of this volume (Donovan & Marlatt, 1988), evidence has also accumulated in support of the efficacy of cognitive-behavioral relapse prevention approaches with cocaine-dependent populations (Carroll et al., 2004; Carroll, Nich, Ball, McCance-Katz, & Rounsaville, 1998; Carroll et al., 2000; Carroll, Rounsaville, Gordon, et al., 1994; Carroll, Rounsaville, Nich, et al., 1994; Epstein, Hawkins, Covi, Umbricht, & Preston, 2003; Maude-Griffin et al., 1998; McKay, Alterman, Cacciola, et al., 1999; Monti, Rohsenow, Michalec, Martin, & Abrams, 1997; Rohsenow, Monti, Martin,

Michalec, & Abrams, 2000). Given the focus of this pair of volumes on relapse prevention and assessment, more detailed discussion of assessment issues specific to cognitive-behavioral therapy (CBT) for cocaine abusers is warranted. CBT approaches focus closely on functional analysis of drug use, that is, understanding patterns of cocaine use, identification of those high-risk situations in which the individual is likely to use cocaine, and development of individualized coping skills to reduce the likelihood of relapse. Thus, instruments that assess specific antecedents of cocaine use or relapse, such as the Inventory of Drug-Taking Situations (IDTS; Turner, Annis, & Sklar, 1997), may be quite useful in treatment planning in CBT (McKay, Alterman, Mulvaney, & Koppenhaver, 1999). For conducting functional analyses and understanding patterns of cocaine and other substance use, the Timeline Followback (TLFB; Sobell & Sobell, 1992; Sobell, Toneatto, & Sobell, 1994) method is excellent for evaluating quantity–frequency information, as well as understanding patterns of drug use (Westerberg, Tonigan, & Miller, 1998). In addition, adaptations of the Situational Confidence Questionnaire (Breslin, Sobell, Sobell, & Agrawal, 2000), originally developed to assess problem drinkers' confidence in their ability to resist urges to use, have been adapted for use with drug-using populations (J. G. Barber, Cooper, & Heather, 1991). The Drug-Taking Confidence Questionnaire (DTCQ), a 50-item self-report developed to assess coping self-efficacy for a number of different types of drug and alcohol use (Sklar, Annis, & Turner, 1997), can be quite helpful in prioritizing among various coping skills and targeting high-risk situations on which to focus in CBT. More recently, a short (8-item) version of the DTCQ has also been developed and has been shown to have good psychometric properties (Sklar & Turner, 1999); thus, it may be quite useful in clinical practice.

An important shortcoming of the CBT literature on treatment of cocaine dependence to date is the relative lack of emphasis on assessment of individuals' levels of coping skills and targeting treatment to individuals' specific coping styles, strengths, weaknesses, and likely relapse precipitants. Comprehensive assessment of an individual's level of coping skills can be done through role-playing tests, which can help pinpoint specific coping deficits and assess whether treatment has had an impact on the individual's ability to cope with specific high-risk situations (e.g., the experience of wanting cocaine, being alone, having cash available, unstructured free time, and strong unpleasant and pleasant effects) (see McKay, Rutherford, Alterman, Cacciola, & Kaplan, 1995). Role-playing instruments that seek to pinpoint specific coping skills include the Cocaine Risk Response Test (CCRT; Carroll, Nich, Frankforter, & Bisighini, 1999), which was adapted from the Situational Competency Test (Chaney, O'Leary, & Marlatt, 1978; Hawkins, Catalano, & Wells, 1986). Acquisition of specific cognitive and behavioral coping skills using the CCRT has been linked to better short- and long-term outcomes among cocaine-dependent populations (Carroll et al., 1999).

Another significant weakness of the CBT/relapse prevention literature is failure to attend to cognitive functioning in treatment planning with cocaine users. Given clear evidence of cognitive impairment among chronic cocaine users (DiSclafani, Tolou-Shams, Price, & Fein, 2002; Gottschalk, Beauvais, Hart, & Kosten, 2001), this omission is particularly significant, because CBT's emphasis on learning and applying complex, abstract, and often novel skills assumes comparatively intact attention, memory, and reasoning skills. Recently, Aharonovich, Nunes, and Hasin (2003) reported that cocaine users with higher levels of neuropsychological impairment were less likely to complete CBT. Thus, effective implementation of CBT may require assessment of cognitive functioning, to enable the clinician to be aware of the individual's pattern of cognitive strengths and weaknesses, and, where indicated, to modify treatment appropriately (e.g., through repeating material, presenting it in different formats) Commonly used tests of drug users' neuropsychological functioning that have reasonable psychometric support include the Trail Making Test (Davies, 1968; Reitan, 1958), the Shipley Institute of Living Scale (Shipley, 1967), and the Mini-Mental Status Examination (Folstein, Folstein, & McHugh, 1975). The Neuropsychological Screening Battery (NSB; Heaton, Thompson, Nelson, Filley, & Franklin, 1990), a compilation of a number of widely used neuropsychological tests, has been demonstrated to discriminate between substance abusers and nonusers (Fals-Stewart, 1996; Fals-Stewart & Bates, 2003; O'Malley, Adamse, Heaton, & Gawin, 1992). As suggested by Fals-Stewart and Bates (2003), the NSB can be supplemented by a number of other tasks to assess four key areas of cognitive functioning frequently affected by drug abuse: executive functioning, verbal ability, memory, and speed. Assessment of impulsivity may also be important in treatment planning and understanding treatment response in cocaine users, and impulsivity may be independent of antisocial personality disorder and aggression (Allen, Moeller, Rhoades, & Cherek, 1998; Moeller et al., 2002).

EVALUATING TREATMENT OUTCOME

There is no uniformly held standard, or even clear consensus, regarding an ideal treatment outcome indicator or definition of treatment success in cocaine abuse treatment. Although definitions of success are broadening beyond requiring complete abstinence from cocaine (Lavori et al., 1999), meaningful reductions in cocaine use remain a central indicator of improvement (McKay, Alterman, et al., 2001). In general, researchers have used two primary indicators of outcome: frequency of substance use and a measure of severity/intensity (Babor et al., 1994). This rough distinction has applied to cocaine use as well, with most reports evaluating outcome in terms of percent days of cocaine use (frequency) and consequences of use (intensity). McKay, Alterman, et al. (2001) conducted a psychometric evaluation of a large number of commonly used cocaine outcome indices; using confirmatory factor analyses, they demonstrated that the majority of the indicators fell into one of two general categories: frequency (e.g., percent days of cocaine use, monetary value of cocaine, abstinence status, time to relapse, results of urine toxicology screens) and severity (e.g., ASI drug or cocaine composite scores, craving measures). They also found that a variable assessing latency to a second relapse episode (i.e. time between a first episode of cocaine use and the start of a second episode) was one variable that was fairly independent of the other, more widely used dimensions and worthy of further study.

Clinicians who treat individuals for cocaine use have access to a readily available, easy to use, rapid-feedback, valid, and highly sensitive assessment of current symptoms and treatment outcome. Because drugs such as cocaine are metabolized and excreted through urine, analysis of urine specimens for metabolites of cocaine, opioids, marijuana, benzodiazepines, and several other drug classes are a practical and accurate strategy of monitoring recent drug use. Depending on the half-life of the particular drug, the clinician can, by varying the frequency with which urines specimens are obtained from a patient, detect almost all new episodes of use (Schwartz, 1988; Hawks & Chiang, 1986). Recent development of rapid (e.g., 5-minute) on-site testing methods, which analyze for specific metabolites within the urine specimen collection cup itself, eliminate the need for the clinician to mix chemicals and make monitoring of drug use simple, reliable, rapid, and comparatively inexpensive, even in office-based settings. Newer technologies for detecting cocaine abuse, including hair testing and sweat patches (Winhusen et al., 2003), are also available but have not yet come into wide clinical use outside of research settings.

Although monitoring of recent drug use through urinalysis is an important strategy of assessing cocaine use and progress in treatment (Calsyn, Saxon, & Barndt, 1991), evaluating the efficacy of treatment (Blaine, Ling, Kosten, O'Brien, & Chiarello, 1994) and predicting treatment outcome (Kampman et al., 2001; Preston et al., 1998) form the backbone of effective behavioral strategies for treating drug dependence, such as contingency management (Higgins et al., 1994; Petry, 2000); evaluation of treatment outcome is much more complex than assessment of recent cocaine use via analysis of urine samples alone. Self-reports of cocaine use, like other types of substance use, can be highly reliable (Babor, Steinberg, Anton, & Del Boca, 2000; Maisto, McKay, & Connors, 1990; Zanis, McLellan, & Randall, 1994), and in many cases may be more sensitive than urine monitoring, which can only detect all new episodes of cocaine use if done very frequently (e.g., two to three times per week) (Preston, Silverman, Schuster, & Cone, 1997).

Regarding outcomes for cocaine users, several investigators have found comparatively strong relationships between achieving even comparatively brief periods of abstinence during treatment and better long-term prognosis (Carroll et al., 2000; Higgins, Wong, Badger, Haug-Ogden, & Dantona, 2000; McKay, Alterman, et al., 2001). Conversely, an initial cocaine-positive urine specimen (a likely marker of severity) has been associated with poor treatment outcome (Alterman et al., 1997; Ehrman, Robbins, & Cornish, 2001; Preston et al., 1998; Sofuoglu, Gonzalez, Poling, & Kosten, 2002).

As emphasized earlier, however, cocaine abusers' problems are multidimensional, and improvements in areas other than cocaine use must be assessed as a component of treatment outcome. Evaluations of multiple dimensions of outcome, including functioning in the medical, legal, psychological, social, and employment domains, are important in determining the efficacy and breadth of treatment effects. Thus, the ASI has become a widely used measure of treatment outcome in clinical trials evaluating a range of treatments for cocaine use disorders (see Crits-Christoph et al., 2001; Silverman et al., 1998), although it was not originally intended to serve as an assessment of treatment outcome (Cacciola, Alterman, O'Brien, & McLellan, 1997).

ISSUES OF SPECIAL CONSEQUENCE IN WORKING WITH COCAINE-USING POPULATIONS

Cocaine Craving

The measurement of cocaine craving is highly complex (Sayette et al., 2000). Accurate and appropriate assessment of craving depends on how craving is defined (e.g., as desire for the drug, intentions to use the drug, anticipation for specific drug effects), the time frame by which it is measured, and the extent to which the individual is aware of craving and can monitor internal states (Sayette et al., 2000). There is also a great deal of debate concerning whether craving is necessary for relapse, and whether drug use can occur in the absence of craving (Tiffany, 1990). Several investigators have noted that relationships between different measures of craving, and between craving and drug use, have tended to be modest (McMillan & Gilmore-Thomas, 1996; Robbins, Ehrman, Childress, Cornish, & O'Brien, 2000; Rohsenow, Niaura, Childress, Abrams, & Monti, 1990/1991; Tiffany, 1990). Experts generally caution against single-item measures, which tend to be less reliable and less sensitive (Sayette et al., 2000; Tiffany, Carter, & Singleton, 2000). Multidimensional craving scales with good psychometric properties have been developed (Tiffany, Singleton, Haertzen, & Henningfield, 1993). Including these measures, when selected on the basis of the specific issues to be addressed in a population or study, in clinical assessment of cocaine users may be quite useful, particularly for clinicians using extinction of craving procedures, evaluating behavioral approaches with a focus on craving, evaluating new pharmacologic approaches (Lavori et al., 1999), and for those seeking to understand mechanisms of action of particular treatments (Weiss et al., 2003).

Alcohol Use

Another problem of great significance among cocaine users is comorbid alcohol use. As many as 60–80% of cocaine abusers in clinical and community samples meet lifetime diagnostic criteria for alcohol abuse or dependence (Carroll, Rounsaville, & Bryant, 1993; McKay, Alterman, Rutherford,

Cacciola, & McLellan, 1999; Mengis, Maude-Griffin, Delucchi, & Hall, 2002; Regier et al., 1990). Although elevated rates of alcohol use are common in drug-using populations (Anthony et al., 1994; Kessler et al., 1997), several lines of evidence suggest special features of the co-occurrence of cocaine abuse and alcoholism that may distinguish it from other forms of alcohol–drug comorbidity. First, although elevated rates of alcoholism would be predicted for cocaine abusers given the base rates of both disorders, epidemiological evidence suggests that the cocaine–alcohol relationship may be particularly strong. Helzer and Pryzbek's (1988) analysis of Epidemiologic Catchment Area (ECA) data showed a higher degree of association between cocaine and alcohol dependence than between alcohol and any other type of drug. Regier and colleagues (1990) reported that 85% of ECA subjects who met criteria for cocaine dependence also met criteria for alcohol abuse or dependence, a rate far higher than that of alcoholism among those meeting criteria for heroin–opioid (65%), cannabis (45%), or sedative–hypnotic–anxiolytic (71%) dependence. A second feature that may distinguish between cocaine–alcohol comorbidity and other forms of coexistent alcohol and drug dependence is the order of onset for the alcohol versus the drug disorder. Alcohol abuse or dependence typically antedates the use of illicit drugs and drops off when regular drug use is established (Anthony & Helzer, 1991; Kandel, 1985; Kandel & Logan, 1984). Furthermore, a diagnosis of abuse or dependence on "harder" drugs is comparatively rare among individuals without a lifetime history of alcohol abuse or dependence (Helzer & Pryzbeck, 1988). In contrast, cocaine use may foster secondary alcohol dependence, because alcohol is often employed by cocaine users to attenuate negative acute effects of cocaine, such as nervousness or sleeplessness. Finally, Jatlow and colleagues have identified cocaethylene, a metabolite of cocaine and alcohol, which may enhance and extend cocaine euphoria (Jatlow et al., 1991; McCance-Katz, Price, Kosten, & Jatlow, 1995). Use of alcohol to potentiate cocaine euphoria may increase cocaine abusers' vulnerability to secondary alcoholism (Carroll, Rounsaville, et al., 1993).

Comorbid alcohol-dependence has been associated with more severe cocaine dependence, poorer retention in treatment, and poorer outcome in several studies (Brady, Sonne, Randall, Adinoff, & Malcolm, 1995; Carroll, Powers, et al., 1993; Heil, Badger, & Higgins, 2001). Alcohol use may confer poorer prognoses among cocaine users, because it is a powerful, conditioned cue for cocaine use, and because alcohol-related disinhibition may interfere with the individual's efforts to remain abstinent. Higgins, Roll, and Bickel (1996) also reported that alcohol use increases cocaine users' preference for cocaine over other reinforcers, such as money. Moreover, alcohol use has frequently been identified as a precipitant of relapse among cocaine users (McKay, Alterman, Rutherford, et al., 1999), and strategies that effectively reduce cocaine users' alcohol use tend to improve cocaine outcomes (Carroll et al., 1998, 2000; Higgins, Budney, Bickel, Hughes, & Foerg, 1993).

CONCLUSIONS

There has been great progress in the understanding and treatment of cocaine use disorders in the past 15 years. In keeping with the general themes of this volume, we have attempted to summarize major issues relevant to clinical assessment of cocaine users, including both those that cut across addictive behaviors and those that are particular to cocaine dependence. While these advancements have been substantial, a number of gaps in the field remain: First is the lack of a general consensus on what constitutes "good outcome" among cocaine abusers, with different researchers using different indicators, which in turn renders cross-study comparisons quite challenging. Second, a number of assessments described here have been borrowed from the assessment of other clinical disorders, with little or no systematic evaluation of their psychometric properties in diverse groups of cocaine abusers. More detailed evaluation of such instruments within and across groups of substance users may greatly enhance our understanding of cocaine abusers and allow clinicians to render precise conclusions regarding the effectiveness of the treatments we offer.

ACKNOWLEDGMENTS

Support for the preparation of this chapter was provided by National Institute on Drug Abuse Grant Nos. K05-DA 00457 (KMC) and P50-DA09241, and by the U.S. Department of Veterans Affairs VISN 1 Mental Illness Research, Education, and Clinical Center. Portions of this chapter appeared in Carroll and Rounsaville (2002). Copyright 2003 by Elsevier. Reprinted by permission.

REFERENCES

Aharonovich, E., Nunes, E. V., & Hasin, D. (2003). Cognitive impairment, retention and abstinence among cocaine abusers in cognitive-behavioral treatment. *Drug and Alcohol Dependence, 71*, 207–211.

Allen, T., Moeller, F. G., Rhoades, H. M., & Cherek, D. R. (1998). Impulsivity and history of drug dependence. *Drug and Alcohol Dependence, 50*, 137–145.

Alterman, A. I., Bovasso, G. B., Cacciola, J. S., & McDermott, P. A. (2001). A comparison of the predictive validity of four sets of baseline ASI summary indices. *Psychology of Addictive Behaviors, 15*, 159–162.

Alterman, A. I., Brown, L. S., Zaballero, A., & McKay, J. R. (1994). Interviewer severity ratings and composite scores of the ASI: A further look. *Drug and Alcohol Dependence, 34*, 201–209.

Alterman, A. I., Kampman, K. M., Boardman, C., Cacciola, J. S., Rutherford, M. J., McKay, J. R., et al. (1997). A cocaine-positive baseline urine predicts outpatient treatment attrition and failure to attain initial abstinence. *Drug and Alcohol Dependence, 46*, 79–85.

Alterman, A. I., McDermott, P. A., Cook, T. G., Cacciola, J. S., McKay, J. R.,

McLellan, A. T., et al. (2000). Generalizability of the clinical dimensions of the Addiction Severity Index to nonopioid-dependent patients. *Psychology of Addictive Behaviors, 14,* 287–294.

Alterman, A. I., McLellan, A. T., & Shifman, R. B. (1993). Do substance abuse patients with more pathology receive more treatment? *Journal of Nervous and Mental Disease, 181,* 576–582.

American Psychiatric Association. (1994). *Diagnostic and statistical manual of mental disorders* (4th ed.). Washington, DC: Author.

Anglin, M. D., Weisman, C. P., & Fisher, D. G. (1989). The MMPI profiles of narcotic addicts: I. A review of the literature. *International Journal of the Addictions, 24,* 867–880.

Anthony, J. C., & Helzer, J. E. (1991). Syndromes of drug use and drug dependence. In L. N. Robins & D. A. Regier (Eds.), *Psychiatric disorders in America* (pp. 116–154). New York: Free Press.

Anthony, J. C., Warner, L. A., & Kessler, R. C. (1994). Comparative epidemiology of dependence on tobacco, alcohol, controlled substances and inhalants: Basic findings from the National Comorbidity Study. *Experimental and Clinical Psychopharmacology, 2,* 244–268.

Appleby, L., Dyson, V., Altman, E., & Luchins, D. J. (1997). Assessing substance use in multiproblem patients: Reliability and validity of the Addiction Severity Index in a mental hospital population. *Journal of Nervous and Mental Disease, 185,* 159–165.

Babor, T. F. (1993). Alcohol and drug use history, patterns and problems. In B. J. Rounsaville, F. M. Tims, A. M. Horton, & B. J. Sowder (Eds.), *Diagnostic source book on drug abuse research and treatment* (NIH Publication No. 93-3508 ed., pp. 19–34). Rockville, MD: National Institute on Drug Abuse.

Babor, T. F., Hoffman, M., DelBoca, F. K., Hesselbrock, V. M., Meyer, R. E., Dolinsky, Z. S., et al. (1992). Types of alcoholics: I. Evidence for an empirically derived typology based on indicators of vulnerability and severity. *Archives of General Psychiatry, 49,* 599–608.

Babor, T. F., Longabaugh, R., Zweben, A., Fuller, R. K., Stout, R. L., Anton, R. F., et al. (1994). Issues in the definition and measurement of drinking outcomes in alcoholism treatment research. *Journal of Studies on Alcohol, 12*(Suppl.), 83–90.

Babor, T. F., Steinberg, K., Anton, R. F., & Del Boca, F. K. (2000). Talk is cheap: Measuring drinking outcomes in clinical trials. *Journal of Studies on Alcohol, 61,* 55–63.

Ball, S. A., Carroll, K. M., Rounsaville, B. J., & Babor, T. F. (1995). Subtypes of cocaine abusers: Support for a Type A/Type B distinction. *Journal of Consulting and Clinical Psychology, 63,* 115–124.

Barber, J. G., Cooper, B. K., & Heather, N. (1991). The Situational Confidence Questionnaire (Heroin). *International Journal of Addiction, 26,* 565–575.

Barber, J. P., Frank, A., Weiss, R. D., & Blaine, J. D. (1996). Prevalence and correlates of personality disorder diagnoses among cocaine dependent outpatients. *Journal of Personality Disorders, 10,* 297–311.

Beck, A. T., Ward, C. H., Mendelson, M., Mock, J., & Erbaugh, J. (1961). An inventory for measuring depression. *Archives of General Psychiatry, 4,* 561–571.

Biener, L., & Abrams, D. (1991). The Contemplation Ladder: Validation of a measure of readiness to consider smoking session. *Health Psychology, 10,* 360–365.

Blaine, J. D., Ling, W., Kosten, T. R., O'Brien, C. P., & Chiarello, R. J. (1994). Establishing the efficacy and safety of medications for the treatment of drug dependence and abuse: Methodological issues. In R. F. Prien & D. S. Robinson (Eds.), *Clinical evaluation of psychotropic drugs* (pp. 593–623). New York: Raven Press.

Bovasso, G. B., Alterman, A. I., Cacciola, J. S., & Cook, T. G. (2001). Predictive validity of the Addiction Severity Index's composite scores in the assessment of 2–year outcomes in a methadone maintenance population. *Psychology of Addictive Behaviors, 15,* 171–176.

Brady, K. T., Sonne, S., Randall, C. L., Adinoff, B., & Malcolm, R. J. (1995). Features of cocaine dependence with concurrent alcohol dependence. *Drug and Alcohol Dependence, 39,* 69–71.

Breslin, F. C., Sobell, L. C., Sobell, M. B., & Agrawal, S. (2000). A comparison of a brief and long version of the Situational Confidence Questionnaire. *Behaviour Research and Therapy, 38,* 1211–1220.

Brownell, K. D., Marlatt, G. A., Lichtenstein, E., & Wilson, G. T. (1986). Understanding and preventing relapse. *American Psychologist, 41,* 765–782.

Budney, A. J., & Higgins, S. T. (1998). *A community reinforcement plus vouchers approach: Treating cocaine addiction.* Rockville, MD: National Institute on Drug Abuse.

Butler, S. F., Newman, F. L., Cacciola, J. S., Frank, A., Budman, S. H., McLellan, A. T., et al. (1998). Predicting Addiction Severity Index (ASI) interviewer severity ratings for a computer-administered ASI. *Psychological Assessment, 10,* 399–407.

Cacciola, J. S., Alterman, A. I., O'Brien, C. P., & McLellan, A. T. (1997). The Addiction Severity Index in clinical efficacy trials of medications for cocaine dependence. In B. Tai, C. N. Chiang, & P. Bridge (Eds.), *Medication development for the treatment of cocaine dependence: Issues in clinical efficacy trials* (pp. 182–191). Rockville, MD: National Institute on Drug Abuse.

Calsyn, D. A., Saxon, A. J., & Barndt, D. C. (1991). Urine screening practices in methadone maintenance clinics: A survey of how the results are used. *Journal of Nervous and Mental Disease, 179,* 222–227.

Carey, K. B., Purnine, D. M., Maisto, S. A., & Carey, M. P. (1999). Assessing readiness to change substance abuse: A critical review of instruments. *Clinical Psychology: Science and Practice, 6,* 245–266.

Carroll, K. M. (1995). Methodological issues and problems in assessment of substance use. *Psychological Assessment, 7,* 349–358.

Carroll, K. M., Ball, S. A., & Rounsaville, B. J. (1993). A comparison of alternate systems for diagnosing antisocial personality disorder in cocaine abusers. *Journal of Nervous and Mental Disease, 181,* 436–443.

Carroll, K. M., Fenton, L. R., Ball, S. A., Nich, C., Frankforter, T. L., Shi, J., et al. (2004). Efficacy of disulfiram and cognitive-behavioral therapy in cocaine-dependent outpatients. *Archives of General Psychiatry, 61,* 264–272.

Carroll, K. M., Nich, C., Ball, S. A., McCance-Katz, E. F., Frankforter, T. F., & Rounsaville, B. J. (2000). One year follow-up of disulfiram and psychotherapy for cocaine-alcohol abusers: Sustained effects of treatment. *Addiction, 95,* 1335–1349.

Carroll, K. M., Nich, C., Ball, S. A., McCance-Katz, E., & Rounsaville, B. J. (1998). Treatment of cocaine and alcohol dependence with psychotherapy and disulfiram. *Addiction, 93,* 713–728.

Carroll, K. M., Nich, C., Frankforter, T. L., & Bisighini, R. M. (1999). Do patients change in the way we intend?: Treatment-specific skill acquisition in cocaine-dependent patients using the Cocaine Risk Response Test. *Psychological Assessment, 11*, 77–85.

Carroll, K. M., Powers, M. D., Bryant, K. J., & Rounsaville, B. J. (1993). One-year follow-up status of treatment-seeking cocaine abusers: Psychopathology and dependence severity as predictors of outcome. *Journal of Nervous and Mental Disease, 181*, 71–79.

Carroll, K. M., & Rounsaville, B. J. (2002). On beyond urine: Clinically useful assessment instruments in the treatment of drug dependence. *Behaviour Research and Therapy, 40*, 1329–1344.

Carroll, K. M., Rounsaville, B. J., & Bryant, K. J. (1993). Alcoholism in treatment seeking cocaine abusers: Clinical and prognostic significance. *Journal of Studies on Alcohol, 54*, 199–208.

Carroll, K. M., Rounsaville, B. J., Gordon, L. T., Nich, C., Jatlow, P. M., Bisighini, R. M., et al. (1994). Psychotherapy and pharmacotherapy for ambulatory cocaine abusers. *Archives of General Psychiatry, 51*, 177–197.

Carroll, K. M., Rounsaville, B. J., Nich, C., Gordon, L. T., Wirtz, P. W., & Gawin, F. H. (1994). One year follow-up of psychotherapy and pharmacotherapy for cocaine dependence: Delayed emergence of psychotherapy effects. *Archives of General Psychiatry, 51*, 989–997.

Chaney, E. F., O'Leary, M. R., & Marlatt, G. A. (1978). Skill training with problem drinkers. *Journal of Consulting and Clinical Psychology, 46*, 1092–1104.

Chen, K., & Kandel, D. (2002). Relationship between extent of cocaine use and dependence among adolescents and adults in the United States. *Drug and Alcohol Dependence, 68*, 65–85.

Community Epidemiology Work Group. (2003). *Epidemiologic trends in drug abuse: Highlights and executive summary* (NIH Publication No. 03–5364). Bethesda, MD: National Institute on Drug Abuse.

Cottler, L. B., Grant, B. F., Blaine, J. D., Vanetsanos, M., Pull, C., Hasin, D., et al. (1997). Concordance of the DSM-IV alcohol and drug disorder criteria and diagnoses as measured by AUDADIS-ADR, CIDI and SCAN. *Drug and Alcohol Dependence, 47*, 195–205.

Cottler, L. B., Shillington, A. M., Compton, W. M., Mager, D., & Spitznagel, E. L. (1993). Subjective reports of withdrawal among cocaine users: Recommendations for DSM-IV. *Drug and Alcohol Dependence, 33*, 97–104.

Crits-Christoph, P., Siqueland, L., McCalmont, E., Weiss, R. D., Gastfriend, D. R., Frank, A., et al. (2001). Impact of psychosocial treatments on associated problems of cocaine-dependent patients. *Journal of Consulting and Clinical Psychology, 69*, 825–830.

Cunningham, J. A., Sobell, L. C., Gavin, D. R., Sobell, M. B., & Breslin, F. C. (1997). Assessing motivation for change: Preliminary development and evaluation of a scale measuring the costs and benefits of changing alcohol or drug use. *Psychology of Addictive Behaviors, 11*, 107–114.

Darke, S. (1998). Self-report among injecting drug users: A review. *Drug and Alcohol Dependence, 51*, 253–263.

Darke, S., Hall, W., Heather, N., Ward, J., & Wodak, A. (1991). The reliability and validity of a scale to measure HIV risk-taking behavior among intravenous drug users. *AIDS, 5*, 181–185.

Davies, A. D. M. (1968). The influence of age on trail making test performance. *Journal of Clinical Psychology, 24,* 96–98.

Derogatis, L. R., & Melisaratos, N. (1983). The Brief Symptom Index: An introductory report. *Psychological Medicine, 13,* 595–605.

DiClemente, C. C., & Hughes, S. O. (1990). Stages of change profiles in outpatient alcoholism treatment. *Journal of Substance Abuse, 2,* 217–235.

DiSclafani, V., Tolou-Shams, M., Price, L. J., & Fein, G. (2002). Neuropsychological performance of individuals dependent on crack cocaine or crack cocaine and alcohol, at 6 weeks and 6 months of abstinence. *Drug and Alcohol Dependence, 66,* 161–171.

Donovan, D. M. (1999). Assessment strategies and measures in addictive behaviors. In B. S. McCrady & E. E. Epstein (Eds.), *Addictions: A comprehensive guidebook* (pp. 187–215). New York: Oxford University Press.

Donovan, D. M., & Marlatt, G. A. (1988). *Assessment of addictive behaviors.* New York: Guilford Press.

Downey, L., Rosengren, D. B., & Donovan, D. M. (2001). Sources of motivation for abstinence: A replication analysis of the Reasons for Quitting Questionnaire. *Addictive Behaviors, 26,* 79–89.

Edwards, G., Arif, A., & Hodgson, R. (1981). Nomenclature and classification of drug and alcohol related problems. *Bulletin of the World Health Organization, 59,* 225–242.

Ehrman, R. N., Robbins, S. J., & Cornish, J. W. (2001). Results of a baseline urine test predict levels of cocaine use during treatment. *Drug and Alcohol Dependence, 62,* 1–7.

Epstein, D. E., Hawkins, W. E., Covi, L., Umbricht, A., & Preston, K. L. (2003). Cognitive behavioral therapy plus contingency management for cocaine use: Findings during treatment and across 12–month follow-up. *Psychology of Addictive Behaviors, 17,* 73–82.

Fals-Stewart, W. (1996). Intermediate length screening of impairment among psychoactive substance-abusing patients: A comparison of two batteries. *Journal of Substance Abuse, 8,* 1–17.

Fals-Stewart, W., & Bates, M. E. (2003). The neuropsychological test performance of drug-abusing patients: An examination of latent cognitive abilities and risk factors. *Experimental and Clinical Psychopharmacology, 11,* 34–45.

Feingold, A., Ball, S. A., Kranzler, H. R., & Rounsaville, B. J. (1996). Generalizability of the Type A/Type B distinction across different psychoactive substances. *American Journal of Drug and Alcohol Abuse, 22,* 449–462.

First, M. B., Spitzer, R. L., Gibbon, M., & Williams, J. B. W. (1995). *Structured Clinical Interview for DSM-IV, Patient Edition.* Washington, DC: American Psychiatric Press.

Folstein, M. F., Folstein, S. E., & McHugh, P. R. (1975). "Mini-Mental State": A practical method for grading the cognitive state of patients for the clinician. *Journal of Psychiatric Research, 12,* 189–198.

Gastfriend, D. R., Filstead, W. J., Reif, S., & Najavits, L. M. (1995). Validity of assessing treatment readiness in patients with substance use disorders. *American Journal on Addictions, 4,* 254–260.

Gossop, M., Best, D., Marsden, J., & Strang, J. (1997). Test–retest reliability of the Severity of Dependence Scale. *Addiction, 92,* 353.

Gossop, M., Darke, S., Griffiths, P., Hando, J., Powis, B., Hall, W., et al. (1995). The Severity of Dependence Scale (SDS): Psychometric properties of the SDS in English and Australian samples of heroin, cocaine and amphetamine users. *Addiction, 90,* 607–614.

Gottschalk, C. H., Beauvais, J., Hart, R., & Kosten, T. R. (2001). Cognitive function and cerebral perfusion during cocaine abstinence. *American Journal of Psychiatry, 158,* 540–545.

Graham, J. R., & Strenger, V. E. (1988). MMPI characteristics of alcoholics: A review. *Journal of Consulting and Clinical Psychology, 56,* 197–205.

Hall, S. M., Havassy, B. E., & Wasserman, D. A. (1991). Effects of commitment to abstinence, positive moods, stress and coping to relapse to cocaine use. *Journal of Consulting and Clinical Psychology, 59,* 526–532.

Hasin, D. S., & Grant, B. F. (1987). Psychiatric diagnosis of patients with substance abuse problems: A comparison of two procedures, the DIS and the SADS-L. *Journal of Psychiatric Research, 21,* 7–22.

Hasin, D. S., Trautman, K. D., Miele, G. M., Samet, S., Smith, M., & Endicott, J. (1996). Psychiatric Research Interview for Substance and Mental Disorders (PRISM): Reliability for substance abusers. *American Journal of Psychiatry, 153,* 1195–1201.

Hatsukami, D. K., & Fischman, M. W. (1996). Crack cocaine and cocaine hydrochloride: Are the differences myth or reality? *Journal of the American Medical Association, 276*(19), 1580–1588.

Hawkins, J. D., Catalano, R. F., & Wells, E. A. (1986). Measuring effects of a skills training intervention for drug abusers. *Journal of Consulting and Clinical Psychology, 54,* 661–664.

Hawks, R. L., & Chiang, C. N. (1986). *Urine testing for drugs of abuse.* Rockville, MD: National Institute on Drug Abuse.

Heaton, R. K., Thompson, L. L., Nelson, L. M., Filley, C. M., & Franklin, G. M. (1990). Brief and intermediate length screening of neuropsychological impairment in multiple sclerosis. In S. M. Rao (Ed.), *Multiple sclerosis: A neuropsychological perspective* (pp. 149–160). New York: Oxford University Press.

Heil, S. H., Badger, G. J., & Higgins, S. T. (2001). Alcohol dependence among cocaine dependent outpatients: Demographics, drug use, treatment outcome and other characteristics. *Journal of Studies on Alcohol, 62,* 14–22.

Helzer, J. E., & Pryzbeck, T. R. (1988). The co-occurence of alcoholism with other psychiatric disorders in the general population and its impact on treatment. *Journal of Studies on Alcohol, 49,* 219–224.

Higgins, S. T., Budney, A. J., Bickel, W. K., Foerg, F. E., Donham, R., & Badger, G. J. (1994). Incentives improve outcome in outpatient behavioral treatment of cocaine dependence. *Archives of General Psychiatry, 51,* 568–576.

Higgins, S. T., Budney, A. J., Bickel, W. K., & Hughes, J. R. (1993). Achieving cocaine abstinence with a behavioral approach. *American Journal of Psychiatry, 150,* 763–769.

Higgins, S. T., Budney, A. J., Bickel, W. K., Hughes, J. R., & Foerg, F. (1993). Disulfiram therapy in patients abusing cocaine and alcohol. *American Journal of Psychiatry, 150,* 675–676.

Higgins, S. T., Roll, J. M., & Bickel, W. K. (1996). Alcohol pretreatment increases preference for cocaine over monetary reinforcement. *Psychopharmacology (Berlin), 123,* 1–8.

Higgins, S. T., Wong, C. J., Badger, G. J., Haug-Ogden, D. E., & Dantona, R. L. (2000). Contingent reinforcement increases cocaine abstinence during outpatient treatment and one year follow-up. *Journal of Consulting and Clinical Psychology, 68,* 64–72.

Hunt, W., Barnet, L., & Branch, L. (1971). Relapse rates in addiction programs. *Journal of Clinical Psychology, 27,* 455–456.

Husband, S. D., Marlowe, D. B., Lamb, R. J., Iguchi, M. Y., Bux, D. A., Kirby, K. C., et al. (1996). Decline in self-reported dysphoria after treatment entry in inner-city cocaine addicts. *Journal of Consulting and Clinical Psychology, 64,* 221–224.

Irwin, M., Schuckit, M. A., & Smith, T. L. (1990). Clinical importance of age of onset in Type 1 and Type 2 primary alcoholics. *Archives of General Psychiatry, 47,* 320–324.

Jatlow, P. M., Ellsworth, J. D., Bradberry, C. W., Winger, G., Taylor, R., & Roth, R. K. (1991). Cocaethylene: A neuropharmacologically active metabolite associated with concurrent cocaine–ethanol ingestion. *Life Sciences, 48,* 1787–1794.

Kampman, K. M., Alterman, A. I., Volpicelli, J. R., Maany, I., Muller, E. S., Luce, D. D., et al. (2001). Cocaine withdrawal symptoms and initial urine toxicology results predict treatment attrition in outpatient cocaine dependence treatment. *Psychology of Addictive Behaviors, 15,* 52–59.

Kampman, K. M., Volpicelli, J. R., McGinnis, D. E., Alterman, A. I., Weinrieb, R. M., D'Angelo, L., et al. (1998). Reliability and validity of the Cocaine Selective Severity Assessment. *Addictive Behaviors, 23,* 449–461.

Kandel, D. B. (1985). Stages in adolescent involvement in drug use. *Science, 190,* 912–914.

Kandel, D. B., & Logan, J. A. (1984). Patterns of drug use from adolescence to young adulthood: I. Periods of risk for initiation, stabilization, and decline in use. *American Journal of Public Health, 74,* 660–666.

Kandel, D. B., Yamaguchi, K., & Chen, K. (1992). Stages of progression in drug involvement from adolescence to adulthood. *Journal of Studies on Alcohol, 53,* 447–457.

Kessler, R. C., Crum, R. M., Warner, L. A., Nelson, C. B., Schulenberg, J., & Anthony, J. C. (1997). Lifetime co-occurence of DSM-III-R alcohol abuse and dependence with other psychiatric disorders in the National Comorbidity Study. *Archives of General Psychiatry, 54,* 313–321.

Kessler, R. C., McGonagle, K. A., Zhao, S., Nelson, C. B., Hughes, M., Eshleman, S., et al. (1994). Lifetime and 12–month prevalence of DSM-III-R psychiatric disorders in the United States: Results from the National Comorbidity Study. *Archives of General Psychiatry, 51,* 8–19.

Kosten, T. R., Rounsaville, B. J., & Kleber, H. D. (1983). Concurrent validity of the Addiction Severity Index. *Journal of Nervous and Mental Disease, 171,* 606–610.

Kosten, T. R., Rounsaville, B. J., & Kleber, H. D. (1987). Multidimensionality and prediction of treatment outcomes in opioid addicts: 2.5 year follow-up. *Comprehensive Psychiatry, 28,* 3–13.

Lavori, P. W., Bloch, D. A., Bridge, P. T., Leiderman, D. B., LoCastro, J. S., & Somoza, E. (1999). Plans, designs, and analyses for clinical trials of anti-cocaine medications: Where are we today? *Journal of Clinical Psychopharmacology, 19,* 246–256.

Leshner, A. I. (1999). Science-based views of drug addiction and its treatment. *Journal of the American Medical Association, 282,* 1314–1316.

Levin, F. R., Evans, S. M., & Kleber, H. D. (1998). Prevalence of adult attention deficit hyperactivity disorder among cocaine abusers seeking treatment. *Drug and Alcohol Dependence, 52,* 15–25.

Maisto, S. A., McKay, J. R., & Connors, G. J. (1990). Self-report issues in substance abuse: State of the art and future directions. *Behavioral Assessment, 12,* 117–134.

Marlatt, G. A., & Gordon, J. R. (Eds.). (1985). *Relapse prevention: Maintenance strategies in the treatment of addictive behaviors.* New York: Guilford Press.

Marlowe, D. B., Husband, S. D., Lamb, R. J., & Kirby, K. C. (1995). Psychiatric comorbidity in cocaine dependence: Diverging trends, Axis II spectrum, and gender differentials. *American Journal on Addictions, 4,* 70–81.

Maude-Griffin, P. M., Hohenstein, J. M., Humfleet, G. L., Reilly, P. M., Tusel, D. J., & Hall, S. M. (1998). Superior efficacy of cognitive-behavioral therapy for crack cocaine abusers: Main and matching effects. *Journal of Consulting and Clinical Psychology, 66,* 832–837.

McCance-Katz, E. F., Price, L. H., Kosten, T. R., & Jatlow, P. M. (1995). Cocaethylene: Pharmacology, physiology, and behavioral effects in humans. *Journal of Pharmacology and Experimental Therapeutics, 274,* 215–223.

McDermott, P. A., Alterman, A. I., Brown, L. S., & Zaballero, A. (1996). Construct refinement and confirmation for the Addiction Severity Index. *Psychological Assessment, 8,* 182–189.

McDowell, D. M., Levin, F. R., Seracini, A. M., & Nunes, E. V. (2000). Venlafaxine treatment of cocaine abusers with depressive disorders. *American Journal of Drug and Alcohol Abuse, 26,* 25–31.

McGue, M., Pickens, R. W., & Svikis, D. S. (1992). Sex and age effects on the inheritance of alcohol problems: A twin study. *Journal of Abnormal Psychology, 101,* 3–17.

McKay, J. R., Alterman, A. I., Cacciola, J. S., O'Brien, C. P., Koppenhaver, J., & Shepard, D. S. (1999). Continuing care for cocaine dependence: Comprehensive 2–year outcomes. *Journal of Consulting and Clinical Psychology, 63,* 70–78.

McKay, J. R., Alterman, A. I., Koppenhaver, J. M., Mulvaney, F. D., Bovasso, G. B., & Ward, K. (2001). Continuous, catergorical and time to event cocaine use outcome variables: Degree of intercorrelation and sensitivity to treatment group differences. *Drug and Alcohol Dependence, 62,* 19–31.

McKay, J. R., Alterman, A. I., Mulvaney, F. D., & Koppenhaver, J. M. (1999). Predicting proximal factors in cocaine relapse and near miss episodes: Clinical and theoretical implications. *Drug and Alcohol Dependence, 56,* 67–78.

McKay, J. R., Alterman, A. I., Rutherford, M. J., Cacciola, J. S., & McLellan, A. T. (1999). The relationship of alcohol use to cocaine relapse in cocaine dependent patients in an aftercare study. *Journal of Studies on Alcohol, 60,* 176–180.

McKay, J. R., Merikle, E., Mulvaney, F. D., Weiss, R. V., & Koppenhaver, J. M. (2001). Factors accounting for cocaine use two years following initiation of continuing care. *Addiction, 96,* 213–225.

McKay, J. R., Rutherford, M. J., Alterman, A. I., Cacciola, J. S., & Kaplan, M. R. (1995). An examination of the cocaine relapse process. *Drug and Alcohol Dependence, 38,* 35–43.

McLellan, A. T., Alterman, A. I., Metzger, D. S., Grissom, G. R., Woody, G. E., Luborsky, L., et al. (1994). Similarity of outcome predictors across opiate, cocaine, and alcohol treatments: Role of treatment services. *Journal of Consulting and Clinical Psychology, 62,* 1141–1158.

McLellan, A. T., Arndt, I. O., Metzger, D., Woody, G. E., & O'Brien, C. P. (1993). The effects of psychosocial services in substance abuse treatment. *Journal of the American Medical Association, 269,* 1953–1959.

McLellan, A. T., Grissom, G. R., Zanis, D., & Randall, M. (1997). Problem-service "matching" in addiction treatment: A prospective study in four programs. *Archives of General Psychiatry, 54,* 730–735.

McLellan, A. T., Hagan, T. A., Levine, M., Meyers, K., Gould, F., Bencivengo, M., et al. (1999). Does clinical case management improve outpatient addiction treatment? *Drug and Alcohol Dependence, 55,* 91–103.

McLellan, A. T., Kushner, H., Metzger, D., Peters, R., Smith, I., Grissom, G., et al. (1992). The fifth edition of the Addiction Severity Index. *Journal of Substance Abuse Treatment, 9,* 199–213.

McLellan, A. T., Luborsky, L., Woody, G. E., & O'Brien, C. P. (1980). An improved diagnostic evaluation instrument for substance abuse patients: The Addiction Severity Index. *Journal of Nervous and Mental Disease, 168,* 26–33.

McLellan, A. T., Luborsky, L., Woody, G. E., O'Brien, C. P., & Druley, K. A. (1983). Predicting response to alcohol and drug treatments: Role of psychiatric severity. *Archives of General Psychiatry, 40,* 620–625.

McLellan, A. T., Luborsky, L., Woody, G. E., O'Brien, C. P., & Kron, R. (1981). Are the addiction-related problems of substance abusers really related? *Journal of Nervous and Mental Disease, 169,* 232–239.

McLellan, A. T., & McKay, J. R. (1998). The treatment of addiction: What can research offer practice? In S. Lamb, M. R. Greenlick, & D. McCarty (Eds.), *Bridging the gap between practice and research: Forging partnerships with community based drug and alcohol treatment* (pp. 147–185). Washington, DC: National Academy Press.

McMillan, D. E., & Gilmore-Thomas, K. (1996). Stability of opioid craving over time as measured by visual analog scales. *Drug and Alcohol Dependence, 40,* 235–239.

Mee-Lee, D. (1988). An instrument for treatment progress and matching: The Recovery Attitude and Treatment Evaluator (RAATE). *Journal of Substance Abuse Treatment, 5,* 183–186.

Mengis, M. M., Maude-Griffin, P. M., Delucchi, K. L., & Hall, S. M. (2002). Alcohol use affects the outcome of treatment for cocaine abuse. *American Journal on Addictions, 11,* 219–227.

Miele, G. M., Carpenter, K. M., Cockerham, M. S., Trautman, K. D., Blaine, J. D., & Hasin, D. S. (2000). Concurrent and predictive validity of the Substance Dependence Severity Scale (SDSS). *Drug and Alcohol Dependence, 59,* 77–88.

Miller, W. R., & Heather, N. (1998). *Treating addictive behaviors, second edition.* New York: Plenum Press.

Miller, W. R., & Rollnick, S. (1991). *Motivational interviewing: Preparing people to change addictive behavior.* New York: Guilford Press.

Miller, W. R., & Tonigan, J. S. (1996). Assessing drinker's motivation for change: The Stages of Change Readiness and Treatment Eagerness Scale (SOCRATES). *Psychology of Addictive Behaviors, 10,* 81–89.

Miller, W. R., Tonigan, J. S., & Longabaugh, R. (1995). *The Drinker Inventory of Consequences (DRIC): An instrument for assessing adverse consequences of alcohol abuse: Test manual* (Vol. 4). Rockville, MD: NIAAA.

Miller, W. R., Zweben, A., DiClemente, C. C., & Rychtarik, R. G. (1992). *Motiva-*

tional enhancement therapy manual: A clinical research guide for therapists treating individuals with alcohol abuse and dependence. Rockville, MD: National Institute on Alcohol Abuse and Alcoholism.

Milligan, C. O., Nich, C., & Carroll, K. M. (2004). Ethnic differences in substance abuse treatment retention, compliance, and outcome: Findings from two randomized clinical trials. Psychiatric Services, 55, 167–173.

Moeller, F. G., Dougherty, D. M., Barratt, E. S., Oderinde, V., Mathias, C. W., Harper, R. A., et al. (2002). Increased impulsivity in cocaine dependent subjects independent of antisocial personality disorder and aggression. Drug and Alcohol Dependence, 68, 105–111.

Monti, P. M., Rohsenow, D. J., Michalec, E., Martin, R. A., & Abrams, D. B. (1997). Brief coping skills treatment for cocaine abuse: Substance abuse outcomes at three months. Addiction, 92, 1717–1728.

Nathan, P. E. (1989). Substance use disorders in the DSM-IV. Journal of Abnormal Psychology, 100, 356–361.

Navaline, H. A., Snider, E. C., Petro, C. J., Tobin, D., Metzger, D., Alterman, A. I., et al. (1994). Preparation for AIDS vaccine trials: An automated version of the Risk Assessment Battery. AIDS Research and Human Retroviruses, 10, 281–291.

Nunes, E. V., Quitkin, F. M., Donovan, S. J., Deliyannides, D., Ocepek-Welikson, K., Koenig, T., et al. (1998). Imipramine treatment of opiate dependent patients with depressive disorders: A placebo-controlled trial. Archives of General Psychiatry, 55, 153–160.

O'Brien, C. P. (1997). A range of research-based pharmacotherapies for addiction. Science, 278, 66–70.

O'Malley, S. S., Adamse, M., Heaton, R. K., & Gawin, F. H. (1992). Neuropsychological impairment in chronic cocaine abusers. American Journal of Drug and Alcohol Abuse, 18, 131–144.

Pantalon, M. V., Nich, C., Frankforter, T., & Carroll, K. M. (2002). The URICA as a measure of motivation to change among treatment-seeking individuals with concurrent alcohol and cocaine problems. Psychology of Addictive Behaviors, 16, 299–307.

Perry, J. C. (1992). Problems and considerations in the valid assessment of personality disorders. American Journal of Psychiatry, 149, 1645–1653.

Peterson, L., & Sobell, L. C. (1994). Introduction to the state-of-the-art review series: Research contributions to clinical assessment. Behavior Therapy, 25, 523–532.

Petry, N. M. (2000). A comprehensive guide to the application of contingency management procedures in clinical settings. Drug and Alcohol Dependence, 58, 9–25.

Petry, N. M., Tedford, J., Austin, M., Nich, C., Carroll, K. M., & Rounsaville, B. J. (2002). Prize reinforcement contingency management for treating cocaine users: How low can we go, and with whom? Addiction, 99, 349–360.

Preston, K. L., Silverman, K., Higgins, S. T., Brooner, R. K., Montoya, I. D., Schuster, C. R., et al. (1998). Cocaine use early in treatment predicts outcome in a behavioral treatment program. Journal of Consulting and Clinical Psychology, 66, 691–696.

Preston, K. L., Silverman, K., Schuster, C. R., & Cone, E. J. (1997). Assessment of cocaine use with quantitative urinalysis and estimation of new uses. Addiction, 92, 717–727.

Prochaska, J. O., & DiClemente, C. C. (1982). Transtheoretical therapy: Toward a more integrative model of change. *Psychotherapy: Theory, Research and Practice, 19,* 276–288.

Prochaska, J. O., DiClemente, C. C., & Norcross, J. C. (1992). In search of how people change: Applications to addictive behaviors. *American Psychologist, 47,* 1102–1114.

Regier, D. A., Farmer, M. E., Rae, D. S., Locke, B. Z., Keith, S. J., Judd, L. L., et al. (1990). Comorbidity of mental disorders with alcohol and other drug abuse. Results from the Epidemiologic Catchment Area (ECA) study. *Journal of the American Medical Association, 264,* 2511–2518.

Reitan, R. M. (1958). Validity of the Trail Making Test as an indicator of organic brain damage. *Perceptual and Motor Skills, 8,* 271–276.

Robbins, S. J., Ehrman, R. N., Childress, A. R., Cornish, J. W., & O'Brien, C. P. (2000). Mood state and recent cocaine use are not associated with levels of cocaine cue reactivity. *Drug and Alcohol Dependence, 59,* 33–42.

Robins, L. N., Helzer, J. E., Croughan, J., & Ratcliff, K. S. (1981). National Institute of Mental Health Diagnostic Interview Schedule: Its history, characteristics, and validity. *Archives of General Psychiatry, 38,* 381–389.

Robins, L. N., Wing, J. K., & Helzer, J. E. (1983). *Composite International Diagnostic Interview (CIDI).* Geneva: World Health Organization.

Rohsenow, D. J., Monti, P. M., Martin, R. A., Michalec, E., & Abrams, D. B. (2000). Brief coping skills treatment for cocaine abuse: 12-month substance use outcomes. *Journal of Consulting and Clinical Psychology, 68,* 515–520.

Rohsenow, D. J., Niaura, R. S., Childress, A. R., Abrams, D. B., & Monti, P. M. (1990/1991). Cue reactivity in addictive behaviors: Theoretical and treatment implications. *International Journal of the Addictions, 25,* 957–993.

Rollnick, S., Heather, N., Gold, R., & Hall, W. (1992). Development of a short "readiness to change" questionnaire for use in brief, opportunistic interventions among excessive drinkers. *British Journal of Addiction, 87,* 743–754.

Rosen, C. S., Henson, B. R., Finney, J. W., & Moos, R. H. (2000). Consistency of self-administered and interview-based Addiction Severity Index composite scores. *Addiction, 95,* 419–425.

Ross, H. E., Glaser, F. B., & Germanson, T. (1988). The prevalence of psychiatric disorders in patients with alcohol and other drug problems. *Archives of General Psychiatry, 44,* 505–513.

Rounsaville, B. J., Anton, S. F., Carroll, K. M., Budde, D., Prusoff, B. A., & Gawin, F. I. (1991). Psychiatric diagnosis of treatment seeking cocaine abusers. *Archives of General Psychiatry, 48,* 43–51.

Rounsaville, B. J., Dolinsky, Z. S., Babor, T. F., & Meyer, R. E. (1987). Psychopathology as a predictor of treatment outcome in alcoholics. *Archives of General Psychiatry, 44,* 505–513.

Rounsaville, B. J., Kosten, T. R., Weissman, M. M., & Kleber, H. D. (1986). Prognostic significance of psychopathology in treated opiate addicts. *Archives of General Psychiatry, 43,* 739–745.

Rounsaville, B. J., Kranzler, H. R., Ball, S. A., Tennen, H., Poling, J., & Triffleman, E. G. (1998). Personality disorders in substance abusers: Relation to substance use. *Journal of Nervous and Mental Disease, 186,* 87–95.

Rounsaville, B. J., Spitzer, R. L., & Williams, J. B. W. (1986). Proposed changes in

DSM-III substance use disorders: Description and rationale. *American Journal of Psychiatry, 143,* 463–468.

Rounsaville, B. J., Tierney, T., Crits-Christoph, T., Weissman, M. M., & Kleber, H. D. (1982). Predictors of outcome in treatment of opiate addicts: Evidence for the multidimensional nature of addicts' problems. *Comprehensive Psychiatry, 23,* 462–478.

Rounsaville, B. J., Weissman, M. M., Kleber, H. D., & Wilber, C. W. (1982). Heterogeneity of psychiatric diagnosis in treated opiate addicts. *Archives of General Psychiatry, 39,* 161–166.

Roy, A., DeJong, J., Lamparksi, D., & Adinoff, B. (1991). Mental disorders among alcoholics: Relationship to age of onset and cerebrospinal fluid neuropeptides. *Archives of General Psychiatry, 48,* 423–427.

Satel, S. L., Kosten, T. R., Schuckit, M. A., & Fischman, M. W. (1993). Should protracted withdrawal from drugs be included in DSM-IV? *American Journal of Psychiatry, 150*(5), 695–704.

Satel, S. L., Price, L. H., Palumbo, J. M., McDougle, C. J., Krystal, J. H., Gawin, F. H., et al. (1991). Clinical phenomenology and neurobiology of cocaine abstinence: A prospective inpatient study. *American Journal of Psychiatry, 148,* 1712–1716.

Sayette, M. A., Shiffman, S., Tiffany, S. T., Niaura, R. S., Martin, C. S., & Shadel, W. G. (2000). The measurement of drug craving. *Addiction, 95*(Suppl. 2), S189–S210.

Schwartz, R. H. (1988). Urine testing in the detection of drugs of abuse. *Archives of Internal Medicine, 148,* 2407–2412.

Shaffer, H. J., & Eber, G. (2002). Temporal progression of cocaine dependence symptoms in the U.S. National Comorbidity Survey. *Addiction, 97,* 543–554.

Shipley, W. C. (1967). *Manual: Shipley—Institute of Living Scale.* Los Angeles: Western Psychological Services.

Silverman, K., Wong, C. J., Umbricht-Schneiter, A., Montoya, I. D., Schuster, C. R., & Preston, K. L. (1998). Broad beneficial effects of cocaine abstinence reinforcement among methadone patients. *Journal of Consulting and Clinical Psychology, 66,* 811–824.

Simpson, D. D., Joe, G. W., Fletcher, B. W., Hubbard, R. L., & Anglin, M. D. (1999). A national evaluation of treatment outcomes for cocaine dependence. *Archives of General Psychiatry, 56,* 507–514.

Sklar, S. M., Annis, H. M., & Turner, N. E. (1997). Development and validation of the Drug-Taking Confidence Questionnaire: A measure of coping self-efficacy. *Addictive Behaviors, 22,* 655–670.

Sklar, S. M., & Turner, N. E. (1999). A brief measure for the assessment of coping self-efficacy among alcohol and other drug users. *Addiction, 94,* 723–729.

Sobell, L. C., & Sobell, M. B. (1992). Timeline Followback: A technique for assessing self-reported alcohol consumption. In R. Z. Litten & J. Allen (Eds.), *Measuring alcohol consumption: Psychosocial and biological methods* (pp. 41–72). Totowa, NJ: Humana Press.

Sobell, L. C., Toneatto, T., & Sobell, M. C. (1994). Behavioral assessment and treatment planning for alcohol, tobacco, and other drug problems: Current status with an emphasis on clinical applications. *Behavior Therapy, 25,* 533–580.

Sofuoglu, M., Dudish-Poulsen, S., Brown, S. B., & Hatsukami, D. K. (2003). Association of cocaine withdrawal symptoms with more severe dependence and enhanced subjective response to cocaine. *Drug and Alcohol Dependence, 69,* 273–282.

Sofuoglu, M., Gonzalez, G., Poling, J., & Kosten, T. R. (2003). Prediction of treatment outcome by baseline urine cocaine results and self-reported cocaine use for cocaine and opioid dependence. *American Journal of Drug and Alcohol Abuse, 29,* 713–727.

Sonne, S. C., & Brady, K. T. (1998). Diagnosis of personality disorders in cocaine-dependence individuals. *American Journal on Addictions, 7,* 1–6.

Sorenson, J., & Copeland, A. L. (2000). Drug abuse treatment as an HIV prevention strategy: A review. *Drug and Alcohol Dependence, 59,* 17–31.

Strain, E. C., Stitzer, M. L., & Bigelow, G. E. (1991). Early treatment time course of depressive symptoms in opiate addicts. *Journal of Nervous and Mental Disease, 179,* 215–221.

Substance Abuse and Mental Health Services Administration. (2003). *Results from the 2002 National Survey on Drug Use and Health: National findings* (NHSDA Series H-22, DHHS Publication No. SMA 03-3836). Rockville, MD: Office of Applied Statistics, Substance Abuse and Mental Health Services Administration.

Tiffany, S. T. (1990). A cognitive model of drug urges and drug use behavior: Role of automatic and nonautomatic processes. *Psychological Review, 97,* 147–168.

Tiffany, S. T., Carter, B. L., & Singleton, E. G. (2000). Challenges in the manipulation, assessment and interpretation of craving relevant variables. *Addiction, 95,* S177–187.

Tiffany, S. T., Singleton, E., Haertzen, C. A., & Henningfield, J. E. (1993). The development of a cocaine craving questionnaire. *Drug and Alcohol Dependence, 34,* 19–28.

Topp, L., & Mattick, R. P. (1997). Choosing a cut-off on the Severity of Dependence Scale (SDS) for amphetamine users. *Addiction, 92,* 839–845.

Turnbull, J. E., George, L. K., Landerman, R., Swartz, M. S., & Blazer, D. G. (1990). Social outcomes related to age of onset among psychiatric disorders. *Journal of Consulting and Clinical Psychology, 58,* 832–839.

Turner, N. E., Annis, H. M., & Sklar, S. M. (1997). Measurement of antecedents to drug and alcohol use: Psychometric properties of the Inventory of Drug-Taking Situations (IDTS). *Behaviour Research and Therapy, 35,* 465–483.

Verheul, R., Ball, S. A., & van den Brink, W. (1998). Substance abuse and personality disorders. In H. R. Kranzler & B. J. Rounsaville (Eds.), *Dual diagnosis and treatment: Substance abuse and comorbid medical and psychiatric disorders.* New York: Marcel Dekker.

Wagner, F. A., & Anthony, J. C. (2002). From first drug use to drug dependence: Developmental periods of risk for dependence upon marijuana, cocaine, and alcohol. *Neuropsychopharmacology, 26,* 479–488.

Weiss, R. D., Griffin, M. L., Mazurick, C., Berkman, B., Gastfriend, D. R., Frank, A., et al. (2003). The relationship between cocaine craving, psychosocial treatment, and subsequent cocaine use. *American Journal of Psychiatry, 160,* 1320–1325.

Weiss, R. D., Mirin, S. M., Griffin, M. L., Gunderson, J. G., & Hufford, C. (1993). Personality disorders in cocaine dependence. *Comprehensive Psychiatry, 34,* 145–149.

Westerberg, V. S., Tonigan, J. S., & Miller, W. R. (1998). Reliability of Form 90D: An instrument for quantifying drug use. *Substance Abuse, 19,* 179–189.

Winhusen, T. M., Somoza, E. C., Singal, B., Kim, S., Horn, P. S., & Rotrosen, J. (2003). Measuring outcome in cocaine clinical trials: A comparison of sweat patches with urine toxicology and participant self-report. *Addiction, 98,* 317–324.

Zanis, D. A., McLellan, A. T., & Corse, S. (1997). Is the Addiction Severity Index a reliable and valid assessment instrument among clients with severe and persistent mental illness and substance abuse disorders? *Community Mental Health Journal, 33,* 213–227.

Zanis, D. A., McLellan, A. T., & Randall, M. (1994). Can you trust patient self-reports of drug use during treatment? *Drug and Alcohol Dependence, 35,* 127–132.

Zimmerman, M. (1994). Diagnosing personality disorders: A review of issues and research methods. *Archives of General Psychiatry, 51,* 225–245.

CHAPTER 6

Assessment of Amphetamine Use Disorders

RICHARD A. RAWSON
RUTHLYN SODANO
MAUREEN HILLHOUSE

Amphetamine and methamphetamine (MA) are the most widely abused illicit drugs globally, second only to marijuana (World Health Organization [WHO], 1997). Over 35 million individuals use and abuse MA on a regular basis worldwide, whereas cocaine use is limited to approximately 15 million people (mostly in North America) and heroin is used by fewer than 10 million (WHO, 1997). However, the cocaine epidemic of the 1980s received far greater attention and research effort than the comparable problem of MA use in the United States during the 1990s (Rawson, Marinelli-Casey, & Huber, 2002). As a result, the research literature on both the nature of cocaine abuse and on the clinical management and assessment of cocaine use is far more developed than that on MA.

MA and cocaine are both powerful psychostimulants that share many similarities in their pharmacology, the pathologies that result from their use and abuse, and the manner in which users should be assessed and treated. Consequently, the principles and methods described by Carroll and Ball (Chapter 5, this volume) for the assessment of cocaine users have considerable application for clinical assessment work with MA users. Chapter 9, this volume, contains essential information relevant to the assessment of individuals with all forms of psychostimulant disorders and should be read in conjunction with this chapter.

Although MA and related compounds have many properties that are similar to those of cocaine, there are some important differences in terms of pharmacology, the populations and geographic areas affected, associated syndromes, and the specific clinical manifestations that are relevant to the proper recognition and assessment of MA use disorders (Brecht, von Mayrhauser, & Anglin, 2000; Castro, Barrington, Walton, & Rawson, 2000; Simon, Domier, Carnell, Brethen, Rawson, & Ling, 2000). This chapter highlights some of the issues that are of particular importance to clinicians faced with the challenge of properly assessing MA users.

WHAT IS METHAMPHETAMINE?

As a specific compound in the larger family of powerful psychoactive stimulants, the amphetamines, MA has become the most popular of the amphetamines for illicit manufacture and use due to its high potency, its ease of manufacture, and the ready availability of its precursor chemicals (Center for Substance Abuse Treatment [CSAT], 1997). Methamphetamine is known by many different names including "crystal," "meth," or "speed." It can be injected, smoked, snorted, or ingested orally. The intensity and duration of the "rush" that accompanies the use of MA is a result of the release of high levels of dopamine into the brain and depends in part on the method of administration. Specifically, the effect is almost instantaneous when smoked or injected, whereas it takes approximately 5 minutes after snorting or 20 minutes after oral ingestion (Anglin, Burke, Perrochet, Stamper, & Dawud-Noursi, 2000). The half-life of methamphetamine is 12 hours, giving a duration of effect ranging from 8 to 24 hours. In contrast, the half-life of cocaine is 1 hour, giving a short-lived high of 20–30 minutes (Gawin & Ellinwood, 1988).

The immediate physiological effects of MA use are similar to those produced by the fight-or-flight response and include increased blood pressure, body temperature, and heart and breathing rates. Negative side effects include stomach cramps, shaking, high body temperature, stroke, and cardiac arrhythmia, as well as increased anxiety, insomnia, aggressive tendencies, paranoia, and hallucinations (Anglin et al., 2000). Subjective effects include euphoria, reduced fatigue, reduced hunger, increased energy, increased sex drive, and increased self-confidence. Prolonged use of MA may result in a tolerance for the drug and increased use at higher dosage levels, which may produce dependence. Such continual use of the drug, which is generally accompanied by little or no sleep, leads to an extremely irritable and paranoid state. In addition, chronic MA use produces a sensitization in some areas of the brain, and for some individuals, this results in an almost immediate, severe paranoia. Discontinuing use of MA often results in a state of depression, as well as irritability, fatigue, anergia, anhedonia, and some types of cognitive impairment that last anywhere from 2 days to several months.

The potential danger arising from the use of amphetamines and MAs is indicated in their placement in the schedules of the Controlled Substances Act (CSA). The CSA addresses the manufacture and distribution of narcotics, stimulants, depressants, hallucinogens, anabolic steroids, and chemicals used in the illicit production of controlled substances. All substances that are regulated under existing federal law are sorted into one of five schedules, based on the substance's medicinal value, harmfulness, and potential for abuse or addiction. Schedule I includes the most dangerous drugs that have no recognized medical use, whereas Schedule V includes the least dangerous drugs. Amphetamines and MAs, along with other amphetamine-type drugs, such as methylphenidate (Ritalin) and phenmetrazine (Preludin), are included in Schedule II (Control Level). Schedule II drugs are considered those with a high abuse potential and severe psychic or physical dependence liability. Other amphetamine-like drugs, such as diethylpropion (Tenuate), benzphetamine (Didrex), and phentermine (Ionamin), are included in Schedules III or IV of the CSA. It is presumed that all of these drugs are capable of producing each of the listed amphetamine-induced disorders (Jaffe, Ling, & Rawson, 2005).

BACKGROUND

Amphetamines were introduced into medical use in the early 1930s as a nasal spray for the treatment of asthma. By the mid-1960s, however, the Food and Drug Administration (FDA) placed the entire class of drugs under regulatory control due to growing concern over their misuse and overuse. Terms including "speed freaks" and "speed kills" left an enduring legacy in the popular vocabulary. Over the next decade, regulatory controls on lawfully made amphetamines were progressively tightened. Some misuse of amphetamines and amphetamine-like drugs persisted in the United States, with much of the supply coming from illicit laboratories. When it became illegal to procure the commonly used precursor phenyl2propanone (P2P), illicit manufacturers devised ways to create MA from ephedrine and/or pseudoephedrine, which were widely available in over the counter medications for colds and asthma (Anglin et al., 2000; Substance Abuse and Mental Health Services Administration [SAMHSA], 1999). The new method of synthesis actually yields a higher percentage of the active disomer of MA and was adopted both by criminal organizations using largescale laboratories and by independent producers whose small laboratories, usually located in remote rural areas, are more difficult to detect and eliminate.

Availability and Epidemiology

In the western and midwestern United States, MA use increased significantly in the 1990s and has resulted in both current and lifetime nonmedical use of amphetamines overtaking cocaine use in these areas (SAMHSA, 1999). Availability of MA is likely to increase in the United States, since production of MA is a relatively simple process, and while access to the necessary precursor chemicals (often common household items) can be reduced, it cannot feasibly be eliminated. Over the last decade, knowledge of how to manufacture MA has spread from a few "biker gang cookers" to two very important new groups. Creative "mom and pop chemists" can now download the recipes for MA from the Internet and produce small amounts for personal and associate use, and organized drug trafficking cartels have moved into the large-scale manufacturing of MA. As the epidemic of MA use has spread within the United States and in other countries, it has been clear that when MA becomes more available in a region, the use of the drug and the negative consequences of its use increase in response (Rawson, Anglin, & Ling, 2002).

Not only is MA likely to remain available, but it is also likely to remain inexpensive. MA users generally spend only about a quarter of the amount of money on MA as cocaine users do in purchasing cocaine, perhaps because the effects of MA are significantly longer lasting (10–12 hours). Nevertheless, MA users use more days per week and spend far more time under the influence than do cocaine users (Rawson et al., 2000). MA's efficacy in reducing fatigue and sustaining attention, as well as its value in weight reduction (primarily to women) are two of the reasons cited by users for their initial attraction to MA. These socially acceptable and valued uses of MA are quite effective for extended periods of time. Unless users begin injecting the drug, it is possible for many individuals to take MA for a period of years before intolerable negative consequences begin to occur. As long as people need to work long hours in tedious, physically demanding jobs, and as long as people want to lose weight, the allure of MA is likely to persist (Rawson, Anglin, & Ling, 2002).

The 2001 National Household Survey on Drug Abuse (NHSDA; SAMHSA, 2002) found that 7.1% of adults (ages 12 and older) reported lifetime nonmedical use of stimulants, which demonstrated a significant increase compared to the 1997 survey (4.5%). The percentage of adults reporting use in the previous 30 days was 1.1% in 2001, compared with 0.3% in 1997. In 1993, the treatment admission rate for primary amphetamine abuse in the United States was 14 admissions per 100,000 persons age 12 or older. By 1999, this rate had increased to 32 per 100,000 persons age 12 or older. Thirteen states had amphetamine admission rates of at least 55 per 100,000, and eight of these had rates of 100 or more per 100,000 (SAMHSA, 2002).

Geography

Continental United States

Epidemiological indicators have recorded the extensive use of MA in California and other western states for over a decade (Finnerty, 2003). This finding was recently underscored in California, when data from the first year of California's Proposition 36 program, which diverts drug use offenders to treatment programs, indicated that 50.4% of all admissions for this program were for individuals with a primary diagnosis of MA abuse or dependence. This is in contrast to cocaine users at 14% and heroin users at 11% (Longshore et al.,

2003). Additionally, rural areas of the western states, including many Indian reservations, have been severely impacted by MA use and its consequences.

Since 1995, Midwestern states, including Missouri and Iowa, have become popular locations for MA use and production due to the availability of secluded areas, ideal for clandestine labs, and access to major transportation routes (Barnes, Boeger, & Huffman, 1998). In addition to the Midwest, there appears to be a trend of increased MA trafficking and use in the Southeast (SAMHSA, 1999). The impact of MA in smaller cities and rural communities has been particularly troubling, since the substance abuse/mental health systems lack the infrastructures necessary to treat patients with such severe substance use and related disorders (Rawson, Anglin, & Ling, 2002; Methamphetamine Interagency Task Force, 2000). Law enforcement officials similarly lack the training and financial resources required to deal with the dismantling and cleanup of clandestine MA laboratories in their communities (Methamphetamine Interagency Task Force, 2000).

Hawaii

A form of MA known as "ice" became a problem in Hawaii in the mid- to late 1980s. Hawaiian users thought it was a new drug, unrelated to speed, and smoked it in glass pipes. Ice had been available in Hawaii since the 1970s, imported from Korea, Taiwan, and the Philippines, but use had been limited to small ethnic gangs. During the 1980s, however, use spread to all areas of the population, regardless of ethnicity, gender, age, or socioeconomic status (Miller, 1991). Ice continues to be a major public health and criminal justice problem in Hawaii.

Japan

Japan has experienced repeated epidemics of MA use. The preferred route of administration is smoking, by inhaling the fumes from powdered MA as it turns to vapor when heated on a piece of aluminum foil. Smoking "speed," or "S," is preferred to injecting, especially among younger users, because of the fears related to injection use and the perception that smoking affords the user more control over drug intake and the reduced likelihood of developing use-related psychosis (Matsumoto et al., 2002). There is also evidence that MA smoking may be utilized as an appetite suppressant among young females.

Thailand

Thailand is also experiencing a sustained epidemic of MA use (Farrell, Marsden, Ali, & Ling, 2002). *Yaa baa* ("crazy pill") is sold in pill form and smoked. The rise in use began in the late 1960s and early 1970s. A retrospective study at the largest addiction treatment hospital in Thailand revealed that

MA admissions increased from 0.4% in 1989 to 10.3% in 1996, then esca-
lated to a high of 51.5% in 1998 (Verachai, Dechongkit, Patarakorn, &
Lukanapichonchut, 2001). A study by Sattah and colleagues (2002) documented that 41.3% of the males and 19.0% of the females in a sample of
1,725 secondary students had previously used methamphetamine MA at some
point in their lives.

Populations of Special Concern

In the United States, MA has historically been associated with white, male,
blue-collar workers. However, the number of groups affected by MA use is
expanding (National Institute on Drug Abuse [NIDA], 1998). Several groups
appear to have elevated levels of risk for MA use and its consequences.

Women

In several large treatment studies (i.e., Brecht, O'Brien, von Mayrhauser, &
Anglin, 2004; Rawson et al., 2000), the number of women who have entered
treatment for MA use disorders has approached or even exceeded the number
of men. This is a particularly unusual finding, because the rates of drug treatment admission are typically two to three times higher for men than for
women. The reasons for the elevated rates of MA use among women are not
clear, although anecdotally, the two reasons that are most widely reported in
treatment samples are that women initially find MA useful as a weight control
method and as a way to manage the fatigue brought on by their multiple responsibilities (parent, spouse, employee, other family roles). In addition, data
suggest that MA may serve as a way of coping with the psychological/emo-
tional sequelae of historical sexual/physical abuse and/or current abusive environments (Cohen et al., 2003).

Individuals with Co-Occurring Psychiatric Disorders

One of the issues of greatest interest to clinicians assessing and treating individuals who are or may be using MA is distinguishing between individuals
with MA-induced psychiatric symptoms and individuals who have coexisting
psychiatric disorders. Co-occurring psychiatric diagnoses frequently accompany MA use/abuse. It is unclear how the disorders are etiologically related,
but epidemiological evidence suggests that disorders such as depression and
other mood disorders, schizophrenia, and antisocial personality disorder increase the likelihood of developing substance abuse or dependence (Jaffe et al.,
2005). Those with antisocial personality disorder are more likely to exhibit
risky behavior and ignore social inhibitions about illicit drug use, and MA
may serve a self-medicating function for those with mood disorders and other
dysfunctional states, such as attention deficit disorder. Drug use can also pre-
date the psychiatric disorders. Individuals taking part in the Epidemiologic

Catchment Area Study (ECA) who reported cocaine or amphetamine/MA use were found to be 8 times more likely to have depression and 14 times more likely to have experienced a panic attack (Jaffe et al., 2005).

Gay Men

Extensive evidence indicates that in many major U.S. cities (especially western and midwestern cities, and New York City), MA is used extensively by gay males and is frequently associated with high-risk sexual behavior, a major factor in the transmission of HIV (Frosch, Shoptaw, Huber, Rawson, & Ling, 1996; Gorman, Morgan, & Lambert, 1995; Shoptaw, Reback, & Freese, 2002). Within this particular group, effective treatment for MA dependence may be one of the most important strategies in reducing the spread of HIV and other, associated communicable diseases (Shoptaw et al., 2002). However, despite the serious consequences of MA and the extremely risky behavior associated with it, the use of MA in combination with sexual activities within some parts of the gay male community has become almost accepted, normative behavior (Reback & Ditman, 1997).

Individuals with Eating Disorders

Eating disordered behavior is often comorbid with substance use. Findings by Wiederman and Pryor (1996) indicated that amphetamine abuse was predictive of more severe restrictive eating behavior, whereas tranquilizer use was associated with higher levels of binge eating, purging, and cigarette, alcohol, and cocaine use. Given the fact that amphetamines inhibit appetite and boost metabolism, it makes sense that those individuals most concerned with having a thin physique would be more likely to engage in amphetamine and methamphetamine MA use to reach this goal (Wiederman & Pryor, 1996). Gritz and Crane (1991) surveyed over 3,000 high school seniors and found that over 8% of females reported amphetamine use in attempts to control weight in the previous 12 months. Only 1.8% of males reported using MA for this reason. Race also was a factor in using MA for weight loss/control, with white females being over 10 times more likely to engage in this behavior than black females.

School-Age Children and Methylphenidate

Nearly 90% of prescriptions for methylphenidate are for the treatment of attention-deficit/hyperactivity disorder (ADHD) among children and adolescents (Goldman, Genel, Bezman, & Slanetz, 1998). Although illegal use of methylphenidate is relatively low, misuse appears to be on the rise among adolescents and young adults (Klein-Schwartz, 2002). Prescriptions increased 600% from 1990 to 1995 for this drug, according to the Drug Enforcement Agency (DEA) (Llana & Crismon, 1999, cited in Klein-Schwartz, 2002).

Prescription drug misuse in general appears to be on the rise, and the increase has been most dramatic among adolescents and young adults. Data from the 1999 NNHSDA (SAMHSA, 1999) seem to suggest that younger and high school age adolescents prefer both prescription painkillers and stimulants, while college-age students appear to prefer painkillers more exclusively, such as oxycodone (Percodan) and hydrocodone (Vicodin). In one study that addressed Canadian high school students with a valid stimulant prescription (Poulin, 2001), 14.7% of students reported that they gave some of their medication to others, and 7.3% sold it. Of these same students, 3.0% had been coerced to provide their medication to others, and 4.3% had experienced theft of their medication. This study also indicated that students who gave away or sold their medication were more likely to engage in illegal stimulant use.

Similar findings were reported by Musser and colleagues (1998, cited in Klein-Schwartz, 2002) in a survey conducted with students who were prescribed methylphenidate: 16% of the 73 students surveyed reported that they had been asked by peers to trade, sell, or give away their medication.

Despite evidence that suggests high school age adolescents are most affected by this trend of methylphenidate abuse, there are data that also suggest an increase in methylphenidate use among older adolescents and young adults. According to the NHSDA (SAMHSA, 2002), between 2000 and 2001, methylphenidate lifetime use in 12- to 17-year-olds decreased slightly, from 2.2 to 2.0%, whereas in the 18–25 age range, lifetime use increased modestly, from 3.6 to 4.7% within the same time frame.

In a survey of 283 predominantly college-age individuals at a small, public liberal arts college, 16.0% reported having used methylphenidate, and 12.7% reported having used it intranasally. A majority of the participants indicated knowing someone who used methylphenidate recreationally (Babcock & Byrne, 2000).

Methylphenidate abuse among adolescents and young adults is an issue of concern, but rates of abuse remain relatively low. Additionally, little or conflicting evidence suggests that individuals prescribed methylphenidate might be at higher risk to become involved with/dependent upon amphetamines as adults or to abuse the medication as adolescents (Klein-Schwartz, 2002).

Children of Methamphetamine Users

Children constitute an increasing percentage of the victims of MA use through exposure both before and after birth. Children are negatively affected (1) when exposed to MA prenatally, (2) through neglect and abuse when a parent is using MA, and (3) when exposed to the dangers of MA manufacturing. Although a paucity of studies have examined the effects of MA use on the developing fetus, research demonstrates that MA crosses the placenta and can cause fetal loss, placental hemorrhage, and decreased intrauterine growth (MacKenzie & Heischober, 1997). Babies born after prenatal MA exposure have suffered from growth retardation, premature birth, developmental disorders and delay, and altered neonatal behavioral patterns (Lukas, 1997; National Institute of Justice, 1999; Rawson, Gonzales, & Brethen, 2002; Smith et al., 2001). Because MA increases body temperature, thermal regulation of the developing child may be compromised, leading to neurological damage. Newborns born addicted to MA may experience physical trembling, feeding problems, and have trouble making eye contact. In a study that followed for 16 years after birth children exposed prenatally to amphetamine (Lukas, 1997), it was found that by the age of 8, these children exhibited higher levels of aggressive behavior, had greater difficulty adjusting to different environments, and had higher rates of school failure than nonexposed children. In addition to the dangers of MA itself to the unborn child are the problems associated with MA use by the pregnant mother that affect the unborn child: dangers from intravenous drug use; risky sexual behaviors and concomitant health issues; violence perpetuated by and against the MA user; accidents; and malnutrition (Lukas, 1997).

After birth, children of MA users may be victims of abuse and neglect (Rawson, Gonzales, & Brethen, 2002), and may also be exposed to the physical dangers that exist in living in an environment in which MA is manufactured. Medical and psychological health consequences of MA use may interfere with a parent's ability to respond to the needs of his or her children. The psychological consequences of MA use, such as psychosis and paranoia, and associated violence, may endanger the user's child directly and indirectly. A parent's mental state has important consequences for the child, and parental incapacitation may lead to adverse consequences for the child's own physical and psychological state. In addition to the effects of neglect, the child may experience fear and anxiety, and may also become a target of the parent's violent behavior. Poor nutrition, grooming, and hygiene, as well as fatigue and mood swings, are commonly observed among children of MA users. One recent study identified the additional risk of inadvertent MA poisoning in children of MA users (Kolecki, 1998).

At most danger are children living in MA manufacturing environments, who are at risk for the dangers inherent in MA labs—the volatility of the cooking process and the odors. In 1998, 208 of the 1,006 laboratories seized by the Bureau of Narcotic Enforcement had 401 children present (United States Senate, 2000). Because MA is easy to produce, many MA users make their supply in their own home lab. In fact, the DEA reports that small-scale laboratories are being operated increasingly in single- and multifamily-residences in urban and suburban neighborhoods. This exposes children living in these homes to the dangers inherent in the chemicals, cooking process, and toxic fumes. The chemicals used in the manufacturing process can be corrosive, explosive, flammable, and toxic (Irvine & Chin, 1991), and are often stored in places accessible to children. There is always the potential for explosion or fire at clandestine laboratories. In California, the three children (ages 1, 2, and 3) of an MA-making woman were killed when the kitchen stove, used to cook MA, exploded (Manning & Vedder, 1998). The lack of proper ventilation also exposes children to the drug and by-product toxicity. Traces of chemicals that can permeate the walls, drapes, carpets, and furniture of a laboratory site and leave a lingering odor that does not easily dissipate can result in adverse effects on the laboratory's inhabitants, particularly children, whose physical systems are still developing. In Hawaii, 25% of all babies tested for MA had traces of it in their system (Little, Snell, & Gilstrap, 1988; Oro & Dixon, 1987). A report of 18 pediatric patients diagnosed with MA poisoning indicated that children have a somewhat different clinical presentation than is typical with adult toxicity. The children often present in a way that is reminiscent of other childhood illnesses, and diagnosis is further complicated by the fact that parents may be less than forthcoming about the child having access to MA. Presenting symptoms were agitation (9 patients), tachycardia (18 patients), inconsolable irritability and crying (6 patients), and protracted vomiting (6 patients) (Kolecki, 1998).

SYSTEMS OF ASSESSMENT:
DIAGNOSTIC CATEGORIES AND CRITERIA

As with other drugs, the crux of the MA assessment quandary is to identify what we need to know about the phenomena of MA use and MA users in order to develop the most effective treatment strategies. Since research has not provided definitive answers, assessment is predicated on a commonsense approach—collecting as much information as possible across multiple domains. Typical areas of assessment include demographic characteristics, drug use history and diagnosis, treatment history, and other life domain problems. Because drug use does not occur in isolation from other behaviors, assessment for treatment purposes may involve consideration of sociocultural and economic setting, family history, personal history, premorbid personality, and psychological and psychiatric disorders. Although treatment planning for drug users does not always include assessment of physical and medical functioning, assessment of physical health status is vital in MA users due to the severity and prevalence of adverse physical health effects related to MA use.

Methods for Assessing Past and Present
Drug Use and Dependence

MA use, abuse, and dependence are diagnosed with clinical tools and nonclinical assessment methods, including biological tests and self-report. Clinical tools are designed to determine whether the client meets the criteria for substance abuse or dependence, as well as other substance-related disorders. Other methods of assessment not intended to determine a clinical diagnosis include both objective and self-report methods of assessing MA use, and have advantages and disadvantages. For example, biological tests offer the ability to ascertain objectively use in the recent past given identified cutoff levels; however, no information about pattern, progression, and severity of use and related behaviors is possible. Conversely, self-reported use allows assessment of an unlimited amount of information about the user and his or her drug use history, but is limited by the unknown reliability and validity of the self-reported information. The assessment of past and present drug use is vital to treatment planning. Understanding the client's pattern of use and vulnerability to relapse are important factors when tailoring a treatment plan to best fit the needs of the client.

Diagnostic and Statistical Manual of Mental Disorders

As with other substance use disorders, the tool most often used to diagnose MA and amphetamine use disorders is the fourth edition of the *Diagnostic and Statistical Manual of Mental Disorders* (DSM-IV; American Psychiatric Association, 1994). MA-related disorders are included in the section addressing amphetamine-related disorders, as are all amphetamine-like substances. The criteria address two groups of disorders, shown in Table 6.1. Sections on substance use disorders provide a check-off of symptoms empirically established as markers of amphetamine/MA substance use disorders. Descriptions contained in each emphasize the drugusing behavior itself, its maladaptive nature, and how the choice to engage in that behavior shifts and becomes more involuntary as a result of interaction with the drug over time. The coding scheme of DSM-IV provides distinct numbers for amphetamine dependence and amphetamine abuse, but the codes for the other amphetamineinduced disorders are common to several other substancerelated disorders (see Table 6.1).

TABLE 6.1. DSM-IV Coding for Amphetamine/MA Use and Induced Disorders

AMPH/MA use disorders		AMPH/MA-induced disorders	
304.40	Dependence	292.89	Intoxication
305.70	Abuse	292.0	Withdrawal
		292.81	AMPH-induced intoxication delirium
		292.11	AMPH-induced psychotic disorder, with delusions
		292.12	AMPH-induced psychotic disorder, with hallucinations
		292.84	AMPH-induced mood disorder
		292.89	AMPH-induced anxiety disorder
		292.89	MPH-induced sexual dysfunction
		292.89	AMPH-induced sleep disorder
		292.9	AMPH-induced disorder not otherwise specified

TABLE 6.2. DSM-IV Diagnostic Criteria for Amphetamine (Methamphetamine) Intoxication

A. Recent use of AMPH/MA or a related substance.

B. Clinically significant maladaptive behavioral or psychological changes.

C. Two or more of the following, developing during, or shortly after, use of AMPH or a related substance:
   1. Tachycardia or bradycardia
   2. Pupillary dilation
   3. Elevated or lowered blood pressure
   4. Perspiration or chills
   5. Nausea or vomiting
   6. Evidence of weight loss
   7. Psychomotor agitation or retardation
   8. Muscular weakness, respiratory depression, chest pain, or cardiac arrhythmias
   9. Confusion, seizures, dyskinesias, dystonias, or coma

D. The symptoms are not due to a general medical condition and are not better accounted for by another mental disorder.

Note. Adapted from American Psychiatric Association (1994, pp. 207–208). Copright 1994 by the American Psychiatric Association. Adapted by permission.

TABLE 6.3. DSM-IV Diagnostic Criteria for Amphetamine (Methamphetamine) Dependence

A maladaptive pattern of AMPH/MA use, leading to clinically significant impairment or distress. Diagnosis of dependence requires the occurrence of three or more of the following, occurring at any time in the same 12-month period:

1. Tolerance, defined by either:
   a. A need for markedly increased amounts of AMPH/MA to achieve intoxication or desired effect
   b. Markedly diminished effect with continued use of the same amount of AMPH/MA

2. Withdrawal, manifested by either:
   a. Reduction or cessation of AMPH/MA use that has been heavy and prolonged, resulting in dysphoric mood and at least two other physiological changes (fatigue; vivid, unpleasant dreams; insomnia or hypersomnia; increased appetite; psychomotor retardation or agitation)
   b. AMPH/MA or closely related substance is taken to relieve or avoid withdrawal symptoms

3. AMPH/MA is often taken in larger amounts or over a longer period than was intended.

4. There is a persistent desire or unsuccessful efforts to cut down or control AMPH/MA use.

5. A great deal of time is spent in activities necessary to obtain the substance, use the substance, or recover from its effects.

6. Important social, occupational, or recreational activities are given up or reduced because of AMPH/MA use.

7. AMPH/MA use is continued despite knowledge of having a persistent or recurrent physical or psychological problem that is likely to have been caused or exacerbated by AMPH/MA.

Note. Adapted from American Psychiatric Association (1994, p. 181). Copright 1994 by the American Psychiatric Association. Adapted by permission.

TABLE 6.4. DSM-IV Diagnostic Criteria for Amphetamine (Methamphetamine) Abuse

A maladaptive pattern of AMPH/MA use leading to clinically significant impairment or distress.

A. The occurrence of one or more of the following, occurring within a 12-month period:
   1. Recurrent AMPH/MA use resulting in a failure to fulfill major role obligations at work, school, or home
   2. Recurrent AMPH/MA use in situations in which it is physically hazardous
   3. Recurrent AMPH/MA-related legal problems
   4. Continued AMPH/MA use despite having persistent or recurrent social or interpersonal problems caused or exacerbated by the effects of AMPH/MA

B. The symptoms have never met criteria for AMPH/MA dependence.

Note. Adapted from American Psychiatric Association (1994, pp. 182–183). Copright 1994 by the American Psychiatric Association. Adapted by permission.

Criteria for the amphetamine/MA-related disorders of intoxication, dependence, abuse, and withdrawal are presented in Tables 6.2 to 6.5. The DSM-IV diagnostic criteria for amphetamine dependence are the same generic criteria applied to other substances. Amphetamine and MA use disorders are divided into two categories on the basis of symptomatology and severity of symptoms. *Amphetamine abuse* describes a pattern of maladaptive use of the drug, leading to clinically significant impairment or distress and occurring within a 12-month period in which the symptoms have never met the criteria for amphetamine dependence. *Amphetamine dependence,* as the more severe diagnosis of the two amphetamine/MA use disorders, is defined as a cluster of physiological, behavioral, and cognitive symptoms that, taken together, indicate that the person continues to use amphetamine-like drugs despite significant problems related to such use. Dependence is distinguished from abuse by

TABLE 6.5. DSM-IV Diagnostic Criteria for Amphetamine (Methamphetamine) Withdrawal

A. Reduction or cessation in amphetamine or related substance use that has been heavy and prolonged.

B. Dysphoric mood and at least two of the following physiological changes developing within a few hours to several days after Criterion A:
   1. Fatigue
   2. Vivid, unpleasant dreams
   3. Insomnia or hypersomnia
   4. Increased appetite
   5. Psychomotor retardation or agitation

C. The symptoms in Criterion B cause clinically significant distress or impairment in social, occupational, or other important areas of functioning.

D. The symptoms are not due to a general medical condition and are not better accounted for by another mental disorder.

Note. Adapted from American Psychiatric Association (1994, p. 204). Copright 1994 by the American Psychiatric Association. Adapted by permission.

the presence of physical factors such as tolerance and withdrawal, and by increasing loss of control over drug use.

Addiction Severity Index

A multitude of self-report measures exist for assessing drug and alcohol use and abuse, as well as consequences of this use; however, few MA-specific measures have been developed. Assessments of MA use typically include either a measure to ascertain a clinical diagnosis or an assessment of problematic use. The Addiction Severity Index (ASI; McLellan, Kushner, & Metzger, 1992) is the most widely utilized standardized, multidimensional measure for assessing problem severity in areas commonly affected by alcohol and drug misuse. These areas include medical, employment, illegal activity, family and social support, legal, psychiatric, and drug and alcohol use. The easy-to-administer format of the measure and its measurement of related life domains have provided treatment providers with a useful tool to assess clients at intake, as well as throughout the treatment episode. The ASI has been used with diverse populations, treatment modalities, and drug classes, and has been found reliable and valid in numerous settings since its construction (McLellan et al., 1992).

Biological Tests

MA can be detected for varying lengths of time in urine—usually several days, depending on frequency of use, amount of dose, and sensitivity of the testing method. Metabolites can also be detected in blood, saliva, and hair. Blood and saliva furnish a better index of current levels, whereas urine provides a longer window of opportunity for detecting use over the previous few days. Hair analysis can reveal drug use over a period of weeks to months but has little applicability in clinical situations. Objective measures of drug use can be used alone to detect the presence of MA or to verify self-reported use. Testing biological samples for the presence of MA provides an objective measure of treatment progress, which may help the client to resist urges and cravings by establishing accountability and reducing the likelihood of client denial (Washton, Stone, & Hendrickson, 1988).

Urine

Traditionally, urinalysis using thin-layer chromatography (TLC) and immunoassays has been the primary means of validating self-reported drug use. The enzyme multiple-immunoassay technique (EMIT) has been a favorite for routine testing, because it can reliably detect the presence of drugs of abuse in urine for up to 72 hours after last use. TLC tests are cheaper but also less sensitive than EMIT, and are therefore more likely to give a negative result for a sample that is actually positive for MA. When treatment planning decisions are based on test results, the accuracy of the test used should be carefully considered. Gas chromatography combined with mass spectroscopy (GC-MS) is superior in accuracy to EMIT or other test methods.

Hair

Recently, radioimmunoassay of hair (RIAH) has been incorporated into some testing protocols. Like urinalysis, RIAH depends on the detection of metabolites created by the body when drugs are ingested (Mieczkowski, Barzelay, Gropper, & Wish, 1991). While hair assay does not increase the types of drugs that can be detected, it does offer an increased time span in which to survey for drug use (Mieczkowski et al., 1991).

Saliva

Due to the ability to collect oral fluid in a noninvasive, directly observable way, as well as the difficulty in adulterating saliva samples, drug testing via saliva is gaining popularity. Test results are available in 15 minutes, and it appears that results from point-of-collection oral fluid drug analysis kits correlate well with laboratory-based urine screening test results. Use of oral fluid testing can reduce the embarrassment that accompanies direct observation, as well as chances of sample adulteration, compared to traditional urine-testing procedures. In addition, no special facilities or special laboratory equipment or reagents are needed (Barrett, Good, & Moore, 2001).

Blood

Until recently, urine samples were the preferred specimen for drug testing because, among other reasons, the concentrations of drugs are higher in urine than in other matrices such as blood, saliva, and sweat. Yet the metabolites of other drugs of abuse often need to be assessed along with, and in some cases instead of, the original drug. In recent years, substantial technological gains have been made in sample preparation, chromatography, and detection methods, making whole blood a viable alternative specimen for drug testing. With whole blood, identification and quantification can be performed in a single sample using one procedure. In most cases, the unchanged drug is detectable in blood, eliminating the need for further testing of drug by-products.

MEDICAL CONSIDERATIONS IN THE ASSESSMENT OF METHAMPHETAMINE USERS

MA increases blood pressure and heart rate, constricts blood vessels, dilates bronchioles (breathing tubes), and increases blood sugar levels as the body prepares for the simulated emergency. These effects can cause irreversible damage to blood vessels in the brain, producing strokes, respiratory problems, irregular heartbeat, and extreme anorexia. MA use can result in cardiovascular collapse and death. Chronic MA abuse can result in inflammation of the heart lining, and among users who inject the drug, damaged blood vessels and skin abscesses. Hyperthermia (elevated body temperature) and convulsions occur with MA overdoses, and if not treated immediately, can result in death.

Importantly, the route of administration affects the potential for adverse reactions and associated medical disorders. Intravenous use may result in illnesses associated with the use or sharing of contaminated drug paraphernalia, including HIV, hepatitis, tuberculosis, lung infections, pneumonia, bacterial or viral endocarditis, cellulites, wound abscesses, sepsis, thrombosis, renal infarction, and thrombophlebitis (Gold & Miller, 1997; Sowder & Beschner, 1993). Nasal insufflation is associated with sinusitis, loss of sense of smell, congestion, atrophy of nasal mucosa, nosebleeds, perforation or necrosis of the nasal septum, hoarseness, problems with swallowing, throat ailments, and a productive cough with black sputum (Gold & Miller, 1997).

Table 6.6 presents adverse effects associated with MA use (Albertson, Derlet, & Van Hoozen, 1999).

Neurological Effects

Investigations of the long-term consequences of MA use in animals indicate that as much as 50% of the dopamine-producing cells in the brain can be damaged even after low levels of MA use, and serotonin-containing nerve cells may be damaged even more extensively (National Institutes of Health, 1998). Numerous studies have addressed the neurotoxic effects of MA on human users. In a recent study of 15 MA-dependent users, Volkow et al. (2001) utilized positron-emission tomography (PET) scans and a neuropsychological test battery to examine differences between the MA and comparison groups. As expected, metabolic differences in the MA group were similar to those reported for laboratory animals administered MA. Importantly, the pattern of brain metabolism of MA users was found to be similar to that seen in patients with atypical Parkinson's disease. Other researchers have also noted adverse neurological effects of MA use, as seen in movement disorders.

Abnormal movements and facial gestures are hallmarks of chronic stimulant abuse (Rhee, Albertson, & Douglas, 1988; Weiner & Lang, 1989), and both acute and chronic use of amphetamine and MA may result in chorea, including orofacial dyskinesia, stereotyped movements, dystonia, and tics (Weiner & Lang, 1989). Abnormal, involuntary movements associated with stimulant use may decrease or end when drug use is ceased; however, chronic amphetamine addicts may demonstrate long-lasting movement disorders that may persist for several years after drug withdrawal. Rhee et al. (1988) documented emergency room admissions of MA overdoses, who were described by medical personnel as "jumping around," writhing, and having involuntary movement of the limbs, mouth, and tongue. Lundh and Tunving (1981) re-

TABLE 6.6. Adverse Effects Associated with Methamphetamine Use

System	Effect
Neurological	Headache Seizures Cerebral infarcts/stroke Cerebral vasculitis Cerebral edema Mydriasis Cerebral hemorrhage Chorea and choreoathetoid (orofacial dyskinesia, involuntary and stereotyped movements, dystonia, and tics)
Cardiovascular	Myocardial infarction Cardiomyopathy Myocarditis Hypertension Arrhythmia and palpitations (rapid and irregular heartbeat) Tachycardia Inflammation of the heart lining Irreversible, stroke-producing damage to small blood vessels in the brain
Respiratory	Pulmonary edema Dyspnea Bronchitis Pulmonary hypertension Hemoptysis Pleuritic chest pain Asthma exacerbation Pulmonary granuloma
Psychiatric	Paranoia Psychosis Depression Anxiety Suicidality Delirium/hallucinations Aggression and violence
Social	Violence Negative effects on children Risky sexual behavior Environmental and health dangers of manufacturing methamphetamine
Other	Skin ulcers and dermatological infections Dental problems Anorexia/weight problems Obstetric complications Ulcers Hyperpyrexia Renal failure Ischemic colitis Rhabdomyolysis Disseminated vasculitis Infectious diseases

ported that efforts to reduce the long-standing abnormal movements of former amphetamine addicts were ineffective, possibly due to an amphetamine-induced plasticity of synaptic transmission in the brain regions controlling extrapyramidal movements.

Cardiovascular Effects

Cardiovascular complications associated with MA abuse have been increasingly reported and include multiple problems: rapid and irregular heartbeat; increased blood pressure; inflammation of the heart lining; and irreversible, stroke-producing damage to small blood vessels in the brain. Pharmacological effects including hypertension, tachycardia, and myocardial ischemia, which may promote the occurrence of cardio- and cerebrovascular diseases (Perez-Reyes et al., 1991; Zhu et al., 2000).

Although adverse cardiovascular effects have been documented, the chronic cardiotoxicity of MA has only recently been addressed in experimental studies. In one study of the cardiovascular effects of MA in rats (He, Matoba, Fujitani, Sodesaki, & Onishi, 1996), cardiovascular effects were clearly seen by day 14; myocytolysis, contraction bands, atrophied myocytes, and spotty fibrosis were patchily distributed throughout the myocardium. These effects were more severe by day 56, such that these myocardial lesions resembled the cardiomyopathy associated with MA abuse in humans.

Respiratory Effects

The respiratory system is also compromised by amphetamine/MA use. Adverse effects to the respiratory system may be increased when smoking or snorting is the route of administration. Pulmonary hypertension has been reported since the 1960s, as a result of amphetamine use (Lewman, 1972), and more recent reports present evidence that chronic obstructive lung disease in MA users may result from thrombosis of small pulmonary vessels, with gradual reduction of the pulmonary vascular bed, pulmonary fibrosis, and granuloma formation (CSAT, 1997). Among "ice" smokers in Hawaii, respiratory problems, including asthma, are commonly reported as medical consequences of MA use (W. Haning, personal communication, January 10, 2000).

Infectious Diseases

There are myriad health problems not directly caused by the drug itself, but by aspects of the MA-using lifestyle. MA users may be at an increased risk of HIV/AIDS and other communicable diseases due to two use factors: (1) MA use has been linked to unsafe sexual activity, particularly in the gay male population; and (2) MA may be used intravenously. Transmission of HIV, hepatitis, and other communicable diseases is often through sexual activity and/or intravenous drug use. Research has documented a particularly strong association between MA use and sexual behaviors, particularly HIV/sexually transmitted disease (STD)-related risk behaviors, and an association between MA use and HIV serostatus (Harris et al., 1993, Klee, 1993; Crofts et al., 1994; Kall, 1994). In the United States, MA has also been associated with hepatitis A outbreaks (Harkess, Gildon, & Istre, 1989; Hutin, Bell, & Marshall, 1999). Hutin and colleagues (1999) found that of the hepatitis A outbreaks occurring in a 7-month period, approximately 26.1% occurred among injection drug users, with the majority of those being MA users. In a study of the association between MA use and hepatitis A (Hutin et al., 2000), 54.1% of those screened for study inclusion reported MA use. In one study in Japan (Wada, Greberman, Konuma, & Hirai, 1999) that assessed seroprevalence of HIV and hepatitis by substance of dependence, approximately 54% of 39 MA users tested positive for hepatitis C virus (HCV) 26% for hepatitis B (Ab), and 2.6% for hepatitis B (Ag). Drug users with a history of injection drug use were significantly more likely than subjects without an intravenous drug use history to be HCV-positive. Finally, the MA-dependent group was 9.8 times more likely to be positive for HCV compared to the alcohol-dependent sample.

Dental Effects

Adverse dental effects of MA use include unusual and accelerated patterns of dental wear in users of amphetamine and amphetamine derivatives (Freire-Garabal et al., 1999; Redfearn, Agrawal, & Mair, 1998; See & Tan, 2003). Di Cugno, Perec, and Tocci (1981) documented that amphetamine-using patients had four times the number of decayed teeth as controls, and parotid salivary flow was reduced to 26.2% of normal. Abnormal damage to teeth in MA users includes caries, erosion, attrition, and abrasion (Richards & Brofeldt, 2000). Amphetamine addiction (Ashcroft, Eccleston, & Waddell, 1965) and use of Ecstasy (Redfearn et al., 1998; Duxbury, 1993) has been found to be associated with accelerated tooth wear from the effect of teeth clenching and grinding. In addition to the general increase in tooth wear and decay seen in MA users, the method of use may also influence accelerated tooth erosion. Richards and Brofeldt (2000) found that patients who regularly snorted MA had significantly more tooth wear in their back teeth than did patients who injected, smoked, or ingested MA.

Dermatological Effects

Skin problems and cutaneous ulcers are also hallmarks of the chronic MA user (MacKenzie & Heischober, 1997). The most common dermatological problems seen with amphetamine/MA drug use include self-inflicted skin lesions and those resulting from intravenous needle use or burns (Cadier & Clarke, 1993). Because one consequence of MA use is stereotypical behavior,

MA users are likely to engage in repetitive, unnecessary behaviors such as skin picking. Additionally, the sensation of something moving under the skin is common and often results in MA users itching or picking at their skin until it bleeds.

METHAMPHETAMINE PSYCHOSIS

MA use can cause a psychotic state that may appear virtually indistinguishable from paranoid schizophrenia (Connell, 1958; Fujii, 2002; Iwanami et al., 1994), and evidence shows that as many as two-thirds of chronic users suffer from delusional psychoses (Satel, Southwick, & Gawin, 1991). Paranoid delusions and transient auditory and visual hallucinations are frequent with this diagnosis. The delusions may be brief; however, clinicians are much more frequently reporting longer episodes, lasting several days to months (Gawin, Khalsa, & Ellinwood, 1996). Among the documented cases are psychotic behaviors that likely resulted from perceptual–cognitive disturbances and enduring disorders resembling the symptoms of chronic schizophrenia. Sekine et al. (2001) found that the severity of psychiatric symptoms was significantly correlated with the duration of MA use, although psychotic symptoms have been documented in clients who have used MA for as little as 3 months (Buffenstein, Heaster, & Ko, 1999) and in users as young as age 17 (Iwanami et al., 1994). Murray (1998) reported that even casual amphetamine/MA use can precipitate psychotic reactions, and research has documented the dangers for even first-time users. Although most improve with the use of neuroleptics, chronic MA users may be resistive to treatment and show continued psychotic symptoms despite extended abstinence (Fujii, 2002). In a study of MA psychosis among 104 Japanese patients, symptoms disappeared in 54 patients within a week after MA abstinence and antipsychotic medication but persisted for more than 3 months in 17 patients (Iwanami et al., 1994). Spontaneous recurrences of amphetamine/MA-induced paranoid–hallucinatory states have been noted in response to stress (Utena, 1966; Yui, Goto, Ikemoto, & Ishiguro, 1996; Yui, Ishiguro, Goto, & Ikemoto, 1997). Of 86 MA users, 52 had previous or persistent episodes of MA psychosis (Yui, Goto, Ikemoto, & Ishiguro, 2000), although no other psychiatric disorder was diagnosed in the absence of MA use.

In studies comparing the psychological effects of various drugs, MA is associated with more negative and damaging effects. In a comparison study of nicotine-, alcohol-, MA-, and inhalant-dependent subjects (Kono et al., 2001), MA produced the most intensive acute psychic disturbance in thinking (delusions), mood (emotional lability and irritability), anxiety (generalized anxiety, fear, panic attacks, and hypochondria), volition (psychomotor agitation), perception (hallucinations), and sleep (insomnia). Self-reported adverse effects of drug use in 158 Ecstasy, cocaine, and amphetamine users included anxiety, depression, mood swings, feelings of paranoia, panic attacks, and sleep and appetite disturbances (Williamson et al., 1997), but amphetamine use was associated with significantly more adverse effects, and more severe effects than Ecstasy or cocaine.

METHAMPHETAMINE WITHDRAWAL

MA withdrawal effects include fatigue, insomnia or restless hypersomnia, unpleasant dreams, hyperphagia, psychomotor agitation–retardation, dysphoria, anhedonia, and fragmented attention span. These symptoms can be intense and may be protracted because of the long duration of action of amphetamines. Withdrawal from MA has aversive psychological qualities, but it is not accompanied by the same degree of physical pain and discomfort as withdrawal from opiates. Withdrawal anhedonia and fatigue may contribute to an urge to use after recent cessation. For individuals who used MA to maintain long working hours and/or high energy, the withdrawal syndrome may be viewed as intolerable, because the lethargy and anergia can be quite severe and can last for several weeks or more. At present, there are no pharmacological agents with demonstrated efficacy for relieving the severity of the withdrawal syndrome. Rest, exercise, and a healthy diet are probably the best recommendations for addressing this syndrome.

METHAMPHETAMINE-RELATED
COGNITIVE IMPAIRMENT

Cognitive deficits associated with chronic MA use include deficits in memory, problem solving, and information manipulation (Simon et al., 2000). Adverse behavioral effects include violence and aggression, and development of stereotypical behavior patterns and repetitive behaviors that appear pointless, such as rearranging or taking objects apart (King & Ellinwood, 1992). Although psychological, cognitive, and behavioral functioning may return to non-dysfunctional levels after abstaining from MA use for a period of time, some damage may be permanent. Appropriate assessment of functioning in these areas has clear applicability for treatment efforts. Because psychological and cognitive dysfunction may interfere with the ability to benefit from treatment, to learn and process new information, to follow directions, and to make rational and logical decisions, it is necessary to assess psychological and cognitive function and dysfunction in the treatment setting. It is important to try to distinguish clients who *will not* from those who *cannot* follow the treatment plan. Psychological and/or cognitive dysfunction may be barriers to treatment compliance, and efforts to assess and address these dysfunctions may lead to effective strategies for making improvements.

CONSIDERATIONS FOR ACHIEVING ABSTINENCE FROM METHAMPHETAMINE

The systematic study of factors that influence the efforts to abstain from MA use is only in its early stages. As discussed earlier, the research literature on MA and the treatment of MA users is at least a decade behind the work that has been done on cocaine. Therefore, the empirical base for discussing factors associated with achieving MA abstinence is very meager. This topic is in great need of research. However, clinical observations do suggest that some issues appear important to achieving initial abstinence from MA.

Withdrawal Discomfort

The most troublesome symptoms of the MA withdrawal syndrome are anergia, difficulty concentrating, and dysphoria/depression. These symptoms can persist for up to several weeks. Although, individuals withdrawing from MA do not experience serious physical discomfort, their distress from the low energy and perceived inability to perform expected daily tasks can be considerable. Frequently, after a number of days of fatigue and perceived subpar functioning, individuals will find that their craving to use MA becomes very severe, which can result in a return to use. The common post hoc analysis is "I needed to be able to [take care of my kids, function at work, think clearly, etc.], so I decided to use."

At present, no medications have been shown to assist individuals with this set of withdrawal symptoms. After long runs of MA use, in which there is substantial sleep deprivation, failure to eat, and frequently substantial musculoskeletal strain from extended drug use postures, the individual is simply worn out, and the needed intervention is a proper diet, rest, and exercise. Certainly, there are depletions of the neurotransmitters that are involved with MA effects (e.g., dopamine, serotonin); however, no pharmacological treatment strategies are currently supported by research evidence. Many MA users are able to recover from this syndrome without medical attention. However, there are individuals whose psychological and physical withdrawal symptoms are so severe that they have to be temporarily housed in a drug-free environment while they achieve an initial 7–10 days of abstinence. This intervention is frequently necessary with individuals who inject MA, those who live in MA laboratories or with other MA users, and/or those who experience severe paranoia and continuing psychotic symptoms during the early stages of their recovery.

Protracted Dysphoria, Low Energy, Anhedonia, Paranoia, and Cognitive Dysfunction

The acute MA withdrawal syndrome is readily identifiable, and the majority of symptoms are typically resolved within several days to 2 weeks. However, although there is disagreement about whether a true "protracted withdrawal" exists following discontinuation of MA use, many users unquestionably experience an array of symptoms that affect their functioning adversely, and these symptoms are often cited as contributing to relapse to MA use. The constellation of symptoms includes dysphoria, low energy, anhedonia, episodic low grade paranoia, and various types of cognitive dysfunction. Those who suffer these symptoms generally are reported to go through intermittent periods of days or weeks in which they are more troublesome, alternating with periods of lower severity. In general, this symptom constellation seems to appear, abate, and reappear over the first 6 months of MA abstinence and possibly longer. Recent PET scan data from London et al. (2004) document the fact that some of the cognitive effects appear to correlate with specific areas of abnormal brain dysfunction, apparently resulting from MA use. There is speculation that the entire array of symptoms may represent a predictable syndrome associated with the recovery of the brain following the discontinuation of MA. More research is clearly needed to define explicitly and measure the nature of this phenomenon.

Sexual Behavior

MA users frequently associate their sexual behavior with MA use (Rawson, Gonzales, & Brethen, 2002). More than with other drugs of abuse, MA use very often becomes an essential and integral part of all sexual behavior for both men and women, and the MA-involved sexual activities often occur at a high frequency. This is especially true with gay men. Discontinuation of MA use is often associated with a decreased sex drive, decreased ability to perform sexually, and/or decreased pleasure derived from sexual behavior. Any or all of these sexual consequences can be the source of a great deal of anxiety for individuals during their early stages of abstinence (as well as during the initial 4–6 months of abstinence). Restriction of sexual activities to avoid high-risk situations (user friends/sexual partners, gay bars, etc.) can be viewed as a tremendous sacrifice for newly abstinent individuals. Reduction in sex drive and/or inability to achieve an erection or reach orgasm are all viewed as catastrophic events and frequently can be cited as reasons for return to use. Educating patients about the inevitable adjustment in sexual activity that occurs as a natural part of discontinuation of MA, and the fact that many of these negative effects are transitory, can be tremendously helpful in relieving anxiety about this issue and in preventing a return to MA use.

CONCLUSION

MA is a widely abused drug worldwide, and its use in the United States is increasing as its production and trafficking migrate from the western to the eastern part of the country. It has many properties in common with the other powerful and far more well-researched psychostimulant, cocaine. For this reason, Chapter 5 (this volume) by Carroll and Ball contains a tremendous amount of information relevant to the assessment and treatment of MA users. Our goal in this chapter was to highlight some of the ways that the clinical disorders associated with MA are distinct and different from those produced by cocaine. Particular attention was given to the geographical regions where MA is found, to the specific groups of individuals who are at risk for MA use, and to the medical and psychiatric symptoms associated with MA use.

ACKNOWLEDGMENTS

Support for the preparation of this chapter was provided by the National Instutute on Drug Abuse through the Methamphetamine Clinical Trials Group (MCTG; N01DA08804); and through the CSAT ATTC Program (UD1TI13594), Pacific Southwest Addiction Technology Transfer Center, and CSAT Methamphetamine Abuse Treatment—Special Studies (270-01-7089).

REFERENCES

Albertson, T. E., Derlet, R. W., & Van Hoozen, B. E. (1999). Methamphetamine and the expanding complications of amphetamines. *Western Journal of Medicine, 170*, 214–219.

American Psychiatric Association. (1994). *Diagnostic and statistical manual of mental disorders* (4th ed.). Washington, DC: Author.

Anglin, M. D., Burke, C., Perrochet, B., Stamper, E., & Dawud-Noursi, S. (2000). History of the methamphetamine problem. *Journal of Psychoactive Drugs, 32*, 137–141.

Ashcroft, G. W., Eccleston, D., & Waddell, J. L. (1965). Recognition of amphetamine addicts. *British Medical Journal, 1*, 57.

Babcock, Q., & Byrne, T. (2000). Student perceptions of methylphenidate abuse at a public liberal arts college. *Journal of American College Health, 49*, 143–146.

Barnes, M. R., Boeger, M. R., & Huffman, T. L. (1998). Illicit methamphetamine production and use in Missouri: How bad is the problem? *Missouri Medicine, 95*(2), 85–89.

Barrett, C., Good, C., & Moore, C. (2001). Comparison of point-of-collection screening of drugs of abuse in oral fluid with a laboratory-based urine screen. *Forensic Science International, 122*, 163–166.

Brecht, M., O'Brien, A., von Mayrhauser, C., & Anglin, M. D. (2004). Methamphetamine use behaviors and gender differences. *Addictive Behaviors, 29*(1), 89–106.

Brecht, M.-L., von Mayrhauser, C., & Anglin, M. D. (2000). Predictors of relapse after treatment for methamphetamine use. *Journal of Psychoactive Drugs, 32*, 211–220.

Buffenstein, A., Heaster, J., & Ko, P. (1999). Chronic psychotic illness from methamphetamine. *American Journal of Psychiatry, 156*, 662.

Cadier, M. A., & Clarke, J. A. (1993). Ecstasy and Whizz at a rave resulting in a major burn plus complications. *Burns, 19*, 239–240.

Castro, F. G., Barrington, E. H., Walton, M. A., & Rawson, R. A. (2000). Cocaine and methamphetamine: Differential addiction rates. *Psychology of Addictive Behaviors, 14,* 390–396.

Center for Substance Abuse Treatment. (1997). *Proceedings of the National Consensus Meeting on the use, abuse, and sequelae of abuse of methamphetamine with implications for prevention, treatment and research* (DHHS Publication No. [SMA] 96-8013). Rockville, MD: Author.

Cohen, J. B., Dickow, A., Horner, K., Zweben, J. E., Balabis, J., Vandersloot, D., & Reiber, C. (2003). Abuse and violence history of men and women in treatment for methamphetamine dependence. *American Journal on Addictions, 12,* 377–385.

Connell, P. H. (1958). *Amphetamine psychosis.* London: Chapman & Hall.

Crofts, N., Hopper, J. L., Milner, R., Breschkin, A. M., Bowden, D. S., & Locarnini, S. A. (1994). Blood-borne virus infections among Australian injecting drug users: Implications or spread of HIV. *European Journal of Epidemiology, 10,* 687–694.

Di Cugno, F., Perec, C. J., & Tocci, A. A. (1981). Salivary secretion and dental caries experience in drug addicts. *Archives of Oral Biology, 26,* 363–367.

Duxbury, A. J. (1993). Ecstasy–Dental implications. *British Dental Journal, 175,* 38.

Farrell, M., Marsden, J., Ali, R., & Ling, W. (2002). Methamphetamine: Drug use and psychoses becomes a major public health issue in the Asia Pacific region. *Addiction, 97,* 771–772.

Finnerty, B. (2003). Monitoring and reporting alcohol and drug use trends in California: The California Substance Abuse Research Consortium meetings. *Journal of Psychoactive Drugs, SARC Suppl. 1,* 119–125.

Freire-Garabal, M., Nunez, J. J., Balboa, J., Rodriguez-Cobo, A., Lopez-Paz, J. M., Rey-Mendez, M., Suarez-Quintanilla, J. A., Millan, J. C., & Mayan, J. M. (1999). Effects of amphetamine on development of oral candidiasis in rats. *Clinical and Diagnostic Laboratory Immunology, 6,* 530–533.

Frosch, D., Shoptaw, S., Huber, A., Rawson, R. A., & Ling, W. (1996). Sexual HIV risk among gay and bisexual male methamphetamine abusers. *Journal of Substance Abuse Treatment, 13*(6), 483–486.

Fujii, D. (2002). Risk factors for treatment-resistant methamphetamine psychosis. *Journal of Neuropsychiatry and Clinical Neurosciences, 14,* 239–240.

Gawin, F., Khalsa, M., & Ellinwood, E. (1996). Stimulants and related drugs. In G. O. Gabbard & S. D. Atkinson (Eds.), *Synopsis of treatments of psychiatric disorders* (pp. 313–328). Washington, DC: American Psychiatric Press.

Gawin, F. H., & Ellinwood, E. H. (1988). Cocaine and other stimulants: Actions, abuse and treatment. *New England Journal of Medicine, 318,* 1173–1182.

Gold, M. S., & Miller, N. S. (1997). Cocaine (and crack): Neurobiology. In J. H. Lowinson, P. Ruiz, R. B. Millman, & J. G., Langrod (Eds.), *Substance abuse: A comprehensive textbook* (3rd ed., pp. 166–181). Baltimore: Williams & Wilkins.

Goldman, L. S., Genel, M., Bezman, R. J., & Slanetz, P. J. (1998). Diagnosis and treatment of attention-deficit/hyperactivity disorder in children and adolescents. *Journal of the American Medical Association, 279,* 1100–1107.

Gorman, E. M., Morgan, P., & Lambert, E. Y. (1995). Qualitative research considerations and other issues in the study of methamphetamine use among men who have sex with other men. In E. Y. Lambert, R. S. Ashery, & R. H. Needle (Eds.), *Qualitative methods in substance abuse and HIV research* (NIDA Research Monograph No. 157, pp. 156–181). Rockville, MD: Department of Health and Human Services.

Gritz, E. R., & Crane, L. A. (1991). Use of diet pills and amphetamines to lose weight among smoking and nonsmoking high school seniors. *Health Psychology, 10*(5), 330–335.

Harkess, J., Gildon, B., & Istre, G. R. (1989). Outbreaks of hepatitis A among illicit drug users Oklahoma, 1984–1987. *American Journal of Public Health, 79,* 463–466.

Harris, N., Thiede, H., McGough, J., & Gordon, D. (1993). Risk factors for HIV infection among injection drug users: Results of blinded surveys in drug treatment centers. King County, Washington, 1998–1991. *Journal on AIDS, 6,* 1275–1282.

He, S., Matoba, R., Fujitani, N., Sodesaki, K., & Onishi, S. (1996). Cardiac muscle lesions associated with chronic administration of methamphetamine in rats. *American Journal of Forensic Medicine and Pathology, 17,* 155–162.

Hutin, Y. J., Bell, B. P., & Marshall, K. L. (1999). Identifying target groups for a potential vaccination program during a hepatitis A community wide outbreak. *American Journal of Public Health, 89,* 918–921.

Hutin, Y. J. F., Sabin, K. M., Hutwagner, L. C., Schaben, L., Shipp, G. M., Lord, D. M., Conner, J. S., Quinlisk, M. P., Shapiro, C. N., & Bell, B. P. (2000). Multiple modes of hepatitis A virus transmission among methamphetamine users. *American Journal of Epidemiology, 152,* 186–192.

Irvine, G. D., & Chin, L. (1991). The environmental impact and adverse health effects of the clandestine manufacture of methamphetamine. In M. A. Miller & N. J. Kozel (Eds.), *Methamphetamine abuse: Epidemiologic issues and implications* (Research Monograph No. 115, pp. 33–46). Rockville, MD: National Institute on Drug Abuse.

Iwanami, A., Sugiyama, A., Kuroki, N., Toda, S., Kato, N., Nakatani, Y., Horita, N., & Kaneko, T. (1994). Patients with methamphetamine psychosis admitted to a psychiatric hospital in Japan: A preliminary report. *Acta Psychiatrica Scandinavica, 89,* 428–432.

Jaffe, J. A., Ling, W., & Rawson, R. A. (2005). Amphetamines. In B. J. Sadock & V. A. Sadock (Eds.), *Kaplan and Sadock's comprehensive textbook of psychiatry* (pp. 1188–1200). Baltimore: Lippincott.

Kall, K. (1994). The risk of HIV infection for noninjecting sex partners of injecting drug users in Stockholm. *AIDS Education, 6,* 351–364.

King, G. R., & Ellinwood, E. H., Jr. (1992). Amphetamines and other stimulants. In J. H. Lowinson, P. Ruiz, R. B. Millman, & J. G. Langrod (Eds.), *Substance abuse: A comprehensive textbook* (pp. 247–270). Baltimore: Williams & Wilkins.

Klee, H. (1993). HIV risks for women drug infectors: Heroin and amphetamine users compared. *Addiction, 88,* 1055–1062.

Klein-Schwartz, W. (2002). Abuse and toxicity of methylphenidate. *Current Opinion in Pediatrics, 14*(2), 219–223.

Kolecki, P. (1998). Inadvertent methamphetamine poisoning in pediatric patients. *Pediatric Emergency Care, 14*(6), 385–387.

Kono, J., Miyata, H., Ushijima, S., Yanagita, T., Miyasato, K., Ikawa, G., & Hukui, K. (2001). Nicotine, alcohol, methamphetamine, and inhalant dependence: A comparison of clinical features with the use of a new clinical evaluation form. *Alcohol, 24,* 99–106.

Lewman, L. V. (1972). Fatal pulmonary hypertension from intravenous injection of methylphenidate (Ritalin) tablets. *Human Pathology, 3,* 67–70.

Little, B. B., Snell, L. M., & Gilstrap, L. C., III. (1988). Methamphetamine abuse during pregnancy: Outcome and fetal effects. *Obstetrics and Gynecology, 72,* 541–544.

Llana, M. E., & Crismon, M. L. (1999). Methylphenidate: Increased abuse or appropriate use? *Journal of the American Pharmaceutical Association, 39,* 526–530.

London, E., Simon, S. L., Berman, S., Mandelkern, M., Lichtman, A. M., Bramen, J., Shinn, A. K., Miotto, K., Learn, J., Dong, Y., Matochik, J. A., Kurian, V., Newton, T., Woods, R., Rawson, R. A., & Ling, W. L. (2004). Regional cerebral dysfunction associated with mood disturbances in abstinent methamphetamine abusers. *Archives of General Psychiatry, 61,* 73–84.

Longshore, D., Evans, L., Urada, D., Teruya, C., Hardy, M., Hser, Y.-I., Prendergast, M., & Ettner, S. (2003). *Evaluation of the Substance Abuse and Crime Prevention Act: 2002 Report.* Prepared for the Department of Alcohol and Drug Programs, California Health and Human Services Agency, Sacramento.

Lukas, S. E. (1997). *Proceedings of the National Consensus Meeting on the Use, Abuse, and Sequelae of Methamphetamine with Implications for Prevention, Treatment and Research* (DHHS Publication No. [SMA] 96-8013). Rockville, MD: U.S. Department of Health and Human Services.

Lundh, H., & Tunving, K. (1981). An extrapyramidal choreiorm syndrome caused by amphetamine addiction. *Journal of Neurology and Neurosurgical Psychiatry, 44,* 728–730.

MacKenzie, R. G., & Heischober, B. (1997). Methamphetamine. *Pediatric Review, 18,* 305–309.

Manning, T., & Vedder, D. (1998). Toxic chemicals: Toxic kids. *Law Enforcement Quarterly, 27,* 20–23.

Matsumoto, T., Kamijo, A., Miyakawa, T., Endo, K., Yabana, T., Kishimoto, H., Okudaira, K., Iseki, E., Sakai, T., & Kosaka, K. (2002). Methamphetamine in Japan: The consequences of methamphetamine abuse as a function of route of administration. *Addiction, 97*(7), 809–817.

McLellan, A. T., Kushner, H., & Metzger, D. (1992). The fifth edition of the Addiction Severity Index. *Substance Abuse Treatment, 9,* 199–213.

Methamphetamine Interagency Task Force. (2000). *Final report.* Washington, DC: Department of Health and Human Services.

Mieczkowski, T., Barzelay, D., Gropper, B., & Wish, E. (1991). Concordance of three measures of cocaine use in an arrestee population: Hair, urine, and self-report. *Journal of Psychoactive Drugs, 23,* 241–249.

Miller, M. A. (1991). Trends and patterns of methamphetamine smoking in Hawaii. *NIDA Research Monograph, 115,* 72–83.

Murray, J. B. (1998). Psychophysiological aspects of amphetamine–methamphetamine abuse. *Journal of Psychology, 132,* 227–237.

Musser, C. J., Ahmann, P. A., Theye, F. W., Mundt, P., Broste, S. K., & Mueller-Rizner, N. (1998). Stimulant use and the potential for abuse in Wisconsin as reported by school administrators and longitudinally followed children. *Journal of Developmental and Behavioral Pediatrics, 19,* 187–192.

National Institute of Justice. (1999). *Annual report of methamphetamine use among arrestees.* Results from the ADAM Program. Retrieved on May 13, 2003, from www.adam-nij.net/files/175660.pdf.

National Institute on Drug Abuse. (1998). *Methamphetamine.* Community Drug Alert Bulletin. Retrieved on May 13, 2003, from www.nida.nih.gov/methalert/methalert.html.

National Institutes of Health. (1998). *Research report series—Methamphetamine abuse and addiction* (Publication No. 98-4210). Washington, DC: Department of Health and Human Services.

Oro, A. S., & Dixon, S. D. (1987). Perinatal cocaine and methamphetamine exposure: Maternal and neonatal correlates. *Journal of Pediatrics, 111*, 571–578.

Perez-Reyes, M., White, W. R., McDonald, S. A., Hicks, R. E., Jeffcoat, A. R., Hill, J. M., & Cook, C. E. (1991). Clinical effects of daily methamphetamine administration. *Clinical Neuropharmacology, 14*, 352–358.

Poulin, C. (2001). Medical and nonmedical stimulant use among adolescents: From sanctioned to unsanctioned use. *Canadian Medical Association Journal, 165*(8), 1039–1044.

Rawson, R. A., Anglin, M. D., & Ling, W. (2002). Will the methamphetamine problem go away? *Journal of Addictive Diseases, 21*, 5–19.

Rawson, R. A., Gonzales, R. G., & Brethen, P. (2002). Methamphetamine: Current research findings and clinical challenges. *Journal of Substance Abuse Treatment 23*, 145–150.

Rawson, R. A., Huber, A., Brethen, P. B., Obert, J. L., Gulati, V., Shoptaw, S., & Ling,W. (2000) Methamphetamine and cocaine users: Differences in characteristics and treatment retention. *Journal of Psychoactive Drugs, 32*, 233–238.

Rawson, R. A., Marinelli-Casey, P., & Huber, A. (2002). A multisite evaluation of treatment of methamphetamine dependence in adults. In J. M. Herrell & R. B. Straw (Eds.), Conducting multiple site evaluations in real-world settings (Special issue). *New Directions in Evaluation, 94*, 73–87.

Reback, C. J., & Ditman, D. (1997). *The social construction of a gay drug: Methamphetamine use among gay and bisexual males in Los Angeles*. Los Angeles: City of Los Angeles.

Redfearn, P. J., Agrawal, N., & Mair, L. H. (1998). An association between the regular use of 3,4 methylenedioxy-methamphetamine (Ecstasy) and excessive wear of the teeth. *Addiction, 92*, 745–748.

Rhee, K. J., Albertson, T. E., & Douglas, J. C. (1988). Choreoathetoid disorder associated with amphetamine-like drugs. *American Journal of Emergency Medicine, 6*, 131–133.

Richards, J. R., & Brofeldt, B. T. (2000). Patterns of tooth wear associated with methamphetamine use. *Journal of Periodontics, 171*, 1371–1374.

Satel, S. L., Southwick, W. M., & Gawin, F. H. (1991). Clinical features of cocaine-induced paranoia. *American Journal of Psychiatry, 148*, 495–498.

Sattah, M. V., Supawitkul, S., Dondero, T. J., Kilmarx, P. H., Young, N. L., Mastro, T. D., Chaikummao, S., Manopaiboon, C., & Griensven, F. (2002). Prevalence of and risk factors for methamphetamine use in northern Thai youth: Results of an audio-computer-assisted self-interviewing survey with urine testing. *Addiction, 97*(7), 801–808.

See, S. J., & Tan, E. K. (2003). Severe amphetamine-induced bruxism: Treatment with botulinum toxin. *Acta Neurologica Scandinavica, 107*, 161–163.

Sekine, Y., Iyo, M., Ouchi, Y., Matsunage, T., Tsukada, H., Okada, H., Yoshikawa, E., Fatatsubashi, M., Takei, N., & Mori, N. (2001). Methamphetamine-related psychiatric symptoms and reduced brain dopamine transporters studied with PET. *American Journal of Psychiatry, 158*, 1206–1214.

Shoptaw, S., Reback, C. J., & Freese, T. E. (2002). Patient characteristics, HIV serostatus, and risk behaviors among gay and bisexual males seeking treatment for methamphetamine abuse and dependence in Los Angeles. *Journal of Addictive Diseases, 21*(1), 91–105.

Simon, S. L., Domier, C., Carnell, J., Brethen, P., Rawson, R., & Ling, W. (2000). Cognitive impairment in individuals currently using methamphetamine. *American Journal on Addictions, 9*, 222–231.

Smith, L. M., Chang, L., Yonekura, M. L., Grob, C., Osborn, D., & Ernst, T. (2001). Brain proton magnetic resonance spectroscopy in children exposed to methamphetamine *in utero. Neurology, 57*, 255–260.

Sowder, B., & Beschner, G. (Eds.). (1993). *Methamphetamine: An illicit drug with high abuse potential* (Unpublished report from NIDA Contract No. 271-90-0002). Rockville, MD: T. Head and Company.

Substance Abuse and Mental Health Services Administration. (1999). Center for Substance Abuse Treatment: Treatment for stimulant use disorders, Treatment Improvement Protocol (TIP) Series No. 33, 29–32.

Substance Abuse and Mental Health Services Administration. (2002). *Summary of the National Household Survey on Drug Abuse for 2001*. Retrieved on May 13, 2003, from www.samhsa.gov/oas/nhsda/2k1nhsda/vol1/toc.htm.

United States Senate. (2000). *Combating methamphetamine proliferation in America* (Hearing before the Committee on the Judiciary, July 28, 1999, Report No. J-106-41). Washington, DC: U.S. Government Printing Office.

Utena, H. (1966). Behavioral aberrations in methamphetamine-intoxicated animals and chemical correlations in the brain. *Progress in Brain Research, 31B*, 192–207.

Verachai, V., Dechongkit, S., Patarakorn, A., & Lukanapichonchut, L. (2001). Drug addicts treatment for ten years in Thanyarak Hospital (1989–1998). *Journal of the Medical Association of Thailand, 84*(1), 24–29.

Volkow, N. D., Chang, L., Wang, G. J., Fowler, J. S., Franceschi, D., Sedler, M. J., Gatley, S. J., Hitzemann, R., Ding, Y-S., Wong, C. H., & Logan, J. (2001). Higher cortical and lower subcortical metabolism in detoxified methamphetamine abusers. *American Journal of Psychiatry, 158*, 383–389.

Wada, K., Greberman, S. B., Konuma, K., & Hirai, S. (1999). HIV and HCV infection among drug users in Japan. *Addiction, 94*, 1063–1069.

Washton, A. M., Stone, N. S., & Hendrickson, E. C. (1988). Cocaine abuse. In D. M. Donovan & G. A. Marlatt (Eds.), *Assessment of addictive behaviors* (pp. 364–389). New York: Guilford Press.

Wiederman, M. W., & Pryor, T. (1996). Substance use among women with eating disorders. *International Journal of Eating Disorders, 20*(2), 163–168.

Williamson, S., Gossop, M., Powis, B., Grifiths, P., Fountain, J., & Strang, J. (1997). Adverse effects of stimulant drugs in a community sample of drug users. *Drug and Alcohol Dependence, 44*, 87–94.

World Health Organization. (1997). *Amphetamine-type stimulants* (Programme on Substance Abuse). Geneva: Division of Mental Health and Prevention of Substance Abuse.

Yui, K., Goto, K., Ikemoto, S., & Ishiguro, T. (1996). Plasma monoamine metabolites and spontaneous recurrence of methamphetamine-induced paranoid–hallucinatory psychosis: Relation of noradrenergic activity to the occurrence of flashbacks. *Psychiatry Research, 63*, 93–107.

Yui, K., Goto, K., Ikemoto, S., & Ishiguro, T. (2000). Stress induced spontaneous recurrence of methamphetamine psychosis: The relation between stressful experiences and sensitivity to stress. *Drug and Alcohol Dependence, 58*, 67–75.

Yui, K., Ishiguro, T., Goto, K., & Ikemoto, S. (1997). Precipitating factors in spontaneous recurrence of methamphetamine psychosis. *Psychopharmacology, 134*,
303–308.

Zhu, B.-L., Oritani, S., Shimotouge, K., Ishida, K., Quan, L., Fujita, M. Q., Ogawa,
M., & Maeda, H. (2000). Methamphetamine-related fatalities in forensic autopsy
during five years in he southern half of Osaka city and surrounding areas. *Forensic Science International, 113*, 443–447.

CHAPTER 7

Assessment of Opioid Use

JAMES WESTPHAL
DAVID A. WASSERMAN
CARMEN L. MASSON
JAMES L. SORENSEN

Opioids are a class of naturally occurring and synthetically derived drugs that act on the enkephalin, dynorphin, and endorphin receptors in the mammalian central nervous system. The prototype drug in this class is morphine, one of the active ingredients in opium, which is derived from the seeds of the opium poppy (*Papaver somniferum*). The term "opiates" is used to refer to the group of drugs derived from opium, such as heroin. Opiates plus synthetically derived drugs that are cross-tolerant with opiates, such as methadone and buprenorphine, are grouped together as opioids. Because opioids are highly effective in the alleviation of pain and anticipatory anxiety, they are used in medicine and surgery. Opioids also produce euphoria, resulting in a high abuse potential (Gold, 1998). Opioid abuse and dependence represent a significant public health problem for the United States in terms of both clinical management and direct medical care costs. For example, in 2001, heroin was a factor in 15% of emergency department drug-related episodes (Substance Abuse and Mental Health Services Administration [SAMHSA, 2002). Furthermore, statistics for that same year indicated that heroin in combination with other drugs was one of the three most frequently mentioned drugs in reported deaths. Other opioids, such as methadone, oxycodone, and hydrocodone, accounted for an additional 9% of drug-related emergency department visits (SAMHSA, 2002). Heroin-related medical care costs were estimated to be approximately $5 billion in the United States in 1996 (Mark, Woody, Juday, & Kleber, 2001). The large economic costs and human suffering that result from heroin addiction highlight the importance of investment in early identification and treatment of this addiction. Table 7.1 provides a list of commonly abused opioids, including both naturally occurring opioids and synthetics.

TABLE 7.1. Naturally Occurring and Synthetic Opioids

Opiates	Synthetically derived
Codeine (sulfate, phosphate)	Methadone (Dolophine)
Heroin	Meperidine (Demerol)
Morphine (sulphate)	Oxycodone (Percodan)
Opium	Oxymorphone (Numorphan)
	Propoxyphene (Darvon)
	Buprenorphine (Subutex)
	Fentanyl (Sublimaze)
	Hydrocodone (Tussionex)
	Hydromorphone (Dilaudid)

In the United States, the treatment of opioid-dependent patients has been highly regulated and generally confined to specialized treatment programs since the passage of the Harrison Act in 1914. Until late 2002, the only legal modalities available to treat opioid dependence were methadone and LAAM (levo-alpha-acetylmethadol) maintenance and detoxification, naltrexone (an opioid antagonist), and "drug-free" modalities, such as residential and intensive outpatient treatment. Methadone maintenance (Marsch, 1998; Mattrick, Kimber, Breen, & Davoli, 2002), buprenorphine maintenance (Mattrick et al., 2002), and contingency management during methadone maintenance have the most evidence supporting their efficacy (Griffith, Rowan-Szal, Roark, & Simpson, 2000). In 2002, sublingual buprenorphine became available in the United States to physicians who had attended training programs in its use. These physicians can prescribe buprenorphine for the treatment of opioid dependence in the context of an outpatient medical practice. Accessibility to counseling services is mandated for patients treated with buprenorphine. The change in regulations will allow increased flexibility in the assessment and treatment of opioid-dependent patients in more geographically and clinically diverse settings.

Opioid-dependent individuals, a heterogeneous population, differ greatly in the severity of their disorder, the presence and extent of coexisting disorders, and in other dimensions (Cacciola, Alterman, Rutherford, McKay, & Mulvaney, 2001). Previous research has demonstrated that a number of client factors, such as drug use severity, psychiatric diagnosis and severity, criminal justice pressure, poor motivation, and employment and family problems, are associated with treatment noncompliance and poor treatment outcomes (McLellan, Luborsky, Woody, O'Brien, & Druley, 1983; McLellan et al., 1994; Backmund, Meyer, Eikenlaub, & Schultz, 2001; Mutasa, 2001). Gaining an understanding of the person's uniqueness, life experiences, general level of function, and how these factors might interact to influence treatment outcomes is a critical first step in developing a comprehensive treatment plan.

Therefore, the clinician should consider the interaction of biological, psycho-logical, and sociocultural factors in assessing the patient's condition and treat-ment placement. Over the past decade, significant advances have been made in the assessment of opioid use, with a greater emphasis on multidimensional as-sessment that informs outcome-oriented, individualized treatment. Our pur-pose in this chapter is to review the assessment of opioid use across biological, psychological, and sociocultural systems of functioning.

DIAGNOSIS AND LEVEL-OF-CARE DETERMINATION

The diagnosis of opioid use disorders is made using criteria similar to those employed for the diagnosis of other drug use disorders. The *Diagnostic and Statistical Manual of Mental Disorders* (DSM-IV-TR; American Psychiatric Association, 2000) defines two diagnostic categories for substance use disor-ders: abuse and dependence. According to DSM-IV-TR, a diagnosis of either substance abuse or dependence requires the presence of specific, substance-related behaviors within a 12-month period. "Substance abuse" is defined as a maladaptive pattern of substance use, characterized by hazardous or compul-sive use or the presence of role impairment or recurrent legal problems, but without evidence of tolerance or withdrawal. "Substance dependence" re-quires a higher level of associated dysfunction that is usually accompanied by the physiological symptoms of tolerance and withdrawal. More information on the DSM-IV-TR criteria used to diagnose opioid dependence is provided in the biological and psychological assessment sections.

Determining the differences among opioid use, opioid abuse, and opioid dependence is critical in deciding whether treatment is indicated and which modality to use. For example, opioid replacement therapies, such as metha-done and buprenorphine, are reserved for opioid-dependent patients and would be inappropriate for patients who abuse or use opioids. The most im-portant criterion dividing use and the abuse/dependence categories is the pres-ence of clinically significant distress or dysfunction. When clinically significant distress or dysfunction is determined and the decision to treat has been made, the American Society of Addiction Medicine Patient Placement Criteria can be used to guide decisions regarding treatment site and modality (Graham et al., 2003). The Patient Placement Criteria are not opioid-specific and can be used to guide treatment planning for any substance use disorder. The criteria define six dimensions to assess (1) acute intoxication and/or withdrawal potential; (2) biomedical conditions and complications; (3) emotional, behavioral or cognitive conditions and complications; (4) readiness to change; (5) recovery/ living environment; and (6) relapse, continued use, or continued problem po-tential. Collection and organization of the relevant information allow the cli-nician to consider appropriate treatment placement from outpatient through hospitalization. Use of these criteria to guide treatment placement may improve treatment outcome and often is important in interactions with third-party payers.

SYSTEMS OF ASSESSMENT

Biological/Physical Systems

The biological and physical assessment of opioid use is addressed first. The primary methods of assessment are the physical examination and the use of laboratory tests. The aims of the assessment are to establish the diagnosis of opioid dependence, determine whether detoxification or maintenance on opioid replacement therapy is necessary, and identify co-occurring physical disorders that may affect treatment.

In the United States, federal (21 of the Code of Federal Regulations Part 291, and 42 of The Code of Federal Regulations Part 8) and state regulations guide the clinical practices used to determine patient eligibility for opioid maintenance and detoxification treatment. In general, federal regulations require a physical examination within 14 days of admission and determination by qualified personnel using medical criteria such as those found in the DSM-IV-TR (American Psychiatric Association, 2000) that the patient currently shows physiological signs and symptoms of dependence on an opioid drug. For maintenance treatment, the patient needs a history of opioid addiction for at least 1 year. The federal regulations are the minimal regulatory standards for opioid detoxification and maintenance using methadone. Each individual state has the ability to use the federal standards or add more stringent regulations. The states do not have the ability to waive the federal regulations.

The DSM-IV-TR criterion for substance dependence is a maladaptive pattern of substance use leading to clinically important distress or impairment within a single 12-month period as shown by three or more of the following symptoms: (1) tolerance, shown by (a) the need for either a markedly increased intake of the substance to achieve the same effect, or (b) with continued use, the markedly decreased effect of the same amount of the substance; (2) withdrawal, shown by either (a) the substance's characteristic withdrawal syndrome, or (b) use of the substance (or one closely related) to avoid or relieve withdrawal symptoms; (3) amount or duration of use that is often greater than intended; (4) the patient's repeated attempts without success to control or reduce substance use; (5) the patient spending much time using the substance, recovering from its effects, or trying to obtain it; (6) the patient reducing or abandoning important social, occupational, or recreational activities because of substance use; and (7) the patient continuing to use the substance, despite knowing that it has probably caused physical or psychological problems (American Psychiatric Association, 2000). The American Psychiatric Association allows the diagnosis of opioid dependence to be made without requiring either tolerance or withdrawal; however, in practice, a patient fitting this profile rarely would be seen. A patient without tolerance or dependence would not fulfill the current criteria for opioid replacement treatment but would be suitable for other types of treatment.

Tolerance/Withdrawal

In clinical assessment, the presence and severity of withdrawal symptoms determine the necessity for detoxification. Withdrawal symptoms are often legally required for the use of opioid replacement therapies. Opioid withdrawal is uncomfortable but not life threatening. When withdrawal symptoms are present, detoxification is not only humane but often also necessary to establish a therapeutic alliance and allow the patient enough physical comfort to engage in the treatment process. Recent research has shown that the presence of withdrawal or tolerance is associated with a more severe form of dependence (Schuckit et al., 1999). Documentation of opioid withdrawal by physical examination is often part of establishing the diagnosis of opioid dependence. Both the DSM-IV-TR (American Psychiatric Association, 2000) and the 10th edition of the *International Classification of Diseases and Related Health Problems* (ICD-10; World Health Organization, 1992) specify a physiological withdrawal state as one of the criteria for diagnosing opioid dependence. The DSM-IV-TR defines opioid withdrawal (292.0) as three or more of the following symptoms occurring after cessation or reduction of prolonged and heavy opioid use or the administration of an opioid antagonist: (1) dysphoric mood; (2) nausea or vomiting; (3) muscle aches; (4) lacrimation or rhinorrhea; (5) pupillary dilation, piloerection, or sweating; (6) diarrhea; (7) yawning; (8) fever; and (9) insomnia. The ICD-10 does not specifically define opioid withdrawal. Withdrawal may be observed naturalistically or induced by administration of an opioid antagonist such as naloxone. Standardized protocols have been established to measure the presence and severity of opioid withdrawal symptoms at specific time intervals (0, 10, 20, and 30 minutes) when a dose of an opioid antagonist (intramuscular naloxone 0.4 mg) is administered (Fudula, Berkow, Fralich, & Johnson, 1991). However, these practices are usually clinically unnecessary and are used in research situations where the severity of withdrawal needs to be precisely documented. A newer and less uncomfortable procedure for the patient uses the administration of naloxone eye drops and measurement of pupillary change to establish withdrawal (Ghodse, Greaves, & Lynch, 1999).

The assessment of withdrawal using DSM-IV-TR criteria focuses on observable signs (vomiting, lacrimation, rhinorrhea, piloerection, sweating, diarrhea, yawning), patient-reported symptoms (dysphoric mood, nausea, muscle aches, and insomnia), and measurable physiological variables (pupillary dilation and fever). However, studies have found that objective and subjective aspects of opioid withdrawal do not correlate (Loimer, Linzmayer, & Grunberger, 1991; Turkington & Drummond, 1989), and that observer-rated and subjective measures of withdrawal do not correlate with measurable physiological parameters such as pulse, temperature, blood pressure, and pupil size. Hence, these studies recommend using both objective and subjective scales in assessing opioid withdrawal.

Opioid withdrawal has been assessed using subjective, observer-rated, and physiological measures. The first two categories of measures are, of course, the most likely to be used by nonmedical clinicians. Two well-validated and psychometrically sound measures of withdrawal are the 16-item, self-administered Subjective Opiate Withdrawal Scale (SOWS) and the 13-item, rater-administered Objective Opiate Withdrawal Scale (OOWS), both developed by Handelsman et al. (1987) (see Table 7.2). A 10-item self-administered scale, the Short Opiate Withdrawal Scale has been described by Gossop (1990). Several other observer-rated withdrawal scales appear in the research literature, such as the modified Himmelsbach (1941) scale described by Eissenberg and associates (1996) and the Clinical Opiate Withdrawal Scale (COWS; Wesson & Ling, 2003). Physiological indicators of withdrawal include systolic and diastolic blood pressure, pulse rate, respiration rate, skin temperature, pupil diameter, and oxygen saturation (Donny, Walsh, Bigelow, Eissenberg, & Stitzer, 2002).

Both the DSM-IV-TR (American Psychiatric Association, 2000) and the ICD-10 (World Health Organization, 1992) specify tolerance as one of the criteria for diagnosing opioid dependence. Clinically, patient self-report usually establishes tolerance by a history of increasing doses used over time. Tolerance has been more difficult to measure objectively. One method is to administer increasing doses of methadone over several hours and observe the patient for signs of opioid intoxication, such as sedation (Arlett, 1982).

Often documentation of physical signs associated with opioid use is part of establishing opioid dependence. The signs can be needle puncture marks, tracks (areas of discoloration or scarring following the course of superficial veins), hand edema, thrombophlebitis (obstructed or inflamed veins), abscesses, skin ulcers, ulceration of the nasal septum from snorting heroin, cigarette burns or scars (from smoking when intoxicated), and cheilosis (cracking of the skin at the corners of the mouth). These signs are mostly associated with intravenous drug use and are not specific for opioid dependence.

Urine Drug Testing

Laboratory testing is often needed to confirm the patient's current opioid use for admission into opioid maintenance and detoxification programs. Unfortunately, there are no universally recommended or accepted drug testing procedures (Cone & Preston, 2002). Testing is most commonly performed on urine in a laboratory with thin-layer chromatography (TLC) because of its economy. TLC is a technique for separating and identifying organic compounds. It involves using a solvent such as acetone and a thin layer of adsorbent (usually silica gel or alumina) coated on a plate. The sample is dissolved in the solvent, which travels up the plate, carrying the sample with it. Any drugs or metabolites will separate on the plate according to how much they absorb on the sil-

TABLE 7.2. Major Domains and Selected Assessments for Opioid-Using Populations

Purpose	Domain/ construct	Instrument(s)	Authors
Diagnosis, assessment of severity	Diagnosis of substance use and psychiatric disorders	Composite International Diagnostic Interview (CIDI)	Robins et al. (1983)
		Structured Clinical Interview for DSM-IV Axis I Disorders—Clinician Version (SCID-CV)	First et al. (1997)
		Diagnostic Interview Schedule (DIS)	Robins et al. (1981)
		Psychiatric Research Interview for Substance and Mental Disorders (PRISM)	Hasin et al. (1996)
	Withdrawal symptoms	Subjective Opiate Withdrawal Scale (SOWS)	Handelsman et al. (1987)
		Objective Opiate Withdrawal Scale (OOWS)	Handelsman et al. (1987)
		Short Opiate Withdrawal Scale	Gossop (1990)
		Clinical Opiate Withdrawal Scales (COWS)	Wesson & Ling (2003)
	Severity of substance dependence	Substance Dependence Severity Scale (SDSS)	Miele et al. (2000)
		Severity of Dependence Scale (SDS)	Gossop et al. (1997)
		Addiction Severity Index (ASI), 5th edition	McLellan et al. (1992)
Treatment planning	Psychosocial functioning	Addiction Severity Index (ASI), 5th edition	McLellan et al. (1992)
		ASAM Patient Placement Criteria	American Society of Addiction Medicine (2003)
	Cognitive impairment	Trail Making Test	Reitan (1958)
		Shipley Institute of Living Scale	Shipley (1967)
		Mini-Mental Status Examination	Folstein et al. (1975)
		Frank Jones Story	Bechtold et al. (2001)
		Executive Interview (EXIT)	Royall et al. (1992)
	Motivation	Outcomes Expectancy Questionnaire	Saunders et al. (1995)
		Thoughts about Abstinence	Wasserman et al. (1998) Hall et al. (1990)

(continued)

TABLE 7.2. (*continued*)

Purpose	Domain/ construct	Instrument(s)	Authors
Identification of risk factors related to relapse, relapse prevention	Craving	Obsessive Compulsive Drug Use Scales (OCDUS)	Franken et al. (2002)
		Desires for Drug Questionnaire (DDQ)	Franken et al. (2002)
		Measurement of Drug Craving	Sayette et al. (2000)
	Expectations of abstinence	Outcomes Expectancy Questionnaire	Saunders et al. (1995)
	High-risk situations	Inventory of Drug-Taking Situations (IDTS)	Turner et al. (1997)
		Social Influences on Abstinence and Drug Use Scale (SIADU)	Wasserman et al. (2001)
	Situational response efficacy	Situational Confidence Questionnaire (SCQ-39)	Annis & Graham (1988)
		Situational Confidence Questionnaire (Heroin Users)	Barber et al. (1991)
		Drug-Taking Confidence Questionnaire (DTCQ)	Sklar et al. (1997)
		Alcohol Abstinence Self-Efficacy Scale (AASE)	DiClemente et al. (1994)
	Emotional states	Profile of Mood States	McNair et al. (1971)

ica gel versus how much they dissolve in the solvent. The drugs or metabolites for which the laboratory is testing are also run, giving a standard to compare with the urine sample's compounds. A positive test indicates that a compound in the urine has traveled a distance identical to that of one of the test drugs or metabolites.

Another type of urine testing is the relatively newer immunologically based testing, such as Testcup and Teststik. Immunologically based testing uses specifically engineered monoclonal mouse antibodies to detect drugs or their metabolites. The immunologically based testing is easy to perform on-site, with results available within 5 minutes. Urine testing, either TLC or immunologically based, is qualitative; it gives a result of drug presence or absence in the urine based on a detection level, usually given in the range of nanograms per milliliter (ng/ml). The currently used methods of urine testing are susceptible to false positives; therefore, urine testing usually requires confirmation of positive results by a more accurate method. Sometimes synthetic opioids are not routinely included in urine drug testing, so false-negative results are also possible. Gas chromatography, high-performance liquid chromatography, and gas chromatography–mass spectrometry are some of the methods used to confirm positive tests. Drug testing methods continue to evolve; reviews of detection levels, false-negative, and false-positive rates of the chosen testing method need to be performed regularly. Descriptions of these testing methods are beyond the scope of this chapter.

Physical Examination and Laboratory Tests

Physical examination and laboratory tests are used to screen for physical disorders associated with opioid and/or injection drug use. Examination by a physician is often necessary before the start of treatment because of the risk of spreading communicable diseases to other treatment participants and to determine whether possible life-threatening complications of intravenous use, such as endocarditis, are present and need immediate treatment. Signs of hepatitis, such as jaundice, or signs of HIV/AIDS, such as opportunistic infections (e.g., monilial infection or thrush), can be found on physical examination. Endocarditis, septicemia, fungal infections, cellulites, and abscesses are complications of poor aseptic injection techniques often associated with intravenous opioid drug use (but not specific to opioids) that can be detected on physical examination (Center for Substance Abuse Treatment, 1993). Other communicable disorders such as, lice, scabies, and venereal warts that can be detected on physical examination are associated with neglect to physical health and hygiene associated with severe alcohol or drug dependence but are not specific to opioid use.

A complementary method of screening for physical disorders is laboratory testing. Recommended laboratory screening often changes as technology improves and diseases evolve. A current assessment battery may include a complete blood count with differential to screen for acute infections, a tuberculin skin test and/or chest X-ray for tuberculosis, an HIV test (with consent of the patient), a Venereal Disease Research Laboratory test for syphilis, and hepatitis antigen and antibody tests for hepatitis A, B, and C (Center for Substance Abuse Treatment, 1993). An electrocardiogram, a urinalysis, and a blood chemistry profile are often added to assess general health status and to screen for metabolic disorders associated with poor nutrition, comorbid physical disorders, and/or symptoms associated with withdrawal, such as diarrhea or vomiting. A pregnancy test for females with reproductive ability is usually performed, especially before the administration of opioid replacement medication.

Psychological Assessment

The presence of physiological symptoms of opioid tolerance and withdrawal alone do not suffice for the diagnosis of opioid dependence. Many medical patients using prescribed opioid medication for chronic pain relief will have symptoms of tolerance and withdrawal but do not meet any of the other diagnostic criteria for dependence (Adriaensen, Vissers, Noorduin, & Meert, 2003). Assessment of the patient's behavior, psychology, and functioning is critical in the determination of opioid dependence. The distinction between abuse and dependence is clinically important for some substances, most notably alcohol. For opioids, abuse is usually a transitory state, rapidly developing into dependence (Ridenour, Cottler, Compton, Spitznagel, & Cunningham-Williams, 2003). Psychological assessment of opioid use also includes assessment for the presence and severity of co-occurring psychiatric disorders and cognitive impairment, and the assessment of treatment readiness.

A number of screening and comprehensive tools designed to assess opioid use disorders and related problems are available for the clinician's use. Many of these instruments have user-friendly features, including favorable psychometric properties, norms for clinical samples, and score reports that directly assist with treatment referral decisions and planning. In busy treatment settings, the use of brief screening instruments may be more cost-effective than full-length batteries. The use of screening tools allows busy programs to identify opioid use disorders and related problems efficiently and accurately. However, when a definitive diagnosis is needed, structured and semistructured interviews provide a precise and reliable means to elicit the information needed. A well-trained layperson can administer most structured interviews with acceptable reliability. In the case of semistructured interviews, more advanced training is required, and there is also a greater reliance on clinical judgment in scoring the responses. However, the use of semistructured interviews allows the clinician to gather more comprehensive information than can be obtained from fully structured interviews. This section focuses on the assessment of dependence.

Multiple strategies can be used to assess the severity of opioid dependence. There are several instruments that assess the severity of dependence across substances, such as the Substance Dependence Severity Scale (SDSS; Miele et al., 2000) and the Severity of Dependence Scale (SDS; Gossop, Best, Marsden, & Strang, 1997). The former takes specialized training and up to 40 minutes to administer. The latter is a brief, 5-item scale. The Severity of Opiate Dependence Questionnaire (SODQ) is opioid-specific, but there is some controversy in the literature about the stability of its psychometric properties (Burgess, Stripp, Pead, & Holman, 1989). One relatively simple approach to assessing severity is counting the number of positive DSM-IV-TR or ICD-10 substance dependence criteria. Another approach is using a nonspecific instrument such as the Addiction Severity Index (ASI), a commonly used treatment planning and outcome measurement instrument, to assess systematically for opioid use and associated dysfunction (McLellan et al., 1992). The ASI, a semistructured interview, evaluates the history, frequency, and consequences of drug and alcohol use, and also problems in five other areas: medical, legal, employment, social/family, and psychological. The ASI provides severity scores in each of the areas.

Psychological Disorders

Drug dependence in general is associated with a higher risk of psychiatric comorbidity, with illicit drug dependence presenting a higher risk of psychiatric comorbidity than dependence on a legal drug. The risks are additive, so that patients with multiple drug dependencies are at the highest risk for psychiatric disorders (Kandel, Huang, & Davies, 2001). One study found that 47% of patients seeking methadone maintenance treatment had additional psychiatric disorders (Brooner, King, Kidorf, Schmidt, & Bigelow, 1997). Although the specific comorbid diagnoses will depend on the location and population studied, the dramatic cluster of personality (antisocial for males, borderline for females), affective, and anxiety disorders has higher prevalence in opioid-dependent populations (Brooner et al., 1997).

Several psychological instruments can be used to screen or to diagnose psychiatric disorders in opioid-dependent patients. The ASI can be used to screen for co-occurring psychiatric disorders (McLellan et al., 1992). An elevated psychological functioning score is likely because of the high rate of psychiatric comorbidity among patients with opioid dependence. Both the Composite International Diagnostic Interview (CIDI; Robins, Wing, & Helzer, 1983) and the Diagnostic Interview Schedule (DIS; Robins, Helzer, Croughan, & Ratkliff, 1981) are structured interviews that can assist in making Axis I psychiatric diagnoses. A specialized instrument for use in substance-using populations is the Psychiatric Research Interview for Substance and Mental Disorders (PRISM; Hasin et al., 1996). The use of these instruments requires experience and skill in distinguishing substance-induced psychiatric symptoms.

There are fewer assessment instruments available for making a DSM-IV-TR Axis II or personality disorder diagnosis in opioid- or substance-using populations in general, compared to making Axis I diagnoses. One study in a cocaine-dependent population found that a self-report personality assessment instrument (Millon Clinical Multiaxial Inventory–II; Millon, 1997) was useful only in screening for personality disorder. A structured interview instrument for personality disorder (Structured Clinical Interview for DSM-IV Axis I Disorders; First, Spitzer, Gibbon, & Williams, 1997) was found to be more reliable in making a specific diagnosis of personality disorder (Marlowe, Husband, Bonieskie, Kirby, & Platt, 1997).

Other Substance Use Disorders

Thorough assessment of other substance use in opioid-dependent patients is clinically necessary. A study on co-occurring disorders found that among most patients seeking opioid maintenance treatment, at least two other substance use disorders could be diagnosed (Brooner et al., 1997). A structured review of other substance use can be obtained when using the ASI. However, the ASI alcohol and drug section does not determine substance use diagnoses. Both the

CIDI (Robins et al., 1983) and the DIS (Robins et al., 1981) have relatively brief computerized substance use disorder diagnostic sections if making precise diagnoses of other substance use disorders is necessary.

Biological testing may be used to confirm information obtained on other substance use. The clinician also needs to remember that substance use is not static and often changes, especially in opioid maintenance patients. Ongoing testing for opioid and other substance use during treatment is federally mandated for opioid maintenance and detoxification programs. Current alcohol use can be monitored with a Breathalyzer, and alcohol use over several weeks can be detected using specialized blood tests, such as carbohydrate-deficient transferrin (Reynaud et al., 2000). Ongoing Breathalyzer tests at dispensing windows are often used to monitor patients who use alcohol. Methadone doses may need to be adjusted or withheld to avoid dangerous levels of sedation in patients who drink.

Currently, the multiple choices for ongoing monitoring for drug use include five biological matrices (urine, plasma, sweat, hair, and oral fluids) and the site of analysis (laboratory-based or on-site kits). The timeliness of on-site testing leads to its use in contingency management programs or counseling approaches that use timely feedback about drug use.

One advantage of testing with hair, saliva, and sweat is that collection is less intrusive. For both sweat and hair, drug use over more extended periods, a week (sweat patch) to months (hair), can be quantitatively monitored; that is, the amount of use over that time period can be determined rather than simply whether specific substance was occurred. The alternative matrices may be more sensitive detectors of drug use, but some studies show no clinical improvement in drug use with more sensitive monitoring (Taylor, Watson, Tames, & Lowe, 1998). The optimal use of the newer testing technologies is yet to be determined.

The choice and parameters of drug testing methodology need to be periodically reassessed by clinicians because of numerous, changing factors, such as the emergence of newer technologies, and changes in local drug supplies and patient drug preferences. The parameters that need to be periodically reviewed are drug detection thresholds, specific drugs detected, the laboratory's false-positive and false-negative rates, and the clinical utility of the information that testing provides.

Cognitive Impairment

Cognitive impairment is a frequent finding in substance-using populations in general and is especially prevalent in opioid replacement therapy populations. Fals-Stewart (1997) found that 43% of patients in detoxification treatment had measurable cognitive impairment. Such cognitive deficits have been shown to retard skills acquisition and to moderate the effects of psychotherapeutic interventions (Smith & McCardy, 1991; Roehrich & Goldman, 1993).

The deficits in opioid replacement therapy populations are usually found across all or multiple testing domains when compared to controls (Darke, Sims, McDonald, & Wickes, 2000; Mintzer & Stitzer, 2002). The cause of the deficits may not be related to the direct effects of opioids on cognition (Mintzer & Stitzer, 2002). One study found that significant independent predictors of cognitive impairment among methadone maintenance patients were co-occurring alcohol dependence and the number of nonfatal heroin overdoses (Darke et al., 2000). The clinical significance of the deficits and their impact on fitness for specific tasks must be determined on an individual basis (Specka et al., 2000). Because of the presence of multiple confounding variables of other substance use and co-occurring psychiatric disorders, the specific effects of chronic opioid use on neuropsychological performance have been difficult to determine. A study of chronic pain patients using daily morphine found significant deficits in vigilance/attention, psychomotor speed, and working memory (Sjogren, Thomsen, & Olsen, 2000).

The individual's level of neuropsychological abilities should be taken into account in determining treatment modality and setting. Several instruments that assess cognitive impairment (Trail Making Test [Reitan, 1958], Shipley Institute of Living Scale [Shipley, 1967], and the Mini-Mental Status Examination [Folstein, Folstein, & McHugh, 1975]) have evidence to support their use in substance-using populations (Carroll & Rounsaville, 2002). Of these instruments, the Mini-Mental Status Examination is briefest and easiest to learn to administer. It tests orientation, recent memory, attention, verbal fluency, naming, figure drawing, and ability to follow a three-step instruction. Possible scores range from 0 to 30. Depending on the educational and literacy level of the patient, a score below 24 usually indicates cognitive impairment and should activate consideration of further neuropsychological evaluation.

"Executive functioning," simply defined, is the patient's ability to organize and sequence tasks toward a goal and is more closely related to problem-solving ability. Executive functioning is more difficult to assess than general cognitive impairment and is less studied in substance-using populations. Executive functioning has been found to be impaired in patients with substance use disorders. Morgenstern and Bates (1999) found that more than 50% of their treatment sample exhibited executive functioning impairment. The authors did not find any significant differences in outcomes of their patients with executive impairment compared to those who had no impairment, but they did find different courses of treatment for the two groups. In dementia and schizophrenia, level of executive functioning is better correlated to functional ability and level of care needed than to standard neuropsychological functioning (Royall, Mahurin, & Gray, 1992). Briefer clinical tests relating to executive functioning are the Frank Jones Story (Bechtold, Horner, Labbate, & Windham, 2001) and the Trail Making Test B (Reitan, 1958). The Frank Jones Story is a story about a person whose feet are so big that he has to put his pants on over his head. The patient's affective response is observed, and he or she is asked if Frank can do it, and also asked why not? The three responses are scored. A perfect score would include an appropriate affective response (smiles or laughs), a "no" answer, and an explanation of the difficulty.

The Trail Making Test B has numbers and letters on a page. The patient is asked to connect the points by alternating numbers in ascending order and letters in alphabetical order. The test is timed, and mistakes in the sequencing are recorded to yield a score. A more extensive test of executive functioning that is still considered a "bedside" test rather than formal neuropsychological testing is the Executive Interview (EXIT; Royall, Mahurin, & Gray, 1992), a 10-minute, 25-item interview scored from 0 to 50. Scores on the EXIT have been found to correlate with the level of care required and amount of disruptive behavior in dementia populations. The EXIT may be useful for assessing substance-using patients with cognitive impairment to determine appropriateness for residential treatment. Any treatment approach that involves learning and applying new information will need to be modified if significant cognitive impairment or executive dysfunction are found.

Other important aspects of psychological assessment and treatment planning are the patient's motivation, and the resources and obstacles relevant to change. Classification of readiness for change (Prochaska & DiClemente, 1983) has been a useful clinical heuristic device. Several instruments have been developed to assess stages of change, but none is specific to opioids. Psychometric support for these instruments is variable, and their predictive validity among patients seeking drug treatment is controversial (Carey, Purnine, Maisto, Carey, & Barnes, 1999). Limited work with techniques, such as motivational interviewing, that use the stages-of-change framework has been done with opioid-dependent populations (Saunders, Wilkinson, & Phillips, 1995).

Determining the patient's expectations of abstinence and goals for treatment is also important in assessment. Annis (1984) developed an Outcomes Expectancies Questionnaire that Saunders et al. (1995) adapted for opioid users. It measures positive versus negative perceptions of abstinence. In Saunders et al., lower outcome expectancy predicted earlier dropout from methadone treatment. A realistic (vs. ideal) goal of permanent absolute abstinence from heroin predicted subsequent continued abstinence in opiate-abstinent methadone maintenance patients (Wasserman, Weinstein, Havassy, & Hall, 1998). Belding, McLellan, Zanis, and Incmikoski (1998) speculated that the absence of characteristics distinguishing methadone maintenance patients in their study who continue to use opiates from those who did not may have reflected a simple lack of desire on the part of the users to quit.

Craving

Craving can be a serious obstacle to continued abstinence. "Craving" has been variously defined as a desire to use a drug, anticipation of a drug's reinforcing effects, and intention to engage in drug use (Sayette et al., 2000). A common synonym for "craving" is "urge." Some theorists have postulated that craving is necessary for relapse to occur, while others argue that craving is difficult to define and is of little import in relapse. Drummond (2000) distinguished between cue-elicited craving and withdrawal craving, and argued that the former is more likely to predict relapse after withdrawal symptoms have subsided. Empirically, the relationship between craving and relapse is not robust.

Measures of craving range from a single item to multifactorial scales. Franken, Hendriks, and van den Brink (2002) recently published two opioid craving questionnaires. The first, the 13-item Obsessive Compulsive Drug Use Scale (OCDUS), was derived from the Yale–Brown Obsessive Compulsive Scale (Goodman et al., 1989) and measures general craving within a time frame of 1 week (sample item: "How much of your time when you are not using is occupied by ideas, thoughts, impulses, or images related to heroin use?"). The second scale, the 14-item Desires for Drug Questionnaire (DDQ), assesses instantaneous craving at the time of assessment (sample item: "I would do almost anything to use heroin now"). Each scale has three subscales. The OCDUS subscales are Thought about Heroin and Interference, Desires and Control, and Resistance to Thoughts and Intention. For the DDQ, the subscales are Desire and Intention, Negative Reinforcement, and Control. The authors recommend attending to subscale scores rather than total scale scores. Evidence for the concurrent and predictive validity of the OCDUS and DDQ is limited.

Visual analogue scales have also been used to assess craving for opioids; for example, patients may indicate their level of craving by making a mark on a 100-mm line (e.g., Franken et al., 2002). In an abstinence reinforcement study of heroin users in methadone maintenance, participants were asked to rate on a 5-point scale, from "not at all" to "extremely,", how much they had wanted heroin during the past week (Preston, Umbricht, & Epstein, 2000).

Social/Cultural Assessment

The psychological aspects of assessment just reviewed involve examining the patient's behavior, cognition, attitudes, and symptoms. The current section focuses on the patient's environment and its effects on opioid use.

Gathering social and cultural data on opioid-using patients can enhance our understanding of the context of their drug-using behavior, help us develop hypotheses about their drug use, and lead to identification of intermediate target variables for treatment, for example, strengthening patients' support network of non-drug users. The technology for social and cultural assessment, however, is not as practical or well-developed as is the case for biological and physical assessment systems. Instead of having a wide array of validated instruments at their disposal, clinicians and researchers must rely on measures that may have been used in only one or a few observational research studies. Often, these studies focus on the deleterious effects of having other drug users in one's social network. Other variables, researched less frequently, include social network variables such as number of social ties, general social support (e.g., emotional support), support specific to abstinence, participation in the drug use economy, and neighborhood and community factors. Investigations of social and cultural variables relevant to needle sharing (rather than to drug use per se) constitute a sizable literature in their own right and, for the most part, are not included in this discussion.

Social and cultural assessment is an ongoing process and cannot be completed in a single interview. Not only is the information potentially vast but also patients may not recall or report important aspects of their social histories at first, may see certain facts as irrelevant, or may choose not to disclose information because of shame, guilt, or fear of repercussions.

There are different ways to categorize the enormous number of sociocultural variables relevant to opioid treatment. One useful grouping is demographic variables, social support, involvement in the drug economy or drug scene, and the nature of the neighborhood environment.

Demographic Variables

Gathering demographic information can help to locate a person in his or her sociocultural context. Important data to collect include age, gender, ethnicity and national origin; acculturation-related variables, such as language(s) spoken at home, education level, vocational skills, current employment status and employment history; current engagement in nonwork meaningful activities, such as volunteering or school attendance; income and income sources; type of housing (or lack thereof); neighborhood environment; involvement with the legal system; and spirituality and religious participation. For variables that may change over time, such as employment, it is important to gather historical data. Often, patients enter treatment when they are experiencing one or more severe downturns in their lives, and they may have been functioning within society at higher levels in the past. The ASI (McLellan, Luborsky, Woody, & O'Brien, 1980; McLellan et al., 1992) described in a prior section on psychological assessment, assesses much of the information just detailed. Other instruments or intake interview sessions may be needed to gather a complete picture.

Although several demographic variables have been shown, albeit inconsistently, to be related to opioid treatment outcomes, the mediating factors are not always clear. Kidorf, Stitzer, and Brooner (1994) offered a helpful analysis of why employment is associated with positive treatment outcomes in methadone maintenance patients. First, the reinforcements inherent in employment may successfully compete with the reinforcing effects of drug use. Second, employment provides structure in one's daily life. Third, in opioid replacement programs, medication take-home incentives, which are usually available only to nonusing patients, may be more valuable to employed patients because of their busy lives.

Social Support

STRUCTURAL SOCIAL SUPPORT

Structural social support, or the quantity and type of social ties, is important to assess in opioid-using individuals in order to ascertain their degree of social integration versus isolation. Although some opioid users are involved in intimate relationships and maintain contact with relatives and friends, others are estranged from most or all of their immediate family members, including their children, and regard themselves as having no close friends, only acquaintances. Distress at their circumstances may impede treatment progress. Structural variables that should be assessed include intimate relationship status (with legal marital status differentiated from other intimate relationships); family constellation (including family of origin); degree of involvement with, versus estrangement from, family members; conflicts with family members; deaths of important others; other types of ruptures in important relationships; number of close friendships and frequency of contact with friends; and involvement with social groups (formal and informal).

Evidence is mixed as to whether stronger structural support predicts better treatment outcomes in opioid users (Havassy, Hall, & Wasserman, 1991; Wasserman, Stewart, & Delucchi, 2001); however, increasing the number of social ties or decreasing social conflict may improve quality of life and increase social support for abstinence. Knight and Simpson (1996), for example, showed that reductions in family conflict during methadone maintenance treatment were associated with lower injection frequency. Assessment instruments for measuring structural support in opioid users include the Social Participation Index and the Social Network Interview (Havassy et al., 1991; Havassy, Wasserman, & Hall, 1995; Wasserman et al., 2001).

Cultural identification and behavior have rarely been studied in opioid users. Ethnographers have published articles describing the mores of drug-using cultures, but studies of opioid users' connections to other cultural and ethnic groups are scarce. Ethnicity can be a strong predictor of drug-related variables, such as route of administration (Havassy et al., 1995). It stands to reason that the degree of embeddedness in various cultural groups influences the demographics of opioid use, the social ties of opioid users, and possibly the prognosis for successful treatment outcomes. For example, in a study of heroin users in the London Bangladeshi community, White (2001) found that heroin use was overwhelmingly more prevalent among men than among women; 96% of Bangladeshis presenting at drug treatment centers were male. Gender-role expectations (e.g., that women should stay indoors) might have minimized women's exposure to heroin and, consequently, their risk of developing drug problems. White also found that many Bangladeshi heroin users experimented with heroin before ever trying alcohol, a likely consequence of the prohibition on alcohol use in the Muslim religion. Finally, relative to a comparison group, Bangladeshis were significantly more likely to report family contact and family support for treatment, to endorse a belief in God, and to report religious involvement. White speculated that the lower levels of social exclusion and higher levels of involvement with religious life reported by Bangladeshis might be associated with a more positive treatment prognosis compared to other cultural groups.

GENERAL FUNCTIONAL SUPPORT

General functional support concerns the availability of specific interpersonal support functions such as affection and instrumental aid. The influence of generic perceived social support on drug use may be minimal. In three studies that measured availability of generic functional support among opioid maintenance patients, no concurrent or prospective effects on abstinence were found (Goehl, Nunes, Quitkin, & Hilton, 1993; Gogineni, Stein, & Friedmann, 2001; Wasserman et al., 2001). Therefore, at this time, it may be less important to assess general functional support than to assess specific social domains.

ABSTINENCE-SPECIFIC STRUCTURAL SUPPORT

Abstinence-specific structural support concerns the level of drug use versus abstinence in one's social network. Numerous studies have demonstrated that having substance users in the social network is associated with drug use. In particular, a substance-using live-in partner is a major risk for continued use or relapse. Darke, Swift, Hall, and Ross (1994) found that having a sexual partner who injected drugs was a strong predictor of injection drug use in methadone maintenance patients. Kidorf et al. (1994) demonstrated that methadone patients who lived with a sexual partner who used illicit drugs were less likely to earn methadone take-home doses. Gogineni et al. (2001) showed that, among methadone maintenance patients, injection drug use was most prevalent among those with a substance-using live-in partner and those who interacted with more substance users. Goehl et al. (1993), in a sample of methadone maintenance patients, discovered that patients reporting a drug user among their close significant others had a subsequently higher percentage of positive toxicology screens for illicit drugs. In a study of 335 out-of-treatment injection drug users, participants with a higher proportion of social network members with whom they had used drugs were less likely to report having ceased heroin and cocaine use at study follow-up approximately 5 months later (Latkin, Knowlton, Hoover, & Mandell, 1999). Silverman et al. (1998) showed that responders, compared to nonresponders, in a voucher-based reinforcement study of cocaine-using methadone patients, scored higher on a measure of lifestyle changes that assessed avoidance of drug users, avoidance of places where drugs were available, and more time spent with people who did not use drugs. In a prospective study of social relationships among opioid maintenance patients, Wasserman et al. (2001) found that having cocaine users in one's social network at study baseline predicted cocaine use at a

3-month follow-up assessment; however, having heroin users in one's network did not predict heroin use. In a rare negative result, Gossop, Stewart, Browne, and Mardsen (2002) found no differences with regard to having a drug-using partner or drug-using friends among heroin users who remained abstinent after residential or inpatient treatment, had a lapse, or relapsed.

The consistent finding that having drug users in the social network predicts negative outcomes suggests that higher numbers of non-drug users in the network may enhance abstinence. Unfortunately, little published research has assessed the richness of non-drug-using networks and the importance of large numbers of nonusers for abstinence.

ABSTINENCE-SPECIFIC FUNCTIONAL SUPPORT

Abstinence-specific functional support refers to perceived behaviors by others, verbal or nonverbal, that focus directly on the person's abstinence, for example, encouraging someone to remain in drug abuse treatment. Negative examples of this type of support include behaviors such as offering drugs. Our University of California, San Francisco, group has published several articles that focus on assessment of abstinence-specific social support in various patient populations (Havassy et al., 1991, 1995; Wasserman et al., 2001). In the most recent of these, we described a new, 41-item self-report instrument, Social Influences on Abstinence and Drug Use (SIADU), that assesses nine behavioral domains. Decreases in three of the negative subscales (Complaints about Drug Use, Drug Exposure, and Demoralization) from study baseline to the 3-month follow-up assessment predicted cocaine abstinence in 128 opioid maintenance patients. Drug Exposure continued to predict, even when the number of cocaine users in the social network was held constant. Notably, none of the subscales we thought would be positively related to abstinence (e.g., Positive Reinforcement) showed significant effects. Although the instrument may be useful in cocaine-abusing opioid maintenance patients, opioid use was not predicted at all by SIADU scores. Overall, the results suggest that negative social influences may be more powerful than positive influences.

Involvement in the Drug Economy or Drug Scenes

Participation in the drug economy, beyond simply being a purchaser and user, may predict a poorer chance of staying in treatment and achieving abstinence. Friedman et al. (1998) discussed various roles that drug users may take in "drug scenes." Participants in their survey of street-recruited drug injectors were more likely to engage in high-risk drug use behaviors if they held roles in the drug scene. In another community sample of heroin and cocaine users, Sherman and Latkin (2002) found that holding at least one role in the drug economy versus none was associated with far higher levels of daily drug use and daily injection of heroin, and also smaller differences in percentage of active drug users in the social network and other network drug use variables.

The implications for assessment of opioid users are clear. As trust builds within treatment relationships, patients should be asked which roles they have played or currently play in the drug economy, such as selling drugs, needles, or syringes; being paid by others to help them inject; copping drugs or buying needles or syringes for others; operating a shooting gallery or allowing others to use drugs in one's home for money or drugs; and engaging in sex work for money or drugs. Participation in these activities that obviously increase proximity to drugs and drug users therefore has implications for future abstinence, not to mention personal safety and involvement with the legal system. Patients may be loath to give up some of these activities because of loss of income.

Nature of the Neighborhood Environment

This domain concerns the drug-related social characteristics of the area where the individual opioid user lives. Neighborhood variables have been little studied, but intriguing findings have been reported. Because it is impossible to assess the actual prevalence of illicit drug use in a community, researchers and clinicians must rely on proxy measures, such as drug-related arrests. For example, in a study of 342 adults with a history of injection drug use, higher levels of drug arrests in the neighborhood predicted continuing drug use, independent of drug use in the social network, although the latter was a stronger predictor (Schroeder et al., 2001).

In summary, most of the research we reviewed shows that contact with the drug culture, such as people and areas where drug use is prevalent, is associated with drug use in people trying to abstain. A thorough understanding and assessment of the patient's social environment is therefore an important factor in treatment planning, especially residential treatment. The social environment is also important in assessing risk factors for relapse.

ASSESSMENT RELATED TO RELAPSE PREVENTION

The clinical course of opioid dependence usually involves multiple detoxification episodes. Brief cessation of opioid use is often easier than staying abstinent. For patients who do not use agonist maintenance therapies, relapse prevention is critical to their treatment. To make the clinical situation more complex, opioid users commonly use multiple substances in addition to heroin—commonly, alcohol, benzodiazepines, cocaine, marijuana, methamphetamine, and nicotine. When discussing relapse prevention in this population, one might well ask: Relapse to which substance(s)? Because this chapter is devoted to opioid dependence, we mostly limit our discussion of relapse to illicit opioid use. Still, some of the information we impart derives from studies of relapse to other substances, primarily cocaine, in opioid-using samples (e.g., Silverman et al., 1998). Other data comes from combined samples of opioid users and users of other drugs (e.g., Hall, Havassy, & Wasserman, 1990;

Sklar & Turner, 1999). Most studies we discuss were conducted with persons in treatment, usually methadone maintenance or detoxification, but a few studies focused on out-of-treatment samples. Variables related to relapse prevention may behave dissimilarly across treatment modalities, for example, agonist treatment, antagonist treatment, inpatient treatment, and residential treatment including therapeutic communities, and also across patients who quit using drugs while in treatment versus no treatment, either in the community or in controlled environments such as jail or prison.

Ideally, factors related to relapse prevention in opioid users should be researched only in those individuals who are abstinent (biochemically verified) and at moderate risk for relapse. Such persons should be followed over time, with associations between relapse factors and drug use examined prospectively. Prospective studies, compared to cross-sectional ones, lead to clearer interpretations of temporal (but not necessarily causal) relationships between potential relapse factors and drug use. The results of cross-sectional or retrospective studies can be difficult to interpret. For example, if negative mood states are assessed in patients who have relapsed versus those who have not, a strong association between relapse and moods may be noted. But, this association may be due to the relapse intensifying the negative mood rather than a dysphoric mood preceding (and possibly causing) the relapse (Hall et al., 1990). Changes in other variables thought to cause relapse (e.g., craving, low commitment to abstinence, even stressful events) may instead be caused by relapse, or the effects could be reciprocal.

Proximal Factors

Many assessment instruments have been described for measuring proximal variables related to relapse prevention. We have identified from the literature the following broad constructs as potentially fruitful areas for assessment: *high-risk situations, conditioned cue reactivity, situational response efficacy,* and *emotional states.* All of these constructs have been posited to be theoretically linked to relapse, and each may have relevance for particular patients. In only a few cases, however, have the links between the constructs and relapse to opioid use been consistently empirically supported, especially among opioid maintenance patients.

An optimal dose of an opioid medication, because of its physiological effects, may reduce the importance of most other variables usually considered important in relapse. This could explain why some studies have failed to find effects for numerous variables on continued illicit opiate use in methadone or LAAM patients (e.g., Belding et al., 1998), while others have found no effects on opiate use for certain variables, such as social relationships, despite strong effects on cocaine use (Wasserman et al., 2001).

Dosing in opioid replacement therapy remains controversial despite studies demonstrating the importance of dosing to clinically relevant outcomes, such as treatment retention, illicit opioid use, other drug use (alcohol and benzodiazepines), and psychiatric symptoms (Maxwell & Shinderman, 1999). An important concern is the presence of a co-occurring Axis I psychiatric disorder. In one study, Maremmani et al. (2000) found that doses needed for stabilization for patients without co-occurring psychiatric disorder (99 ± 49 mg) were significantly lower than the patients with co-occurring disorders (154 ± 84 mg).

High-Risk Situations

High-risk situations that may lead to relapse to opioid use are perhaps too numerous to mention. Marlatt (1985) created a well-known categorization of eight types of situations that may lead to relapse. This scheme formed the conceptual basis for the 50-item Inventory of Drug-Taking Situations (Turner, Annis, & Sklar, 1997), which the authors suggest may be used as a treatment planning tool. Some major categories of high-risk situations suggested by the empirical literature are *encounters with other drug users*, *exposure to drugs and drug-related cues*, and *use of other substances*. As noted in the section on social and cultural assessment, associating with other drug users is a robust predictor of relapse. Contact may occur by necessity, by chance, or by choice. Often it is for financial reasons (e.g., staying in an intimate relationship for economic security, letting a drug-using acquaintance stay at one's residence in exchange for money). Social pressure to buy and use drugs may occur when ex-users run into former drug-using partners or "connections." In a retrospective study conducted in India, the most prevalent reasons for a first lapse to heroin use after treatment entry was "saw others using and felt like using" (Maulik, Tripathi, & Pal, 2002).

Exposure to drugs and drug-related cues may be the result of poor planning or a function of lack of resources. Some former users may neglect to empty their residences of all drugs and drug-related paraphernalia. Individuals may wander unthinkingly into neighborhoods where they once used drugs, perhaps rationalizing the necessity of going into such areas to do errands. Clinically, we have noted that leaving a protected environment, such as an inpatient unit, halfway house, or prison, often results in rapid relapse, possibly because the individual returns to cue-rich environments. Sometimes, dangerous areas cannot be avoided. Most drug users have few resources and can afford to live only in those neighborhoods where drug use is prevalent. The 41-item SIADU (Wasserman et al., 2001) includes a 7-item Drug Exposure subscale (e.g., "In the past 4 weeks, how often did people you spent time with leave their drugs, outfit, pipe, etc., where you could see them?") that may be useful for assessing exposure to drugs and drug-related cues. Among opioid maintenance patients, the subscale appears to be a better predictor of cocaine use than of opioid use.

In opioid maintenance patients, the use of substances other than opiates increases the risk of opiate use. Darke et al. (1994), surveying a sample of 222 methadone maintenance patients, discovered that current injection drug use was more likely among cocaine and benzodiazepine users. In a prospective study of heroin-abstinent opioid maintenance patients, where participants were drug-tested and interviewed about their drug use weekly, marijuana use predicted subsequent relapse to heroin (Wasserman et al., 1998).

Conditioned Cue Reactivity

Conditioned cue reactivity may be defined as the occurrence of symbolic–expressive, physiological, and behavioral responses occurring after exposure to drug-related stimuli. The stimuli may be exteroceptive or interoceptive (Drummond, 2000). Usual measures of cue reactivity include changes in self-rated craving, withdrawal, moods, and changes in heart rate, skin conductance, and body temperature. Whether cue-reactivity resembles unconditioned drug withdrawal, unconditioned drug effects, or opposes the unconditioned drug effect is a matter of debate (Drummond, 2000). Also unknown is the extent to which cue reactivity in abstinent opioid users, although demonstrable, predicts relapse. A decrease in cue reactivity is the goal of cue exposure treatments for relapse prevention.

Situational Response Efficacy

Published studies have demonstrated the usefulness of self-efficacy ratings in predicting continued opioid use among treatment patients (e.g., Reilly et al., 1995). Several published measures assess self-efficacy in handling specific situations that may result in relapse, either by increasing the desire to use opioids (craving) or by exposing the individual to cues previously paired with drug use. Self-efficacy measures for opioid users have tended to be modeled on measures developed with other substance-using populations. Annis (1982), for example, designed a 100-item Situational Confidence Questionnaire (SCQ) for alcohol users that assesses beliefs about one's ability to cope with difficult situations without drinking. A briefer version, the SCQ-39 (Annis & Graham, 1988), followed. The SCQ has eight subscales corresponding to Marlatt's (1985) classification of high-risk situations (e.g., coping with negative emotional states and social pressure). The SCQ was later the basis for several self-efficacy measures for opioid users. Lower scores on a 20-item adaptation described by Saunders et al. (1995) predicted earlier treatment dropout from methadone maintenance. Barber, Cooper, and Heather (1991) used Annis's SCQ as the basis for a 22-item Situational Confidence Questionnaire for heroin users. Sklar et al. (1997) reported data from a 50-item Drug-Taking Confidence Questionnaire (DTCQ) developed on a broad range of substance users (only 53 of the 713 patients in the development sample were heroin users). Like the SCQ, the DTCQ assesses the eight types of high-risk situations posited by Marlatt and Gordon (1985). Confirmatory factor analysis showed that a three-factor model (negative situations, positive situations, and temptation situations) provided a good fit to the data. A final example of self-efficacy measures, the Alcohol Abstinence Self-Efficacy Scale (AASE), asks respondents to rate 20 situations according to "how confident you are that you would not use alcohol" (DiClemente, Carbonari, Montgomery, & Hughes, 1994). The AASE has now been adapted for general substance users (Hiller, Broome, Knight, & Simpson, 2000). The original 20-item AASE has four 5-item subscales: Negative Affect, Social/Positive, Physical and Other Concerns, and Withdrawal and Urges. A confirmatory factor analysis of the newer version for drug users suggested that four subscales (or factors) similar to those on the AASE provided a good fit to the data; however, the item composition of the subscales was slightly different compared to the original AASE, with only 15 of the original 20 items assigned to subscales (Hiller et al., 2000).

Emotional States

Negative emotional states and, to a far lesser extent, positive states have long been theorized to be important antecedents of relapse. In Marlatt and Gordon's (1985) taxonomy of relapse determinants, "coping with negative emotional states" and "enhancement of positive emotional states" are both included. Negative affect may stimulate drug-related responses. For example, in a laboratory study, Childress et al. (1994) demonstrated that hypnotically induced depression led to increases in drug craving and self-rated withdrawal in newly opioid-abstinent patients. Actual subsequent use was not examined. Unfortunately, most of the research data suggesting a role for negative mood states in relapse are retrospective. Some prospective studies of mood states and relapse have not found a relationship (e.g., Hall et al., 1990; Wasserman et al., 1998). In these studies, moods measurement may not have been close enough to the relapse event. One well-known instrument for assessing moods is the 65-item Profile of Mood States (POMS; McNair, Lorr, & Droppelman, 1971), which assesses six dimensions of affect or mood: Tension–Anxiety, Depression–Dejection, Anger–Hostility, Vigor–Activity, Fatigue–Inertia, and Confusion–Bewilderment. The short form of this instrument contains 30 items.

Distal Factors

Distal factors affecting relapse can be personality related, such as coping styles, or biologically related, such as differences in drug metabolism.

Biological Factors

An example of a biological factor would be concurrent physical disease, especially a disorder that can produce chronic or acute pain. Managing pain in opioid-dependent patients on replacement therapies or in remission is a controversial area with limited empirical support (Friedman, Li, & Mehrotra, 2003). Often, management of those patients is a team effort, with addiction medicine, pain management and other relevant medical or surgical specialties involved. Even the time-limited use of medically necessary opioids in controlled settings can be a risk factor for relapse. Careful relapse prevention planning and education is often necessary with opioid-dependent patients who have concurrent medical disorders.

Another distal biological factor related to relapse in patients using opioid maintenance therapies is genetically based drug metabolism. Individual differences in metabolism can affect the adequacy of the opioid maintenance dose. The repetitive assessment of the severity of opioid withdrawal and craving can be performed using scales to determine the adequacy of dosing (Hiltunen et al., 1995). Another method to assist in dose determination is to measure peak and trough plasma methadone levels. A range of 150 to 200 ng/ml is usually considered adequate to prevent craving and withdrawal, and 400 ng/ml is considered adequate to block other opioids. A peak to trough ratio of 2 or less indicates a normal metabolism. Indications for ordering a plasma methadone level are suspected drug interactions, to ensure adequacy of dosing, to document need for doses above regulatory limits, and to determine whether a patient has a fast metabolism and may benefit from split dosing (Loimer & Schmid, 1992).

General Coping Skills

The importance of coping skills is supported in many studies that have assessed the processes involved in relapse to illicit opioid use. Individuals who are quicker to describe coping responses, use coping responses, use more coping responses, and have better coping skills are less likely to relapse. Gossop et al. (2002) studied 242 heroin users treated in inpatient or residential programs. Coping responses were assessed using 10 items selected from a processes of change questionnaire (Prochaska, Velicer, DiClemente, & Fava, 1988). Items were combined into three categories: avoidance, cognitive, and distraction. Participants rated the frequency with which they used the responses on a 5-point, Likert-type scale. Patients who remained abstinent after treatment reported increased use of all forms of coping strategies at follow-up compared to intake. Furthermore, they used more coping responses than did patients who relapsed.

Avant, Warburton, and Margolin (2000), in a study of 307 methadone maintenance patients, found that patients who attained abstinence from other opioid use after a 12-week coping skills training intervention decreased their use of avoidant coping strategies. Belding, Iguchi, Lamb, Latkin, and Terry (1996), in a cross-sectional study of 276 black and white methadone maintenance patients, found that across ethnic groups, avoidant coping was associated with the use of drugs or alcohol to cope. For blacks, but not for whites, the use of religion as a coping strategy was inversely related to the use of substances to cope. Conversely, active coping was negatively associated with the use of substances only for whites. Finally, for whites, but not blacks, lesser use of active coping strategies and greater use of substances to cope were positively related to concurrent opioid use.

Clinical application of research on coping skills still remains limited. Patients may have particular coping skills yet decide not to use them (Gossop et al., 2002). Relatedly, there is a difference between coping skills and coping styles (Belding et al., 1996). Whereas the term "coping skills" denotes abilities, or what one knows how to do, "coping styles" suggests one's usual or typical strategies for handling stress. Finally, causality cannot be inferred from most coping studies, since the studies are observational rather than experimental. Although specific coping behaviors, or their absence, may lead to relapse, drug use may complicate the learning and practice of more successful coping (Belding et al., 1996).

CONCLUSIONS

As the treatment of opioid dependence extends beyond the specialized, traditional treatment modalities of methadone maintenance and residential treatment, more clinicians will become involved in the assessment and treatment of opioid-dependent patients. However, the expansion of opioid dependence treatment (i.e., maintenance pharmacotherapies) to nontraditional settings also raises some important concerns. Clinicians may lack the necessary experience and training needed to assess effectively and treat opioid-dependent clients. Another concern is the large and ever-growing number of opioid-dependent persons presenting with dual diagnoses in treatment settings (Mason et al., 1998). Clinicians working in practice-based or community settings may not be fully qualified to diagnose psychiatric conditions in complex, polysubstance-dependent patients (Vignau et al., 2001). As a consequence, some psychiatric disorders may remain unrecognized, and therefore untreated. However, training programs can assist clinicians in acquiring the skills necessary to assess effectively and treat opioid use disorders (Lintzeris, Ritter, Dunlop, & Muhleisen, 2002).

In this chapter, we have reviewed the determination of opioid dependence, including the assessment of tolerance and withdrawal; the evaluation of co-occurring physical, psychiatric, substance use, and cognitive disorders; determination of treatment readiness; evaluation of social environment; and relapse risk factors. The information from these domains can be developed into a comprehensive treatment plan, with or without the use of opioid replacement therapy. The treatment of opioid-dependent patients in nontraditional settings is one of the most exciting challenges that substance use disorder and mental health clinicians face.

ACKNOWLEDGMENTS

Preparation of this chapter was supported in part by National Institute on Drug Abuse Grant Nos. K01DA00408, P50DA09253, R01DA14922, and U10DA15815. We appreciate the support of the San Francisco General Hospital Department of Psychiatry's

Division of Substance Abuse and Addiction Medicine, including the administrative assistance of Ms. Remy Hammel.

REFERENCES

Adriaensen, H., Vissers, K., Noorduin, H., & Meert, T. (2003). Opioid tolerance and dependence: An inevitable consequence of chronic treatment? *Acta Anaesthesiologica Belgica, 54,* 37–47.

American Psychiatric Association. (2000). *Diagnostic and statistical manual of mental disorders* (4th ed., text rev.). Washington, DC: Author.

Annis, H. M. (1982). *Situational Confidence Questionnaire.* Toronto: Addiction Research Foundation of Ontario.

Annis, H. M. (1984). *Outcome Expectancies Questionnaire.* Toronto: Addiction Research Foundation of Ontario.

Annis, H. M., & Graham, J. M. (1988). *Situational Confidence Questionnaire (SCQ-39): User's guide.* Toronto: Addiction Research Foundation of Ontario.

Arlett, P. (1982). Methadone dose assessment in heroin addiction. *International Journal of the Addictions, 17,* 1329–1336.

Avant, S. K., Warburton, L. A., & Margolin, A. (2000). The influence of coping and depression on abstinence from illicit drug use in methadone–maintained patients. *American Journal of Drug and Alcohol Abuse, 26,* 399–416.

Backmund, M., Meyer, K., Eichenlaub, D., & Schultz, C. G. (2001). Predictors for completing an inpatient detoxification program among intravenous heroin users, methadone substituted and codeine substituted patients. *Drug and Alcohol Dependence, 64,* 173–180.

Barber, J. G., Cooper, B. K., & Heather, N. (1991). The Situational Confidence Questionnaire (heroin). *International Journal of the Addictions, 26,* 565–575.

Bechtold, K. T., Horner, M. D., Labbate, L. A., & Windham, W. K. (2001). The construct validity and clinical utility of the Frank Jones story as a brief screening measure of cognitive dysfunction. *Psychosomatics, 42,* 146–149.

Belding, M. A., Iguchi, M. Y., Lamb, R. J., Lakin, M., & Terry, R. (1995). Stages and processes of change among polydrug users in methadone maintenance treatment. *Drug and Alcohol Dependence, 39,* 45–53.

Belding, M. A., Iguchi, M. Y., Lamb, R. J., Lakin, M., & Terry, R. (1996). Coping strategies and continued drug use among methadone maintenance patients. *Addictive Behaviors, 21,* 389–401.

Belding, M. A., McLellan, A. T., Zanis, D. A., & Incmikoski, R. (1998). Characterizing "nonresponsive" methadone patients. *Journal of Substance Abuse Treatment, 15,* 485–492.

Brooner, R. K., King, V. L., Kidorf, M., Schmidt, C. W., Jr., & Bigelow, G. E. (1997). Psychiatric and substance use comorbidity among treatment-seeking opioid abusers. *Archives of General Psychiatry, 54,* 71–80.

Burgess, P. M., Stripp, A. M., Pead, J., & Holman, C. P. (1989). Severity of opiate dependence in an Australian sample: Further validation of the SODQ. *British Journal of Addiction, 84,* 1451–1459.

Cacciola, J. S., Alterman, A. I., Rutherford, M. J., McKay, J. R., & Mulvaney, F. D. (2001). The relationship of psychiatric comorbidity to treatment outcomes in methadone maintained patients. *Drug and Alcohol Dependence, 61,* 271–280.

Carey, K. B., Purnine, D. M., Maisto, S. A., Carey, M. P., & Barnes, K. L. (1999). Decisional balance regarding substance use among persons with schizophrenia. *Community Mental Health Journal, 35,* 289–299.

Carroll, K. M., & Rounsaville, B. J. (2002). On beyond urine: Clinically useful assessment instruments in the treatment of drug dependence. *Behaviour Research and Therapy, 40,* 1329–1344.

Center for Substance Abuse Treatment. (1993). *Screening for infectious diseases among substance abusers* (TIP 6, Department of Health and Human Services Publication No. [SMA] 93–2048, Treatment Improvement Protocol [TIP] Series No. 6). Rockville, MD: U.S. Department of Health and Human Services.

Childress, A. R., Ehrman, R., McLellan, A. T., MacRae, J., Natale, M., & O'Brien, C. P. (1994). Can induced moods trigger drug-related responses in opiate abuse patients? *Journal of Substance Abuse Treatment, 11,* 17–23.

Cone, E. J., & Preston, K. L. (2002). Toxicologic aspects of heroin substitution treatment. *Therapeutic Drug Monitoring, 2,* 193–198.

Darke, S., Sims, J., McDonald, S., & Wickes, W. (2000). Cognitive impairment among methadone maintenance patients. *Addiction, 95,* 687–695.

Darke, S., Swift, W., Hall, W., & Ross, M. (1994). Predictors of injecting and injecting risk-taking behavior among methadone maintenance clients. *Addiction, 89,* 311–316.

DiClemente, C. C., Carbonari, J. P., Montgomery, R. P., & Hughes, S. O. (1994). The Alcohol Abstinence Self-Efficacy Scale. *Journal of Studies on Alcohol, 55,* 141–148.

Donny, E. C., Walsh, S. L., Bigelow, G. E., Eissenberg, T., & Stitzer, M. L. (2002). High-dose methadone produces superior opioid blockade and comparable withdrawal suppression to lower doses in opioid-dependent humans. *Psychopharmacology, 161,* 202–212.

Drummond, D. C. (2000). What does cue-reactivity have to offer clinical research? *Addiction, 95*(Suppl. 2), S129–S144.

Eissenberg, T., Greenwald, M. K., Johnson, R. E., Liebson, I. A., Bigelow, G. E., & Stitzer, M. L. (1996). Buprenorphine's physical dependence potential: Antagonist-precipitated withdrawal in humans. *Journal of Pharmacology and Experimental Therapeutics, 276,* 449–459.

Fals-Stewart, W. (1997). Detection of neuropsychological impairment among substance-abusing patients: Accuracy of the neurobehavioral cognitive status examination. *Experimental and Clinical Psychopharmacology, 5,* 269–276.

First, M. B., Spitzer, R. L., Gibbon, M., & Williams, J. B. W. (1997). *Structured Clinical Interview for DSM-IV Axis I Disorders—Clinician Version* (SCID-CV). Washington, DC: American Psychiatric Press.

Folstein, M. F., Folstein, S. E., & McHugh, P. R. (1975). "Mini-mental state": A practical method for grading the cognitive state of patients for the clinician. *Journal of Psychiatric Research, 12,* 189–198.

Franken, I. H. A., Hendriks, V. M., & van den Brink, W. (2002). Initial validation of two opiate craving questionnaires: The Obsessive Compulsive Drug Use Scale and the Desires for Drug Questionnaire. *Addictive Behaviors, 27,* 675–685.

Friedman, R., Li, V., & Mehrotra, D. (2003). Treating pain patients at risk: Evaluation of a screening tool in opioid-treated pain patients with and without addiction. *Pain Medicine, 4,* 182–185.

Friedman, S. R., Furst, T., Jose, B., Curtis, R., Neaigus, A., Des Jarlais, D. C., et al. (1998). Drug scene roles and HIV risk. *Addiction, 93,* 1403–1416.

Fudala, P. J., Berkow, L. C., Fralich, J. L., & Johnson, R. E. (1991). Use of naloxone in the assessment of opiate dependence. *Life Sciences, 49*, 1809–1814.

Ghodse, A. H., Greaves, J. L., & Lynch, D. (1999). Evaluation of the opioid addiction test in an out-patient dependence unit. *British Journal of Psychiatry, 175*, 158–162.

Goehl, L., Nunes, E., Quitkin, F., & Hilton, I. (1993). Social networks and methadone treatment outcome: The costs and benefits of social ties. *American Journal of Drug and Alcohol Abuse, 19*, 251–262.

Gogineni, A., Stein, M. D., & Friedmann, P. D. (2001). Social relationships and intravenous drug use among methadone maintenance patients. *Drug and Alcohol Dependence, 64*, 47–53.

Gold, M. S. (1998). The pharmacology of opioids. In A. W. Graham, T. K. Schultz, & B. B. Wilford (Eds.), *Principles of addiction medicine, second edition* (pp. 131–136). Chevy Chase, MD: American Society of Addiction Medicine.

Goodman, W. K., Price, L. H., Rasmussen, S. A., Mazure, C., Fleischman, R. L., Hill, C. L., et al. (1989). The Yale–Brown Obsessive Compulsive Scale: I. Development, use, and reliability. *Archives of General Psychiatry, 46* 1006–1011.

Gossop, M. (1990). The development of a Short Opiate Withdrawal Scale (SOWS). *Addictive Behaviors, 15*, 487–490.

Gossop, M., Best, D., Marsden, J., & Strang, J. (1997). Test–retest reliability of the Severity of Dependence Scale (SDS). *Addiction, 92*, 353.

Gossop, M., Stewart, D., Browne, N., & Marsden, J. (2002). Factors associated with abstinence, lapse, or relapse to heroin use after residential treatment: Protective effect of coping responses. *Addiction, 97*, 1259–1267.

Graham, A. W., Shultz, T. K., Mayo-Smith, M. F., Ries, R. K., & Wilford, B. B. (Eds.). (2003). *Crosswalks of the ASAM Patient Placement Criteria, Second Edition—Revised (ASAM PPC-2R)*. Chevy Chase: American Society of Addiction Medicine.

Griffith, J. D., Rowan-Szal, G. A., Roark, R. R., & Simpson, D. D. (2000). Contingency management in outpatient methadone treatment: A meta-analysis. *Drug and Alcohol Dependence, 58*, 55–66.

Hall, S. M., Havassy, B. E., & Wasserman, D. A. (1990). Commitment to abstinence and acute stress in relapse to alcohol, opiates, and nicotine. *Journal of Consulting and Clinical Psychology, 58*, 175–181.

Handelsman, L., Cochrane, K. J., Aronson, M. J., Ness, R., Rubinstein, K. J., & Kanof, P. D. (1987). Two new rating scales for opiate withdrawal. *American Journal of Drug and Alcohol Abuse, 13*, 293–308.

Hasin, D. S., Trautman, K. D., Miele, G. M., Samet, S., Smith, M., & Endicott, J. (1996). Psychiatric Research Interview for Substance and Mental Disorders (PRISM): Reliability for substance abusers. *American Journal of Psychiatry, 153*, 1195–1201.

Havassy, B. E., Hall, S. M., & Wasserman, D. A. (1991). Social support and relapse: Commonalities among alcoholics, opiate users, and cigarette smokers. *Addictive Behaviors, 16*, 235–246.

Havassy, B. E., Wasserman, D. A., & Hall, S. M. (1995). Social relationships and abstinence from cocaine in an American treatment sample. *Addictions, 90*, 699–710.

Hiller, M. L., Broome, K. M., Knight, K., & Simpson, D. D. (2000). Measuring self-efficacy among drug-involved probationers. *Psychological Reports, 86*, 529–538.

Hiltunin, A. J., Lafolie, P., Martel, J., Ottosson, E. C., Boreus, L. O., Beck, O., et al. (1995). Subjective and objective symptoms in relation to plasma methadone concentration in methadone patients. *Psychopharmacology, 118,* 122–126.

Himmelsbach, C. K. (1941). The morphine abstinence syndrome, its nature and treatment. *Annals of Internal Medicine, 15,* 829–839.

Kandel, D. B., Huang, F. Y., & Davies, M. (2001). Comorbidity between patterns of substance use dependence and psychiatric syndromes. *Drug and Alcohol Dependence, 1,* 233–241.

Kidorf, M., Stitzer, M. L., & Brooner, R. K. (1994). Characteristics of methadone patients responding to take-home incentives. *Behavior Therapy, 25,* 109–121.

Knight, D. K., & Simpson, D. D. (1996). Influences of family and friends on client progress during drug abuse treatment. *Journal of Substance Abuse, 8,* 417–429.

Latkin, C. A., Knowlton, A. R., Hoover, D., & Mandell, W. (1999). Drug network characteristics as a predictor of cessation of drug use among adult injection drug users: A prospective study. *American Journal of Drug and Alcohol Abuse, 25,* 463–473.

Lintzeris, N., Ritter, A., Dunlop, A., & Muhleisen, P. (2002). Training primary health care professionals to provide buprenorphine and LAAM treatment. *Substance Abuse, 23,* 245–254.

Loimer, N., Linzmayer, L., & Grunberger, J. (1991). Comparison between observer assessment and self rating of withdrawal distress during opiate detoxification. *Drug and Alcohol Dependence, 28,* 265–268.

Loimer, N., & Schmid, R. (1992). The use of plasma levels to optimize methadone maintenance treatment. *Drug and Alcohol Dependence, 30,* 241–246.

Maremmani, I., Zolesi, O., Aglietti, M., Marini, G., Tagliamonte, A., Shinderman, M., & Maxwell, S. (2000). Methadone dose and retention during treatment of heroin addicts with Axis I psychiatric comorbidity. *Journal of Addictive Diseases, 19,* 29–41.

Mark, T. L., Woody, G. E., Juday, T., & Kleber, H. D. (2001). The economic costs of heroin addiction in the United States. *Drug and Alcohol Dependence, 61,* 195–206.

Marlatt, G. A. (1985). Situational determinants of relapse and skill-training interventions. In G. A. Marlatt & J. R. Gordon (Eds.), *Relapse prevention: Maintenance strategies in the treatment of addictive behaviors* (pp. 71–127). New York: Guilford Press.

Marlowe, D. B., Husband, S. D., Bonieskie, L. M., Kirby, K. C., & Platt, J. J. (1997). Structured interview versus self-report test vantages for the assessment of personality pathology in cocaine dependence. *Journal of Personality Disorders, 11,* 177–190.

Marsch, L. A. (1998). The efficacy of methadone maintenance interventions on reducing illicit opiate use, HIV risk behavior and criminality: A meta-analysis. *Addiction, 93,* 515–532.

Mason, B. J., Kocsis, J. H., Melia, D., Khuri, E. T., Sweeney, J., Wells, A., et al. (1998). Psychiatric comorbidity in methadone maintained patients. *Journal of Addictive Diseases, 17,* 75–89.

Mattrick, R. P., Kimber, J., Breen, C., & Davoli, M. (2002a). Methadone maintenance therapy versus no opioid replacement therapy for opioid dependence. *Cochrane Database of Systematic Reviews (Online: Update Software),* CD002209.

Mattrick, R. P., Kimber, J., Breen, C., & Davoli, M. (2002b). Buprenorphine maintenance versus placebo or methadone maintenance for opioid dependence. *Cochrane Database of Systematic Reviews (Online: Update Software),* CD002207.

Maulik, P. K., Tripathi, M., & Pal, H. R. (2002). Coping behaviors and relapse precipitants in opioid dependence: A study from North India. *Journal of Substance Abuse Treatment, 22,* 135–140.

Maxwell, S., & Shinderman, M. (1999). Optimizing response to methadone maintenance treatment: Use of higher-dose methadone. *Journal of Psychoactive Drugs, 31,* 95–102.

McLellan, A. T., Kushner, H., Metzger, D., Peters, R., Smith, I., Grissom, G., et al. (1992). The fifth edition of the Addiction Severity Index. *Journal of Substance Abuse Treatment, 9,* 199–213.

McLellan, A. T., Luborsky, L., Woody, G. E., & O'Brien, C. P. (1980). An improved diagnostic evaluation instrument for substance abuse patients: The Addiction Severity Index. *Journal of Nervous and Mental Disease, 168,* 26–33.

McLellan, A. T., Luborsky, L., Woody, G. E., O'Brien, C. P., & Druley, K. A. (1983). Predicting response to alcohol and drug treatments: Role of psychiatric severity. *Archives of General Psychiatry, 40,* 620–625.

McLellan, A. T., Metzger, D. S., Grissom, G. R., Woody, G. E., Luborsky, L., & O'Brien, C. P. (1994). Similarity of outcome predictors across opiate, cocaine, and alcohol treatments: Role of treatment services. *Journal of Consulting and Clinical Psychology, 62,* 1141–1158.

McNair, D., Lorr, M., & Droppelman, L. F. (1971). *Profile of mood states.* San Diego: Educational and Industrial Services, Medicine, Inc.

Miele, G. M., Carpenter, K. M., Smith Cockerham, M. S., Trautman, K. D., Blaine, J. D., & Hasin, D. S. (2000). Concurrent and predictive validity of the Substance Dependence Severity Scale (SDSS). *Drug and Alcohol Dependence, 59,* 77–88.

Millon, T. (1997). *Manual for the MCMI-II.* Minneapolis: National Computer Systems.

Mintzer, M. Z., & Stitzer, M. L. (2002). Cognitive impairment in methadone maintenance patients. *Drug and Alcohol Dependence, 67,* 41–51.

Morgenstern, J., & Bates, M. E. (1999). Effects of executive function impairment on change processes and substance use outcomes in 12–step treatment. *Journal of Studies on Alcohol, 60,* 846–855.

Mutasa, H. C. (2001). Risk factors associated with noncompliance with methadone substitution therapy (MST) and relapse among chronic opiate users in an outer London community. *Journal of Advanced Nursing, 35,* 97–107.

Preston, K. L., Umbricht, A., & Epstein, D. H. (2000). Methadone dose increase and abstinence reinforcement for treatment of continued heroin use during methadone maintenance. *Archives of General Psychiatry, 57,* 125–137.

Prochaska, J. O., Velicer, W. F., DiClemente, C. C., & Fava, J. (1988). Measuring processes of change: Applications to the cessation of smoking. *Journal of Consulting and Clinical Psychology, 56,* 520–528.

Prochaska, J. O., & DiClemente, C. C. (1983). Stages and processes of self-change of smoking: toward an integrative model of change. *Journal of Consulting and Clinical Psychology, 51,* 390–395.

Reilly, P. M., Sees, K. L., Shopshire, M. S., Hall, S. M., Delucchi, K . L., Tusel, D. J., et al. (1995). Self-efficacy and illicit opioid use in a 180–day methadone detoxification treatment. *Journal of Consulting and Clinical Psychology, 63,* 158–162.

Reitan, R. M. (1958). Validity of the Trail Making Test as an indicator of organic brain damage. *Perceptual and Motor Skills, 8,* 271–276.

Reynaud, M., Schellenberg, F., Loisequx-Maunier, M. N., Schwan, R., Maradeix, B., Planche, F., et al. (2000). Objective diagnosis of alcohol abuse: Compared values of carbohydrate-deficient transferrin (CDT), gamma-glutamyl transferase (GGT), and mean corpuscular volume (MCV). *Alcoholism, Clinical and Experimental Research, 24,* 1414–1419.

Ridenour, T. A., Cottler, L. B., Compton, W. M., Spitznagel, E. L., & Cunningham-Williams, R. M. (2003). Is there a progression from abuse disorders to dependence disorders? *Addiction, 98,* 635–644.

Robins, L. N., Helzer, J. E., Croughan, J., & Ratkliff, K. S. (1981). National Institute of Mental Health Diagnostic Interview Schedule: Its history, characteristics, and validity. *Archives of General Psychiatry, 38,* 381–389.

Robins, L. N., Wing, J. K., & Helzer, J. E. (1983). *Composite International Diagnostic interview (CIDI).* Geneva: World Health Organization.

Roehrich, L., & Goldman, M. S. (1993). Experience-dependent neuropsychological recovery and the treatment of alcoholism. *Journal of Consulting and Clinical Psychology, 61,* 812–821.

Royall, D. R., Mahurin, R. K., & Gray, K. F. (1992). Bedside assessment of executive cognitive impairment: The executive interview. *Journal of the American Geriatric Society, 40,* 1221–1226.

Saunders, B., Wilkinson, C., & Phillips, M. (1995). The impact of a brief motivational intervention with opiate users attending a methadone program. *Addiction, 90,* 415–424.

Sayette, M. A., Shiffman, S., Tiffany, S. T., Niaura, R. S., Martin, C. S., & Shadel, W. G. (2000). The measurement of drug craving. *Addiction, 95*(Suppl. 2), S189–S210.

Schroeder, J. R., Latkin, C. A., Hoover, D. R., Curry, A. D., Knowlton, A. R., & Celentano, D. D. (2001). Illicit drug use in one's social network and in one's neighborhood predicts individual heroin and cocaine use. *Annals of Epidemiology, 11,* 389–394.

Schuckit, M. A., Daeppen, J. B., Danko, G. P., Tripp, M. L., Smith, T. L., Li, T., et al. (1999). Clinical implications for four drugs of the DSM-IV distinction between substance dependence with and without a physiological component. *American Journal of Psychiatry, 156,* 41–49.

Sherman, S. G., & Latkin, C. A. (2002). Drug users' involvement in the drug economy: Implications for harm reduction and HIV prevention programs. *Journal of Urban Health, 79,* 266–277.

Shipley, W. C. (1967). *Manual: Shipley–Institute of Living Scale.* Los Angeles: Western Psychological Services.

Silverman, K., Wong, C. J., Umbricht-Schneiter, A., Montoya, I. D., Schuster, C. R., & Preston, K. L. (1998). Broad beneficial effects of cocaine abstinence reinforcement among methadone patients. *Journal of Consulting and Clinical Psychology, 66,* 811–824.

Sjogren, P., Thomsen, A. B., & Olsen, A. K. (2000). Impaired neuropsychological performance in chronic nonmalignant pain patients receiving long-term oral opioid therapy. *Journal of Pain and Symptom Management, 19,* 100–108.

Sklar, S. M., Annis, H. M., & Turner, N. E. (1997). Development and validation of the drug-taking confidence questionnaire: A measure of coping self-efficacy. *Addictive Behaviors, 22,* 655–670.

Sklar, S. M., & Turner, N. E. (1999). A brief measure for the assessment of coping self-efficacy among alcohol and other drug users. *Addiction, 94,* 723–729.

Smith, D. E., & McCardy, B. S. (1991). Cognitive impairment among alcoholics: Impact on drink refusal skill acquisition and treatment outcome. *Addictive Behaviors, 16,* 265–274.

Specka, M., Finkbeiner, T., Lodemann, E., Leifert, K., Kluwig, J., & Gastpar, M. (2000). Cognitive–motor performance of methadone-maintained patients. *European Addiction Research, 6,* 8–19.

Substance Abuse and Mental Health Services Administration, Office of Applied Studies. (2002). *Emergency department trends from the Drug Abuse Warning Network,* final estimates 1992–2001 (DAWN Series D-21, DHHS Publication No. [SMA] 02-3635). Rockville, MD: Author.

Taylor, J. R., Watson, I. D., Tames, F. J., & Lowe, D. (1998). Detection of drug use in a methadone maintenance clinic: Sweat patches versus urine testing. *Addiction, 93,* 847–853.

Turkington, D., & Drummond, D. C. (1989). How should opiate withdrawal be measured? *Drug and Alcohol Dependence, 24,* 151–153.

Turner, N. E., Annis, H. M., & Sklar, S. M. (1997). Measurement of antecedents to drug and alcohol use: Psychometric properties of the Inventory of Drug-Taking Situations (IDTS). *Behaviour Research and Therapy, 35,* 465–483.

Vignau, J., Duhamel, A., Catteau, J., Legal, G., Pho, A. H., Grailles, I., et al. (2001). Practice-based buprenorphine maintenance treatment (BMT): How do French healthcare providers manage the opiate-addicted patients? *Journal of Substance Abuse Treatment, 21,* 135–144.

Wasserman, D. A., Stewart, A .L., & Delucchi, K. L. (2001). Social support and abstinence from opiates and cocaine during opioid maintenance treatment. *Drug and Alcohol Dependence, 65,* 65–75.

Wasserman, D. A., Weinstein, M. G., Havassy, B. E., & Hall, S. M. (1998). Factors associated with lapses to heroin use during methadone maintenance. *Drug and Alcohol Dependence, 52,* 183–192.

Wesson, D. R., & Ling, W. (2003). The Clinical Opiate Withdrawal Scales (COWS). *Journal of Psychoactive Drugs, 35,* 253–259.

White, R. (2001). Heroin use, ethnicity and the environment: The case of the London Bangladeshi community. *Addiction, 96,* 1815–1824.

World Health Organization. (1992). *International statistical classification of diseases and related health problems* (10th rev.). Geneva: Author.

CHAPTER 8

Assessment of Cannabis Use Disorders

ROBERT S. STEPHENS
ROGER A. ROFFMAN

Cannabis is the most commonly used illicit substance in the United States. According to the 2002 National Household Survey on Drug Abuse, there were 14.6 million cannabis users who had smoked in the past month and about 2.6 million new users in each of the last several years (Substance Abuse and Mental Health Services Administration [SAMHSA], 2003). About 4.8 million people, or one-third of the current users, used cannabis on 20 or more days in the past month. Data from a national survey of high school students indicated that more than one-third of high school seniors used cannabis in 2002, and 6% reported daily use (Johnston, O'Malley, & Bachman, 2003). These data show that frequent cannabis use by high school students has been at near record levels for the past several years.

Although most cannabis users with moderate recreational use do not develop problems, a subset develops a chronic use pattern, with symptoms of dependence and adverse consequences. Both the Epidemiological Catchment Area Survey (Anthony & Helzer, 1991) and the National Comorbidity Study (Anthony, Warner, & Kessler, 1994) estimated that slightly more than 4% of the population developed dependence on cannabis. Approximately 9% of those who had ever used cannabis met criteria for a diagnosis of dependence at some time (Anthony et al., 1994). The risk of dependence may be as high as 20–30% for those who have used cannabis more than a few times (Hall, Solowij, & Lemon, 1994). The rate of current cannabis dependence, given any smoking in the past year, is estimated to be 8% among adults (Kandel, Chen, Warner, Kessler, & Grant, 1997), whereas the comparable rates for cocaine and alcohol use are 12 and 5%, respectively. Thus, a large number of cannabis smokers are dependent, some of whom may need treatment.

In 2000, 14% of treatment admissions for substance abuse reported cannabis as the primary drug of concern, more than for any illicit drug other than heroin (15%) and more than twice the percentage reported in 1992 (SAMHSA, 2002). Recent controlled treatment–outcome research shows that these users' response to treatment is similar to that of persons with other substance abuse problems (e.g., Marijuana Treatment Project Research Group [MTPRG], 2004; Budney, Higgins, Radonovich, & Novy, 2000; Stephens, Roffman, & Simpson, 1994; Stephens, Roffman, & Curtin, 2000). In this chapter, we review the assessment of marijuana use, antecedents and consequences of use, and processes related to use. The chapter is organized around particular biological, behavioral, and cognitive targets of assessment, and we begin with commentary on the applicability of the biospsychosocial model (e.g., Donovan, 1988) to cannabis use and abuse. Commentary on the use of assessment data in treatment planning and delivery is provided throughout.

APPLICABILITY OF A BIOPSYCHOSOCIAL MODEL FOR CANNABIS USE DISORDERS

Until relatively recently, many may have thought that only the psychosocial part of the biopsychosocial model applied to cannabis. Cannabis was often described as a soft drug that might produce psychological dependence but not physical addiction. However, the biopsychosocial model that guides much of the thinking and research regarding the nature of addiction now clearly seems to apply to cannabis as well. In addition to long-established social and psychological influences on the initiation, escalation, and maintenance of marijuana use, we now have a greater understanding of neuropharmacology underlying the reinforcing effects of the drug and an awareness of the potential for tolerance and withdrawal phenomena that may contribute to dependence. Consideration of these multiple factors in the assessment process informs treatment, and feedback from the assessment may affect clients' decisions to make changes.

Psychosocial Factors in Cannabis Use and Abuse

The risk factors for initiation and escalation of drug use during adolescence are well established and include psychosocial variables such as peer pressure, low self-esteem, and deficient life skills competencies (e.g., Hawkins, Catalano, & Miller, 1992; Jessor, Van Den Bos, Vanderryn, Costa, & Turbin, 1995; Newcomb, Maddahian, & Bentler, 1986). We also know that cognitive variables such as expectancies for reinforcing effects are related to marijuana use (e.g., Schafer & Brown, 1991), and cognitive processes such as self-efficacy may be important in understanding response to treatment (Stephens, Wertz, & Roffman, 1995). Similarly, relapse to cannabis use following treatment occurs most frequently in situations characterized by negative affect, direct social pressure from peers, and desire for positive reinforcement (Stephens, Curtin, Simpson, & Roffman, 1994). The psychosocial consequences of chronic heavy use are also apparent (e.g., Budney & Moore, 2002) and play a key role in decisions to enter treatment and make changes in marijuana use. Thus, the importance of assessing and understanding a variety of psychosocial variables as they relate to the individual user is clear.

Biological and Health Factors in Cannabis Use and Abuse

The neuropharmacological processes through which cannabinoids exert their psychoactive effects were poorly understood until the early 1990s. In 1990, several investigators converged on the finding of specific neuronal receptors for cannabinoids (see Earleywine, 2002, for review). High densities of the receptors have been identified in the cerebral cortex, hippocampus, cerebellum, and basal ganglia. It is noteworthy that the functions served by those portions of the brain with the highest concentration of cannabinoid receptors correspond to long-established effects of marijuana on fragmented thought (cortex), memory (hippocampus), and motor coordination (cerebellum). Furthermore, the euphoria produced by marijuana appears to be related to the cannabinoid receptor's modulation of the mesolimbic dopaminergic pathways in the brain (Gardner, 1992). This dopaminergic pathway partially mediates the experience of reward or reinforcement produced by nearly all drugs that are typically abused. Tetrahydrocannabinol (THC), the primary active ingredient in cannabis, is known to modulate the endogenous opioid system, which then interacts with the dopaminergic system to produce euphoria (Gardner, 1992; Tanda, Pontieri, & DiChiara, 1997).

Both animal and human laboratory studies have demonstrated that tolerance and withdrawal develop with daily use of large doses of cannabis or THC (e.g., Jones & Benowitz, 1976; Haney, Ward, Comer, Foltin, & Fischman, 1999a, 1999b; Kouri & Pope, 2000; Lichtman & Martin, 2002). Chronic cannabis exposure produces neuroadaptive changes in the limbic system, which may explain withdrawal and craving phenomena associated with abstinence (Lichtman & Martin, 2002). About 15% of moderate to heavy users reported a withdrawal syndrome comprising symptoms of nervousness, sleep disturbance, and appetite change (Wiesbeck, Schuckit, Kalmijn, Tipp, Bucholz, & Smith, 1996), and most cannabis dependent adults presenting for treatment reported affective symptoms and craving during periods of abstinence (Budney, Novy, & Hughes, 1999). Recent studies have further described the onset and time course of cannabis withdrawal in adults (Budney, Hughes, Moore, & Novy, 2001; Budney, Moore, Vandrey, & Hughes, 2003). We are only beginning to understand the role of these factors in the dependence process, but assessment seems imperative, because they present a potential obstacle to cessation or reduction efforts for some users.

There are adverse health and physiological consequences to heavy cannabis use. Cannabis smoking has been shown to increase chronic and acute bronchitis, cause functional alterations in the respiratory system, and produce morphological changes in the airways that may precede malignant change (see Tashkin, 1999, for a review). These adverse effects appear to occur with fewer cannabis cigarettes per day and at earlier ages than with tobacco (e.g., Taylor, Poulton, Moffit, Ramankutty, & Sears, 2000). In addition, concurrent tobacco smoking augments many of the effects of cannabis smoking in an additive fashion. Although there is little evidence of substantial damage to the brain from chronic cannabis use, recent evidence suggests altered brain function and subtle impairments of memory, attention, and higher cognitive function related to cannabis use (e.g., Bolla, Brown, Eldreth, Tate, & Cadet, 2002; Pope, Gruber, Hudson, Huestis, & Yurgelun-Todd, 2001; Solowij, 1998; Solowij, Stephens, Roffman, Babor, Kadden, Miller, Christiansen, McRee, Vendetti, & the Marijuana Treatment Project Research Group, 2002). Thus, the potential physiological consequences of chronic, heavy cannabis use should also be assessed, because they may provide important motivation for making changes.

ASSESSING THE EXTENT AND PATTERN OF USE

Assessment of the extent and pattern of cannabis use is fundamental to decisions regarding the need for treatment and specific aspects of treatment planning. While there are no generally accepted cutoffs for the amount of cannabis use that constitutes a threat to the individual's health or well-being, more frequent use, or use in close temporal proximity to specific activities (e.g., driving, working, etc.), likely increases the chances of negative consequences. The identification of hazardous levels of use is hampered by difficulties in assessing the quantity of the plant and the concentration of THC consumed. Route of administration (i.e., smoking vs. oral consumption), preparation of the plant (e.g., marijuana, hashish, hash oil), and mechanism of delivery (e.g., joints, pipes, baked goods) all affect both the quantity of cannabis consumed and the amount of THC that reaches the bloodstream. Awareness of these issues is important in communicating knowledgably and assessing risks with users. Many of THC's effects on performance are dose dependent, and some health risks associated with smoking cannabis may increase with the quantity of the plant consumed.

Marijuana, the most common preparation of cannabis used in the United States, consists of a mixture of the flowering tops, leaves, and stems of the dried cannabis plant. THC is concentrated most highly in the flowering tops, then in the upper leaves, then the lower leaves, and finally in the stems and seeds. A particularly potent variety of marijuana, sinsemilla, consists largely of the flowering tops of female plants that have not been fertilized because male plants were removed from the growing area. Differences in the genetics of particular plants, and other aspects of growing conditions and storage of the dried plant, can also affect potency. Hashish is a potent cannabis preparation created by shaking, squeezing, or otherwise extracting the yellowish resin from the flowering tops of the plant. It turns dark brown or black as it dries and is pressed into small rocks that may be smoked in a pipe or baked in cookies or other confections for oral consumption (e.g., "hash brownies"). In hash oil, a purified variation of hashish, THC and other cannabinoids are extracted and concentrated through the use of an organic solvent. The oily substance is typically black or red and may be added to tobacco and smoked or heated on a piece of foil or in a pipe and inhaled. A rough ordering of the various preparations by percentage of THC typically is marijuana (0.5–14%), hashish (2–20%), and hash oil (15–60%) (Earleywine, 2002; Hall et al., 1994). Therefore, knowing the type of preparation consumed can suggest something about the actual amount of THC consumed. However, even within a type of preparation there is great variability in potency that further complicates an accurate assessment of THC consumed.

The large variability in the concentration of THC in marijuana and related preparations makes it difficult to establish the dose typically consumed by the average user. Only 2–3 mg of intravenous THC is needed to produce the desired effects (Perez-Reyes, Timmons, & Wall, 1974). A single marijuana cigarette or "joint" may have between 5 mg and 150 mg of THC, but anywhere between 30 and 80% of the THC may be lost in the combustion process or through sidestream smoke that is never inhaled. Furthermore, the fraction of inhaled THC that actually reaches the bloodstream may be as low as 5–24% (Hall et al., 1994). It is estimated that the average daily user in the United States may consume 50 mg of THC per day (Hall et al., 1994). There is some evidence that cannabis users titrate or adjust the amount they smoke to compensate for the varying concentrations of THC (Perez-Reyes, DiGuiseppi, Davis, Shindler, & Cook, 1982), but the data are mixed, and learned smoking habits may play a larger role (Wu, Tashkin, Rose, & Djahed, 1988).

Smoking is by far the most common route of administration of cannabis. Marijuana is typically rolled in cigarette papers to make "joints." It may also be smoked in pipes, as are hashish and hash oil. Recently, it has become popular in some regions to roll marijuana in cigar wrappers, which are called "blunts." Water pipes ("bongs") force the smoke through a chamber of water prior to inhalation and are used by some individuals to cool the smoke and filter unwanted constituents. Oral consumption of marijuana and hashish is less common and is accomplished by baking the substance in cookies, brownies, or cakes. When consumed orally, the effects are delayed by about 1 hour and are typically not as intense (Agurell, Lindgren, Ohlsson, Gillespie, & Hollister, 1984). On the other hand, oral consumption prolongs the effects, which are experienced for several hours or more depending upon the amount consumed. The inability to titrate the dose when consumed orally and the prolonged duration of effects may increase the likelihood of anxiety and panic reactions. Route of administration may affect health consequences independent of the amount of THC. Whereas some of the negative consequences may be associated with the amount of THC consumed (e.g., cognitive or occupational impairment), negative effects on the respiratory system are related to tars and other constituents in smoked preparations only.

Frequency of Use

Perhaps because of the difficulties in quantifying the amount of cannabis consumed, most assessment has focused on the frequency of use or the number of days of any use during a specified period. Frequency of use can be assessed with simple summary questions (e.g., "During the past month, on how many days did you use marijuana?"), prospective diaries or logs, or time-line follow-back (TLFB) techniques (Sobell & Sobell, 1992). A number of more comprehensive drug use surveys embed summary-style questions about the frequency of marijuana use among items assessing use of other drugs (e.g., Customary Drinking and Drug Use Record [CDDR]; Brown, Myers, Lippke, Tapert, Stewart, & Vik, 1998; Addiction Severity Index [ASI]; McLellan et al., 1992). Single-item summary questions lend themselves well to initial screening because of their brevity, whereas TLFB and self-monitoring techniques may be used to obtain more detailed information on the pattern of use once the user is engaged and adequate time is available. TLFB procedures have been thoroughly described for the assessment of alcohol and other drugs (Sobell & Sobell, 1992) and modified for use with cannabis (Stephens, Babor, Kadden, Miller, & MTPRG, 2004). An advantage to both TLFB and self-monitoring approaches is that changes in patterns of use can be seen during relatively brief periods (within a week, across several weeks, etc.) and may provide clues to specific antecedents for use or evidence of cyclical patterns that need to be further assessed.

The time frame or window for assessment of cannabis use frequency can be as long as the past year or as short as the past week and depends on the goals of the assessment. Use patterns closer to contact with clinical services are more likely to be relevant to current functioning and decision making regarding the need for treatment. We have typically used a 90-day window to capture recent use. Additional questions can be asked about how the assessed pattern compares to use at more distal time points in order to get a longer history of use. Both general summary questions (Stephens, Roffman, et al., 1994; Stephens et al., 2000) and TLFB methods (Fals-Stewart, O'Farrell, Freitas, McFarlin, & Rutigliano, 2000; MTPRG, 2004) have been shown to be valid ways of collecting cannabis use frequency information at least in the context of treatment–outcome studies. We are unaware of any published data on the reliability or validity of self-monitoring cannabis use through prospective logs but suspect, based on studies of alcohol use and other behaviors, that it would yield valid data (see Korotitsch & Nelson-Gray, 1999).

The use of marijuana can also be detected via the presence of metabolites in the urine. However, THC is lipid-soluble and may be stored and excreted from fat cells for extended periods of time after the acute administration. Cannabis use may be detected via urinalysis as much as 30 days after the last administration in regular users (Smith-Kielland, Skuterud, & Morland, 1999). Therefore, a single urine test is a relatively poor indicator of recency of use. Cannabis metabolites in urine can be quantified, but large interindividual differences in excretion over time make these values uninterpretable as a measure of either extent or recency of use. Within a given individual, the level of metabolites would be expected to decrease over successive days of abstinence, and comparison of quantitative values from successive urine samples may be used to determine whether new smoking has occurred (Huestis & Cone, 1998). However, the accuracy of these methods across a range of users with varying histories of cannabis use has yet to be determined.

Quantity or Intensity of Use

As noted earlier, assessing the quantity of cannabis consumed is more difficult because of varying potencies and modes of consumption. Currently there is little information on the reliability and validity of self-reports of quantity consumed. Single-item questions have been used to assess the typical quantity of cannabis consumed per week (e.g., in ounces) and the typical number of joints smoked per day of use, but these data provided only gross estimates of consumption and generally were not as sensitive to the effects of treatment because of large interindividual differences in reporting (e.g., MTPRG, 2004). In cultures where the use of "bongs" or water pipes predominates as the method of smoking cannabis, items have been created to assess the number of "bongs" smoked per day (Lang, Engelander, & Brooke, 2000). Such reports of quantity consumed could also be collected on a day-by-day basis using either TLFB or self-monitoring approaches, but we are unaware of any systematic evaluations of this technique.

Focusing on the pattern or intensity of use during a day may be more clinically meaningful than quantity per se. For instance, the psychoactive effects of a single dose typically will peak after about 30–60 minutes, but lingering effects on mood, cognition, and performance may last several hours depending upon the size of the dose and individual tolerance. Therefore, individuals who smoke multiple times per day may feel the effects for most of their waking hours and may be at greater risk of negative social, occupational, and health consequences and dependence symptoms than users who smoke only once on a typical day. Again, single-item questions can and have been used to assess the pattern of smoking on a typical day (e.g., "On a typical day, how many times do you smoke?" or "On a typical day, how many hours are you high or under the influence of cannabis?"). However, these types of questions have some inherent ambiguity and sometimes are confusing to clients who want to know what defines a discrete episode of smoking versus continuous use. We modified the TLFB interview to collect cannabis use information for the quarterly periods of each day (i.e., 6:00 A.M.–12:00 P.M.; 12:00 P.M.–6:00 P.M.; 6:00 P.M.–12:00 A.M.; 12:00 A.M.–6:00 A.M.). The quarters roughly correspond to typical notions of morning, afternoon, evening, and night. For each day of cannabis use, the interviewer prompts the individual to report whether any use occurred in each specific quarter. The information is recorded on the calendar in a separate box for each quarter of the day. The total number of daily quarters of use can then be calculated for a given period of time, further differentiating daily users. Although formal reliability and validity studies of this technique have not been conducted, our data show moderate-to-large correlations between single-item measures of typical number of times used per day, or hours "high" per day, and the TLFB quarters per day method, and it was sensitive to the effects of treatment (Stephens et al., 2002; MTPRG, 2004).

ASSESSING THE SEVERITY OF DEPENDENCE, WITHDRAWAL, AND CRAVING

Dependence

Assessment of dependence has obvious relevance for treatment planning. Dependent users may be more likely to need intervention, and perhaps need more intensive intervention in order to make changes. The conceptualization of drug dependence as a syndrome defined by the high salience of drug use in the user's life, difficulty quitting or controlling use, a narrowing of the drug-using repertoire, and rapid reinstatement of dependence after abstinence clearly seems to apply to cannabis (Edwards, Arif, & Hodgson, 1981; Edwards & Gross, 1976). The dependence syndrome concept has influenced the diagnostic criteria for cannabis dependence found in the *Diagnostic and Statistical Manual of Mental Disorders* (DSM-IV-R; American Psychiatric Association, 1994) and in the *ICD-10 Classification of Mental and Behavioural Disorders* (ICD-10; World Health Organization, 1993a). Psychometric studies of these dependence criteria in a variety of samples indicate that they provide a coherent description of cannabis dependence across multiple cultures (e.g., Kosten, Rounsaville, Babor, Spitzer, & Williams, 1987; Nelson, Rehm, Ustun, Grant, & Chatterji, 1999; Morgenstern, Langenbucher, & Labouvie, 1994; Newcomb, 1992; Rounsaville, Bryant, Babor, Kranzler, & Kadden, 1993). There is also evidence that the syndrome described by these diagnostic criteria is applicable to adolescent cannabis users, although more work needs to be done in characterizing potential differences in the manifestation of dependence in adolescents (Winters, Latimer, & Stinchfield, 1999).

The most comprehensive method to assess cannabis dependence is structured or semistructured clinical or research interview protocols. Examples of such interviews include the Structured Clinical Interview for DSM-IV Axis I Disorders (SCID; First, Spitzer, Gibbon, & Williams, 1996), the Composite International Diagnostic Interview (CIDI; World Health Organization, 1997), the Schedule for Clinical Assessment in Neuropsychiatry (SCAN; World Health Organization, 1993b), and the Adolescent Diagnostic Interview (ADI; Winters & Henley, 1993). These interviews map directly onto the DSM and ICD diagnostic criteria and are considered the gold standard in the diagnosis of dependence. Although they require a lengthier assessment and some training in administration, they also offer more detail regarding the nature and experience of cannabis use, and can be useful in both research and clinical contexts. These structured interviews are known to possess good interrater and test–retest reliability with trained interviewers.

According to current diagnostic systems, endorsement of three or more dependence criteria yields the diagnosis of cannabis dependence. Recent research indicates that use of such arbitrary cutoffs yields "diagnostic orphans," individuals who report some dependence systems but do not meet the cutoff. Examination of the characteristics of members of this group suggests that they may be similar to those who meet the cutoff in terms of cannabis use patterns, and that strict adherence to the cutoff may overlook some individuals with significant problems (Degenhardt, Lynskey, Coffey, & Patton, 2002). Researchers often count the number of dependence criteria met and use it as an indicator of the severity of dependence, but there is little research with cannabis users on the validity of this approach. Reductions in cannabis dependence symptoms appear to covary with reductions in use following treatment, lending some convergent validity to dependence severity indices (MTPRG, 2004; Stephens et al., 2000).

There has been little systematic effort to develop shorter, self-report questionnaire measures of cannabis dependence. Such measures would be useful in clinical screening, and as dependent and predictor variables in research that cannot afford the time and cost of the lengthier structured interviews. Stephens, Roffman, and Simpson (1993, 1994) adapted the Drug Abuse Screening Test (DAST; Skinner, 1982; Gavin, Ross, & Skinner, 1989) for use as an outcome measure and found that 88% of those seeking treatment for marijuana use exceeded the cutoff of 5 for identifying drug abuse. Significant reductions in this problem indicator were seen with treatment, but no attempt was made to validate it in relation to formal diagnoses. Another recently published instrument designed to screen for cannabis use disorders uses a format similar to the DAST and other screening test predecessors. The Marijuana Screening Inventory (MSI) consists of 39 items, answered primarily in a yes–no format, that survey the occurrence of dependence-related symptoms and negative consequences from cannabis use (Alexander, 2003). This preliminary study has examined the internal structure of the instrument but has not addressed its validity in identifying diagnosable dependence.

Other researchers have systematically looked at the optimal cutoffs for detecting cannabis dependence by comparing interview-derived diagnoses with scores on three short, self-report measures in a sample of long-term users (Swift, Copeland, & Hall, 1998). They found that all three measures showed good sensitivity and specificity in detecting "moderate" levels of dependence, but the optimal cutoff point on one scale, the Severity of Dependence Scale (SDS; Gossop, Griffiths, Powis, & Strang, 1992), had to be modified downward from the cutoff recommended for other drugs in order to achieve optimal detection and discrimination. The SDS also has been shown to be sensitive to the effects of treatment (Copeland, Swift, Roffman, & Stephens, 2001). These findings suggest that a variety of existing short scales developed to detect dependence on other drugs have some validity for cannabis as well. However, cutoff points may need to be adjusted, if the goal is to detect diagnosable disorder. Furthermore, the ability of these measures to discriminate milder levels of dependence has not been determined, in part because the studied samples have generally included a preponderance of heavier users, who tend to meet many diagnostic criteria. Studies are needed that examine the utility of brief measures in detecting and assessing dependence among a wider range of use patterns and for time frames shorter than the past 12 months. It is also important to note that severity of dependence has not yet been reported as a predictor of response to treatment and, as such, the importance of the construct in guiding the need for more or less intensive treatments is not yet known.

Withdrawal

In the dependence syndrome, withdrawal symptoms and tolerance are seen as co-occurring aspects of the disorder. Although they are neither necessary nor sufficient for diagnosis, the presence of withdrawal symptoms may signal the need for interventions to target these potential obstacles to behavior change. Two recent controlled studies that followed daily users in the natural environment during periods of regular use and then abstinence suggest a consistent pattern of withdrawal symptoms that includes irritability, restlessness, anger, aggression, sleep difficulty, decreased appetite, and weight loss (Budney et al., 2001, 2003). Onset of most symptoms occurred within the first few days of abstinence, and most lasted about 2 weeks (Budney et al., 2003). The authors suggest that the syndrome is comparable in severity to nicotine withdrawal. These studies make significant progress toward answering questions about the existence and clinical significance of a cannabis withdrawal syndrome that have been raised, but additional studies are needed to estimate the number and the characteristics of users who are affected (cf. Smith, 2002). Although some users approaching treatment clearly report and express concern about withdrawal phenomena, others do not, and the contribution of physical dependence to chronic cannabis use and a dependence syndrome is not yet fully understood. Several research groups have developed withdrawal questionnaires or checklists that range in length from 14 to 50 items (e.g., Budney et al., 2003; Haney et al., 1999b; Kouri & Pope, 2000).

Craving

The phenomenon of craving has been explained from a variety of perspectives and can be understood as both positive expectancies for drug effects and expected relief from withdrawal symptoms. Many conceptualizations of dependence assume that craving is related to an underlying pathophysiological process that occurs in the dependent individual. Attempts to assess craving and urges to use cannabis have begun to appear, and they mimic the earlier work on the assessment of craving for tobacco and cocaine (Tiffany & Drobes, 1991; Tiffany, Singleton, Haertzen, & Henningfield, 1993).

Comprehensive assessment typically involves several subscales that reflect the multidimensional nature of craving. Budney and colleagues (2001, 2003), in their work on withdrawal symptoms, have directly adapted a 10-item tobacco craving questionnaire with two subscales that roughly correspond to anticipated positive effects and anticipated relief from negative affect or withdrawal, as well as an overall total score. Scores on their Marijuana Craving Questionnaire (MCQ) scales increased in daily cannabis users during periods of abstinence (Budney et al., 2001). However, in another study, they did not see a spike in craving with abstinence, but rather found that craving scores diminished gradually with prolonged abstinence. Another 45-item Marijuana Craving Questionnaire (MCQ) has four subscales defined by a 17-item subset of the original questionnaire (Heishman, Singleton, & Liguori, 2001; Singleton, Trotman, Zavahir, Taylor, & Heishman, 2002). These scales demonstrate good reliability and convergent validity with measures of related constructs, but they have not yet been systematically linked to cannabis use or response to treatment.

ASSESSING NEGATIVE CONSEQUENCES

The assessment of negative consequences associated with cannabis use can be distinguished from the assessment of dependence. Whereas the diagnosis of dependence is predicated on notions of loss of control, compulsive use, increased salience of use, and associated tolerance and withdrawal, negative consequences may befall users who do not show these signs of the dependence. The DSM and ICD diagnostic symptoms acknowledge the distinction with the diagnostic category of cannabis abuse. Individuals who acknowledge either recurrent interference with major role obligations, use in hazardous situations, legal problems, or interpersonal problems related to use meet criteria for cannabis abuse. Although cannabis abuse is technically a residual diagnosis to be used only when individuals do not meet the dependence diagnosis, there are other reasons for assessing negative consequences associated with use. Information on the specific types of negative consequences, their number, frequency, and severity is useful in assessing the nature and extent of impact on the person's life and, consequently, their likely motivations for making changes. Consistent with harm reduction approaches, targeting and monitoring changes in negative consequences may be a valid goal in cases in which the user is not interested in complete abstinence. Although the assessment of negative consequences is included in the same structured interviews discussed earlier in relation to the diagnosis of dependence, several self-report questionnaires have been developed specifically for this purpose.

Initial studies of negative consequences in daily cannabis users who were approaching treatment supplemented existing drug abuse screening tests with additional items (Stephens, Roffman, et al., 1993, 1994). Subsequently, the most frequently endorsed items were incorporated into a 19-item Marijuana

Problem Scale (MPS) that has been used in at least two treatment-outcome studies to document the impact of treatment (Stephens et al., 2000, MTPRG, 2004). A three-response option format was incorporated to increase sensitivity and minimize underreporting. Respondents indicate whether each listed consequence was a major problem, minor problem, or no problem during the past 90 days. The number of items endorsed as either a minor or major problem can be summed to create an overall index of negative consequences with good internal consistency and sensitivity to treatment effects. A weighted total score is also possible by assigning higher values to problems endorsed as "major." The scale includes several items tapping effects of cannabis use on self-perceptions (i.e., feeling bad about using, lowered self-esteem, lacking self-confidence) that are some of the most frequently endorsed items, along with perceived impacts on energy level and procrastination, and concerns about memory loss (Stephens et al., 2002). Negative effects on finances, family, and sleep were reported by 40–60% of those seeking treatment and constitute the next most frequently endorsed consequences. These findings suggest that more subtle effects on motivation and self-evaluation may be important in understanding cannabis's impact on heavy users. In one study assessing the reasons participants gave for seeking treatment, cannabis users were most motivated by issues of self-control rather than negative impacts on health or social functioning (McBride, Curry, Stephens, Wells, Roffman, & Hawkins, 1994).

A longer and more comprehensive self-report measure of negative consequences, the Cannabis Problems Questionnaire (CPQ; Copeland, Swift, & Rees, 2001; Copeland, Swift, Roffman, et al., 2001), is a 53-item questionnaire that contains more specific items concerning use in inappropriate situations, interpersonal problems, psychological concerns, physical health, finances, and neglect of other activities. A number of items on the scale may tap more into the dependence syndrome concept rather than into negative consequences. This measure is still under development, but findings in a sample of users seeking treatment indicated frequent cannabis use during inappropriate situations (e.g., driving, at work), and negative affective and psychological reactions to use, in addition to the types of problems reported for the MPS. A decrease in the proportion of endorsed problems on the CPQ was shown following treatment (Copeland, Swift, Roffman, et al., 2001).

When cannabis-related negative consequences are assessed in users who are not seeking treatment, the rate of problem identification is lower, even though their frequency of cannabis use does not appear to differ much from that of the treatment-seeking samples (e.g., Reilly, Didcott, Swift, & Hall, 1998; Swift, Hall, & Copeland, 1998; Stephens, Roffman, Fearer, Williams, Picciano, & Burke, 2004). These discrepancies highlight issues in the reporting of cannabis-related negative consequences. It may that there are particular patterns of cannabis use (e.g., using multiple times per day) that are more likely to lead to problems, or that characteristics of users moderate the experience of problems. For instance, a finding that home ownership (rather than renting) predicted fewer self-reported negative consequences following treatment, but was not related to posttreatment frequency of cannabis use, is consistent with this hypothesis (Stephens, Wertz, & Roffman, 1993). It may be that individuals with greater socioeconomic resources are either better able or more motivated to use marijuana in ways that do not interfere with other areas of functioning. In addition, awareness of the problems or readiness to acknowledge them may vary across individuals and affect self-reporting. Future research with samples that show wider variation in their use patterns, problem recognition, and sociodemographic characteristics are needed to disentangle these issues.

The ASI (McLellan et al., 1992), a standardized and structured interview with known reliability and validity, has also been used to assess the negative psychosocial impacts of cannabis use in at least two treatment outcome studies. The ASI assesses the nature and severity of problems in seven areas: alcohol use, drug use, medical status, psychiatric problems, employment, family/social relationships, and legal status. An advantage to the ASI is that it assesses psychosocial functioning more objectively and without requiring the drug user to make attributions about the role of drug use in causing problems. Such an approach avoids the issue of problem awareness or acknowledgment but does not allow for an unambiguous connection between use and functioning. Perhaps as a result, the ASI scales may lack sensitivity to more subtle forms of dysfunction and be less sensitive to changes in use (e.g., Budney et al., 2000; MTPRG, 2004). Informal (Stephens et al., 2002) and formal (Budney, Radonovich, Higgins, & Wong, 1998) comparisons of primary cannabis users with other drug users on the ASI scales at intake suggest that the psychosocial dysfunction of cannabis users may be somewhat less. Studies are needed that assess psychosocial functioning objectively and comprehensively to understand the extent of the link between cannabis use and particular negative consequences. In the meantime, users' reports of cannabis-related problems are our most sensitive and clinically useful indices of negative consequences.

ASSESSING COGNITIVE IMPAIRMENT

Concerns about memory and attention are some of the negative consequences most commonly reported by cannabis users seeking treatment. Although both early and recent reviews of the literature have concluded that there is no evidence of major cognitive dysfunction associated with cannabis use (e.g., Wert & Raulin, 1986a, 1986b; Grant, Gonzalez, Carey, Natarajan, & Wolfson, 2003), several recent studies indicate that impairment is evident in some heavy users (Pope & Yurgelin-Todd, 1996; Pope et al., 2001; Solowij, 1998; Solowij et al., 2002). However, the degree of impairment may be subtle, and detection appears to require sensitive neuropsychological assessment. There is ongoing debate about the cause and duration of the effects (Pope, 2002), with some findings suggesting a return of full cognitive function within a month of abstinence (Pope et al., 2001), and other data suggesting that recovery, if it occurs, may be prolonged (Bolla et al., 2002; Solowij, 1998). A review of the specific neuropsychological tests that have been sensitive to cannabis-related impairment is beyond the scope of this chapter; the interested reader is referred to the references given earlier. In general, tests specifically designed to test learning and memory (e.g., Rey Auditory Verbal Learning Test [RAVLT]: Rey, 1964; Buschke Selective Reminding Test [BSRT]: Buschke, 1973) and frontal lobe function (e.g., Stroop test: Stroop, 1935; Wisconsin Card Sorting Test [WCST]: Heaton, 1981) have been the most sensitive to cannabis use.

ASSESSING HIGH-RISK SITUATIONS, SELF-EFFICACY, AND COPING SKILLS

Cognitive-behavioral treatment (CBT) models for substance use place heavy emphasis on the concepts of high-risk situations, self-efficacy, and coping skills (e.g., Marlatt & Gordon, 1985; Monti, Kadden, Rohsenow, Cooney, & Abrams, 2002); these concepts are relevant for the assessment and treatment of cannabis use disorders. CBT emphasizes that the risk for substance use is greatest in user-specific situations, commonly referred to as high-risk situations or triggers. Failure to have or to employ alternative coping responses in these situations increases the probability of drug use by decreasing the individual's self-efficacy or confidence in being able to avoid using. Identification of high-risk situations, assessment of relevant coping skills, and knowledge of situation-specific self-efficacy for avoiding use, therefore, are central in treatment planning. CBT has been tested in several studies with cannabis users, and some have assessed and examined the importance of these proposed mediating processes.

Although high-risk situations for cannabis use may be idiosyncratic, common precipitants of relapse to many addictive behaviors are negative emotional states, interpersonal conflict, and social pressure to use (e.g., Marlatt & Gordon, 1985). In one study of cannabis users, open-ended descriptions and attributions of causality for relapse events were coded using a categorical scheme employed in earlier studies of relapse to alcohol, tobacco, and heroin. The results confirmed that negative emotional states (33%) and direct pressure to use (24%) accounted for the majority of slips back into cannabis use, with positive emotional states (22%) a close third (Stephens, Curtin, et al., 1994). These findings highlight both commonalities in vulnerability to relapse between cannabis and other psychoactive substances and potential differences. In addition to the commonly reported role of drugs in coping with negative affect and the influence of social pressure to use, cannabis may serve important functions for users who wish to enhance already positive intrapersonal states. Assessment of users' particular relapse vulnerabilities is essential, but a self-report assessment tool for cannabis high-risk situations has not been developed yet. Future research might profitably focus on developing an inventory of situations similar to ones for alcohol users that could be completed by cannabis users to aid in the identification of high-risk situations (e.g., Annis, Graham, & Davis, 1987).

The assessment of situation-specific self-efficacy for avoiding drug use is closely related to the identification of high-risk situations. Self-efficacy is commonly operationalized as confidence in one's ability to avoid substance use in specific situations. It is proposed to be the central mediating pathway of behavior change according to the social-cognitive model that underlies CBT (Bandura, 1997). Self-efficacy judgments theoretically incorporate information from past experiences, new vicarious learning, verbal encouragement, as well as mood and arousal. Thus, they should be one of the strongest predictors of behavior change. Situation-specific low self-efficacy may guide the focus of coping skills training during treatment. The teaching and practice of coping skills is proposed to increase self-efficacy in these situations through both vicarious and *in vivo* learning, and subsequently to decrease the probability of drug use (Marlatt & Gordon, 1985). Stephens, Wertz, et al. (1993, 1995) created a Self-Efficacy (SE) scale for avoiding cannabis use based on a 19-item inventory of high-risk situations adapted from prior research with other drug users. Using a 7-point scale, respondents indicate their confidence that they can avoid cannabis use in each situation. Item responses typically have been averaged to create an overall index of degree or level of self-efficacy across situations.

Research has shown pretreatment self-efficacy to be one of the strongest predictors of reduced cannabis use after treatment, although it did not mediate the effects of hypothesized sources of efficacy judgments or other contextual variables (Stephens, Wertz, et al., 1993). Subsequent analyses comparing pretreatment and posttreatment self-efficacy judgments indicated that posttreatment self-efficacy may be better informed by recent attempts at quitting and, hence, a better predictor of subsequent cannabis use (Stephens, Wertz, et al., 1995). Posttreatment self-efficacy judgments were higher following CBT in comparison with a nonbehavioral treatment and were a moderately strong predictor of cannabis use during the follow-up period. Posttreatment efficacy judgments appeared to partially mediate the influence of the hypothesized sources of efficacy judgments on future use (i.e., prior frequency of use, temptation, coping skills utilization, stress, and contact with other users). Thus, results generally support the predictive validity of self-efficacy judgments and partially support theoretically implied relationships with other predictors.

The assessment of coping skills ideally should occur concomitantly with the identification of high-risk situations. However, there has been little work in this area with cannabis users. The self-reported likelihood of using various cognitive and behavioral coping strategies in each of three high-risk situations was assessed in one study and showed theoretically consistent positive relationships, with self-efficacy for avoiding cannabis use and the expected negative relationships with the frequency of actual cannabis use following treatment (Stephens, Wertz, et al., 1995). However, the Coping Strategies (CS) measure was not differentially changed by participation in a CBT treatment compared to a nonbehavioral treatment. In fact, the likelihood of using coping strategies actually decreased following both treatments, perhaps because of a decrease in temptation to use. The measure was not validated in relation to actual coping skills. In the treatment of alcohol problems, more attention has centered on the assessment of coping using audiotaped vignettes and expert judgments of client responses (see Monti, Rohsenow, Colby, & Abrams, 1995, for a review of measures), but even here, the role of coping in successful outcomes following CBT is unclear (Longabaugh & Morgenstern, 1999; Morgenstern & Longabaugh, 2000).

ASSESSING EXPECTANCIES AND ATTRIBUTIONAL BIASES

The expected effects of drugs may mediate the relationship between early learning and the onset and severity of later alcohol abuse. For example, particular types of expected effects may relate to drinking for specific reasons and, consequently, to the likelihood of developing drinking problems. These expectancy effects can be understood as the result of normal learning processes, and their effects on future behavior may be related to how memories are stored (see Goldman, Brown, Christiansen, & Smith, 1991). They also appear to be amenable to systematic manipulation (Darkes & Goldman, 1993, 1998). Expectancies regarding cannabis effects have been assessed with the Marijuana Expectancy Effects Questionnaire (MEEQ; Schafer & Brown, 1991). The original MEEQ contained 70 items reflecting possible effects of smoking cannabis that were endorsed as either present or absent in a college sample. Subsequent factor analysis identified six domains or factors that were defined by 57 of the items and labeled as follows: Cognitive and Behavioral Impairment; Relaxation and Tension Reduction, Social and Sexual Facilitation, Perceptual and Cognitive Enhancement, Global Negative Effects, and Craving and Physical Effects. Scores on the factor-based subscales discriminated between levels of recent cannabis use, with a general tendency for negative effects to be endorsed more by infrequent or nonusers and for positive effects to be endorsed by more frequent users. Both similarities and differences between the types of effects expected for cannabis versus alcohol and other drugs were noted (Schafer & Brown, 1991). The MEEQ administered with a Likert-type response format also discriminated between nonusers and current users in a clinical sample (Galen & Henderson, 1999). In a longitudinal study with both clinical and community samples of adolescents, a 48-item version of the MEEQ predicted drug preference, and initiation and desistance of cannabis use (Aarons, Brown, Stice, & Coe, 2001). Thus, the expected effects of cannabis appear to relate to present and future drug use across several populations. These findings suggest that assessment of cannabis expectancies could be useful in identifying those at risk for initiation or escalation of use. Interventions might profitably target expected effects to prevent initiation or to encourage quitting, but systematic studies have not yet been conducted to test these hypotheses.

There has been at least one attempt to assess the attributional biases that may increase the probability of a full-blown relapse following an initial use. The abstinence violation effect (AVE), more recently and more generally referred to as the rule violation effect, is proposed to occur when individuals make internal, stable, and global attributions for the cause of an initial use of a substance following a period of abstinence (Marlatt & Gordon, 1985). In this situation, the user is saying that something about him- or herself that will not change, and that affects everything he or she does, is responsible for the initial drug use. This particular constellation of attributions predicts that little effort will be made to control use. Subsequently, the user may experience a sense of loss of control and feelings of guilt that further undermine efforts to regain abstinence. Indeed, one study with cannabis users showed that those who made such attributions for a lapse following treatment were more likely to report increased use of cannabis both concurrently and at future follow-ups (Stephens, Curtin, et al., 1994). AVE attributions were assessed with single-item scales adapted from previous research with tobacco relapse (Curry, Marlatt, & Gordon, 1987), and the development of multi-item scales would benefit future research in this area by providing more reliable assessment and distinguishing between alternative meanings of internal attributions (i.e., effort vs. ability). Also, the tendency to experience the AVE was not differentially affected by CBT versus nonbehavioral treatment, despite the inclusion of cognitive restructuring techniques specifically targeting this attributional style. Although there appears to be some predictive validity to the AVE, modification of AVE responses may take more intensive cognitive therapy than was provided in this study.

THE ROLE OF ASSESSMENT IN TREATMENT

Assessment informs treatment and may be used to decide on the type, duration, and focus of therapy. Assessment also may have direct effects on behavior. During the assessment process, clients must systematically and thoroughly review their history of drug use and associated consequences. This process may lead to changes in awareness of adverse impacts that motivate behavior change. Motivational enhancement treatment (MET) systematically combines the delivery of feedback based on assessment data with motivational interviewing processes to increase readiness to change (Miller & Rollnick, 2002; Miller, Zweben, DiClemente, & Rychtarik, 1992). Feedback from the assessment is typically presented to the client by the therapist during the first session, using a printed feedback report that is then systematically reviewed with the therapist. Data presented on the report vary both in terms of what is presented and in the visual style (e.g., text-based reports vs. graphical presentation) but usually include information on frequency of use, number and nature of negative consequences reported, presence of dependence symptoms, and specific low-self-efficacy situations. Whenever possible, data are presented in relation to norms or cutoff points for disorder that allow the user to see where he or she stands. Therapists use reflective listening techniques to encourage consideration of the meaning of assessment results. Several treatment–outcome studies that have tested this approach with cannabis users generally found it to be effective in promoting reduced use, both in combination with CBT and as a stand-alone brief intervention (Budney et al., 2001; MTPRG, 2004; Stephens et al., 2000). Therefore, incorporating assessment feedback into the treatment intervention makes full use of the assessment process and is quickly becoming standard practice.

CONCLUSIONS

Interest in the assessment and treatment of cannabis problems has grown dramatically since the first edition of this book was published. Fifteen years ago, there were no controlled treatment studies for cannabis use disorders. The relative lack of clinical interest in cannabis users was likely fueled by beliefs that cannabis was a benign drug and not addictive. We now know that the biopsychosocial factors associated with alcohol and other drug abuse are relevant to the assessment and treatment of cannabis use disorders. Issues remain in assessing the nature and severity of the consequences associated with cannabis use, but there is little doubt that a subset of users develops signs of dependence and perceives significant problems as a consequence of use.

Table 8.1 summarizes the cannabis assessment measures reviewed in this chapter. The growth in assessment tools provides clinicians and researchers with a starting point for measuring most domains, but it is important to note that there is much work to be done. With few exceptions, most of the existing measures are adaptations of alcohol, tobacco, or other drug assessments whose reliability and validity have received limited direct testing in relation to cannabis use.

Psychometric studies are needed, some of which might profitably start with an original item pool generated by experts in cannabis use problems, rather than relying on items from other drug measures. In general, future research must be conducted with a wider range of users in order to develop measures that identify and predict hazardous levels of use. Research with clinical populations is needed to develop sound measures of proposed mediating processes that can be tested in treatment–outcome studies in order to understand how treatment works. We must not lose sight of the fact that reliable and valid assessment is the foundation of knowledge and, therefore, a worthy enterprise in and of itself.

TABLE 8.1. Cannabis Use Assessment Measures

Purpose	Domain/construct	Instrument (s)	Author(s)
Cannabis use	Frequency, quantity, and pattern of cannabis use	TLFB	Sobell & Sobell (1992)
		Modified TLFB	Stephens et al. (2002)
		CDDR	Brown et al. (1998)
		ASI	McLellan et al. (1992)
		"Bongs per day"	Lang et al. (2000)
		"Joints per day"	Marijuana Treatment Project Research Group (2004)
		"Times per day"	Stephens et al. (2000, 2002)
Diagnosis of dependence, screening, assessment of problem severity	Dependence, abuse, severity	CIDI	WHO (1997)
		SCID	First et al. (1996)
		SCAN	WHO (1993b)
		ADI	Winters & Henley (1993)
		DAST	Gavin et al. (1989)
		MSI	Alexander (2003)
		SDS	Gossop et al. (1992)
	Negative consequences	MPS	Stephens et al. (2000, 2002)
		CPQ	Copeland et al. (2001)
		ASI	McLellan et al. (1992)
Dependence-related phenomena	Withdrawal	MWC	Budney et al. (2003)
		Daily diaries	Kouri & Pope (2000)
		Visual analogue scales	Haney et al. (1999)
	Craving	MCQ	Budney et al. (2001, 2003)
		MCQ	Heishman et al. (2001)
Cognitive impairment	Neuropsychological functioning	RAVLT	Rey (1964)
		BSRT	Buschke (1973)
		Stroop	Stroop (1935)
		WCST	Heaton (1981)
Mediating Processes	Self-efficacy	SE	Stephens, Wertz, et al. (1993, 1995)
	Coping strategies	CS	Stephens et al. (1995)
	Marijuana effect expectancies	MEEQ	Schafer & Brown (1991)
	Attributional biases for lapses	AVE— Questionnaire	Stephens, Curtin, et al. (1994)

REFERENCES

Aarons, G. A., Brown, S. A., Stice, E., & Coe, M. T. (2001). Psychometric evaluation of the marijuana and stimulant effect expectancy questionnaires for adolescents. *Addictive Behaviors, 26,* 219–236.

Agurell, S., Lindgren, J., Ohlsson, A., Gillispie, H. K., & Hollister, L. (1984). Recent studies on the phannacokinetics of delta-1-tetrahydrocannabinol in man. In S. Agurell, W. L. Dewey, & R. E. Willett (Eds.), *The cannabinoids; Chemical, pharmacological, and therapeutic aspects* (pp. 165–184). Orlando, FL: Academic Press.

Alexander, D. (2003). A Marijuana Screening Inventory (Experimental Version): Description and preliminary psychometric properties. *American Journal of Drug and Alcohol Abuse, 29,* 619–646.

American Psychiatric Association. (1994). *Diagnostic and statistical manual of mental disorders* (4th ed., rev.). Washington, DC: Author.

Annis, H. M., Graham, J. M., & Davis, C. S. (1987). *Inventory of Drinking Situations (IDS) user's guide.* Toronto: Addiction Research Foundation.

Anthony, J. C., & Helzer, J. E. (1991). Syndromes of drug abuse and dependence. In L. N. Robins & D. A. Regier (Eds.), *Psychiatric disorders in America* (pp. 116–154). New York: Free Press.

Anthony, J. C., Warner, L. A., & Kessler, R. C. (1994). Comparative epidemiology of dependence on tobacco, alcohol, controlled substances, and inhalants: Basic findings from the National Comorbidity Survey. *Experimental and Clinical Psychopharmacology, 2,* 244–268.

Bandura, A. (1997). *Self-efficacy: The exercise of control.* New York: Freeman.

Bolla, K. I., Brown, K., Eldreth, D., Tate, K., & Cadet, J. L. (2002). Dose-related neurocognitive effects of marijuana use. *Neurology, 59,* 1337–1343.

Brown, S., Myers, M. G., Lippke, L., Tapert, S. F., Stewart, D. G., & Vik, P. W. (1998). Psychometric evaluation of the Customary Drinking and Drug Use Record (CDDR): A measure of adolescent alcohol and drug involvement. *Journal of Studies on Alcohol, 59,* 427–438.

Budney, A. J., Higgins, S. T., Radonovich, K. J., & Novy, P. L. (2000). Adding voucher-based incentives to coping skills and motivational enhancement improves outcomes during treatment for marijuana dependence. *Journal of Consulting and Clinical Psychology, 68,* 1051–1061.

Budney, A. J., Hughes, J. R., Moore, B. A., & Novy, P. L. (2001). Marijuana abstinence effects in marijuana smokers maintained in their home environment. *Archives of General Psychiatry, 58,* 917–924.

Budney, A. J., & Moore, B. A. (2002). Development and consequences of cannabis dependence. *Journal of Clinical Psychopharmacology, 42,* 28S–33S.

Budney, A. J., Moore, B. A., Vandrey, R. G., & Hughes, J. R. (2003). The time course and significance of cannabis withdrawal. *Journal of Abnormal Psychology, 112,* 393–402.

Budney, A. J., Novy, P. L., & Hughes, J. R. (1999). Marijuana withdrawal among adults seeking treatment for marijuana dependence. *Addiction, 94,* 1311–1322.

Budney, A. J., Radonovich, K. J., Higgins, S. T., & Wong, C. J. (1998). Adults seeking treatment for marijuana dependence: A comparison to cocaine-dependent treatment seekers. *Experimental and Clinical Psychopharmacology, 6,* 1–8.

Buschke, H. (1973). Selective reminding for analyses of memory and learning. *Journal of Verbal Learning and Verbal Behavior, 12*, 543–550.

Copeland, J., Swift, W., & Rees, V. (2001). Clinical profile of participants in a brief intervention program for cannabis use disorder. *Journal of Substance Abuse Treatment, 20*, 45–52.

Copeland, J., Swift, W., Roffman, R., & Stephens, R. (2001). A randomized controlled trial of brief cognitive-behavioral interventions for cannabis use disorder. *Journal of Substance Abuse Treatment, 21*, 55–64.

Curry, S., Marlatt, G. A., & Gordon, J. R. (1987). Abstinence violation effect: Validation of an attributional construct with smoking cessation. *Journal of Consulting and Clinical Psychology, 2*, 145–149.

Darkes, J., & Goldman, M. S. (1993). Expectancy challenge and drinking reduction: Experimental evidence for a mediational process. *Journal of Consulting and Clinical Psychology, 61*, 344–353.

Darkes, J., & Goldman, M. S. (1998). Expectancy challenge and drinking reduction: Process and structure in the alcohol expectancy network. *Experimental and Clinical Psychopharmacology, 6*, 64–76.

Degenhardt, L., Lynskey, M., Coffey, C., & Patton, G. (2002). "Diagnostic orphans" among young adult cannabis users: Persons who report dependence symptoms but do not meet diagnostic criteria. *Drug and Alcohol Dependence, 67*, 205–212.

Donovan, D. M. (1988). Assessment of addictive behaviors: Implications of an emerging biopsychosocial model. In D. M. Donovan & G. A. Marlatt (Eds.), *Assessment of addictive behaviors* (pp. 3–48). New York: Guilford Press.

Earleywine, M. (2002). *Understanding marijuana: A new look at the scientific evidence.* New York: Oxford University Press.

Edwards, G., Arif, A., & Hodgson, R. (1981). Nomenclature and classification of drug- and alcohol-related problems: A WHO memorandum. *Bulletin of the World Health Organization, 59*, 225–242.

Edwards, G., & Gross, M. M. (1976). Alcohol dependence: Provisional description of a clinical syndrome. *British Medical Journal, 1*, 1058–1061.

Fals-Stewart, W., O'Farrell, T. J., Freitas, T. T., McFarlin, S. K., & Rutigliano, P. (2000). The timeline followback reports of psychoactive substance use by drug-abusing patients: Psychometric properties. *Journal of Consulting and Clinical Psychology, 68*, 134–144.

First, M. B., Spitzer, R. L., Gibbon, M., & Williams, J. B. (1996). *Structured Clinical Interview for DSM-IV, Axis I Disorders—Patient Edition (SCID-I/P, Version 2.0).* New York: Biometrics Research Department, New York State Psychiatric Institute.

Galen, L. W., & Henderson, M. J. (1999). Validation of cocaine and marijuana effect expectancies in a treatment setting. *Addictive Behaviors, 24*, 719–724.

Gardner, E. L. (1992). Cannabinoid interactions with brain reward systems—the neurobiological basis of cannabinoid abuse. In L. Murphy & A. Bartke (Eds.), *Marijuana/cannabinoids neurology and neurophysiology* (pp. 275–336). Boca Raton, FL: CRC Press.

Gavin, D. R., Ross, H. E., & Skinner, H. A. (1989). Diagnostic validity of the Drug Abuse Screening Test in the assessment of DSM-III drug disorders. *British Journal of Addiction, 84*, 301–307.

Goldman, M. S., Brown, S. A., Christiansen, B. A., & Smith, G. T. (1991). Alcoholism and memory: Broadening the scope of alcohol-expectancy research. *Psychological Bulletin, 110,* 137–146.

Gossop, M., Griffiths, P., Powis, B., & Strang, J. (1992). Severity of dependence and route of administration of heroin, cocaine, and amphetamines. *British Journal of Addiction, 87,* 1527–1536.

Grant, I., Gonzalez, R., Carey, C. L., Natarajan, L., & Wolfson, T. (2003). Non-acute (residual) neurocognitive effects of cannabis use: A meta-analytic study. *Journal of the International Neuropsychological Society, 9,* 679–689.

Hall, W., Solowij, N., & Lemon, J. (1994). *The health and psychological consequences of cannabis use* (National Drug Strategy Monograph Series No. 25). Canberra: Australian Government Publishing Service.

Haney, M., Ward, A. S., Comer, S. D., Foltin, R. W., & Fischman, M. W. (1999a). Abstinence symptoms following oral THC administration in humans. *Psychopharmacology, 141*(4), 385–394.

Haney, M., Ward, A. S., Comer, S. D., Foltin, R. W., & Fischman, M. W. (1999b). Abstinence symptoms following smoked marijuana in humans. *Psychopharmacology, 141*(4), 395–404.

Hawkins, D. J., Catalano, R. F., & Miller, J. Y. (1992). Risk and protective factors for alcohol and other drug problems in adolescence and early adulthood: Implications for substance abuse prevention. *Psychological Bulletin, 112,* 64–105.

Heaton, R. K. (1981). *Wisconsin Card Sorting test manual.* Odessa, FL: Psychological Assessment Resources.

Heishman, S. J., Singleton, E. G., & Liguori, A. (2001). Marijuana Craving Questionnaire: Development and initial validation of a self-report instrument. *Addiction, 96,* 1023–1034.

Huestis, M. A., & Cone, E. J. (1998). Differentiating new marijuana use from residual drug excretion in occasional marijuana users. *Journal of Analytical Toxicology, 22,* 445–454.

Jessor, R., Van Den Bos, J., Vanderryn, J., Costa, F. M., & Turbin, M. S. (1995). Protective factors in adolescent problem behavior: Moderator effects and developmental change. *Developmental Psychology, 6,* 923–933.

Jones, R. T., & Benowitz, N. (1976). The 30–day trip: Clinical studies of cannabis tolerance and dependence. In M. C. Braude & S. Szara (Eds.), *Pharmacology of marijuana* (Vol. 2, pp. 627–642). Orlando, FL: Academic Press.

Johnston, L. D., O'Malley, P. M., & Bachman, J. G. (2003). *Monitoring the Future national results on adolescent drug use: Overview of key findings, 2002* (NIH Publication No. 03-5374). Bethesda, MD: National Institute on Drug Abuse.

Kandel, D. B., Chen, K., Warner, L., Kessler, R., & Grant, B. (1997). Prevalence and demographic correlates of symptoms of dependence on cigarettes, alcohol, marijuana and cocaine in the U.S. population. *Drug and Alcohol Dependence, 44,* 11–29.

Korotitsch, W. J., & Nelson-Gray, R. (1999). An overview of self monitoring research in assessment and treatment. *Psychological Assessment, 11*(4), 415–425.

Kosten, T. R., Rounsaville, B. J., Babor, T. F., Spitzer, R. L., & Williams, J. B. W. (1987). Substance-use disorders in DSM-III-R. *British Journal of Psychiatry, 151,* 834–843.

Kouri, E. M., & Pope, H. G., Jr. (2000). Abstinence symptoms during withdrawal from chronic marijuana use. *Experimental and Clinical Psychopharmacology, 8,* 483–492.

Lang, E., Engelander, M., & Brooke, T. (2000). Report of an integrated brief intervention with self-defined problem cannabis users. *Journal of Substance Abuse Treatment, 19*, 111–116.

Lichtman, A. H., & Martin, B. R. (2002). Marijuana withdrawal syndrome in the animal model. *Journal of Clinical Pharmacology, 42*, 20S–27S.

Longabaugh, R., & Morgenstern, J. (1999). Cognitive-behavioral coping skills therapy for alcohol dependence: Current status and future directions. *Alcohol Research and Health, 23*, 78–87.

Marijuana Treatment Project Research Group. (2004). Brief treatments for cannabis dependence: Findings from a randomized multisite trial. *Journal of Consulting and Clinical Psychology, 72*, 455–466.

Marlatt, G. A., & Gordon, J. R. (1985). *Relapse prevention: Maintenance strategies in the treatment of addictive behaviors.* New York: Guilford Press.

McBride, C. M., Curry, S. J., Stephens, R. S., Wells, E. A., Roffman, R., & Hawkins, J. D. (1994). Intrinsic and extrinsic motivation for change in cigarette smokers, marijuana smokers and cocaine users. *Psychology of Addictive Behaviors, 8*, 243–250.

McLellan, A., Kushner, H., Metzger, D., Peters, R., Smith, I., Grissom, G., Pettinati, H., & Argeriou, M. (1992). The fifth edition of the Addiciton Severity Index. *Journal of Substance Abuse Treatment 9*(3), 199–213.

Miller, W. R., & Rollnick, S. (2002). *Motivational interviewing: Preparing people to change addictive behavior.* New York: Guilford Press.

Miller, W. R., Zweben, A., DiClemente, C. C., & Rychtarik, R. G. (1992). *Motivational enhancement therapy manual: A clinical research guide for therapists treating individuals with alcohol abuse and dependence* (DHHS Publication No. ADM 92-1894). Washington, DC: U.S. Government Printing Office.

Monti, P. M., Kadden, R. M., Rohsenow, D. J., Cooney, N. L., & Abrams, D. B. (2002). *Treating alcohol dependence: A coping skills training guide.* New York: Guilford Press.

Monti, P. M., Rohsenow, D. J., Colby, S. M., & Abrams, D. B. (1995). Coping and social skills training. In R. K. Hester & W. R. Miller (Eds.), *Handbook of alcoholism treatment approaches: Effective alternatives* (2nd ed., pp. 221–241). Boston: Allyn & Bacon.

Morgenstern, J., Langenbucher, J., & Labouvie, E. W. (1994). The generalizability of the dependence syndrome across substances: An examination of some properties of the proposed DSM-IV dependence criteria. *Addiction, 89*, 1105–1113.

Morgenstern, J., & Longabaugh, R. (2000). Cognitive-behavioral treatment for alcohol dependence: A review of evidence for its hypothesized mechanisms of action. *Addiction, 95*, 1475–1490.

Newcomb, M. D. (1992). Understanding the multidimensional nature of drug use and abuse: The role of consumption, risk factors and protective factors. In M. Glantz & R. Pickens (Eds.), *Vulnerability to drug abuse* (pp. 255–297). Washington, DC: American Psychological Association.

Newcomb, M. D., Maddahian, E., & Bentler, P. M. (1986). Risk factors for drug use among adolescence: Concurrent and longitudinal analyses. *American Journal of Public Health, 76*, 525–531.

Nelson, C. B., Rehm, J., Ustun, T. B., Grant, B., & Chatterji, S. (1999). Factor structures for DSM-IV substance disorder criteria endorsed by alcohol, cannabis, cocaine, and opiate users: Results from the WHO reliability and validity study. *Addiction, 94*, 843–855.

Perez-Reyes, M., DiGuiseppi, S., Davis, K. H., Schindler, V. H., & Cook, C. E. (1982). Comparison of effects of marihuana cigarettes of three different potencies. *Clinical Pharmacology and Therapeutics, 31*, 617–624.

Perez-Reyes, M., Timmons, M. C., & Wall, M. E. (1974). Long-term use of marijuana and the development of tolerance or sensitivity to 9Tetrahydrocannabinol. *Archives of General Psychiatry, 31*, 89–91.

Pope, H. G. (2002). Cannabis, cognition, and residual confounding. *Journal of the American Medical Association, 287*, 1172–1174.

Pope, H. G., Gruber, A. J., Hudson, J. I., Huestis, M. A., & Yurgelun-Todd, D. (2001). Neuropsychological performance in long-term cannabis users. *Archives of General Psychiatry, 58*, 909–915.

Pope, H. G., & Yurgelun-Todd, D. (1996). The residual cognitive effects of heavy marijuana use in college students. *Journal of the American Medical Association, 275*, 521–527.

Reilly, D., Didcott, P., Swift, W., & Hall, W. (1998). Long-term cannabis use: Characteristics of users in an Australian rural area. *Addiction, 93*, 837–846.

Rey, A. (1964). *L'examen clinique en psychologie.* Paris: Presses Universitaires de France.

Rounsaville, B. J., Bryant, K., Babor, T., Kranzler, H., & Kadden, R. (1993). Cross-system agreement for substance use disorders. *Addiction, 88*, 337–348.

Schafer, J., & Brown, S. A. (1991). Marijuana and cocaine effect expectancies and drug use patterns. *Journal of Consulting and Clinical Psychology, 59*, 558–565.

Singleton, E. G., Trotman, A. J.-M., Zavahir, M., Taylor, R. C., & Heishman, S. J. (2002). Determination of the reliability and validity of the Marijuana Craving Questionnaire using imagery scripts. *Experimental and Clinical Psychopharmacology, 10*, 47–53.

Skinner, H. A. (1982). The Drug Abuse Screening Test. *Addictive Behaviors, 7*, 363–371.

Smith, N. T. (2002). A review of the published literature into cannabis withdrawal symptoms in human users. *Addiction, 97*, 621–632.

Smith-Kielland, A., Skuterud, B., & Morland, J. (1999). Urinary excretion of 11–nor-9–carboxy-Δ^9-tetrahydrocannabinol and cannabinoids in frequent and infrequent users. *Journal of Analytical Toxicology, 23*, 323–332.

Solowij, N. (1998). *Cannabis and cognitive functioning.* Cambridge, UK: Cambridge University Press.

Solowij, N., Stephens, R. S., Roffman, R. A., Babor, T., Kadden, R., Miller, M., Christiansen, K., McRee, B., Vendetti, J., & the Marijuana Treatment Project Research Group. (2002). Cognitive functioning of long term heavy cannabis users seeking treatment. *Journal of the American Medical Association, 287*, 1123–1131.

Sobell, L.C., & Sobell, M.B. (1992). Timeline Follow-Back, a technique for assessing self-reported alcohol consumption. In R. Litten & J. Allen (Eds.), *Measuring alcohol consumption* (pp. 41–72). Totowa, NJ: Humana.

Stephens, R. S., Babor, T. F., Kadden, R. A., Miller, M., & the Marijuana Treatment Project Research Group. (2002). The Marijuana Treatment Project: Rationale, design, and participant characteristics. *Addiction, 97*, 109–124.

Stephens, R. S., Curtin, L., Simpson, E. E., & Roffman, R. A. (1994). Testing the abstinence violation effect construct with marijuana cessation. *Addictive Behaviors,
19*, 23–32.

Stephens, R. S., Roffman, R. A., & Curtin, L. (2000). Comparison of extended versus
brief treatments for marijuana use. *Journal of Consulting and Clinical Psychology, 68*, 898–908.

Stephens, R. S., Roffman, R. A., Fearer, S., Williams, C., Picciano, J., & Burke, R.
(2004). The Marijuana Check-Up: Reaching users who are ambivalent about
change. *Addiction, 99*, 1323–1332.

Stephens, R. S., Roffman, R. A., & Simpson, E. E. (1993). Adult marijuana users seeking treatment. *Journal of Consulting and Clinical Psychology, 61*, 1100–1104.

Stephens, R. S., Roffman, R. A., & Simpson, E. E. (1994). Treating adult marijuana
dependence: A test of the relapse prevention model. *Journal of Consulting and
Clinical Psychology, 62*, 92–99.

Stephens, R. S., Wertz, J. S., & Roffman, R. A. (1993). Predictors of marijuana treatment outcomes: The role of self-efficacy. *Journal of Substance Abuse, 5*, 341–
354.

Stephens, R. S., Wertz, J. S., & Roffman, R. A. (1995). Self-efficacy and marijuana cessation: A construct validity analysis. *Journal of Consulting and Clinical Psychology, 63*, 1022–1031.

Stroop, J. R. (1935). Studies of interference in serial verbal reactions. *Journal of Experimental Psychology, 18*, 643–662.

Substance Abuse and Mental Health Services Administration. (2002). *Treatment Episode Data Set (TEDS): 1992–2000: National admissions to substance abuse
treatment services* (DASIS Series: S-17, DHHS Publication No. [SMA] 02-3727).
Rockville, MD: Office of Applied Studies.

Substance Abuse and Mental Health Services Administration. (2003). *Results from the
2002 National Survey on Drug Use and Health: National findings* (NHSDA Series H-22, DHHS Publication No. SMA 03–3836). Rockville, MD: Office of Applied Studies.

Swift, W., Copeland, J., & Hall, W. (1998). Choosing a diagnostic cut-off for cannabis
dependence. *Addiction, 93*, 1681–1692.

Swift, W., Hall, W., & Copeland, J. (1998). Characteristics of long-term cannabis users in Sydney, Australia. *European Addiction Research, 4*, 190–197.

Tanda, G., Pontieri, F. E., & DiChiara, G. (1997). Cannabinoid and heroin activation
of mesolimbic dopamine transmission by a common μ_1 opioid receptor mechanism. *Science, 276*, 2048–2050.

Tashkin, D. P. (1999). Cannabis effects on the respiratory system. In H. Kalant, W.
Corrigall, W. Hall, & R. Smart (Eds.), *The health effects of cannabis* (pp. 313–
345). Toronto: Addiction Research Foundation.

Taylor, D. R., Poulton, R., Moffitt, T. E., Ramankutty, P., & Sears, M. R. (2000). The
respiratory effects of cannabis dependence in young adults. *Addiction, 95*, 1169–
1677.

Tiffany, S. T., & Drobes, D. J. (1991). The development and initial validation of a
questionnaire on smoking urges. *British Journal of Addiction, 86*, 1467–1476.

Tiffany, S. T., Singleton, E., Haertzen, C. A., & Henningfield, J. E. (1993). The development of a cocaine craving questionnaire. *Drug and Alcohol Dependence, 34*,
19–28.

Wert, R. C., & Raulin, M. L. (1986a). The chronic cerebral effects of cannabis use: I.

Methodological issues and neurological findings. *International Journal of the Addictions, 21,* 605–628.

Wert, R. C., & Raulin, M. L. (1986b). The chronic cerebral effects of cannabis use: II. Psychological findings and conclusions. *International Journal of the Addictions, 21,* 629–642.

Wiesbeck, G. A., Schuckit, M. A., Kalmijn, J. A., Tipp, J. E., Bucholz, K. K., & Smith, T. L. (1996). An evaluation of the history of a marijuana withdrawal syndrome in a large population. *Addiction, 91,* 1469–1478.

Winters, K. C., & Henley, G. A. (1993). *Adolescent Diagnostic Interview Schedule and manual.* Los Angeles: Western Psychological Services.

Winters, K. C., Latimer, W., & Stinchfield, R. D. (1999). The DSM-IV criteria for adolescent alcohol and cannabis use disorders. *Journal of Studies on Alcohol, 60,* 337–344.

World Health Organization. (1993a). *The ICD-10 classification of mental and behavioural disorders: Diagnostic criteria for research.* Geneva: Author.

World Health Organization. (1993b). *Schedules for clinical assessment in neuropsychiatry.* Washington, DC: American Psychiatric Press.

World Health Organization. (1997). *Composite International Diagnostic Interview, Core Version 2.1, 12 Month Version.* Geneva: Author.

Wu, T. C., Tashkin, D. P., Rose, J. E., & Djahed, B. (1988). Influence of marijuana potency and amount of cigarette consumed on marijuana smoking pattern. *Journal of Psychoactive Drugs, 20,* 43–46.

CHAPTER 9

Assessment of Club Drug, Hallucinogen, Inhalant, and Steroid Use and Misuse

JASON R. KILMER
REBEKKA S. PALMER
JESSICA M. CRONCE

The results of the 2000 National Household Survey on Drug Abuse (NHSDA; U.S. Department of Health and Human Services, 2001) suggested that 14 million Americans endorsed past-month illicit drug use, representing 6.3% of the population over the age of 12. An estimated 1 million Americans were current users of hallucinogens; 6.4 million had tried Ecstasy at least once in their lifetime (an increase of 1.3 million since the 1999 interviews), and 2.1 million youth under the age of 18 reported having used inhalants at some point in their life. Johnston, O'Malley, and Bachman's (2002) Monitoring the Future study identified Ecstasy and anabolic–androgenic steroids as the two substances increasing in use during 2001. While their 2003 release of the 2002 data noted that Ecstasy use had started to decline, it is still at rates higher than the 1999 survey and all preceding years, with 7.4% of 12th graders, 4.9% of 10th graders, and 2.9% of 8th graders reporting past-year use (Johnston, O'Malley, & Bachman, 2003). Furthermore, steroid use has held steady, though, as they note, at "historically high levels" (p. 4), with past-30-day use reaching 1.4% of high school seniors and lifetime use reported by 4.0% of seniors. While these numbers pale in comparison to the 104 million Americans identified through the NHSDA as current consumers of alcohol, these substances are associated with potentially severe consequences that are leading to increasing exposure in the media.

Accurately describing and understanding substance use itself and the associated consequences is essential to treatment planning and to measuring outcome. This chapter explores assessment issues with a range of substances not already addressed in this book: club drugs, hallucinogens, inhalants, and anabolic–androgenic steroids.

"Club" or "rave" drugs, including Ecstasy (3,4-methylenedioxymethamphetamine [MDMA]), ketamine, and gamma-hydroxybutyrate (GHB), are often associated with the club or rave scene, a party culture characterized by a style of music known as "house" music and attended by numbers that, at times, go into the thousands. While some trace the roots of this scene to 1985 Chicago (e.g., Tyler, 1986), it is widely acknowledged that these parties have spread to even the smallest communities. Efforts to draw large numbers to raves in larger cities often lead to advertising in surrounding, smaller areas. The continued popularity of raves and the documented potential negative consequences of use of the club drugs (Ecstasy in particular) suggest that these substances are and will continue to be targets of prevention and intervention efforts.

The 2002 Monitoring the Future study data suggest that past-year lysergic acid diethylamide (LSD) use significantly decreased from rates reported during 2001, while use of all other hallucinogens has not significantly changed since 1999 (Johnston et al., 2002, 2003). The differential diagnosis issues facing providers working with clients or patients who report LSD or hallucinogen use and/or who demonstrate symptoms associated with schizophrenia raise noteworthy issues in their assessment. Additionally, the extraordinary difficulty in documenting doses of hallucinogen use (particularly with mushrooms) contributes to assessment difficulties.

The rate of more than one in six eighth-grade students reporting that they have used inhalants in their lifetime suggests that this is a behavior for which assessment and, as part of assessment, screening efforts will need to be developed, implemented, and evaluated. Given this rate, routine screening by medical providers could possibly be part of an early detection and prevention program.

Finally, steroid use continues to be a behavior that brings athletes under scrutiny, both in professional and collegiate realms. Steroids can be taken orally or be injected, and in addition to potential negative consequences associated with steroids themselves, the injection practices of an individual can potentially be very dangerous (particularly if needle sharing occurs).

There are a number of valid and reliable measures for the assessment of alcohol use (i.e., patterns, quantity, frequency), consequences, and risk factors. Furthermore, there are a number of measures for the use of drugs in general (e.g., Timeline Followback [TLFB] for Drugs from Sobell et al. [1996]; Drug History Questionnaire [DHQ] from Sobell, Kwan, & Sobell, [1995]; the Drug Abuse Screening Test [DAST] from Skinner [1982]; and the Customary Drinking and Drug Use Record [CDDR] from Brown et al. [1998]). However, surveys, questionnaires, or measures exclusively targeting the substances discussed in this chapter, if they do exist, have been created by altering existing measures for the purposes of particular research projects, without detailed measurement analysis of the measures' psychometrics. This does not, however, mean that the assessment of the use of these substances, the consequences associated with their use, and factors affecting treatment or counseling cannot take place. To do so, one must understand the domains for assessment, the limitations inherent to these domains, and alternative approaches to assessment.

Substance abuse and substance dependence are the diagnostic categories described in the *Diagnostic and Statistical Manual of Mental Disorders* (fourth edition, text revision) (DSM-IV-TR; American Psychiatric Association, 2000). The criteria for substance abuse involve meeting one (or more) of four criteria over a 12-month period. These criteria include (1) recurrent substance use resulting in a failure to fulfill role obligations at work, school, or home; (2) recurrent substance use in situations in which it is physically hazardous; (3) recurrent substance-related legal problems; and (4) continued substance use despite having persistent or recurrent social or interpersonal problems caused or exacerbated by the effects of the substance.

Dependence involves a set of seven criteria; for diagnosis, three or more of the following must occur at any time during the same 12-month period: (1) tolerance; (2) withdrawal; (3) taking the substance over a longer period of time or in larger amounts than was intended; (4) a persistent desire or unsuccessful efforts to cut down or control use; (5) a great deal of time spent in activities to get, use, or recover from the effects of the substance; (6) giving up or reducing important social, occupational, or recreational activities because of the activity; and (7) continuing use despite having persistent or recurrent physical or psychological problems caused or exacerbated by use of the substance. If three or more criteria are met, the provider specifies whether the client or patient meets criteria for dependence with physiological dependence (evidenced by experiencing tolerance or withdrawal) or dependence without physiological dependence (with no evidence of tolerance or withdrawal). If no criteria have been met for at least 1 month, one of four course specifiers describing remission status is selected (early full, early partial, sustained full, or sustained partial). Two remaining course specifiers are used if the client or patient is on agonist therapy (e.g., methadone maintenance) or in a controlled environment (restricting access to substances, such as a locked hospital unit) such that, again, no criteria are met in the month preceding assessment. Issues in assessment and diagnosis with the drugs reviewed in this chapter are discussed, including instances in which the previous criteria may be met (e.g., withdrawal, tolerance), as are substance-induced psychological problems for consideration when ruling in or ruling out other diagnoses.

The assessment of alcohol use differs dramatically from the assessment of other drug use, primarily along the dimension of specifying dose and amount. While the percentage of alcohol by volume can be easily determined, and while standard drinks for dosing purposes can be determined with similar ease, identifying and describing the dose of a drug for which dosing cannot be determined (percentage of tetrahydrocannabinol [THC] in marijuana, potency of Ecstasy, amount of gas inhaled, etc.) are significant limitations to trying to determine quantity of use. Frequency of use, on the other hand, can be described. Interview approaches and published measures for detailing substance use are described. Additionally, we examine approaches to assessing drug-related negative consequences.

Also important to assessment of substance use is an assessment of the context in which that use occurs. Are there major life events that have played a part in the development of a person's substance use, including initiating use, contributing to relapse, or promoting cessation of use? What is the person's family history related to substance use? Is the person currently dealing with other issues? What does the person expect the drug will do for him or her? Answers to these questions are essential to treatment planning and therapy. Additionally, in the midst of assessing behaviors that can feel overwhelming and that seem to review content largely associated with negative connotations, it is important to evaluate an individual's strengths and what is going well for him or her. What coping skills does the person already have in place? Has he or she already made significant changes in their use or experienced past successes in attempting to quit or alter behavior? We discuss approaches to this assessment as well.

Alternatives to surveys, measures, and interviews that involve detecting recent and past substance use enter the biological and physical realm. Blood tests and urinalysis to detect the substances discussed in this chapter are examined, and any additional physiological screens are described.

Finally, assessment of predictors of, or barriers to, treatment success can be made primarily in the area of assessing risk factors for relapse. We describe the assessment of motivation, high-risk situations, cue reactivity, cravings/urges, and one's support system as a component of treatment planning and measuring treatment outcome.

CLUB DRUGS, HALLUCINOGENS, INHALANTS, AND ANABOLIC–ANDROGENIC STEROIDS

There are a number of factors to consider when assessing the quantity and frequency of drug use, including the names by which participants and clients know the substances, the possible routes of administration and dosing information, and how long a given substance can be detected in blood or urine. A substance may have any number of trade or street names associated with it, which can complicate assessment of use. For example, individuals may report frequent use of MDMA, commonly known as *Ecstasy*, when what they have actually used is GHB, also known as *liquid Ecstasy*, or use of *Blue Vials* (LSD) when what they meant was *Blue Nile* (MDMA). Dosing information is important, since two individuals who both report using a particular substance on 5 occasions during the past month may have consumed vastly different quantities of the drug. Operationalizing quantity can be very difficult given that individuals rarely carefully measure their doses, and the concentration or purity of a particular substance may change from use to use (e.g., all capfuls of GHB do not contain the same concentration of the drug, nor do all MDMA tablets have the same ratio of MDMA to adulterants). Therefore, using alternative methods to self-report, such as the analysis of concentrations in blood and urine, may be necessary to get an accurate picture of use. But this too is problematic, since many drugs are completely evacuated from the system within a matter of hours and are not tested for in standard drug screens. When assessing negative consequences associated with the use of a particular substance, it is also important to know other substances with which it might interact. Many assessments do not take into account use of multiple substances when assessing negative consequences associated with a single drug. For example, individuals may report several consequences associated with their GHB use, but the severity of some of these consequences may be due to their use of GHB in combination with alcohol or other central nervous system depressants. Thus, assessing not only the number and type of consequences associated with the substance of interest but also the larger drug use context within which they occurred may be important when developing treatments and interventions. The notion of shifting focus in clinical trials research (and, in turn, assessment) from a single drug toward the possibility of a wide range of psychoactive substance use has been raised by Rounsaville, Petry, and Carroll (2003). All of the drugs discussed here are described at greater length in Kilmer, Cronce, and Palmer (2005).

MDMA is most widely known as Ecstasy but goes by more than 150 pseudonyms, some of which include Adam, Batmans, Blue Nile, Care Bears, Clarity, Doctor, E, Four Leaf Clover, Hug Drug, Kleenex, Lover's Speed, Mercedes, Playboy Bunnies, Scooby Snacks, Smurfs, Stars, Supermans, Wheels, X, and XTC (Office of National Drug Control Policy, 2004a). MDMA acts as a central nervous system stimulant. Ecstasy is distributed in tablets of various shapes and colors, and on average, users report consuming 1 to 2 tablets per occasion (Parrott & Lasky, 1998; Parrott et al., 2002). Tablets are typically consumed orally, although they may be used as a suppository; they can also be ground into powder and snorted, added to drugs that are smoked or dissolved in a solution and injected (Parrott, 2001; Drug Enforcement Administration, 2004a). The amount of MDMA in each tablet is generally assumed to be approximately 100 mg (Drug Enforcement Administration, 2004a); however, the exact concentration of MDMA and drug content in each tablet is highly variable and often unknown to the user. An Ecstasy tablet can include a number of different drugs (e.g., dextromethorphan, ketamine, methylenedioxyamphetamine and paramethoxyamphetamine), in addition to or in the absence of MDMA (Cole, Bailey, Sumnall, Wagstaff, & King, 2002; DanceSafe, 2004; Parrott, 2004). A recent review suggested that the vast majority (between 80% to 100%) of Ecstasy tablets currently in circulation are at least *partially* composed of MDMA, but this estimate may be biased due to nonrandom sampling procedures (Parrott, 2004). Whenever possible, self-reported Ecstasy use should not be used as the only means of quantifying MDMA use. MDMA has a half-life of approximately 9 hours (de la Torre et al., 2000), and the presence of MDMA in bodily fluids may return a positive result for amphetamines on a standard toxicology screen, especially if a lower threshold (300 ng/ml) is used (Dupont & Verebey, 1994). Reports vary in terms of how long MDMA can be detected in blood and urine, with most estimates somewhere in the range of 1 to 3 days (Johnson, 2003; Kalant, 2001; Verebey, Alrazi, & Jaffee, 1988; Verstraete, 2004; Wolff et al., 1999). Use of MDMA in combination with monoamine oxidase inhibitors (MAOIs) or HIV-1 protease inhibitors, ritonavir in particular, may result in a serious and potentially lethal adverse reaction (Antoniou & Tseng, 2002; Gahlinger, 2001; Harrington, Woodward, Hooton, & Horn, 1999).

Ketamine hydrochloride (ketamine) is known by a number of different names including Cat Valium, Jet, Ket, Kit Kat, Purple, Green, Super C, Special K, Vitamin K, Ketalar, Ketajet, Ketaset, Ketavet, and Vetelar (Office of National Drug Control Policy, 2002b; Gahlinger, 2001; Siegel, 1978). Ketamine, a dissociative anesthetic with hallucinogenic properties, is commonly sold as a liquid or powder, and sometimes in the form of capsules and tablets (Diversion Control Program, 2004a; Johnson, 2003). Ketamine can be snorted, injected, swallowed, or smoked (Drug Enforcement Administration, 2004b). A dose is typically 40 mg when snorted (Diverson Control Program, 2004a), or between 1 and 2 mg/kg when injected (Siegel, 1978); multiple smaller doses may be taken until the desired effect is reached. Ketamine has a half-life of approximately 2–3 hours (Facts and Comparisons, 2004; Persson et al., 2002), and it can be detected in urine for 1 to 2 days (Norchem, 2004). Ketamine use may also be detected by the presence of its metabolites, norketamine and dehydronorketamine, in urine (Moore, Sklerov, Levine, & Jacobs, 2001). Concurrent use of ketamine and certain antiretroviral drugs that may potentially interfere with its metabolism could lead to an accumulation of ketamine in the body and unexpected reactions or overdose (Antoniou & Tseng, 2002).

GHB is known by over 25 names, some of which include Cherry Meth, Easy Lay, Goop, Georgia Home Boy, Grievous Bodily Harm, Liquid E, Liquid Ecstasy, Liquid X, Salty Water, Vita G, and Scoop (Office of National Drug Control Policy, 2002c). GHB, a central nervous system depressant, is distributed in liquid, powder, or tablet form (Nicholson & Balster, 2001; Center for Disease Control, 1991). Individual doses are usually sold by the teaspoon- or capful; however, it is hard to establish a standard dose given variable concentration, the potential presence of adulterants, and imprecise measurement (Chin, Kreutzer, & Dyer, 1992; Freese, Miotto, & Reback, 2002; Schwartz, Milteer, & Le Beau, 2000). Sedative effects can be felt at doses as low as 10 mg/kg (Chin et al., 1992). GHB is rapidly metabolized and has a half-life of approximately 20–30 minutes (Li, Stokes, & Woeckener, 1998; Smith et al., 2002). It can be detected in blood and urine for five and twelve hours, respectively (Verstraete, 2004), and in a hair sample several weeks after a single use (Kintz, Cirimele, Jamey, & Ludes, 2003). Use of GHB with methamphetamine may result in seizures and/or coma, and combination with alcohol may potentiate the depressant effects (Johnson, 2003). Concomitant use of GHB and the HIV-1 protease inhibitors ritonavir and saquinavir has been associated with serious adverse reactions (Harrington et al., 1999).

LSD is commonly called Acid but is associated with over 175 terms describing the drug, its use, and its users. Some of these include Blotter, Blue Heaven, Blue Vials, Chocolate Chips, Coffee, Conductor, Cupcakes, Dots, Electric Kool Aid, Microdot, Pane, South Parks, Strawberry Fields, Sugar Cubes, Sunshine, Superman, White Lightning, and Zen (Office of National Drug Control Policy, 2002d). LSD, a powerful hallucinogen, is sold in gelatin squares (window pane), blotter paper, microdots, capsules, sugar cubes, and liquid (Drug Enforcement Administration, 2004c; Johnson, 2003; Kuhn, Swartzwelder, & Wilson, 2003; National Institute on Drug Abuse, 2004a). Recreational doses can range from 20 to 300 micrograms, with each unit of distribution (i.e., individual microdot or blotter paper square) representing a single dose (Drug Enforcement Administration, 2004c; Kuhn et al., 2003l Ungerleider & Pechnick, 1999). Depending on the size of the dose, LSD can typically be detected in urine for 8 to 24 hours (Johnson, 2003; Verstraete, 2004; Wolffe, 1999). Use of marijuana or Prozac, a selective serotonin reuptake inhibitor (SSRI), may trigger flashbacks in heavy LSD users (Kuhn et al., 2003). LSD may also have harmful interactions with certain antiretroviral medications (Antoniou & Tseng, 2002).

Dextromethorphan, a cough suppressant commonly in over-the-counter (OTC) medications that has dissociative effects when misused (National Institute on Drug Abuse, 2004b), is sometimes known as DM, DXM, Robo, Velvet, or Rojo (Diversion Control Program, 2004b; Gahlinger, 2001). It is also sold in powder, pill, and capsule form, and is sometimes a constituent in Ecstasy tablets (Diversion Control Program, 2004b). The concentration of dextromethorphan varies from 1 to 5 mg/ml between cough syrups (Darboe, 1996), and the average therapeutic dose is 15–30 mg, repeated every 3–4 hours (Diversion Control Program, 2004b). Recreational doses are typically much higher, upwards of 240 mg (Darboe, 1996; Diversion Control Program, 2004b). Depending on the dosage used and individual differences in metabolism, dextromethorphan may be detected in urine up to 72 hours after administration (Schadel, Wu, Otton, Kalow, Sellers, 1995).

Inhalants encompass a wide range of volatile solvents, anesthetic gases, and nitrites. Some of the names by which inhalants are known refer to all inhalants, such as Air Blast, Bullet Bolt, Hippie Crack, Huff, Oz, Poor Man's Pot, and Spray, whereas other terms refer to particular chemicals that are abused as inhalants, including Aimies or Amys (amyl nitrite), Poppers (amyl or butyl nitrite), Texas Shoe Shine or Tolly (toluene), and Laughing Gas or Whippets (nitrous oxide) (Office of National Drug Control Policy, 2002e).

Still other terms can refer to specific inhalants or broadly to all inhalants, such as Locker Room, Quicksilver, or Whiteout (Office of National Drug Control Policy, 2002e). Chemicals used as inhalants can be found in a number of common household items, including felt-tip markers, correction fluid, cooking sprays, glue, air fresheners, nail polish removers, and whipped cream dispensers. Inhalants can be sniffed, snorted, huffed (i.e., inhaling vapors from a chemical soaked rag placed over the nose and mouth), or bagged (i.e., placing an inhalant in a plastic bag, and then putting the bag over the nose and mouth, and inhaling the fumes). Most inhalants act as central nervous system depressants, the effects of which are rapid and transient but can be maintained through repeated, successive use (Meredith, Ruprah, Liddle, & Flanagan, 1989). Nitrites, the exception, act as vasodilators (National Institute on Drug Abuse, 2003). Given the number of substances in this category and individual differences in lung capacity, it would be impossible to quantify the amount of specific chemicals that are inhaled in a single dose (i.e., one sniff). Users may have a preference for a single inhalant or utilize several different inhalants; thus it is important to probe for the exact substances used and their chemical composition (Dinwiddie, 1994; Sharp & Rosenberg, 1997). Depending on the dose inhaled, it may be possible to detect inhalant use by a chemical smell on a user's breath up to 24 hours after last use (Meredith et al., 1989). Estimates for how long inhalant use can be detected in bodily fluids vary by dose and substance. Use of many inhalants may no longer be detectable in blood after 10 hours; however, samples have tested positive for the presence of certain inhalants or their metabolites (i.e., toluene or 2, 2, 2-trichloroethanol, a metabolite of trichloroethylene) up to 48 hours after use (Meredith et al., 1989). Use of certain inhalants can also be detected by the presence of their metabolites in urine (Ramsey, Anderson, Bloor, & Flanagan, 1989). Using inhalants with alcohol, opiates, barbiturates, quaaludes, benzodiazepines, and some OTC cold medications may lead to serious health consequences (Kuhn et al., 2003).

Anabolic–androgenic steroids are known by an assortment of street names including Juice, Roids, Arnolds, Gym Candy, and Pumpers (Galloway, 1997; Office of National Drug Control Policy, 2002f). Steroids are also referred to by specific trade names, such as Anadrol, Maxibolin, or Proviron (administered orally), Deca-Duabolin, Dep-Testosterone or Trophobolene (administered through injection) (Office of National Drug Control Policy, 2002f). Anabolic–androgenic steroids are synthetic hormones that promote increases in muscle mass (anabolic) and masculine characteristics (androgenic). Users may take several different steroids in the same time period (i.e., stacking) or alternate use of individual drugs; users often cycle on and off of a given drug, using it only for a few weeks or months at a time (Brower, Blow, Young, & Hill, 1991). The period of detection of steroid use in urine is widely variable (from 3 weeks to 9 months; Onsite Drug Testing, 2004), and is dependent on both the specific substance or substances used and the route of administration.

DIAGNOSIS

When using the *Diagnostic and Statistical Manual of Mental Disorders* (fourth edition, text revision) (DSM-IV-TR), a clinician should not only use the code that applies to the class of substance but also list the name of the specific substance rather than the class of drugs to which it belongs (American Psychiatric Association, 2000). Hallucinogen use disorders and hallucinogen-induced disorders (MDMA is listed in this section), inhalant use disorders and inhalant-induced disorders, and phencyclidine or phencyclidine-related disorders (ketamine is listed as a related substance) are established diagnostic categories within DSM-IV-TR. Under other (or unknown) substance-related disorders, anabolic steroids, nitrite inhalants, and nitrous oxide are listed (American Psychiatric Association, 2000).

In most studies' discussion of dependence issues, the presence of a withdrawal syndrome when the drug leaves the body is often highlighted as a possible symptom of dependence. However, some studies have looked at specific issues around dependence and, for the substances described in this chapter, we will describe ways in which criteria for abuse and dependence may be met when published examples are available.

Anabolic–Androgenic Steroids

After describing what the authors believed was the first published case report of anabolic–androgenic steroid dependence (Brower, Blow, Beresford, & Fuelling, 1989), Brower, Blow, et al. (1991) have detailed the ways in which the criteria for substance dependence, detailed earlier, can be met by users of anabolic–androgenic steroids. They looked at the self-report of DSM-III-R criteria endorsed by 49 steroid users in a questionnaire modifying two existing structured diagnostic measures. At least one symptom of dependence was endorsed by 94% of the sample. Three or more symptoms, required for a diagnosis of dependence, were endorsed by 57% of the participants. Complaints of withdrawal symptoms once abstinence was initiated were endorsed by 84% of the sample. Common signs of steroid withdrawal include fatigue, dysphoria, restlessness, anorexia, headaches, inability to sleep, an urge to take more anabolic–androgenic steroids, and lowered libido. The most commonly endorsed symptoms related to withdrawal were a desire to take more steroids (52%), fatigue (43%), dissatisfaction with body image (42%), and depressed mood (41%). The three dependence criteria most frequently endorsed after withdrawal were (1) taking more of the substance than was intended (endorsed by 51%), (2) expending a great deal of time toward getting, using, or recovering from the effects of the substance (endorsed by 40%), and (3) continued use of steroids despite problems caused or exacerbated by use (37%). These three, along with withdrawal, are still utilized as criteria for dependence in DSM-IV-TR.

To corroborate these data, an earlier study by Brower, Eliopulos, Blow, Catlin, and Beresford (1990) showed that all eight steroid users in a pilot study reported symptoms consistent with DSM-III-R substance dependence criteria. All eight participants in this study reported continued use despite adverse consequences, and every participant reported withdrawal symptoms. Gruber and Pope (2000) found that 76% of a sample of 25 women who used steroids reported at least one adverse medical effect due to steroid use, and 64% reported at least one adverse psychological effect attributed to steroid use.

Brower, Catlin, Blow, Elipulos, and Beresford (1991) explained that individuals may present for care with either side effects or consequences of use as their presenting problem, while not reporting their steroid use. They suggest that urine tests can be important to assessment and treatment planning to rule out causes of related complaints. They report that tests may be indicated when the clinical history and physical, mental status, and laboratory examinations are indicative of steroid use while the patient denies use, and as an adjunct to treatment to monitor the course of abstinence.

Finally, because steroid users may not see their use as a substance abuse problem, they may have many different issues related to treatment once a diagnosis is made. For example, Hays, Littleton, and Stillner (1990) described the case of a 22-year-old male who, they concluded, was dependent on anabolic steroids and did not feel that he "fit in with the alcoholics and addicts" on their chemical dependence unit.

Of course, even when not a dependence or abuse issue, there are clinical signs of possible use that can prompt a more thorough assessment. Brower (1992) explained that the presence of one or more of the following physical signs should signal the possibility of steroid use: high blood pressure; rapid weight gain, with maintenance of or increase in lean body mass; acne; needle marks in large muscle groups; male pattern baldness; hirsutism in females (excessive hair); jaundice; jaundiced eyes; deepened voice in females; gynecomastia in males (breast development); atrophied breasts in females; abdominal tenderness in the right upper quadrant; hepatomegaly (enlargement of the liver); testicular atrophy; prostatic hypertrophy (enlarged prostate) in males; clitoral hypertrophy in females; muscular hypertrophy; disproportionate development of the upper torso; and edema (swelling) in the extremities.

Steroid users who exhibit one or more of the following signs may require therapeutic attention: reduced attention or distractibility, as with delirium or mania; psychomotor agitation or retardation, consistent with manic or depressive disorders; euphoria; irritability; depression; anxiety; labile affect, with abrupt mood shifts; slowed thought process, with depressive states; rapid or disorganized thought process with manic states or delirium; suicidal or homicidal thoughts; and grandiose or persecutory thoughts, delusions, or hallucinations.

Brower (1992) suggested that laboratory tests be conducted with persons suspected of steroid use to examine the possible physical impact, including tests of liver function, muscle enzymes, cholesterol profile, hematocrit and hemoglobin, endocrine tests of the pituitary–gonadal axis, semen analysis, and cardiac function tests.

Inhalants

Keriotis and Upadhyaya (2000) described a case of a 14-year-old boy whose withdrawal symptoms from inhalant use were described as intense craving, increased irritability, poor attention and concentration, bilateral hand tremors, cold sweats, diarrhea, increased tension and anxiety, constant hand wringing, and general restlessness. After 7 days in the hospital, his physical symptoms improved, but he continued to have intense cravings. They noted that there were no inhalant-specific withdrawal scales to quantify his experiences formally, so scales for alcohol were utilized. Keriotis and Upadhyaya concluded that their case supported withdrawal symptoms despite the lack of a formal inhalant withdrawal diagnostic category in DSM-IV, and reported that withdrawal symptoms can mimic symptoms of anxiety and affective disorder. Kono and colleagues (2001) demonstrated, in a sample of six participants meeting criteria for inhalant dependence, that withdrawal from inhalants produced symptoms with a mild intensity. Symptoms endorsed by at least one of the six participants on subjective measures of symptom intensity included craving, anxiety, restlessness, inattentiveness, insomnia, tachycardia, perspiration, shivering, appetite increases, appetite loss, and tremors. Shah, Vankar, and Upadhyaya (1999) suggested that gasoline withdrawal symptoms are similar to alcohol and sedative/hypnotic withdrawal syndromes. While there are DSM-IV-TR criteria for inhalant dependence and inhalant abuse, Beauvais and Oetting (1987) suggest making a distinction that classifies users of inhaled substances, with "inhalant" as the descriptor for patterns of use of volatile hydrocarbons, and establishes specific labels for abuse of anesthetic gases and nitrites.

Club Drugs (MDMA/Ecstasy, Ketamine, and GHB)

Jansen (1999) described three case studies in which criteria for dependence on Ecstasy were met. In the first case description, a 19-year-old male routinely stayed awake almost continuously for an "80-hour weekend" and recovered the remaining part of the week. He spent almost all of his disposable income on MDMA and amphetamine, developed tolerance, and described extreme fatigue and low mood after use stopped. In a second case example, a 30-year-old male who became highly tolerant to MDMA was severely depressed, saw his Ecstasy use as a cause of his depression but nevertheless continued using, lost his job, his residence, and saw a relationship end. He was also dependent on opiates and benzodiazepines, and reported drinking heavily. Finally, a third case example involved a 25-year-old male with posttraumatic stress disorder, who sold "everything he owned" to buy MDMA, went without sleeping or eating for days at a time, drank one bottle of whiskey almost nightly (noting that the Ecstasy prevented him from becoming drunk), developed tolerance, and continued using despite evidence of harm to himself. Jansen concluded that all three cases experienced a strong desire to take the drug, difficulty controlling behavior, tolerance, neglecting alternative activities, continued use of a drug despite having problems caused or exacerbated by MDMA use, and withdrawal evidenced and manifested by fatigue, depression, anxiety, and sleep disturbances.

Jansen and Darracot-Cankovic (2001) reported that tolerance to ketamine develops quickly and can be very pronounced, yet also state that there is little evidence of physical dependence and no evidence of a physical withdrawal syndrome.

Price (2000) described what he believes to be the first reported case of in-patient detoxification from GHB, and Galloway et al. (1997) reported on cases of GHB dependence, with withdrawal symptoms including anxiety, tremors, muscular cramping, insomnia, and "feelings of doom." Galloway and colleagues noted that physical dependence may develop after use of high doses, and that the illicit manufacturing of GHB leads to doses and purity that are likely unknown. McDaniel and Miotto (2001) described five case reports of GHB and/or GBL users; all five cases reported tolerance, craving, and withdrawal symptoms upon cessation of use, and resolution of craving and symptoms upon returning to use. Withdrawal symptoms developed within 2–8 hours of the last ingested dose, and the withdrawal syndrome continued for 3–13 days. In general, mild withdrawal was associated with anxiety, tremor, insomnia, tachycardia, mild blood pressure elevation, and aspartate aminotransferase (AST) elevation. Severe withdrawal symptoms included 3–4 days of autonomic instability, psychosis, and delirium. As vital signs from severe withdrawal normalized, mental status improved over the following 4–7 days. McDaniel and Miotto conclude that withdrawal from GHB is similar to withdrawal from alcohol and benzodiazepines.

Hallucinogens

The prevalence of hallucinogen abuse and dependence with LSD appears low in population studies. In a research project examining the role of genetic and environmental factors in a group 1,934 female twins (500 monozygotic pairs, 326 dizygotic pairs, and 282 women whose twin was not interviewed), the lifetime prevalence of hallucinogen use was 10.4%, with a low .9% meeting DSM-IV criteria for abuse, and .2% meeting criteria for dependence (Kendler, Karkowski, & Prescott, 1999).

Polysubstance Use

Polysubstance use needs to be evaluated with clients or patients reporting use of any of the drugs described in this chapter. Sharp and Rosenberg (1997) noted that alcohol is a common secondary drug of abuse for those who abuse inhalants, so assessing alcohol consumption and use of other drugs will help to put inhalant use into a sharper context. Dinwiddie, Reich, and Cloninger (1991) reported that in a sample of 130 solvent abusers, only one participant reported exclusive use of solvents but no other class of illicit drug, with over two-thirds of their sample reporting use of every class of drug assessed in their study (i.e., cannabis, opioids, stimulants, depressants, and hallucinogens). Additionally, alcohol use preceded inhalant use for the majority of participants. While they acknowledge limitations to generalizability from their sample, the study conducted by Dinwiddie and colleagues highlights the potential polysubstance use practices of inhalant users.

Additional Diagnostic Issues

While abuse or dependence can be diagnosed, there are also other disorders related to the use of the substances discussed in this chapter. First, we discuss issues in the diagnosis of flashbacks, or hallucinogen persisting perception disorder (292.89 in DSM-IV-TR).

Hallucinogen Persisting Perception Disorder

Hallucinogen persisting perception disorder (HPPD) is characterized by re-experiencing one or more of the perceptual symptoms experienced while intoxicated with a hallucinogen, once use of the hallucinogen has stopped. These can include seeing trails behind moving images, halos around objects (anecdotally, several clients complain of seeing halos around lights), false perceptions of movement in the peripheral visual fields, and so on. While these disturbances may subside after several months, many report episodes persisting for much longer (American Psychiatric Association, 2000). To meet criteria for HPPD, these symptoms cannot be due to a general medical condition or be better accounted for by another mental disorder, and the "flashbacks" must cause distress or impairment in an individual's functioning. Abraham and Mamen (1996) explained that in their work with three people reporting problems with HPPD, each individual knew that the visual disturbances were "not real." When these individuals were treated with risperidone, the visual symptoms related to HPPD were intensified and symptoms of panic suddenly developed. Morehead (1997) agreed with their findings, describing a fourth case example in which HPPD symptoms were worsened with risperidone treatment.

Lerner, Finkel, Oyffe, Merenzon, and Sigal (1998) suggested that clonidine be used to treat HPPD given the potential for abuse of benzodiazepines, and, from the same research group, Lerner, Oyffe, Isaacs, and Sigal (1997) also suggest that naltrexone can be useful in some patients, because of the lack of consistent effectiveness with benzodiazepine treatment. Recently, Lerner, Skladman, Kodesh, Sigal, and Shufman (2001) described two cases in which clonazepam resulted in significant improvement. Lerner's team concluded that controlled trials are needed to evaluate the various pharmacological approaches to treating HPPD. Aldurra and Crayton (2001) presented a case study in which improvement in HPPD was seen following a treatment combining fluoxetine (e.g., Prozac) and olanzapine (i.e., Zyprexa).

Substance-Induced Psychotic Disorder
(with Specific Type of Substance Specified in the Diagnosis)

Dewhurst and Hatrick (1972) analyzed case histories of 19 LSD users who were patients in British mental hospitals, and described a wide variety of psychiatric symptoms in the sample, ranging from apathy in only 3 of the 19 patients to thought disorder in 16 of the 19 patients. They concluded that the frequency of thought disorder, auditory hallucinations, disturbed behavior, and paranoid delusions in their population of LSD users makes it difficult to distinguish substance-induced psychotic problems from schizophrenia. Acute hallucinogen-induced psychosis can be difficult to distinguish from an acute schizophrenic reaction; however, Ungergleider and Pechnick (1999) reported that hallucinations in schizophrenic psychosis are predominantly auditory, in contrast to the predominantly visual hallucinations stemming from hallucinogen use.

The use of inhalants containing toluene (e.g., paint remover, paint thinners, correction fluid) seems to play a particularly important role in the experience of inhalant-induced psychotic problems (Hernandez-Avila, Ortega-Soto, Jasso, Hasfura-Buenaga, & Kranzler, 1998), so the client's reported history of inhalant use will be important to determining the nature of his or her symptoms. Complicating differential diagnosis with the inhalant user is the observation that users have more severe and chronic psychopathology when compared to polydrug users and controls (Korman, Trimboli, & Semler, 1980).

As a drug with both hallucinogenic and stimulant properties, Ecstasy also can lead to both persistent flashbacks and drug-induced psychosis (Creighton, Black, & Hyde, 1991). Van Kampen and Katz (2001) described the case of an 18-year-old female for whom psychotic symptoms, including disorganized thought form, delusional ideation, and ideas of reference, emerged following a single use of MDMA and persisted for 12 weeks. Additionally, Galloway and colleagues (1997) described the case of a 22-year-old female who used GHB in combination with MDMA, became agitated and delusional, and appeared to suffer from a drug-induced psychosis.

Substance-Induced Mood Disorder
(with Specific Type of Substance Specified in the Diagnosis)

Abraham and Fava (1999) evaluated 374 consecutive outpatients with major depression to determine whether specific types of drug abuse preceded or followed the onset of depression. Across all drug categories, drug-dependent individuals had a mean age for first depression of 17.6 years, compared to 24.8 years in non-drug-dependent patients. Sedatives, opioids, and cannabis were associated with a mean of 3.7 lifetime depressive episodes compared to 12.2 episodes in polydrug, LSD, and cocaine users. Of note is that the age of onset of drug use was consistently later than the age of onset for depression, with the exception of LSD. The emergence of depressive symptoms with the onset of LSD use complicates differential diagnosis.

Duggal, Sinha, and Nizamie (2000) described the case of an 18-year-old male with a dual diagnosis of bipolar disorder with comorbid dependence on gasoline inhalation who was initially diagnosed with inhalant-induced psychotic disorder. A key to diagnosing this man with a dual diagnosis was a second admission, during which he remained symptomatic despite having achieved 1 month's abstinence. The authors noted the importance of observing symptoms during abstinence for at least 1 month when a dual diagnosis is approached.

Substance-Induced Anxiety Disorder (with Specific Type of Substance Specified in the Diagnosis)

There is little published in the area of anxiety disorder induced by the substances discussed in this chapter. However, Windhaber, Maierhofer, and Dantendorfer (1998) described the case of a 21-year-old male who had a panic attack while using Ecstasy and later developed panic disorder that the authors described as MDMA induced. Additional research on this particular diagnosis is warranted.

Polysubstance Dependence

Criteria for polysubstance dependence are met if at least three groups of substances, excluding caffeine and nicotine, are used during the same 12-month period, with dependence criteria met for the substances as a group but not for any specific substance (American Psychiatric Association, 2000).

Ruling Out Concurrent Psychiatric Disorders

With so many consequences of use mimicking the symptoms or contributing to the problems experienced with other disorders, properly understanding and diagnosing the presenting problems involve exploring the involvement, or lack thereof, of the person's substance use.

With steroid users, ruling out bipolar disorder based on presenting symptoms may be needed. In steroid users, manic-like features may be present, including a sense of power and invincibility, hostility and aggressiveness, increased sexual appetite, unpredictable and restless behavior (including tics), poor impulse control, mood problems, and insomnia (Rashid, 2000; Leckman & Scahill, 1990). Supporting the reports of manic-like features, Pope and Katz (1988) also stated that 12.2% of their sample met criteria for a manic episode during steroid exposure, with an additional 19.5% narrowly missing a diagnosis of a manic episode (i.e., they met all but one of the first three DSM criteria).

Ruling out depressive disorders may also be necessary. Allnutt and Chaimowitz (1994) described the case of a 20-year-old male presenting with depression and suicidal ideation that were related to discontinuing anabolic steroids 2 months earlier.

A number of symptoms that can accompany steroid use highlights the need for differential diagnosis. Pope and Katz (1988) reported that serious psychiatric problems can be an effect of steroid use, including depression, paranoid ideation, audible thoughts, euphoria, irritability, racing thoughts, or hyperactivity, and found that 12.2% of a sample of steroid users met DSM-III-R criteria for psychotic symptoms during periods of steroid use. None of these five had psychotic symptoms during periods of no steroid exposure. Similarly, Annitto and Layman (1980) described the case of a 17-year-old male diagnosed with schizophrenia, paranoid type. While the authors concluded that they could not rule out an organic cause to his problems, the development of symptoms in an acute schizophrenic episode appeared to have been temporally related to his anabolic steroid use.

USE AND CONSEQUENCES

The focus of the chapter is on use of club drugs, hallucinogens, inhalants, and steroids; however, a paucity of assessment methods with established psychometrics, either interview or self-report measures, specifically address these drugs and negative consequences. However, there is information on interview approaches or self-report measures that can be used to obtain information about these substances, and we review these here.

Interview Approaches

Typically, interview assessments can be categorized in one of two ways: structured or semistructured (Winters, Latimer, & Stinchfield, 2002). Structured interview assessments require that the administrator read each question word for word. If the symptom is endorsed, specific follow-up questions are asked that assess the "nature, duration, and clinical impact of the symptoms and related problems" (Winters et al., 2002, p. 1448). Usually, structured interviews can be administered with good reliability contingent on appropriate training with the instrument. Semistructured assessment interviews demand a higher level of mastery, such that the administrator must assess the presence or absence of a symptom, and additional questions tailored to the client may be needed to determine the appropriate diagnosis (Winters et al., 2002).

Some interview assessment methods may have sections that are appropriate in assessing the use of these drugs. The Comprehensive Drinker Profile (CDP; Marlatt & Miller, 1984) is an 88-item, structured clinical interview designed to assess patterns of alcohol and drug use, the biopsychosocial context within which these behaviors occur, and related negative consequences. The interview typically takes between 1 and 2 hours to complete and is divided into three major sections: demographic information, drinking history, and motivational information. Included in the drinking history section is a brief assessment of other drug use that specifically assesses inhalant and hallucinogen use and can be readily modified to assess the other drugs addressed in this chapter (i.e., club drugs and steroids). In the motivational information section are items that assess the presence of other life problems, such as depression, anxiety, aggression, and impaired social contact; the weight the individual gives to the problem (on a scale from least to most important); and whether the problem is associated with the individual's alcohol use. This item could easily be adapted to assess negative life consequences related to use of drugs discussed in this chapter, and help place an individual's drug use within a broader context. The Brief Drinker Profile (Miller & Marlatt, 1987), an abbreviated, 40-item version of the CDP, also includes the specific items described earlier.

The Individual Assessment Profile (Flynn et al., 1995), a structured assessment interview, also has a section that assesses age of initial drug use for specific drugs, frequency of use in past month and past year, as well as frequency during the highest period of use, money spent on drugs within the past month, and family history of alcohol and drug use. Developed by Miller and colleagues (Miller & Del Boca, 1994; Tonigan, Miller, & Brown, 1997), the Form 90 Drug Use Assessment is a comprehensive structured interview that also allows for the assessment of hallucinogens, steroids, inhalants, and other drugs. Although these measures assess drug use overall, they also allow clinicians to assess use of the drugs that are the focus of this chapter.

Brower (1992) explained that clinical assessment of steroid use can take the form of gathering historical information through an interview, identifying signs possibly associated with steroid use through physical examinations, identifying through a mental status examination those who may need therapeutic intervention, and looking for abnormalities in laboratory tests.

While not necessarily a strategy unique to assessing steroid use, the client or patient's defensiveness around use and way in which it is often concealed can possibly be minimized by first asking about use of legal substances and inquiring about nutrition and legal performance aids. The clinician could then ask patients if they know other people who have used or are using steroids, if they have ever used steroids and, if not, if they have ever considered using. If the clients or patients report that they have or are using steroids, their specific subjective complaints about effects associated with steroid use and withdrawal can be assessed. As far as documenting use itself, the clinician can collect information about the specific drug or drugs used, dosages, time of last use, duration of use, frequency of use, routes of administration, and possible needle sharing. Finally, criteria related to dependence and abuse can be evaluated.

Self-Report Measures

A number of self-report measures assess drug use; however, we focus on measures that specifically address the use of club drugs, hallucinogens, inhalants, and steroids. Two measures that assess issues related to what are often considered "other drugs" by most classification systems and researchers are the Drug Abuse Screening Test (DAST) and the Customary Drinking and Drug Use Record (CDDR). The DAST-10, a shortened version of the original 25-item DAST developed by Skinner (1982), asks about drug abuse within the previous year, defining "abuse" as any use of prescribed or OTC drugs that exceeds the specified amount in the instrument's directions, as well as any "nonmedical" use of drugs. The instrument's directions explain that drug use includes a number of different classes of drugs and explicitly name solvents and hallucinogens in addition to other drugs. Although club drugs or steroids are not referred to, use of these drugs can be assessed due to the definition of drug abuse in the directions. The DAST-10 focuses more specifically on the negative consequences due to the use of these drugs, rather than the amount or frequency of use. The CDDR addresses the use of hallucinogens (under which Ecstasy is included), inhalants, and other drugs, and assesses any intravenous drug use (Brown et al., 1998). Steroid use is not included in this measure; however, it is possible with the CDDR to assess steroid use through the other drug or intravenous drug use sections, because steroids can be taken orally or injected.

Assessment of Negative Consequences

The assessment of negative consequences can play a major role for a clinician attempting to discuss possible reasons for an individual to change the frequency or manner of use. The Inventory of Drug Use Consequences (InDUC) assesses negative consequences that individuals may have experienced for any drinking or drug use, although not specific to club drugs, hallucinogens, inhalants or steroids (Tonigan & Miller, 2002). However, the InDUC does tap into a broad range of negative life consequences, such as physical harm, relationship consequences, and loss of financial or social standing. The InDUC has different versions available to assess recent use, past use, or use since last interview assessment. The ability to assess at differing time points is important for monitoring decreases or increases of negative consequences. Sample items include "The quality of my work has suffered because of my drinking or drug use" and "My family has been hurt by my drinking or drug use." Overall, the InDUC is a very comprehensive assessment tool for determining negative consequences of drug use; it is also versatile enough to fit well with the drugs focused upon in this chapter. While making modifications to the instructions in order to specifically target a particular drug would alter the psychometrics of this scale, such adaptation could be an informative and necessary first step in developing more drug-specific measures.

The already mentioned CDDR (Brown et al., 1998) primarily assesses recent and lifetime drug use within the context of an interview format. Questions at the end of the assessment pertain specifically to negative consequences of use within the domains of possible legal, employment, or relationship consequences. The CDDR does assess negative consequences due to drug use more generally; sample questions include "Have you often taken drugs in larger amounts or more often than you planned to" and "Have you stopped any activity (sport, hobby, recreational activity) so you can get or use drugs?"

As acknowledged earlier, altering the measure to fit one's clinical or research needs, while impacting the measure's existing reliability and validity, could nevertheless establish a foundation for more drug-specific consequence measures once data are collected.

BIOLOGICAL/PHYSICAL SYSTEMS OF ASSESSMENT

Urine Screens

Gold and Dackis (1986) described ways in which drug testing can be used to make a differential diagnosis and eliminate substances from consideration as a cause of a range of psychological disorders. The use of oral fluid, sweat, and hair are among the least invasive methods of collecting biological samples. Testing of these matrices has rapidly become much more common and is the direction in which the field is headed, although, due to a number of factors discussed later in this chapter, their use is currently limited. Urine has become the most frequently used sample due in part to greater ease of handling samples and reduced physical intrusiveness compared to blood samples (Wolff et al., 1999). Drug tests or screens are often conducted on urine initially by enzyme immunoassay through different tests (i.e., radioimmunoassay [RIA] or enzyme multiplied immunoassay [EMIT]), and secondarily, if a positive result is found, through gas–liquid chromatography or gas chromatography–mass spectrometry (GC-MS) (Verebey & Buchan, 1997; Wolff et al., 1999).

DuPont and Verebey (1994) highlighted the importance of screening for LSD, MDMA, psilocybin, and other designer drugs that are often used recreationally yet were rarely tested for in previous years. LSD can be difficult to detect, because only low doses are needed to obtain desired pharmacological effects; nevertheless, both LSD and MDMA can be detected in blood and urine using immunoassay screens followed by confirmation using GC-MS technology (Dupont & Verebey, 1994). The cost of these tests, however, is high, in large part because of the infrequent use of the tests.

Blood Screens

Blood, which is considered to be a very useful type of sample to determine the presence of a drug, is very frequently used to assess recent drug use, and therapeutic, toxic, and lethal dose levels can be determined from the presence of the drug or drug metabolites (Wolff et al., 1999).

Liquid chromatography (LC) is one of the most useful and multipurpose tests for detecting drugs in blood, primarily due to its ability to identify a range of drugs simultaneously (Wolff et al., 1999). Another utilized technique is GC-MS; however, further testing may be needed to enhance the sensitivity of the test, and it is considered one of the more expensive tests (Verebey & Buchan, 1997). One advantage of using blood is that with the rapid elimination of some drugs from the urine; the concentration of the drug can quickly fall below detectable levels in the urine while still being able to be detected in blood. Once a drug has fallen below 5–7 half-lives, the amount of time taken for a drug to reach half of the original ingested dose, it is typically no longer detectable in the blood (Wolff et al., 1999).

Hair Analysis

Another possible biological method of testing for the use of drugs is through hair analysis. Typically, hair is collected from the head, although testing of hair from other areas, such as the arm or pubic area is possible (Cone, 1997). There are a number of advantages and disadvantages to hair analysis. Two primary advantages are that one can test for drug use as far back as 6 months, and retest samples can be easily obtained. However, there are disadvantages: The exact process of drug incorporation into hair is not fully understood, and there is some debate regarding the possible contamination of hair by the environment (Cone, 1997). As well, an important issue to consider in hair analysis is the effect of possible racial bias specific to differing levels of drugs found within the hair of Caucasians and non-Caucasians (Harkey, 1995; Cone, 1997). A study by Henderson, Harkey, Zhou, Jones, and Jacob (1998), utilizing cocaine and testing for its presence within hair across ethnic groups, found a large degree of variability between the dose given and the level of cocaine found within the analyzed hair samples. Studies conducted on the link between hair color (black and brown hair, with higher melanin content) and the presence of a drug, suggest that high levels of melanin result in greater incorporation of the drug into hair (Cone, 1996). Therefore, although hair analysis is a valuable tool in assessing long-term drug use and false-positive drug screens, the literature suggests that the results be interpreted with caution (Kintz, Cirimele, & Ludes, 2000; Cone, 1996; Henderson et al., 1998; Harkey, 1995).

In regard to hair testing and the drugs of abuse discussed in this chapter, the detection of steroid use/abuse is difficult to interpret, although it is possible, and gives the additional benefit of being able to identify the parent compound used (Kintz & Samyn, 2002). Newer hair analysis techniques have resulted in reduced costs of testing and in tests able to detect the presence of MDMA, hallucinogens, and anabolic steroids (Lachenmeier, Kroener, Musshoff, & Madea, 2003).

The Substance Abuse and Mental Health Services Administration (SAMHSA) drug testing guidelines are under evaluation for the use of oral fluid (saliva) and sweat, as well as hair, to assess workplace illicit drug use. Currently, there is a greater amount of research on the use of hair for drug testing, and as mentioned previously, although it has a number of advantages, there are also limitations to its use. Oral fluid is showing promise due to being noninvasive; swabs to collect saliva are easily used in various situations, from the laboratory to the side of the road, and have a reduced likelihood of being adulterated (Kintz & Samyn, 2002). The use of saliva to detect MDMA has been documented in the literature, although there is a paucity of research testing its use with inhalants, steroids, or hallucinogens (Kintz & Samyn, 2002; Rivier, 2000). One of the drawbacks to the use of saliva is the rapid elimination of many drugs, such that they are no longer detectable (Rivier, 2000). As well, agents such as citric acid or sour candies that may be used to increase saliva production have resulted in altered pH levels, thereby impacting the saliva–plasma ratio and the concentrations of certain drugs in the saliva (Kintz & Samyn, 2002; Rivier, 2000).

Drug testing using sweat is also noninvasive, easily obtained, and typically collected via a sweat patch that is later tested. A sweat patch may be a useful tool for ongoing monitoring of substance use; however, it would not be appropriate for an immediate drug screen (Rivier, 2000). Although the literature contains research indicating the use of a sweat patch to detect levels of MDMA and other drugs, there is little information regarding the use of a sweat patch to assess the use of hallucinogens, inhalants, or steroids (Samyn et al., 2002; Rivier, 2000). Samyn and colleagues (2002) reported that only very low concentrations of MDMA were found in forehead swipes in comparison to oral fluid concentrations, which were high enough to be detected for 5 hours.

NATIONAL SURVEYS

Even though the focus of the chapter thus far has been on clinical tools for use with an individual client or patient, it is important to be aware of national trends with particular drugs of abuse, as well as changes within these trends over time. Additionally, having accurate information about norms of actual use could be an important part of an intervention. Consequently, we briefly describe sources of this information and the assessment strategies these national resources utilize.

The Monitoring the Future study (Johnston, O'Malley, Bachman, & Schulenberg, 2004), formerly called the National High School Senior Survey, which began in 1975, is coordinated by the faculty and staff of the University of Michigan Survey Research Center. Funded by the National Institute on Drug Abuse (NIDA), the study has both cross-sectional and longitudinal components, and uses self-report measures to assess attitudes toward drugs, perceived availability of drugs, and the temporally proximal and distal drug use behaviors of thousands of adolescents and adults every year. The survey is administered each spring to three age cohorts (8th, 10th, and 12th graders) in about 400 schools nationwide; thus, individuals who are absent on the day of data collection or have dropped out of school are not included. A subsample ($n = 2,400$) is drawn from each year's group of 12th graders and randomly assigned to one of two groups (odd year or even year) for longitudinal follow-up. The 1,200 individuals from each graduating class assigned to the odd-year group are invited to complete the mailed follow-up survey in years ending with an odd number over a 12- to 14-

year period. Thus, all 2,400 individuals are invited to complete the follow-up survey a total of six to seven times. Findings on current prevalence rates and trends in drug use are published in two volumes annually.

The National Survey on Drug Use and Health (Substance Abuse and Mental Health Services Administration, 2003), previously known as the National Household Survey on Drug Abuse, began in 1971. Funded by SAMHSA, the study collects cross-sectional data on the drug use behaviors of approximately 70,000 individuals each year. The survey includes both structured interview and self-report components, and is administered in the individual's place of residence. Households and group living quarters (such as college dormitories and homeless shelters) are randomly selected from all 50 states and the District of Columbia, and within each household or group, individuals age 12 or older are randomly selected to participate in the survey. While educational status does not affect who is included in the sample, active members of the armed services, individuals in mental health and medical institutions or corrections facilities, and homeless individuals not residing in a shelter at the time of the survey are not eligible for inclusion. It is also important to note that due to changes in the content of the survey, researchers should be careful when drawing conclusions from a comparison of data obtained in the 2002 survey and previous years.

The Youth Risk Behavior Surveillance System survey (Centers for Disease Control, 2004), initiated in 1990 by the Centers for Disease Control, assesses drug and other health risk behaviors (including diet, exercise, and sexual behaviors) biannually in a nationally representative, cross-sectional sample of thousands of students (grades 9 through 12) drawn from both public and private high schools. Participants complete the self-report assessments in their classrooms during the spring. As with other school-based assessments, individuals who were not present on the day that the survey was administered were not eligible for participation.

ASSESSMENT RELATED TO RELAPSE PREVENTION AND TREATMENT

Assessment of factors besides substance use itself can be important to both treatment planning and various interventions discussed throughout treatment. Briefly, these include readiness to change, assessment of high-risk situations, and cravings and urges. While some existing measures describe "drug use" or "substance use" generically, several specifically target alcohol or tobacco use, and may seem less relevant to the drugs described in this chapter. It should be noted that if existing measures are changed to accommodate and fit the particular drug pattern of a client, the psychometrics (e.g., reliability, validity) of these measures change as well, and their meaning could be compromised. That said, adaptation may be the first step in scale development, and subsequent psychometric studies could be conducted.

A client's readiness to change or motivation to change can impact the tone, style, and content of a session, and opportunities to assess this information prior to or upon working with a client exist. Prochaska and DiClemente's stages-of-change model posits that change occurs in a progression through various stages (see Prochaska & DiClemente, 1986, for a summary). A slower pace, patience, and the ability to roll with resistance may be required with the person who does not see his or her use as problematic (e.g., someone in the "precontemplation" stage), while a person already taking steps to make changes in his or her use (i.e., the "action" stage) may be ready to hear specific strategies and suggestions. Fortunately, the assessment of readiness to change and motivation can be made through a variety of measures. These include, for example, the Stages of Change Readiness and Treatment Eagerness Scale (SOCRATES; Miller & Tonigan, 1996), the University of Rhode Island Change Assessment Scale (URICA; see McConnaughy, Prochaska, & Velicer, 1983), and the Readiness-to-Change Questionnaire (see Rollnick, Heather, Gold, & Hall, 1992, for information on development and Heather, Rollnick, & Bell, 1993 for validity data). Most relevant to the substances described in this chapter is the SOCRATES.

The SOCRATES (Miller & Tonigan, 1997) does not assign an individual to one of the stages of change, but instead provides information about recognition of a problem, ambivalence, or uncertain thoughts about one's substance use and its impact, and whether steps are being taken to make changes in one's substance use. A version for use with "drug" as the topic is available. Ratings are made relative to one's agreement or disagreement with a particular statement and reflect the categories of recognition (e.g., "If I don't change my drug use soon, my problems are going to get worse"), ambivalence (e.g., "Sometimes I wonder if I am in control of my drug use"), and taking steps (e.g., "I am actively doing things now to cut down or stop my use of drugs"). Only 19 items, this measure can be administered in a time-efficient manner prior to the initiation of counseling or treatment, and/or later in counseling or treatment to assess one's motivation.

Assessment of high-risk situations, and one's confidence when in these situations, can also be used to identify areas in which coping skills training may be needed, stimuli to be initially avoided, or possible threats to one's treatment goal. Starting with past situations, the Inventory of Drug Taking Situations (IDTS; Annis, Turner, & Sklar, 1997) collects information on situations in which a client has used drugs in the past year. Respondents are presented with 50 situations and indicate their frequency of drug use (from "never" to "almost always") in each of these situations. Information from these items are divided into two classes of drug-using situations: personal states and situations involving other people. These classes are further divided into specific categories. The class of personal states is divided into categories of unpleasant emotions, physical discomfort, pleasant emotions, testing personal control, and urges/temptations to use. The class of situations involving other people is divided into categories of conflict with others, social pressure to use, and pleasant times with others.

To explore one's confidence that he or she would be able to resist the urge to use a particular substance, the Drug-Taking Confidence Questionnaire (DTCQ) can be administered (Annis, Sklar, & Turner, 1997). Utilizing of the same items from the IDTS, the DTCQ asks respondents to rate from "0" for "not at all confident" to "100" for "very confident" (in increments of 20) their perception of their ability to resist the urge to use as they imagine themselves in each situation. The same classes and categories described earlier are utilized here.

While the DTCQ provides information about one's perceived ability to resist the urge to use a substance, an adjunct to this formal measure can include daily ratings of the intensity of cravings (Daley & Marlatt, 1997). Daily ratings allow one to examine certain patterns, strongest periods of cravings, and potential decreases in cravings over time. Additionally, one can further examine particular behaviors or situations associated with days of high and low craving, to apply to subsequent efforts.

CONCLUSIONS

A recurrent theme throughout this chapter has been the lack of assessment approaches tailored specifically to the substances we address here. However, the implication of this involves less the need for measures with greater specificity and more the need to be flexible with what does exist. If attention turns fully to developing measures to address substances reviewed here, it is only a matter of time before new drugs, or new trends with existing drugs, that emerge are no longer captured by an assessment approach.

The difficulty in detailing whether a problem exists involves the definition of a problem. Focusing on the impact to the individual, particularly when there is difficulty describing the pattern, quantity, and frequency, allows one's substance use to be placed into a larger context. Pope and Katz (1988) noted that an additional difficulty in identifying reports of problems in the scientific literature is that doses used in natural settings (e.g., particularly with steroids) may be dramatically outside of the realm of what is studied in medical settings. Furthermore, adulterants can impact what a person is actually taking. Future research could continue to document the impact of the use of these substances, so that signs of risky use and information relevant to treatment planning can be used for more efficient and effective screening of clients, patients, and research participants.

Absence of information about one's involvement in a range of drug use does not mean this use is not occurring: The right questions to shed light on this information must be asked. Following up a brief screen of alcohol, tobacco, or marijuana use with questions about other substances (including questions that identify other drugs and are answered by the respondent or interviewee in open-ended form) provides not only more information to better serve the individual but also a more thorough assessment of the factors at play in that person's life.

REFERENCES

Abraham, H. D., & Fava, M. (1999). Order and onset of substance abuse and depression in a sample of depressed outpatients. *Comprehensive Psychiatry, 40*(1), 44–50.

Abraham, H. D., & Mamen, A. (1996). LSD-like panic from risperidone in post-LSD visual disorder. *Journal of Clinical Psychopharmacology, 16*(3), 238–241.

Aldurra, G., & Crayton, J. W. (2001). Improvement of hallucinogen persisting perception disorder by treatment with a combination of fluoxetine and olanzapine: Case report. *Journal of Clinical Psychopharmacology, 21*(3), 343–344.

Allnutt, S., & Chaimowitz, G. (1994). Anabolic steroid withdrawal depression: A case report. *Canadian Journal of Psychiatry, 39*(5), 317–318.

American Psychiatric Association. (2000). *Diagnostic and statistical manual of mental disorders* (4th ed., text rev.). Washington, DC: Author.

Annitto, W. J., & Layman, W. A. (1980). Anabolic steroids and acute schizophrenic episode. *Journal of Clinical Psychiatry, 41*(4), 143–144.

Annis, H. M., Sklar, S. M., & Turner, N. E. (1997). *Drug-Taking Confidence Questionnaire, user's guide.* Toronto: Addiction Research Foundation.

Annis, H. M., Turner, N. E., & Sklar, S. M. (1997). *Inventory of Drug-Taking Situations, user's guide.* Toronto: Addiction Research Foundation.

Antoniou, T., & Tseng, A. L. (2002). Interactions between recreational drugs and antiretroviral agents. *Annals of Pharmacotherapy, 36,* 1598–1613.

Beauvais, F., & Oetting, E. R. (1987). Toward a clear definition of inhalant abuse. *International Journal of the Addictions, 22*(8), 779–784.

Brower, K. J. (1992). Clinical assessment and treatment of anabolic steroid users. *Psychiatric Annals, 22*(1), 35–40.

Brower, K. J., Blow, F. C., Beresford, T. P., & Fuelling, C. (1989). Anabolic–androgenic steroid dependence. *Journal of Clinical Psychiatry, 50*(1), 31–33.

Brower, K. J., Blow, F. C., Young, J. P., & Hill, E. M. (1991). Symptoms and correlates of anabolic–androgenic steroid dependence. *British Journal of Addiction, 86,* 759–768.

Brower, K. J., Catlin, D. H., Blow, F. C., Eliopulos, G. A., & Beresford, T. P. (1991). Clinical assessment and urine testing for anabolic–androgenic steroid abuse and dependence. *American Journal of Drug and Alcohol Abuse, 17*(2), 161–171.

Brower, K. J., Eliopulos, G. A., Blow, F. D., Catlin, D. H., & Beresford, T. P. (1990). Evidence for physical and psychological dependence on anabolic androgenic steroids in eight weight lifters. *American Journal of Psychiatry, 147*(4), 510–512.

Brown, S. A., Meyers, M. G., Lippke, L., Tapert, S. F., Stewart, D. G., & Vik, P. W. (1998). Psychometric evaluation of the Customary Drinking and Drug Use Record (CDDR): A measure of adolescent alcohol and drug involvement. *Journal of Studies on Alcohol, 59*(4), 427–438.

Centers for Disease Control. (1991). Multistate outbreak of poisoning associated with illicit use of gamma hydroxybutyrate. *Journal of the American Medical Association, 265,* 447–448.

Centers for Disease Control. (2004). *About the Youth Risk Behavior Surveillance System.* Retrieved March 23, 2005, from http://www.cdc.gov/HealthyYouth/YRBS/about_yrbss.htm.

Chin, M. Y., Kreutzer, R. A., & Dyer, J. E. (1992). Acute poisoning from gamma-hydroxybutyrate in California. *Western Journal of Medicine, 156,* 380–384.

Cole, J. C., Bailey, M., Sumnall, H. R., Wagstaff, G. F., & King, L. S. (2002). The content of ecstasy tablets: Implications for the study of their long-term effects. *Addiction, 97,* 1531–1536.

Cone, E. J. (1996). Mechanisms of drug incorporation into hair. *Therapeutic Drug Monitoring, 18*, 438–443.

Cone, E. J. (1997). New developments in biological measures of drug prevalence. In L. Harrison & A. Hughes (Eds.), *The validity of self-reported drug use: Improving the accuracy of survey estimates* (NIDA Research Monograph No. 167, pp. 108–129). Rockville, MD: National Institute on Drug Abuse.

Creighton, F. J., Black, D. L., & Hyde, C. E. (1991). "Ecstasy" psychosis and flashbacks. *British Journal of Psychiatry, 159*, 713–715.

Daley, D. C., & Marlatt, G. A. (1997). *Managing your drug or alcohol problem*. San Antonio, TX: Harcourt Brace.

DanceSafe. (2004). *Ecstasy*. Retrieved March 26, 2004, from www.da.ncesafe.org/documents/druginfo/ecstasy.php.

Darboe, M. N. (1996). Abuse of dextromethorphan-based cough syrup as a substitute for licit and illicit drugs: A theoretical framework. *Adolescence, 31*, 239–245.

de la Torre, R., Farré, M., Roset, P. N., Hernándes-Lópes, C., Mas, M., Ortuño, J., Menoyo, E., Pizzarro, N., Segura, J., & Cami, J. (2000). Pharmacology of MDMA in humans. *Annals of the New York Academy of Sciences, 914*, 225–237.

Dewhurst, K., & Hatrick, J. A. (1972). Differential diagnosis and treatment of lysergic acid diethylamide induced psychosis. *Practitioner, 209*, 327–332.

Dinwiddie, S. H. (1994). Abuse of inhalants: A review. *Addiction, 89*, 925–939.

Dinwiddie, S. H., Reich, T., & Cloninger, C. R. (1991). The relationship of solvent use to other substance use. *American Journal of Drug and Alcohol Abuse, 17*(2), 173–186.

Diversion Control Program. (2004a). *Drugs and chemicals of concern: Ketamine*. Retrieved March 29, 2004, from www.deadiversion.usdoj.gov/drugs_concern/ketamine/summary.htm.

Diversion Control Program. (2004b). *Drugs and chemicals of concern: Dextromethorphan*. Retrieved March 31, 2004, from www.deadiversion.usdoj.gov/drugs_concern/dextro_m/summary.htm.

Drug Enforcement Administration. (2004a). *MDMA facts*. Retrieved March 26, 2004, from www.usdoj.gov/dea/concern/mdma/mdma_factsheet.html.

Drug Enforcement Administration. (2004b). *Ketamine facts*. Retrieved March 28, 2004, from www.usdoj.gov/dea/concern/ketamine_factsheet.html.

Drug Enforcement Administration. (2004c). *LSD facts*. Retrieved March 31, 2004, from www.usdoj.gov/dea/concern/lsd_factsheet.html.

Duggal, H. S., Sinha, B. N. P., & Nizamie, S. H. (2000). Gasoline inhalation dependence and bipolar disorder. *Australian and New Zealand Journal of Psychiatry, 34*(3), 531–532.

DuPont, R. L., & Verebey, K. (1994). The role of the laboratory in the diagnosis of LSD and Ecstasy psychosis. *Psychiatric Annals, 24*(3), 142–144.

Facts and Comparisons. (2004). *A to Z drug facts* (5th ed.). St. Louis, MO: Author.

Flynn, P. M., Hubbard, R. L., Luckey, J. W., Forsyth, B. H., Smith, T. K., Phillips, C. D., Fountain, D. L., Hoffman, J. A., & Koman, J. J. (1995). Individual Assessment Profile: Standardizing the assessment of substance abusers. *Journal of Substance Abuse Treatment, 12*(3), 213–211.

Freese, T. E., Miotto, K., & Reback, C. J. (2002). The effects and consequences of selected club drugs. *Journal of Substance Abuse Treatment, 23*, 151–156.

Gahlinger, P. M. (2001). *Illegal drugs: A complete guide to their history, chemistry, use and abuse*. Salt Lake City, UT: Sagebrush Press.

Galloway, G. P. (1997). Anabolic–androgenic steroids. In J. H. Lowinson, P. Ruiz, R.

B. Millman, & J. G. Langrod (Eds.), *Substance abuse: A comprehensive textbook* (3rd ed., pp. 308–318). Baltimore: Williams & Wilkins.

Galloway, G. P., Frederick, S. L., Staggers, F. E., Gonzales, M., Stalcup, S. A., & Smith, D. E. (1997). Gamma-hydroxybutyrate: An emerging drug of abuse that causes physical dependence. *Addiction, 92*(1), 89–96.

Gold, M. S., & Dackis, C. A. (1986). Role of the laboratory in the evaluation of suspected drug use. *Journal of Clinical Psychiatry, 47*(1), 17–23.

Gruber, A. J., & Pope, H. G., Jr. (2000). Psychiatric and medical effects of anabolic–androgenic steroid use in women. *Psychotherapy and Psychosomatics, 69*(1), 19–26.

Harkey, M. R. (1995). Technical issues concerning hair analysis for drugs of abuse. *National Institute on Drug Abuse Research Monograph, 154*, 218–234.

Harrington, R. D., Woodward, J. A., Hooton, T. M., & Horn, J. R. (1999). Life-threatening interactions between HIV-1 protease inhibitors and the illicit drugs MDMA and gamma-hydroxybutyrate. *Archives of Internal Medicine, 159*, 2221–2224.

Hays, L. R., Littleton, S., & Stillner, V. (1990). Anabolic steroid dependence. *American Journal of Psychiatry, 147*(1), 122.

Heather, N., Rollnick, S., & Bell, A. (1993). Predictive validity of the Readiness to Change Questionnaire. *Addiction, 88*, 1667–1677.

Henderson, G. L., Harkey, M. R., Zhou, C., Jones, R. T., & Jacob, P. (1998). Incorporation of isotopically labeled cocaine into human hair: Race as a factor. *Journal of Analytical Toxicology, 22*, 156–165.

Hernandez-Avila, C. A., Oretega-Solo, H. A., Jasso, A., Hasfura-Buenaga, C. A., & Kranzler, H. R. (1998). Treatment of inhalant-induced psychotic disorder with carbamazepine versus haloperidol [Special Issue]. *Psychiatric Services, 49*(6), 812–815.

Jansen, K. L. R. (1999). Ecstasy (MDMA) dependence. *Drug and Alcohol Dependence, 53*, 121–124.

Jansen, K. L. R., & Darracot-Cankovic, R. (2001). The nonmedical use of ketamine: Part 2. A review of problem use and dependence. *Journal of Psychoactive Drugs, 33*(2), 151–158.

Johnson, S. L. (2003). *Therapist's guide to substance abuse intervention.* Fresno, CA: Academic Press.

Johnston, L. D., O'Malley, P. M., & Bachman, J. G. (2002). *Monitoring the Future national survey results on adolescent drug use: Overview of key findings, 2001* (NIH Publication No. 02-5105). Bethesda, MD: National Institute on Drug Abuse.

Johnston, L. D., O'Malley, P. M., & Bachman, J. G. (2003). *Monitoring the Future national survey results on adolescent drug use: Overview of key findings, 2002* (NIH Publication No. 03-5374). Bethesda, MD: National Institute on Drug Abuse.

Johnston, L. D., O'Malley, P. M., Bachman, J. G., & Schulenberg, J. E. (2004). *Monitoring the Future national results on adolescent drug use: Overview of key findings, 2003* (NIH Publication No. 04-5506). Bethesda, MD: National Institute on Drug Abuse.

Kalant, H. (2001). The pharmacology and toxicology of "Ecstasy" (MDMA) and related drugs. *Canadian Medical Association Journal, 165*, 917–928.

Kendler, K. S., Karkowski, L., & Prescott, C. A. (1999). Hallucinogen, opiate, sedative and stimulant use and abuse in a population-based sample of female twins. *Acta Psychiatrica Scandinavica, 99*, 368–376.

Keriotis, A. A., & Upadhyaya, H. P. (2000). Inhalant dependence and withdrawal symptoms. *Journal of the American Academy of Child and Adolescent Psychiatry, 39*(6), 679–680.

Kilmer, J. R., Cronce, J. M., & Palmer, R. S. (2005). Relapse prevention for abuse of club drugs, hallucinogens, inhalants, and steroids. In G. A. Marlatt & D. Donovan (Eds.), *Relapse prevention* (2nd ed., pp. 208–247). New York: Guilford Press.

Kintz, P., Cirimele, V., Jamey, C., & Ludes, B. (2003). Testing for GHB in hair by GC/MS/MS after a single exposure: Application to document sexual assault. *Journal of Forensic Science, 48,* 1–6.

Kintz, P., Cirimele, V., & Ludes, B. (2000). Pharmacological criteria that can affect the detection of doping agents in hair. *Forensic Science International, 107,* 325–334.

Kintz, P., & Samyn, N. (2002). Use of alternative specimens: Drugs of abuse in saliva and doping agents in hair. *Therapeutic Drug Monitoring, 24,* 239–246.

Kono, J., Miyata, H., Ushijima, S., Yanagita, T., Miyasato, K., Ikawa, G., & Hukui, K. (2001). Nicotine, alcohol, methamphetamine, and inhalant dependence: A comparison of clinical features with the use of a new clinical evaluation form. *Alcohol, 24,* 99–106.

Korman, M., Trimboli, F., & Semler, I. (1980). A comparative evaluation of 162 inhalant users. *Addictive Behaviors, 5*(2), 143–152.

Kuhn, C., Swartzwelder, S., & Wilson, W. (2003). *Buzzed: The straight facts about the most used and abused drugs from alcohol to Ecstasy.* New York: Norton.

Lachenmeier, D. W., Kroener, L., Musshoff, F., & Madea, B. (2003). Application of tandem mass spectrometry combined with gas chromatography and headspace solid-phase dynamic extraction for the determination of drugs of abuse in hair samples. *Rapid Communication in Mass Spectrometry, 17,* 472–478.

Leckman, J. F., & Scahill, L. (1990). Possible exacerbation of tics by androgenic steroids. *New England Journal of Medicine, 322*(23), 1674.

Lerner, A. G., Finkel, B., Oyffe, I., Merenzon, I., & Sigal, M. (1998). Clonidine treatment for hallucinogen persisting perception disorder. *American Journal of Psychiatry, 155*(10), 1460–1461.

Lerner, A. G., Oyffe, I., Isaacs, G., & Sigal, M. (1997). Naltrexone treatment of hallucinogen persisting perception disorder. *American Journal of Psychiatry, 154*(3), 437.

Lerner, A. G., Skladman, I., Kodesh, A., Sigal, M., & Shufman, E. (2001). LSD-induced hallucinogen persisting perception disorder treated with clonazepam: Two case reports. *Israel Journal of Psychiatry and Related Sciences, 38*(2), 133–136.

Li, J., Stokes, S. A., & Woeckener, A. (1998). A tale of novel intoxication: A review of the effects of gamma-hydroxybutyric acid with recommendations for management. *Annals of Emergency Medicine, 31,* 729–736.

Marlatt, G. A., & Miller, W. R. (1984). *Comprehensive Drinker Profile.* Odessa, FL: Psychological Assessment Resources.

McConnaughy, E. A., Prochaska, J. O., & Velicer, W. F. (1983). Stages of change in psychotherapy: Measurement and sample profiles. *Psychotherapy: Theory, Research, and Practice, 20,* 368–375.

McDaniel, C. H., & Miotto, K. A. (2001). Gamma hydroxybutyrate (GHB) and gamma butyrolactone (GBL) withdrawal: Five case studies. *Journal of Psychoactive Drugs, 33*(2), 143–149.

Meredith, T. J., Ruprah, M., Liddle, A., & Flanagan, R. J. (1989). Diagnosis and treatment of acute poisoning with volatile substances. *Human Toxicology, 8,* 277–286.

Miller, W. R., & Del Boca, F. K. (1994). Measurement of drinking behavior using the Form 90 family of instruments. *Journal of Studies on Alcohol, 55*(Suppl. 12), 112–118.

Miller, W. R., & Marlatt, G. A. (1987). *The Brief Drinker Profile.* Odessa, FL: Psychological Assessment Resources.

Miller, W. R., & Tonigan, J. S. (1997). Assessing drinkers' motivation for change: The

Stages of Change Readiness and Treatment Eagerness Scale (SOCRATES). *Psychology of Addictive Behaviors, 10*(2), 81–89.

Moore, K. A., Sklerov, J., Levine, B., & Jacobs, A. J. (2001). Urine concentrations of ketamine and norketamine following illegal consumption. *Journal of Analytical Toxicology, 25*, 583–588.

Morehead, D. B. (1997). Exacerbation of hallucinogen-persisting perception disorder with risperidone. *Journal of Clinical Psychopharmacology, 17*(4), 327–328.

National Institute on Drug Abuse. (2003). *Research report series: Inhalant abuse.* Retrieved October 23, 2003, from www.drugabuse. gov/researchreports/inhalants/inhalants2.html.

National Institute on Drug Abuse. (2004a). *InfoFacts: LSD.* Retrieved March 31, 2003, from www.drugabuse.gov/infofax/lsd.html.

National Institute on Drug Abuse. (2004b). *Research report series: Hallucinogens and dissociative drugs.* Retrieved March 31, 2003, from www.drugabuse.gov/researchreports/hallucinogens/halluc2.html.

Nicholson, K. L., & Balster, R. L. (2001). GHB: A new and novel drug of abuse. *Alcohol and Dependence, 63*, 1–22.

Norchem. (2004). *Drug testing information: Club drug panel.* Retrieved March 30, 2004, from www.norchemlab.com/reference/dt-clubdrugs.htm.

Office of National Drug Control Policy. (2002a). *Street terms: Drugs and the drug trade. Drug type: Ecstasy (methylenedioxymethamphetamine; MDMA).* Retrieved April 3, 2004, from www.whitehousedrugpolicy.gov/streetterms/bytype.asp?inttypeid=7.

Office of National Drug Control Policy. (2002b). *Street terms: Drugs and the drug trade. Drug type: Ketamine.* Retrieved April 3, 2004, from wwww.whitehousedrugpolicy.gov/streetterms/bytype.asp?inttypeid=32.

Office of National Drug Control Policy. (2002c). *Street terms: Drugs and the drug trade. Drug type: GHB (gamma hydroxybutyrate).* Retrieved April 5, 2004, from wwww.whitehousedrugpolicy.gov/streetterms/bytype.asp?inttypeid=48.

Office of National Drug Control Policy. (2002d). *Street terms: Drugs and the drug trade. Drug type: LSD (Lysergic acid diethylamide).* Retrieved April 4, 2004, from wwww.whitehousedrugpolicy.gov/streetterms/bytype.asp?inttypeid=6.

Office of National Drug Control Policy. (2002e). *Street terms: Drugs and the drug trade. Drug type: Inhalants.* Retrieved April 4, 2004, from wwww. whitehousedrugpolicy.gov/streetterms/bytype.asp?inttypeid=34.

Office of National Drug Control Policy. (2002f). *Street terms: Drugs and the drug trade. Drug type: Steroids.* Retrieved April 4, 2004, from wwww. whitehousedrugpolicy.gov/streetterms/bytype.asp?inttypeid=46.

Onsite Drug Testing. (2004). *Commonly abused drugs.* Retrieved March 30, 2004, from www.onsitedrugtesting.com/files/common.pdf.

Parrott, A. C. (2001). Human psychopharmacology of Ecstasy (MDMA): A review of 15 years of empirical research. *Human Psychopharmacology, 16*, 557–577.

Parrott, A. C. (2004). Is Ecstasy MDMA?: A review of the proportion of ecstasy tablets containing MDMA, their dosage levels, and the changing perceptions of purity [Electronic version]. *Psychopharmacology, 173*, 234–241.

Parrott, A. C., Buchanan, T., Scholey, A. B., Heffernan, T., Ling, J., & Rodgers, J. (2002). Ecstasy/MDMA attributed problems reported by novice, moderate and heavy recreational users. *Human Psychopharmacology, 17*, 309–312.

Parrott, A. C., & Lasky, J. (1998). Ecstasy (MDMA) effect upon mood and cognition:

Before, during, and after a Saturday night dance. *Psychopharmacology, 139,* 261–268.

Persson, J., Hasselström, J., Maurset, A., Öye, I., Svensson, J. O., Almqvist, O., Scheinin, H., Gustafsson, L. L., & Almqvist, O. (2002). Pharmacokinetics and non-analgesic effects of S- and R-ketamines in healthy volunteers with normal and reduced metabolic capacity. *European Journal of Clinical Pharmacology, 57,* 869–875.

Pope, H. G., & Katz, D. L. (1988). Affective and psychotic symptoms associated with anabolic steroid use. *American Journal of Psychiatry, 145*(4), 487–490.

Price, G. (2000). In-patient detoxification after GHB dependence. *British Journal of Psychiatry, 177,* 181.

Prochaska, J. O., & DiClemente, C. C. (1986). Toward a comprehensive model of change. In W. R. Miller & N. Heather (Eds.), *Treating addictive behaviors: Processes of change* (pp. 3–27). New York: Plenum Press.

Ramsey, J., Anderson, H. R., Bloor, K., & Flanagan, R. J. (1989). An introduction to the practice, prevalence and chemical toxicology of volatile substance abuse. *Human Toxicology, 8,* 261–269.

Rashid, W. (2000). Testosterone abuse and affective disorders. *Journal of Substance Abuse Treatment, 18*(2), 179–184.

Rivier, L., (2000). Techniques for analytical testing of unconventional samples. *Balliere's Clinical Endocrinology and Metabolism, 14*(1), 147–165.

Rollnick, S., Heather, N., Gold, R., & Hall, W. (1992). Development of a short "Readiness to Change" Questionnaire for use in brief opportunistic interventions. *British Journal of Addictions, 87,* 743–754.

Rounsaville, B. J., Petry, N. M., & Carroll, K. M. (2003). Single versus multiple drug focus in substance abuse clinical trials research. *Drug and Alcohol Dependence, 70,* 117–125.

Samyn, N., De Boeck, G., Wood, M., Lamers, C., De Waard, D., Brookhuis, K. A., Verstraete, A. G., & Riedel, W. J. (2002). Plasma, oral fluid and sweat swipe Ecstasy concentrations in controlled and real life conditions. *Forensic Science International, 128,* 90–97.

Schadel, M., Wu, D., Otton, S. V., Kalow, W., & Sellers, E. M. (1995). Pharmacokinetics of dextromethorphan and metabolites in humans: Influence of the CYP2D6 phenotype and quinidine inhibition. *Journal of Clinical Psychopharmacology, 15,* 263–269.

Schwartz, R. H., & Miller, N. S. (1997). Ecstasy and the rave: A review. *Pediatrics, 100,* 705–708.

Schwartz, R. H., Milteer, R., & LeBeau, M. A. (2000). Drug-facilitated sexual assault ("date rape"). *Southern Medical Journal, 94,* 655–656.

Shah, R., Vankar, G. K., & Upadhyaya, H. P. (1999). Phenomenology of gasoline intoxication and withdrawal symptoms among adolescents in India: A case series. *American Journal on Addictions, 8,* 254–257.

Sharp, C. W., & Rosenberg, N. L. (1997). Inhalants. In J. H. Lowinson, P. Ruiz, R. B. Millman, & J. G. Langrod (Eds.), *Substance abuse: A comprehensive textbook* (3rd ed., pp. 246–264). Baltimore: Williams & Wilkins.

Siegel, R. K. (1978). Phencyclidine and ketamine intoxication: A study of four populations of recreational users. In R. C. Peterson & R. C. Stillman (Eds.), *Phencyclidine (PCP) abuse: An appraisal* (NIDA Research Monograph No. 21, pp. 119–147). Rockville, MD: National Institute on Drug Abuse, Division of Research.

Skinner, H. A. (1982). The Drug Abuse Screening Test. *Addictive Behaviors* 7(4), 363–371.

Smith, K. M., Larive, L. L., & Romanelli, F. (2002). Club drugs: Methylenedioxymethamphetamine, flunitrazepam, ketamine hydrochloride, and y-hydroxybutyrate. *American Journal of Health System Pharmacy*, 59, 1067–1076.

Sobell, L. C., Kwan, E., & Sobell, M. B. (1995). Reliability of a drug history questionnaire (DHQ). *Addictive Behaviors, 20*(2), 233–241.

Sobell, L. C., Sobell, M. B., Buchan, G., Cleland, P. A., Fedoroff, I., & Leo, G. I. (1996, November). *The reliability of the Timeline Followback method applied to drug, cigarette, and cannabis use*. Paper presented at the 30th annual meeting of the Association for Advancement of Behavior Therapy, New York, NY.

Steroid World. (2004). *Anabolic steroids detection times*. Retrieved March 30, 2004, from www.steroidworld.com/detect.htm.

Substance Abuse and Mental Health Services Administration. (2001). Summary of *Findings from the 2000 National Household Survey on Drug Abuse* (NHSDA Series H-13, DHHS Publication No. [SMA] 01-3549). Rockville, MD: Office of Applied Studies.

Substance Abuse and Mental Health Services Administration (2003). *The National Survey on Drug Use and Health* (NSDUH). Retrieved on March 23, 2005 from www.oas.samhsa.gove/2k3/NSDUH/nsduh.pdf.

Tonigan, J. S., & Miller, W. R. (2002). The inventory of drug use consequences (InDUC): Test–retest stability and sensitivity to detect change. *Psychology of Addictive Behaviors, 16*(2), 165–168.

Tonigan, J. S., Miller, W. R., & Brown, J. M. (1997). The reliability of Form 90: An instrument for assessing alcohol treatment outcome. *Journal of Studies on Alcohol, 58*(4), 358–364.

Tyler, A. (1986). *Street drugs*. London: Hodder & Stoughton.

Ungerleider, J. T., & Pechnick, R. N. (1999). Hallucinogens. In M. Galanter & H. D. Kleber (Eds.), *The American Psychiatric Press textbook of substance abuse treatment* (2nd ed., pp. 195–203). Washington, DC: American Psychiatric Press.

Van Kampen, J., & Katz, M. (2001). Persistent psychosis after a single ingestion of "Ecstasy." *Psychosomatics: Journal of Consultation Liasion Psychiatry, 42*(6), 525–527.

Verebey, K., Alrazi, J., & Jaffee, J. H. (1988). The complications of "Ecstasy" (MDMA). *Journal of the American Medical Association, 259*, 1649–1650.

Verebey, K., & Buchan, B. J. (1997). Diagnostic laboratory: Screening for drugs of abuse. In H. Lowinson, R. Ruiz, R. B. Millman, & J. G. Langrod (Eds.), *Substance abuse: A comprehensive textbook* (3rd ed., pp. 369–377). Baltimore: Williams & Wilkins.

Verstraete, A. G. (2004). Detection times of drugs of abuse in blood, urine, and oral fluid. *Therapeutic Drug Monitoring, 26*, 200–205.

Windhaber, J., Maierhofer, D., & Dantendorfer, K. (1998). Panic disorder induced by large doses of 3,4–methylenedioxymethamphetamine resolved by paroxetine. *Journal of Clinical Psychopharmacology, 18*(1), 95–96.

Winters, K. C., Latimer, W. W., & Stinchfield, R. (2002). Clinical issues in the assessment of adolescent alcohol and other drug use. *Behaviour Research and Therapy, 40*, 1443–1456.

Wolff, K., Farrell, M., Marsden, J., Monteiro, M. G., Ali, R., Welch, S., & Strang, J. (1999). A review of biological indicators of illicit drug use, practical considerations and clinical usefulness. *Addiction, 94*(9), 1279–1298.

CHAPTER 10

Assessment of Eating Disorders and Obesity

R. LORRAINE COLLINS
LINA A. RICCIARDELLI

Researchers and clinicians assess and diagnose eating disorders for a variety of reasons. Some may be interested in collecting data to enhance understanding of the precursors and consequences of disordered eating. Others may use assessment and/or diagnosis as an important first step in planning treatment. Regardless of the purpose to which assessment is applied, it is an important component of many different types of interactions with individuals who manifest eating disorders. For the purposes of this chapter, eating disorders include bulimia nervosa, anorexia nervosa, obesity, and binge-eating. Although these disorders share the common focus on food and eating, they also represent problems ranging from excessive intake of food (bulimia nervosa, binge-eating, obesity) to overregulation of food intake (anorexia nervosa). The designation of eating disorders is somewhat controversial. For example, the text revision of the fourth edition of the *Diagnostic and Statistical Manual of Mental Disorders* (DSM-IV-TR) of the American Psychiatric Association (2000) includes only anorexia nervosa and bulimia nervosa as meeting criteria for eating disorders. Although obesity occurs in increasingly large proportions of the general population, it is not included in DSM-IV-TR, because it is considered a general medical condition that is not consistently associated with a psychological or behavioral disorders.

Eating disorders are complex and include a variety of biological, psychological, and social antecedents, correlates, and consequences. Thus, the comprehensive assessment of eating disorders includes biological (e.g., body

305

weight, medical effects of weight fluctuations and purging behaviors), cognitive (e.g., cognitions related to body image, depression, and anxiety), and behavioral (e.g., eating behavior) components. Assessment often occurs in the context of a multidisciplinary team approach that includes information on medical, nutritional, psychological, behavioral, and social aspects of eating. Regardless of the specifics, it is useful to assess eating disorders systematically to better inform case conceptualization and the selection of interventions, as well as to track treatment efficacy over time.

In describing the assessment of eating disorders we focus on psychometrically sound measures published since 1988, when the previous edition of this book was published. Although we touch on medical issues and disorders such as depression and substance abuse, as well as various psychiatric and personality disorders that can co-occur with eating disorders (e.g., O'Brien & Vincent, 2003), these topics are beyond the purview of this chapter and are discussed in other chapters in this volume. We focus on behavioral and psychological assessment of eating disorders in adults and adolescents, for whom assessment tends to be similar. Where relevant, we highlight the use of specific measures to assess children.

There are a variety of approaches (e.g., cognitive, restrained eating, behavioral) to conceptualizing eating disorders. The clinician's conceptualization of the factors that contribute to the etiology and maintenance of eating disorders is an important determinant of the approach to and content of assessment. Currently, a cognitive-behavioral model has gained acceptance among many researchers and clinicians. Within this model, assessment is integrated with treatment to address the nature, frequency, and severity of cognitive and behavioral symptoms of specific eating disorders. For example, a cognitive model of bulimia nervosa begins with social pressures for women to be thin. Women with low self-esteem may place more and more value on weight and shape, and so they restrict their food intake. Eventually they lose control over eating and develop maladaptive eating habits such as binge-eating and purging (Fairburn, Marcus, & Wilson, 1993; Wilson, Fairburn, Agras, Walsh, & Kraemer, 2002). In using this model to plan treatment, each of these components (e.g., the valuing of weight and shape, restrained eating, bingeing and purging frequency) would need to be assessed. For some clinicians, the need to diagnose eating disorders may mean that assessment focuses on the criteria outlined in DSM-IV-TR (American Psychiatric Association, 2000). In each case, the conceptualization and purpose of the assessment is likely to influence the specific content (e.g., cognitions, behaviors, or both) and format (e.g., self-report vs. clinical interview), as well as the measure(s) that are administered. Similarly, the type of client (e.g., age, nature of eating disorder) also must be considered. For example, as the diagnosis of eating disorders moves to younger ages, there is now recognition of the need for, and development of, child-specific measures (see Maloney, McGuire, Daniels, & Specker, 1989; Ohzeki, Ontahara, Hanaki, Motozumi, & Shiraki, 1993). Other factors that can influence the nature and content of the assessment of eating disorders are the type of treatment facility (e.g., inpatient vs. outpatient), the medical/physical condition of the client (e.g., some anorexics may need to be stabilized medically and so must begin treatment in a hospital), and the presence of co-occurring disorders such as depression.

In most cases, assessments are based on self-reports. Self-monitoring, a special form of self-report, is discussed later in the chapter. Self-report data often are easier to collect than other types of information, such as biological samples or behavioral observations. In addition, self-report may be the only way to gather certain kinds of information, such as cognitions or affect. Even so, the limitations of self-reports must always be considered. They include the reliance on retrospection, which can lead to forgetting the occurrence of particular events, the aggregation of information across time, and biases that the client may bring to the situation. For example, even with the structure provided by the use of a calendar on which to retrospectively self-report binge-eating episodes, college women tended to underreport the frequency with which they had binged during the past 12 weeks, which suggests forgetting and/or aggregation over time (Bardone, Krahn, Goodman, & Searles, 2000). Given these and other limitations, it is useful to validate self-reports by conducting behavioral observations as is done in experiments (cf. Heatherton, Polivy, Herman, & Baumeister, 1993) or collecting other types of information. In many cases, gathering information from collaterals may not be viable, because disordered eating behaviors, such as bingeing or purging, often take place in secret.

The context in which the assessment occurs can determine the client's reactions to the assessment and the quality of the information that is collected. The best assessments are collaborative, because such collaboration can contribute to the development of a strong therapeutic alliance (Ackerman & Hilsenroth, 2003; Wilson & Vitousek, 1999). In addition, to enhance engagement in assessment and treatment, many researchers and clinicians assess factors such as the client's readiness and motivation to change his or her eating disorder (cf. Geller, Cockell, & Drab, 2001). The key is for clinicians to use their therapeutic skills to create a context in which their clients feel safe about disclosing sensitive information and are motivated to work collaboratively to change maladaptive symptoms and behaviors. In the best situations, the ingredients that create a cooperative therapeutic relationship are in place, from intake through assessment, and into treatment and maintenance. These ingredients include therapist characteristics such as warmth, flexibility, and respectfulness, and use of techniques such as attending to the client's experiences and being supportive (Ackerman & Hilsenroth, 2003). Thus, along with assessment of specific symptoms and behaviors, it also is important for the clinician to have an understanding of the client's background and history; current life circumstances, including relationships with family and significant others; and work and leisure activities, interests, and life goals.

DIAGNOSTIC CRITERIA AND THE PREVALENCE OF EATING DISORDERS

Diagnostic criteria for anorexia nervosa and bulimia nervosa provide useful starting points for understanding the characteristics of eating disorders. The DSM-IV-TR criteria for anorexia include (1) underweight, with refusal to maintain a normal body weight for age and height; (2) intense fear of gaining weight, even while underweight; (3) body image disturbance, including body weight or shape influencing one's self-evaluation; and (4) amenorrhea, which involves the absence of at least three consecutive menstrual cycles (American Psychiatric Association, 2000). Anorexics tend to restrict their food intake, to binge and purge, or in some cases purge even after eating small amounts of food. Other features of this primarily female (approximately 90% of cases) disorder include depression (secondary to reducing food intake) and food-related obsessive–compulsive cognitions and behaviors. The current prevalence of clinical cases of anorexia nervosa is approximately 1% of females in late adolescence and early adulthood (American Psychiatric Association, 2000). However, rates of this disorder are said to be rising.

Persons who meet the DSM-IV-TR criteria for bulimia (1) engage in episodes of binge-eating; (2) try to prevent weight gain by purging, fasting, or engaging in excessive exercise; and (3) are preoccupied with their body weight and shape, such that it influences their self-evaluation (American Psychiatric Association, 2000). Other features of this primarily female (approximately 90% of cases) disorder are depression, anxiety disorders, and in some cases abuse and/or dependence on alcohol and stimulants. The current prevalence of clinical cases of bulimia nervosa is approximately 1–3% of females in late adolescence and early adulthood, and rates of this disorder are said to be rising. In addition to the DSM-IV-TR criteria, research on individuals diagnosed with bulimia and other eating disorders has led to the identification of different subtypes, etiological models, and maintenance factors related to specific combinations of eating disorder symptoms (cf. Grilo, Masheb, & Wilson, 2001; Stice, 2001).

Relative to the preponderance of female cases of anorexia and bulimia, fewer adolescent and adult males develop eating disorders (American Psychiatric Association, 2000; Andersen & Holman, 1997; Carlat & Camargo, 1991; Carlat, Camargo, & Herzog, 1997). It is estimated that adolescent and adult males together make up approximately 10% of the clinically diagnosed cases of eating disorders (e.g., Andersen, 1984; American Psychiatric Association, 2000; Carlat & Camargo, 1991; Garfinkel et al., 1995). The main cases of eating disorders diagnosed in males are bulimia nervosa (Carlat & Camargo, 1991) and binge-eating disorder (Spitzer et al., 1992, 1993). However, it is difficult to obtain accurate estimates, because different diagnostic criteria have been used by clinicians and researchers (e.g., Carlat & Camargo, 1991; Steiger, 1989). It also is more difficult to diagnose eating disorders in men because they are less likely to use extreme weight loss methods, and many of the binge-eating patterns that are seen as abnormal or inappropriate in women are socially sanctioned for men (Carlat & Camargo, 1991; Carlat et al., 1997). Finally, men are generally less likely to seek treatment than women (Braun, Sunday, Huang, & Halmi, 1999; Olivardia, Pope, Mangweth, & Hudson, 1995). Thus, although there is growing interest in disordered eating among males (Ricciardelli & McCabe, 2004), much of the focus of this chapter is research on women.

Currently in the United States, diagnostic criteria for obesity are based on guidelines developed by the National Heart, Lung, and Blood Institute (NHLBI) of the National Institutes of Health (NIH). These criteria focus on the individual's body mass index (BMI), which is calculated as relative weight in kilograms (kg) for height squared (m^2). "Overweight" is defined as a BMI of 25.0 to 29.9 kg/m^2, and obesity is a BMI ≥ 30 kg/m^2. In addition, waist circumference can be measured to assess excess fat in the abdominal area, which is correlated with total body fat. Psychological correlates of obesity share similarities with the other eating disorders, and include depression and maladaptive eating behaviors, including binge-eating. In contrast to anorexia and bulimia, which are predominantly female disorders and have a relatively low prevalence in the general population, obesity now is said to occur in over 55% of adult men and women in the United States, and rates continue to rise.

ASSESSMENT OF BIOLOGICAL ASPECTS OF EATING DISORDERS

Each of the eating disorders is associated with medical conditions. The starvation that occurs in anorexia can produce medical conditions that include mild anemia, abnormal liver function, fluid and electrolyte imbalances, decreased estrogen levels, and cardiac arrhythmia (American Psychiatric Association, 2000). The cycles of binge-eating and purging that occur in bulimia are associated with loss of dental enamel (from recurrent vomiting); menstrual irregularity, including amenorrhea; fluid and electrolyte disturbances; and cardiac arrhythmia (American Psychiatric Association, 2000). The elevated BMI of an obese individual is correlated with total body fat and as such is seen as indicative of risk for medical conditions such as coronary heart disease, sleep apnea and respiratory problems, and type 2 diabetes (NHLBI, 1998). Given the variety of medical conditions associated with each of the eating disorders, a comprehensive assessment of persons with eating disorders should include a complete medical examination, as well as continued monitoring of biological/medical changes. This topic is beyond the purview of this chapter, which focuses on behavioral and psychological assessment. However, we mention biological/medical factors because of their importance, and because they highlight the need for a multidisciplinary team approach to the assessment and treatment of eating disorders.

ASSESSMENT OF BEHAVIORAL, PSYCHOLOGICAL, AND SOCIAL ASPECTS OF EATING DISORDERS

Assessment of psychological factors tends to encompass self-report, either in the context of a structured or semistructured interview or a questionnaire. Some measures are comprehensive and designed to assess multiple dimensions of eating disorders, while others focus on a single aspect of a specific disorder. All measures are listed in Table 10.1.

Measures of Multiple Dimensions (Cognitions and Behaviors) of Eating Disorders: Interviews

The following measures are designed to be administered by clinicians as part of structured or semistructured interviews. Here, we describe commonly used measures that have been published since 1988. In describing each measure, we highlight contents, usefulness for treatment planning, and psychometric characteristics.

Yale–Brown–Cornell Eating Disorder Scale

The Yale–Brown–Cornell Eating Disorder Scale (YBC-EDS; Mazure, Halmi, Sunday, Romano, & Einhorn, 1994) is an 85-item, semistructured, clinician-administered interview that assesses the illness severity of preoccupations and rituals associated with eating disorders. One of the main advantages of the YBC-EDS is that it allows the clinician to use an idiosyncratic list of target symptoms for each person. A wide range of preoccupations and rituals are targeted. Preoccupations include "any food, eating, weight, appearance, or exercise-related 'thoughts, images, or impulses' that repeatedly occur to the patient," while rituals include "any 'behaviors or acts' related to food, eating, weight, appearance, or exercise that the patient feels driven to perform" (Mazure et al., 1994, p. 435). The scale also assesses an individual's motivation for changing his or her preoccupations and rituals, which is useful for planning treatment and assessing progress.

The YBC-EDS has only been validated with women diagnosed with an eating disorder. Interrater reliability for the YBC-EDS total score and subscale scores is excellent: .99 for total score, > .99 preoccupations total, .98 for rituals total, and .81 to > .99 for items that assess motivation for change (Mazure et al., 1994). High levels of internal consistency as assessed by Cronbach's alpha also have been reported for the YBC-EDS total score (.87–.90), preoccupations total (.81–.84), rituals total (.78–.88), and motivation total (.82) (Mazure et al., 1994; Sunday, Halmi, & Einhorn, 1995). However, test–retest reliability data on the YBC-EDS are not available. The YBC-EDS has demonstrated satisfactory convergent validity. Total scores from the YBC-EDS have been found to correlate moderately and significantly ($r = .42$) with scores from the Dutch Eating Behavior Questionnaire (DEBQ) and the Drive for Thinness,

Bulimia, and Body Dissatisfaction subscales from the Eeating Disorders Inventory (r = .47–.60).

Eating Disorder Examination

Since its original publication (Cooper & Fairburn, 1987), the Eating Disorder Examination (EDE) has gone through numerous refinements and is now in its 12th edition (Fairburn & Cooper, 1993). The EDE is a semistructured interview designed to provide information about either the frequency or severity of eating behaviors and attitudes during the past 4 weeks. Interviewers receive training concerning the concepts covered by the EDE, which then allows them to probe client responses in order to rate frequency and severity dimensions on a 6-point scale. Frequency ratings are based on the number of days the behavior/attitude is present (0 = absent, 6 = present every day). Severity ratings are based on the degree of the occurrence of the behavior/attitude (0 = absent, 6 = present to an extreme degree). The current EDE consists of four subscales (the fifth subscale, Bulimia, was dropped because it did not add additional useful information). The four subscales are (1) Restraint (e.g., food avoidance, restraint over eating, dietary rules); (2) Eating Concern (e.g., eating in secret, fear of losing control over eating); (3) Shape Concern (e.g., preoccupation with shape, fear of weight gain); and (4) Weight Concern (e.g., desire to lose weight, importance of weight). Scores on items within subscales are summed to derive a subscale score. A global score that reflects the overall severity of the eating disorder can be derived by summing across the subscale scores and dividing by four, the number of subscales. Internal consistencies of the subscales are good to excellent (alphas = .68–.89), depending on the subscale and the specific study. Although there have been no tests of the test–retest reliability of the EDE, interrater reliability is good to excellent (correlations and kappas ranging from .70–.99 for specific items and subscales). Validity studies indicate that the EDE can discriminate between persons with eating disorders and normal controls (Fairburn & Cooper, 1993).

A questionnaire designed to self-report eating disorder symptoms has been derived from the EDE. The Eating Disorder Examination—Questionnaire (EDE-Q; Fairburn & Beglin, 1994) parallels the EDE, including the focus on behaviors and attitudes during the past 28 days. It uses similar rating format and probe questions, but it does not include the definitions that are part of the EDE. The EDE-Q can be completed in about 15 minutes. It has good psychometric properties; internal consistency alpha = .85 and test–retest reliability (over 3 weeks) = .87 (Black & Wilson, 1996; Fairburn & Beglin, 1994). In a direct comparison of the two versions of the EDE for assessing binge-eating disorder, the two measures showed modest-to-good significant correlations (r's = .63–.69; Wilfley, Schwartz, Spurrell, & Fairburn, 1997). These relationships were lower than those found in previous research (Black & Wilson, 1996; Fairburn & Beglin, 1994). These studies also indicate that the two versions of the EDE show less agreement for binge-eating disorder than for other eating disorders, such as anorexia nervosa and bulimia nervosa. Interestingly, in all direct comparisons of the two versions of the EDE, the EDE-Q produces higher subscale scores than the EDE. Even so, the EDE interview is seen as the better version for making decisions regarding clinical diagnosis (Wilfley et al., 1997).

Measures of Multiple Dimensions (Cognitions and Behaviors) of Eating Disorders: Self-Report Inventories

Two self-report inventories that were reviewed in the previous edition of this volume (Polivy, Herman, & Garner, 1988) have since been revised: the Eating Disorder Inventory (EDI; Garner & Olmsted, 1984) and the Bulimia Test (BULIT; Smith & Thelen, 1984). An update of one of the other self-report questionnaires reviewed by Polivy et al. (1988), the Eating Attitudes Test (EAT), is also provided; the EAT continues to be a widely used instrument. Other measures reviewed in this section are newer instruments that were not reviewed in the earlier edition.

Eating Disorder Inventory–2

The Eating Disorder Inventory–2 (EDI-2; Garner, 1991) is a self-report inventory designed to assess symptoms commonly associated with anorexia nervosa and bulimia nervosa. It was not designed to yield an eating disorder diagnosis, but rather to provide a standardized measurement of the severity of symptomatology that is clinically relevant to eating disorders (Garner, 1991). In the clinical setting, the EDI-2 can provide useful background information for understanding the client, planning treatment, and assessing progress. In nonclinical populations, the EDI-2 can be used as a screening instrument for identifying individuals who have subclinical eating problems or those who may be at risk of developing eating disorders.

The EDI-2 consists of 91 questions, 64 of which are from the original version of the EDI. They form 11 subscales. Three subscales assess attitudes and behaviors concerning eating, weight, and shape: Drive for Thinness, Bulimia, and Body Dissatisfaction. The remaining eight subscales assess psychological characteristics that have been found to be clinically relevant to eating disorders: Ineffectiveness, Perfectionism, Interpersonal Distrust, Interoceptive Awareness, Maturity Fears, Asceticism, Impulse Regulation, and Social Insecurity. The EDI and/or EDI-2 have been validated with both clinical and nonclinical groups across different cultures. Nonclinical groups have included female and male samples of adults and adolescents. In addition, the EDI and/or EDI-2 also have been translated into several languages, including Arabic, Bulgarian, Chinese, Dutch, German, Hebrew, Portuguese, Spanish, and Swedish (Garner, 1991; Niv, Kaplan, Mitrani, & Shiang, 1998; Lee, Lee, Leung, & Hong, 1997; Machado, Gonçalves, Martins, & Soares, 2001).

The majority of the EDI-2 subscales have moderate-to-high levels of internal consistency as assessed by Cronbach's alpha (.70–.93; Garner, 1991). However, the Asceticism subscale has been found to be unreliable in a nonclinical sample of women (alpha = .40). Lower levels of internal consistency also have been found for Bulimia, Maturity Fears, Perfectionism, and Interpersonal Distrust among adolescent girls and boys (alpha = .65–.70). Test–retest reliability is only available for original EDI subscales. Test–retest reliability over 1-week and 3-week periods was found to be high for the majority of the scales (.80–.97). Lower test–retest reliability has been found for Interoceptive Awareness (.67) and Maturity Fears (.65). Satisfactory to good levels of test–retest reliability over a 1-year period also have been found for Drive for Thinness, Body Dissatisfaction, Ineffectiveness, Perfectionism, and Interpersonal Distrust (.55–.75). Lower long-term stability has been found for the other subscales (.41–.48); however, the attitudes and behaviors assessed in these subscales (e.g., Bulimia) are more likely to fluctuate over time (Garner, 1991).

Although there is extensive validity for the original EDI, less validity data has been provided for the EDI-2 (Garner, 1991). All items in the EDI and the additional items in the EDI-2 have been found to discriminate between a clinical group of female anorexics and a control group of college women. The original EDI subscales also have demonstrated satisfactory concurrent and convergent validity. Overall, the subscales have been found to correlate moderately with clinician ratings (.43–.68). The main three EDI subscales, which assess attitudes and behaviors concerning eating, weight, and shape (Drive for Thinness, Bulimia, and Body Dissatisfaction), on the whole have been found to correlate moderately with the EAT (.26–.71) and the Restraint Scale (.44–.61). In addition, a factor analysis of the original EDI items has confirmed the structure of the eight subscales in a clinical sample (Welch, Hall, & Norring, 1990). However, the factors were found to be less well identified in a nonclinical sample (Welch, Hall, & Walkey, 1988).

Bulimia Test—Revised

The Bulimia Test—Revised (BULIT-R; Thelen, Farmer, Wonderlich, & Smith, 1991) is a self-report inventory that was specifically designed to assess bulimic symptomatology according to the DSM-III-R criteria. However, the BULIT-R also has been validated with the DSM-IV criteria for bulimia nervosa (Thelen, Mintz, & Vander Wal, 1996). It consists of 28 scored items and an additional eight unscored items that provide information about radical weight control methods. The BULIT-R has been validated in samples of women with and without eating disorders (Brelsford, Hummel, & Barrios, 1992; Thelen et al., 1991, 1996), and with adolescent girls and boys (Vincent, McCabe, & Ricciardelli, 1999).

Internal consistency of the BULIT-R as assessed by Cronbach's alpha is high in adult women (.92–.98) and in both adolescent girls (.90) and boys

(.88). Test–retest reliability over a 2-month period in a nonclinical adult sample has also been found to be very high (.95). Each of the 28 scored items of the BULIT-R has been found to discriminate between a group of women with bulimia nervosa and a control group consisting of college women. The BULIT-R also was found to be a good predictor of group membership in two independent samples, as indicated by sensitivity (.62 and .83), specificity (.96), the positive predictive value (.73 and .82), and negative predictive value (.89–.97; Thelen et al., 1991, 1996).

The BULIT-R has further demonstrated high concurrent and convergent validity in both adult women and adolescents. It correlated highly with the Binge Scale (.85) of the original BULIT (.99), and a self-monitored diary of binge-eating (.65) and purging (.60) over a 3-week period. Moderate correlations between the BULIT-R and a total score from five items measuring binge-eating as specified by DSM-IV criteria also have been found for adolescent girls (.58) and boys (.43). Although the development of the BULIT-R was based on the premise of a single dimension, and the measure is primarily used in this way (Thelen et al., 1996), a multiple factor structure has been identified with samples of bulimic and nonclinical college women. Specifically, the BULIT-R was found to consist of five factors: (1) Bingeing and Control, (2) Radical Weight Loss and Body Image (3) Laxative and Diuretic Use, (4) Self-Induced Vomiting, and (5) Exercise (Thelen et al., 1991). A somewhat different factor structure was found using a 23-item version of the BULIT-R in adolescent girls and boys: (1) Bingeing, (2) Control, (3) Normative Weight Loss Behaviors, and (4) Extreme Weight Loss Behaviors (Vincent et al., 1999). Unlike that for adult women, the factor structure in adolescents separated between binge-eating and control, which may be in part attributable to adolescents' limited experience with binge-eating and attempts to control eating. Moreover, not all adolescents are familiar with the term "binge-eating" (Neumark-Sztainer & Story, 1998); therefore, caution needs to be exercised when using the BULIT-R with adolescent samples.

Eating Attitudes Test

Although originally developed in 1979, we discuss the EAT here because it continues to be a widely used measure to assess eating disorder symptoms (Mintz & O'Halloran, 2000). Different versions of the EAT consist of varying numbers of items and are designated as such. There is a 40-item version (EAT-40; Garner & Garfinkel, 1979), a 26-item version (EAT-26; Garner, Olmsted, Bohr, & Garfinkel, 1982), and a 12-item version (EAT-12; Lavik, Clausen, & Pedersen, 1991). The EAT also has been modified for use with children. One version is the Children's Eating Attitude Test (ChEAT; Maloney et al., 1989) and another version for children is the Simplified Eating Attitudes Test (s-EAT; Ohzeki et al., 1993). In addition, the EAT has been translated into at least seven foreign languages (Mintz & O'Halloran, 2000).

The EAT recently has been validated with DSM-IV criteria (Mintz & O'Halloran, 2000). Both the EAT-40 and the EAT-26 were found to have a high overall accuracy rate, 91% and 90%, respectively, in correctly diagnosing individuals with and without a DSM-IV eating disorder. Sensitivities (.77), specificities (.95, .94), positive predictive values (.82, .79) and negative predictive values (.93, .94) also were all found to be high. These results indicate that the EAT can be reliably used as a general screening measure of undifferentiated DSM-IV eating disorders, because the majority of missed cases, false-negatives, were eating disorders not otherwise specified (EDNOS). However, follow-up interviews would be needed to eliminate false positives and for specific diagnoses.

Although researchers frequently compute a total EAT score, factor analyses have consistently identified at least three main dimensions of eating disturbance that the instrument assesses: dieting and purging behaviors, bingeing and food preoccupation, and social pressures to eat. These dimensions have been verified in different cultures, in adult males, in adolescent girls and boys, and in preadolescent girls and boys (Engelsen & Hagtvet, 1999; Lee, 1993; Kelly, Ricciardelli, & Clarke, 1999; Smolak & Levine, 1994; Wells, Coope, Gabb, & Pears, 1985).

Eating Questionnaire—Revised

The Eating Questionnaire—Revised (EQR; Williamson, Davis, Goreczny, McKenzie, & Watkins, 1989) is a 15-item, self-report inventory developed as a symptom checklist to screen for bulimia and binge-eating in accordance with the DSM-III criteria. The inventory has been validated in women with and without eating disorders; however, it has yet to be validated using DSM-IV criteria.

Over a 2-week interval, the EQR's internal consistency (.87) and test–retest reliability (.90) were high. Mean scores on the EQR did not discriminate among groups of persons with eating disorders (i.e., anorexia nervosa, bulimia, binge-eating disorder), but they did discriminate between those with eating disorders and either an obese sample or a nonclinical sample. The latter two samples had lower mean EQR scores than the eating-disordered samples. Concurrent validity for the EQR is satisfactory; EQR scores correlate moderately with scores from the EAT ($r = .59$) and the BULIT ($r = .80$).

Survey for Eating Disorders

The Survey for Eating Disorders (SEDs; Götestam & Agras, 1995) is a self-report scale for diagnosing anorexia nervosa, bulimia nervosa, and binge-eating disorder according to DSM-IV criteria. The SEDs consists of 39 questions, 18 of which are used for diagnoses; four items provide demographic information, and the remaining items provide additional information on age of onset for dieting and binge-eating, and both antecedents and triggers of dieting and binge-eating. Ghaderi and Scott (2002) provided preliminary reliability and validity data for the scale using both a clinical and a university sample of adult women. Reliability was established by finding identical diagnostic classifications obtained from the SEDs on two occasions over a 2-week interval. The SEDs also had a high level of concordance with the EDE in diagnosing an eating disorder. All women classified with an eating disorder on the EDE were identified by the SEDs, and only 4% of women diagnosed with an eating disorder using the SEDs were not classified with an eating disorder by the EDE. However, the SEDs demonstrated only a moderate degree of convergent validity in correctly classifying women (69%) with a specific eating disorder as diagnosed by the EDE. For example, seven women diagnosed with binge-eating disorder on the SEDs received an EDNOS diagnosis on the EDE, while two other women diagnosed with binge-eating disorder on the SEDs received a bulimia nervosa diagnosis on the EDE. Overall, these findings suggest that the SEDs may be better used as a general screening instrument of undifferentiated DSM-IV eating disorders, like the EDI and EAT.

Questionnaire for Eating Disorder Diagnoses

The Questionnaire for Eating Disorder Diagnoses (Q-EDD; Mintz, O'Halloran, Mulholland, & Schneider, 1997) is a 50-item, self-report scale based on the Weight Management Questionnaire (Mintz & Betz, 1988). The revised scale was designed to diagnose individuals with DSM-IV eating disorders, to differentially diagnose bulimia and anorexia, and to distinguish those who do not meet DSM-IV criteria for an eating disorder but display symptoms of eating disorders (symptomatic group). The Q-EDD yields both frequency data for individual behaviors (e.g., self-induced vomiting) and diagnostic categories. The categories include asymptomatic (no eating disorder symptoms), symptomatic (some eating disorder symptoms but no DSM-IV diagnosis), bulimia, anorexia, subthreshold bulimia, menstruating anorexia, nonbingeing bulimia, and binge-eating disorder. The Q-EDD has been validated in women with and without eating disorders. Test–retest reliability of diagnoses over a 2-week period as assessed using kappa values was high (.85–.94). Test–retest reliability of diagnoses over a 3-month interval was stable (.54–.64). The Q-EDD has been found to have a high accuracy rate (98%) in correctly classifying women with and without a DSM-IV eating disorder as diagnosed by structured interviews. Sensitivity, specificity, and positive and negative predictive values were all above .94. The accuracy rate for differentiating between symptomatic and asymptomatic groups was 90%, and 100% for differentiating between anorexia and bulimia. Convergent validity for the scales has been demonstrated by the correspondence between Q-EDD diagnoses and scores on the BULIT-R and the EAT. The BULIT-R scores of Q-EDD-defined bulimics were significantly higher than the nonbulimics. Similarly, the EAT scores of the Q-EDD-defined anorexics and menstruating anorexics were significantly higher than those of women without eating disorders.

Eating Disorder Diagnostic Scale

The Eating Disorder Diagnostic Scale (EDDS; Stice, Telch, & Rizvi, 2000) is a 22-item, self-report scale designed to diagnose eating disorders. Items were specifically selected and designed to assess all of the DSM-IV diagnostic symptoms for anorexia nervosa, bulimia nervosa, and binge-eating disorder. The instrument has been validated in women with and without eating disorders, ages 13–61 years. Internal consistency (.89) and test–retest reliability over a 1-week interval (.87) for the composite EDDS were high. Test–retest reliability has also been found to be high for anorexia nervosa diagnoses (.95) and moderate for bulimia nervosa (.71) and binge-eating disorder (.75) diagnoses.

The EDDS has a high accuracy rate in correctly classifying women with DSM-IV eating disorder as diagnosed by structured interviews. The overall accuracy rate was 99% for anorexia nervosa, 96% for bulimia nervosa, and 93% for binge-eating disorder. Sensitivity, specificity, and positive and negative predictive values were all above .83 for anorexia nervosa, above .81 for bulimia nervosa, and above .77 for binge-eating disorder. Convergent validity for the composite EDDS has been found to be satisfactory. Total EDDS scores were found to correlate moderately with all subscales from the EDE and the YBC-EDS, and two subscales, Hunger and Disinhibition, from the Three-Factor Eating Questionnaire (.36–.63). Only the correlation between the composite EDDS and the Cognitive Restraint, one of the other subscales from the Three-Factor Eating Questionnaire, was found to be low and nonsignificant (.10).

Bulimic Investigatory Test

The Bulimic Investigatory Test (BITE; Henderson & Freeman, 1987) is a 33-item, self-report scale designed to identify individuals with symptoms of bulimia nervosa or binge-eating, as defined by DSM-III. The BITE also assesses the severity of bulimic symptoms. It has been validated in women with eating disorders, and in male and female adults and adolescents (Henderson & Freeman, 1997; Ricciardelli, Williams, & Kiernan, 1999). However, it has yet to be evaluated using DSM-IV criteria. Ricciardelli et al. (1999) examined the BITE factor structure in adolescent girls and boys. Consistent with the scale's conceptualization, one factor describing overall bulimic symptoms was found for girls. However, two factors were required to more fully summarize the boys' symptoms, which tended to separate problem from nonproblem binge-eating (Fairburn, 1995). Internal consistency of the BITE as assessed by Cronbach's alpha is high for the symptom subscale (.96) but low for the severity subscale (.62). Test–retest reliability over a 1-week period is low (.68; Henderson & Freeman, 1997). The BITE accurately discriminated between a sample of female bulimics and normal controls. The BITE has also demonstrated adequate concurrent validity; BITE scores correlate moderately with Drive for Thinness, Bulimia, and Body Dissatisfaction from the EDI, and the Dieting and Bulimia subscales from the EAT (.35–.68).

Stirling Eating Disorder Scales

The Stirling Eating Disorder Scales (SEDS; Williams & Power, 1992; Williams et al., 1994) is an 80-item, self-report inventory designed for comprehensive assessment of cognitions and behaviors associated with eating disorders. It consists of eight subscales: Anorexic Dietary Cognitions, Anorexic Dietary Behavior, Bulimic Dietary Cognitions, Bulimic Dietary Behavior, Low Assertiveness, Low Self-Esteem, Self-Directed Hostility, and Perceived External Control. The SEDS has been validated in women with eating disorders, and both women and men without eating disorders.

Internal consistency of the SEDS subscales as assessed by both Cronbach's alpha and split-half correlations has been found to be high (.84–.99). Test–retest reliability over a 3-week interval is high (.90–.97). All subscales differentiated between normal controls and an anorexic and bulimic group. In addition, anorexic patients scored significantly higher than bulimic patients on the scales of Anorexic Dietary Behavior and Anorexic Dietary Cognitions, while bulimic patients scored significantly higher than the anorexics on the scales of Bulimic Dietary Cognitions and Bulimic Dietary Behavior. Concurrent validity for the subscales also has been found to be good. The SEDS subscales correlate highly with the EAT and the BITE (.83–.90; Williams & Power, 1992; Williams et al., 1994). However, the factor structure of the eight subscales has not been verified by factor analysis.

Measures of Eating-Related Cognitions

Mizes Anorectic Cognitions Questionnaire—Revised

The Mizes Anorectic Cognitions Questionnaire—Revised (MAC-R; Mizes et al., 2000) is a 24-item self-report inventory designed to assess cognitions associated with eating disorders. The MAC-R, like the original version, specifically assesses three dimensions of eating disorder cognitions: strict weight regulation and the fear of weight gain, self-control as the basis of self-esteem, and weight and eating behavior as the basis of approval. The revised version has only been validated with a clinical sample of adults that also included a small percentage (2.9%) of males. However, the original version was validated with nonclinical samples consisting of both adult females and males (Mizes & Klesges, 1989; Mizes, 1991). High levels of internal consistency for the total MAC-R (.90) and its three subscales (.82–.85) have been found. Although test–retest reliability for the revised version has yet to be provided, that for the original version over a 2-month period was moderate (.78). Construct validity for the three dimensions has been demonstrated by principal component analysis, which identified three robust factors corresponding to the inventory's three subscales, Weight Regulation, Approval, and Self-Control. Concurrent validity for the MAC-R is satisfactory. The total MAC-R score and subscale scores correlate in the moderate-to-high range with the EDI (.56–.69) and the

Restraint Scales (.40–.70). In addition, two of the subscales, Weight Regulation and Self-Control, discriminated between patients diagnosed with anorexia nervosa and those with bulimia nervosa.

Eating Expectancy Measures

Three instruments have been developed to assess outcome expectancies associated with dieting and other eating behaviors: the Weight Loss Expectancy Scale (Allen, Thombs, Mahoney, & Daniel, 1993), the Eating Expectancy Inventory (Hohlstein, Smith, & Atlas, 1998), and the Thinness and Restricting Expectancy Inventory (Hohlstein et al., 1998).

Weight Loss Expectancy Scale

The Weight Loss Expectancy Scale (WLES; Allen et al., 1993) is a 33-item self-report instrument designed to assess both positive and negative outcomes of dieting practices and losing weight. The scale has been validated with adolescent girls and boys (Allen et al., 1993), and adult women (Thombs, Rosenberg, Mahoney, & Daniel, 1996). Five factors were identified using principal component analysis: Social Confidence, Social Approval, Self-Worth, Positive Performance, and Negative Consequences. These factors possess adequate-to-high levels of internal consistency (Cronbach's alpha = .69–.94). In addition, two of the factors, Social Approval and Self-Worth, were found to discriminate among adolescents who frequently dieted, occasionally dieted, or did not diet. Two of the factors, Self-Worth and Social Confidence, also were found to be moderately related to the BULIT-R in a sample of adult women.

Eating Expectancy Inventory

The Eating Expectancy Inventory (EEI; Hohlstein et al., 1998), a 34-item self-report scale designed to assess cognitive expectations for eating, has been validated in adult women with and without eating disorders (Hohlstein et al., 1998) and adolescent females (Simmons, Smith, & Hill, 2002). The EEI consists of five subscales that have been validated via factor analysis: (1) Eating helps manage negative affect; (2) eating is pleasurable and useful as a reward; (3) eating leads to feeling out of control; (4) eating enhances cognitive competence; and (5) eating alleviates boredom. Levels of internal consistency for the EEI scales as assessed by Cronbach's alpha, range between .78 and .94. The EEI subscales correlate moderately with the BULIT-R, the Restraint Scale, and the Disinhibition subscale from the Three-Factor Eating Questionnaire (.28–.64). In addition, the EEI has been found to differentiate between anorexics and bulimics, and between both groups and psychiatric and normal controls.

Thinness and Restricting Expectancy Inventory

The Thinness and Restricting Expectancy Inventory (TREI; Hohlstein et al., 1998) is a 44-item self-report scale designed to assess cognitive expectations for the consequences of thinness and restricting food intake. Factor analysis has revealed that the scale assesses a unitary dimension that reflects a broad expectation for overgeneralized life improvement from dieting and thinness, such as feeling more capable, confident, and in control. Internal consistency is very high (.98). The TREI correlates moderately with the BULIT-R, the Restraint Scale, the Restraint and Disinhibition subscales from the Three-Factor Eating Questionnaire and the Drive for Thinness subscale from the EDI-2 (.40–.64). In addition, both bulimic and anorexic patients were found to endorse more frequently expectancies assessed by the TREI than normal and psychiatric controls.

Dietary Restraint

Although the measures of dietary restraint currently are in use were developed prior to 1988, we include them here because the measurement of dietary restraint has received considerable attention in the field (Heatherton, Herman, Polivy, King, & McGree, 1988; Lowe, 1993; Williamson et al., 1995) and highlights refinements and new psychometric information. Restrained eaters are an interesting population that has been found to "vacillate between periods of intense caloric restriction and bouts of disinhibited eating" (Heatherton, Polivy & Herman, 1991, p. 78). Although many restrained eaters describe themselves as current dieters, and "restrained eating" and "dieting" are terms often used interchangeably, such a definition would exclude a large proportion of individuals who score high on measures of eating restraint but do not report current dieting (Lowe, 1993). More characteristically, restrained eaters are persons who have dieted and failed many times (Heatherton et al., 1998; Lowe, 1993). Interestingly, a rapid change in dietary restraint was recently identified as the primary mediator of posttreatment improvement in binge-eating and vomiting for bulimics treated using cognitive-behavioral therapy (Wilson et al., 2002).

Restraint Scale

The Restraint Scale (Herman & Mack, 1975), a 10-item self-report measure of dietary restraint (Lowe, 1993), has been shown to predict disinhibition, binge-eating, counterregulated eating, and salivary output (Lowe, 1993). The scale also has been subjected to factor analysis with results consistently revealing two factors, Concern for Dieting and Weight Fluctuations (Allison, Kalinsky, & Gorman, 1992; Heatherton et al., 1988). However, studies have not demonstrated the predictive superiority of one factor over the other; thus, Heatherton et al. recommended the use of a total score over its subscales. The

Restraint Scale has been criticized because it refers to overeating and weight fluctuations (Heatherton et al., 1988; Stice, Ozer, & Kees, 1997).

In order to address the limitations of the Restraint Scale, two other restraint scales were developed: the 10-item Restrained Eating Scale from the Dutch Eating Behavior Questionnaire—Revised (DEBQ-R; van Strien, Frijters, Bergers, & Defares, 1986) and the 21-item Factor Eating Questionnaire—Revised Cognitive Restraint factor (TFEQ-R; Stunkard & Messick, 1985). Factor analyses of the DEBQ-R have consistently shown that it is measuring a unitary dimension of restraint (Allision et al., 1992; Ogden, 1993), while factor analyses of the TFEQ-R have been more equivocal. Some studies have suggested that the cognitive restraint items of the TFEQ assess a unidimensional construct (Collins, Lapp, Helder, & Saltzberg, 1992; Ganley, 1988; Hyland, Irvine, Thacker, Dann, & Dennis, 1989), while others have found support for two dimensions, Cognitive Restraint and Behavioral Restraint (Allison et al., 1992; Ricciardelli & Williams, 1997).

Consistent with the scales' conceptualizations, the TFEQ-R and the DEBQ-R predict reduced caloric intake and correlate only weakly with binge-eating in some studies (Lowe, 1993; van Strien, 1996). These results have led researchers to conclude that the TFEQ-R and DEBQ-R may better describe actual and current dieting, while the Restraint Scale assesses chronic and unsuccessful dieting (Allison et al., 1992; Heatherton et al., 1988; Lowe, 1993; Williamson et al., 1995). However, other studies have found more similarities than differences among the three scales. For example, the Restraint Scale, the TFEQ-R, and the DEBQ-R are moderately intercorrelated (Laessle, Tuschl, Kotthaus, & Pirke, 1989). Similarly, both the Restraint Scale and the TFEQ-R, along with an index of current dieting, load on a single factor (Beebe, Holmbeck, Albright, Noga, & Decastro, 1995). In another study, the DEBQ-R was found to predict bulimic symptoms prospectively, including binge-eating (Stice, 2001).

Body Image/Appearance

DSM-IV diagnostic criteria, as well as cognitive-behavioral models of the etiology of eating disorders, include concern about one's appearance, body image, or shape as important characteristics of eating disorders. Thus, measures of body image are useful in comprehensive assessment of eating disorders. Body image is a multidimensional construct. Controversies exist concerning the nature of body image disturbances related to eating disorders, the operational definition of a body image disturbance, and the methods for measuring it (Cash & Deagle, 1997). Typically, body image dysfunction is said to be characterized by either cognitive evaluation dissatisfaction or distortion in the perception of one's body size. There is inconsistent support for an association between these two constructs. Below, we present examples of two self-report measures designed to assess the cognitive and evaluative aspects of body image related to eating disorders. We also describe methods used to assess the perception of body size and highlight research on body image and eating disorders among men. Additional information on these topics is presented in Thompson and van den Berg's (2002) review of attitudinal measures that assess body image, Thompson and Gardner's (2002) review of the measurement of perceptual body image, and Ricciardelli and McCabe's (2001) review of measures designed to assess eating disturbance and body image concerns among children.

Beliefs About Appearance Scale

The Beliefs About Appearance Scale (BAAS; Spangler & Stice, 2001) is a 20-item self-report measure designed to assess dysfunctional beliefs about the implications of one's appearance. Such beliefs encompass the domains of interpersonal, achievement, self-view, and feelings. Psychometric analysis using three predominantly female samples recruited from universities, a junior college, and private high schools indicated that the 20 items of the BAAS constitute a single factor. The measure is internally consistent (alphas = .94–.96), and has excellent test–retest reliability r's = .73 (over 10 months) and .83 (over 3 weeks). With regard to validity, the BAAS has good discriminant, concurrent, and predictive validity. With regard to discriminant validity, it was not associated with physical health, body weight, or fitness. The BAAS showed concurrent validity with measures of body satisfaction, dieting, and eating disorder symptoms, to which it is conceptually related. In addition, females score higher on the BAAS than do males. Scores on the BAAS accounted for additional variance in eating disorder symptoms and dietary restraint, even after controlling for measures of those constructs. In one study, scores on the BAAS decreased after three 1-hour intervention sessions designed to change body image, thereby indicating its potential usefulness in cognitive-behavioral treatment of eating disorders.

Multidimensional Body–Self Relations Questionnaire

The Multidimensional Body–Self Relations Questionnaire (MBSRQ; Brown, Cash, & Mikulka, 1990; Cash, 1994). The MBSRQ is a self-report inventory that assesses body image attitudes. Its 69 items form 10 subscales (e.g., Appearance Evaluation, seven items that measure degree of satisfaction with one's overall physical appearance; Body Areas Satisfaction, eight items that measure degree of satisfaction with specific parts of the body [e.g., face, torso]; Overweight Preoccupation, four items that measure anxiety about fat and vigilance about weight; Fitness Evaluation, three items that measure the perception of one's physical fitness). Each subscale contains different numbers of items. However, level of agreement with each of the scale items is rated on a 5-point scale (1 = "definitely disagree," 5 = "definitely agree"). Each of the MBSRQ subscales is internally consistent (e.g., Cronbach's alphas generally range from .70 to .90) and has good (range from .70 to .90) test–retest reliability over a 1-month period (Cash, 1994).

Perceptual methods to assess body image focus on either having individuals estimate the size (e.g., width, depth) of specific body parts/sites or use techniques that focus on or distort the whole body. The latter techniques include the use of adjustable mirrors or video technology for estimating body size. In both cases, the nature and size of the distortion of the individual's body can be compared to his or her actual body size (Cash & Deagle, 1997; Thompson & Gardner, 2002).

Muscle Dysmorphia

Although this chapter focuses on women, the area of body image is one in which the effects of men's disordered eating may manifest themselves (Ricciardelli & McCabe, 2004). Pope, Katz, and Hudson (1993) coined the term "reverse anorexia" and described it as a disorder "characterized by a fear of being too small, and by perceiving oneself as small and weak, even when one is actually large and muscular" (p. 406). More recently, it has been renamed "muscle dysmorphia" (Phillips, O'Sullivan, & Pope, 1997) and is recognized as a subcategory of body dysmorphic disorder. Although the formal criteria for diagnosing muscle dysmorphia are still being developed, the current diagnosis involves three criteria (Olivardia, 2001; Pope, Phillips, & Olivardia, 2000): (1) a "preoccupation with the idea that one's body is not sufficiently lean and muscular" (Pope et al., 2000, p. 248); (2) the preoccupation causes clinically significant distress or impairment in social, occupational or other important areas of functioning; and (3) "the primary focus of the preoccupation and behaviors is on being too small or inadequately muscular" (p. 248). However, this focus needs to be "distinguished from fear of being fat as in anorexia nervosa, or primary preoccupation only with other aspects of appearance as in other forms of body dysmorphic disorder" (p. 248).

Self-Monitoring of Eating Behaviors

Many measures of eating behavior are based on retrospective recall. While such information can be helpful in painting a general picture of eating behaviors, as stated earlier, retrospection suffers from limitations related to forgetting the occurrence of particular events and the aggregation of information across time. More specific information collected in close proximity to the behavior of interest can elucidate patterns and highlight relationships that might not be apparent when relying on the averages that retrospective data typically represent. In cases where more specific, prospective information is warranted, ongoing self-monitoring is the assessment approach of choice.

When applied to the assessment of eating disorders, self-monitoring can be useful for collecting information on behavioral (e.g., bingeing, purging), affective (e.g., moods), cognitive (e.g., urges), and environmental (e.g., social activities, eating locations) aspects of eating. Basic information about food intake includes the number and timing of meals/snacks, the types of food being consumed, and estimates of caloric intake. In addition, assessment of various antecedents (e.g., environmental, cognitive, and affective cues), correlates (e.g., type and duration of physical activity), and consequences of eating (e.g., cognitions, affect) can provide a comprehensive picture of the factors that maintain maladaptive eating behaviors.

Self-monitoring is traditionally done using paper-and-pencil methods in which the participant is instructed to maintain a detailed record of a target behavior such as food intake, thoughts (about food or body image), responses to environmental cues, and so on. It is most accurate when recordings are made in close proximity to the target behavior, when recording is not too intrusive or difficult, and when the behavior to be monitored is clearly specified. The integrating of self-monitoring data in planning of treatment or maintenance can be very reinforcing for the client who has collected the data. Self-monitoring is an integral part of cognitive-behavioral treatment of eating disorders (Wilson & Vitousek, 1999). It is a widely used and relatively effective method for measuring eating-related behaviors, and research suggests that its limited reactivity can be used to enhance treatment outcome; that is, increasing clients' awareness of the factors associated with their maladaptive eating may enhance their ability to change certain eating-related behaviors. It also can serve as a useful indicator of compliance with and response to interventions and homework assignments between treatment sessions. Self-monitoring on a daily basis, or even multiple times per day, can provide useful information. Requiring that such diaries be mailed on a daily basis enhances compliance with the self-monitoring protocol (e.g., Rebert, Stanton, & Schwartz, 1991).

To enhance behavioral treatment, Wilson and Vitousek (1999) recommend that self-monitoring be presented in a collaborative fashion that contributes to the development of a strong therapeutic alliance. These benefits are balanced by limitations that are specific to the assessment of eating behavior. They include (1) a tendency for patients to underreport food intake; (2) influence by a variety of contextual factors; and (3) reinforcement of some anorexic and bulimic clients' preoccupation with food. More general limitations of self-monitoring include (1) the relative unreliability of certain kinds of self-report; (2) deficient data (e.g., missing data, ambiguous responses); (3) the possibility of poor compliance or faked data (e.g., failure to complete assessments as instructed); and (4) the inability to provide base-rate data as a context for understanding the target behavior being monitored (Shiffman & Stone, 1998). This last issue is important in establishing associations between potential antecedents (e.g., mood) and the target behavior. Thus, despite a long tradition of paper-and-pencil self-monitoring, more technically sophisticated methods are being developed and/or applied to collecting self-monitoring data on eating.

More than 20 years ago, Johnson and Larson (1982) pioneered the use of technology to enhance the collection of self-monitoring data. To obtain reports on samples of the behavior of 15 bulimic women, they provided the women with pagers and then randomly signaled them to complete a self-monitoring card. During 1 week of self-monitoring, the participants completed multiple reports (mean of 6.4 per person, per day) on items such as their activities, cognitions, mood, and the occurrence of binge-eating and purging. Their results indicated significant differences between bulimics and a control sample of nonbulimic women. Bulimic women reported more negative and fluctuating moods and spent more time either alone or in food-related activities.

Years later, Greeno, Wing, and Shiffman (2000) used small, hand-held computers to prospectively sample the experiences of obese women. During 6 days of self-monitoring, the women interacted with the computers when randomly prompted, just before and just after an episode of eating. They reported on their affect (positive and negative mood), appetite, setting, and the occurrence of binge-eating. Although this study did not include specific data about compliance with the self-monitoring procedures, the vast majority (89%) of the participants completed all 6 days of self-monitoring. They generated over 4,000 observations and provided useful data for identifying binge antecedents.

Bardone and colleagues (2000) used interactive voice response (IVR) technology to collect college women's reports of binge-eating. During each day of a 12-week period, the women called an IVR system and answered questions about binge-eating during the previous day. Participants were provided with the DSM-IV definition of a binge and were trained in the use of a toll-free number and the IVR system to provide their daily reports. They received a financial incentive of 50 cents per day, plus a $10 bonus per uninterrupted week of reports, for a possible total of $162 for the 12 weeks. Compliance was moderately good; 82.4% of the possible 3,612 reports were completed. The 12 weeks of prospective IVR data were compared to the participants' retrospective self-reports of binge-eating during the same 12-week period. The retrospective reports were collected using the structured format of the Timeline Follow-Back method (TLFB; Sobell & Sobell, 1992). The results indicated that the daily IVR reports were discrepant with the TLFB reports, with the latter leading to underestimates of binge-eating frequency.

These innovative studies (summarized in Table 10.1) illustrate the use of state-of-the-art methods for collecting reliable and valid self-monitoring data concerning eating behavior and a variety of related phenomena. As enhancements to traditional self-monitoring, each of these technologies also has the potential to serve as useful adjuncts to cognitive-behavioral approaches for changing eating habits and treating eating disorders (cf. Delichatsios et al., 2001; Latner & Wilson, 2002; Wilson & Vitousek, 1999).

TABLE 10.1. Summary of Eating Disorders Assessment Measures

Purpose	Domain/construct	Instrument(s)	Author(s)
Diagnostic interview	Assess severity of eating preoccupations and rituals	YBC-EDS	Mazure et al. (1994)
	Frequency and severity of eating behaviors and attitudes	EDE, 12th edition	Cooper & Fairburn (1987); Fairburn & Cooper (1993)
Self-report of behavioral symptoms	Frequency and severity of eating behaviors and attitudes	EDE-Q	Fairburn & Beglin (1994)
	Severity of symptoms associated with anorexia nervosa and bulimia nervosa	EDI-2	Garner (1991)
	Bulimia symptoms, DSM-III and DSM-IV criteria	BULIT-R	Thelen et al. (1991, 1996)
	Symptoms of eating disorders, DSM-IV criteria	EAT (versions based on number of items; EAT-40, EAT-26, EAT-12)	Garner & Garfinkle (1979); Garner et al. (1982); Lavik et al. (1991)
	Children's symptoms of eating disorders	ChEAT s-EAT	Maloney et al. (1989) Ohzeki et al. (1993)
	Symptom checklist for bulimia and binge-eating	EQR	Williamson et al. (1989)
	DSM-IV criteria for diagnosing anorexia nervosa, bulimia nervosa, and binge-eating disorder	SEDs	Götestam & Agras (1995)
	DSM-IV criteria for diagnosing eating disorders	Q-EDD	Mintz et al. (1997)
	DSM-IV criteria for diagnosing anorexia nervosa, bulimia nervosa, and binge-eating disorder	EDDS	Stice et al. (2000)
	DSM-III criteria and symptom severity for bulimia nervosa and binge-eating	BITE	Henderson & Freeman (1987)
	Eating disorder cognitions and behaviors	SEDS	Williams & Power (1992); Williams et al. (1994)
	Cognitions associated with eating disorders	MAC-R	Mizes et al. (2000)

(continued)

TABLE 10.1. *(continued)*

Purpose	Domain/construct	Instrument(s)	Author(s)
Assess expectancies	Expectancies related to dieting practices and losing weight	WLES	Allen et al. (1993)
	Cognitive expectancies for eating	EEI	Hohlstein et al. (1998)
	Cognitive expectancies for dieting and thinness	TREI	Hohlstein et al. (1998)
Assess dietary restraint	Caloric restriction and disinhibited eating	Restraint Scale	Herman & Mack (1975)
	Cognitive aspects of restrained eating	DEBQ-R	van Strien et al. (1986)
	Cognitive aspects of restrained eating	TFEQ-R	Stunkard & Merrick (1985)
Assess body image	Dysfunctional beliefs about implications of one's appearance	BAAS	Spangler & Stice (2001)
	Body image attitudes	MBRSQ	Brown et al. (1990); Cash (1994)

REFERENCES

Ackerman, S. J., & Hilsenroth, M. J. (2003). A review of therapist characteristics and techniques positively impacting the therapeutic alliance. *Clinical Psychology Review, 23,* 1–33.

Allen, K. M., Thombs, D. L., Mahoney, C. A., & Daniel, E. L. (1993). Relationships between expectancies and adolescent dieting behaviours. *Journal of School Health, 63,* 176–181.

Allison, D. A., Kalinsky, L. B., & Gorman, B. S. (1992). A comparison of the psychometric properties of three measures of dietary restraint. *Psychological Assessment, 4,* 391–398.

American Psychiatric Association. (2000). *Diagnostic and statistical manual of mental disorders* (4th ed., text rev.). Washington, DC: Author.

Andersen, A. E., & Holman, J. E. (1997). Males with eating disorders: Challenges for treatment and research. *Psychopharmacology Bulletin, 33,* 391–397.

Bardone, A. M., Krahn, D. D., Goodman, B. M., & Searles, J. S. (2000). Using interactive voice response technology and timeline follow-back methodology in studying binge eating and drinking behavior: Different answers to different forms of the same question? *Addictive Behaviors, 25,* 1–11.

Beebe, D. W., Holmbeck, G. N., Albright, J. S., Noga, K., & Decastro, B. (1995). Identification of "binge-prone" women: An experimentally and psychometrically validated cluster analysis in a college population. *Addictive Behaviors, 20,* 451–462.

Black, C. M. D., & Wilson, G. T. (1996). Assessment of eating disorders: Interview versus questionnaire. *International Journal of Eating Disorders, 20,* 43–50.

Braun, D. L., Sunday, S. R., Huang, A., & Halmi, K. A. (1999). More males seek treatment for eating disorders. *International Journal of Eating Disorders, 25,* 415–424.

Brelsford, T. N., Hummel, R. M., & Barrios, B. A. (1992). The Bulimia Test—Revised: A psychometric investigation. *Psychological Assessment, 4,* 399–401.

Brown, T. A., Cash, T. F., & Milulka, P. J. (1990). Attitudinal body image assessment: Factor analysis of the Body–Self Relations Questionnaire. *Journal of Personality Assessment, 55,* 135–144.

Carlat, D. J., & Camargo, C. A. (1991). Review of bulimia nervosa in males. *American Journal of Psychiatry, 148,* 831–843.

Carlat, D. J., Camargo, C. A., & Herzog, D. B. (1997). Eating disorders in males: A report on 135 patients. *American Journal of Psychiatry, 154,* 1127–1132.

Cash, T. F. (1994). *Users manual for the Multidimensional Body–Self Relations Questionnaire.* Norfolk, VA: Old Dominion University.

Cash, T. F., & Deagle, E. A. (1997). The nature and extent of body image disturbances in anorexia nervosa and bulimia nervosa: A meta analysis. *International Journal of Eating Disorders, 22,* 107–125.

Collins, R. L., Lapp, W. M., Helder, L., & Saltzberg, J. A. (1992). Cognitive restraint and impulsive eating: Insights from the Three-Factor Eating Questionnaire. *Psychology of Addictive Behaviors, 6,* 47–53.

Cooper, Z., & Fairburn, C. G. (1987). The Eating Disorder Examination: A semistructured interview for the assessment of the specific psychopathology of eating disorders. *International Journal of Eating Disorders, 6,* 1–8.

Delichatsios, H. K., Friedman, R. H., Glanz, K., Tennstedt, S., Smigelski, C., Pinto, B. M., Kelley, H., & Gillman, M. W. (2001). Randomized trial of a "talking computer" to improve eating habits. *American Journal of Health Promotion, 15,* 215–224.

Engelsen, B. K., & Hagtvet, K. A. (1999). The dimensionality of the 12–item version of the Eating Attitudes Test: Confirmatory factor analyses. *Scandinavian Journal of Psychology, 40,* 293–300.

Fairburn, C. G. (1995). *Overcoming binge-eating.* New York: Guilford Press.

Fairburn, C. G., & Beglin, S. J. (1994). Assessment of eating disorders: Interview or self-report questionnaire? *International Journal of Eating Disorders, 16,* 363–370.

Fairburn, C. G., & Cooper, Z. (1993). The eating disorder examination (12th ed.). In C. G. Fairburn & G. T. Wilson (Eds.), *Binge-eating: Nature, assessment, and treatment* (pp. 317–360). New York: Guilford Press.

Fairburn, C. G., Marcus, M. D., & Wilson, G. T. (1993). Cognitive-behavioral therapy for binge-eating and bulimia nervosa: A comprehensive treatment manual. In C. G. Fairburn & G. T. Wilson (Eds.), *Binge-eating: Nature, assessment, and treatment* (pp. 361–404). New York: Guilford Press.

Ganley, R. M. (1988). Emotional eating and how it relates to dietary restraint, disinhibition, and perceived hunger. *International Journal of Eating Disorders, 7,* 635–647.

Garfinkel, P. E., Kin, E., Goering, P., Spegg, C., Goldbloom, D. S., Kennedy, S., Kaplan, A. S., & Woodside, D. B. (1995). Bulimia nervosa in a Canadian community sample: Prevalence and comparison of subgroups. *American Journal of Psychiatry, 152,* 1052–1058.

Garner, D. M. (1991). *The Eating Disorder Inventory–2: Professional manual.* Odessa, FL: Psychological Assessment Resources.

Garner, D. M., & Garfinkel, P. E. (1979). The Eating Attitudes Test: An index of symptoms of anorexia nervosa. *Psychological Medicine, 9,* 273–279.

Garner, D. M., & Olmsted, M. P. (1984). *The Eating Disorder Inventory manual.* Odessa, FL: Psychological Assessment Resources.

Garner, D. M., Olmsted, M. P., Bohr, Y., & Garfinkel, P. E. (1982). The Eating Attitudes Test: Psychometric features and clinical correlates. *Psychological Medicine, 12,* 872–878.

Geller, J., Cockell, S. J., & Drab, D. L. (2001). Assessing readiness for change in the eating disorders: The psychometric properties of the Readiness and Motivation Interview. *Psychological Assessment, 13,* 189–198.

Ghaderi, A., & Scott, B. (2002). The preliminary reliability and validity of the Survey for Eating Disorders (SEDs): A self-report questionnaire for diagnosing eating disorders. *European Eating Disorders Review, 10,* 61–76.

Götestam, K. G., & Agras, W. S. (1995). General population-based epidemiological study of eating disorders in Norway. *International Journal of Eating Disorders, 18,* 119–126.

Greeno, C. G., Wing, R. R., & Shiffman, S. (2000). Binge antecedents in obese women with and without binge-eating disorder. *Journal of Consulting and Clinical Psychology, 68,* 95–102.

Grilo, C. M., Masheb, R. M., & Wilson, G. T. (2001). Subtyping binge eating disorder. *Journal of Consulting and Clinical Psychology, 69,* 1066–1072.

Heatherton, T. F., Herman, C. P., Polivy, J., King, G. A., & McGree, S. T. (1988). The (mis)measurement of restraint: An analysis of conceptual and psychometric issues. *Journal of Abnormal Psychology, 97,* 19–28.

Heatherton, T. F., Polivy, J., & Herman, C. P. (1991). Restraint, weight loss, and variability in body weight. *Journal of Abnormal Psychology, 100,* 78–83.

Heatherton, T. F., Polivy, J., Herman, C. P., & Baumeister, R. F. (1993). Self-awareness, task failure, and disinhibition: How attentional focus affects eating. *Journal of Personality, 61,* 49–61.

Henderson, M., & Freeman, C. P. L. (1987). A self-rating scale for bulimia: The BITE. *Journal of Psychiatry, 150,* 18–24.

Herman, C. P., & Mack, D. (1975). Restrained and unrestrained eating. *Journal of Personality, 43,* 647–660.

Hohlstein, L. A., Smith, G. T., & Atlas, J. G. (1998). An application of expectancy theory to eating disorders: Development and validation of measures of eating and dieting expectancies. *Psychological Assessment, 10,* 49–58.

Hyland, M. E., Irvine, S. H., Thacker, C., Dann, P. L., & Dennis, I. (1989). Psychometric analysis of the Stunkard–Messick Eating Questionnaire (SMEQ) and comparison with the Dutch Eating Behavior Questionnaire (DEBQ). *Current Psychology Research and Reviews, 8,* 228–233.

Johnson, C., & Larson, R. (1982). Bulimia: An analysis of moods and behavior. *Psychosomatic Medicine, 44,* 341–351.

Kelly, C., Ricciardelli, L. A., & Clarke, J. D. (1999). Problem eating attitudes and behaviors in young children. *International Journal of Eating Disorders, 25,* 281–286.

Laessle, R. G., Tuschl, R. J., Kotthaus, B. C., & Pirke, K. M. (1989). A comparison of the validity of three scales for the assessment of dietary restraint. *Journal of Abnormal Psychology, 98*, 504–507.

Latner, J. D., & Wilson, G. T. (2002). Self-monitoring and the assessment of binge eating. *Behavior Therapy, 33*, 465–477.

Lavik, N. J., Clausen, S. P., & Pedersen, W. (1991). Eating behavior, drug use, psychopathology and parental bonding in adolescents in Norway. *Acta Psychiatrica Scandinavica, 84*, 387–390.

Lee, S. (1993). How abnormal is the desire for slimness?: A survey of eating attitudes and behaviour among Chinese undergraduates in Hong Kong. *Psychological Medicine, 23*, 437–451.

Lee, S., Lee, M. A., Leung, T., & Hong, Y. (1997). Psychometric properties of Eating Disorder Inventory (EDI-I) in a nonclinical Chinese population in Hong Kong. *International Journal of Eating Disorders, 21*, 187–194.

Lowe, M. R. (1993). The effects of dieting on eating behavior: A three-factor model. *Psychological Bulletin, 114*, 100–121.

Machado, P. P. P., Gonçalves, S., Martins, C., & Soares, I. C. (2001). The Portuguese version of the Eating Disorders Inventory: Evaluation of its psychometric properties. *European Eating Disorders Review, 9*, 43–52.

Maloney, M. J., McGuire, J., Daniels, S. R., & Specker, B. (1989). Dieting behavior and eating attitudes in children. *Pediatrics, 84*, 482–489.

Mazure, C. M., Halmi, K. A., Sunday, S. R., Romano, S. J., & Einhorn, A. M. (1994). The Yale–Brown–Cornell Eating Disorder Scale: Development, use, reliability and validity. *Journal of Psychiatric Research, 28*, 425–445.

Mintz, L. B., & Betz, N. E. (1988). Prevalence and correlates of eating disordered behavior among undergraduate women. *Journal of Counseling Psychology, 35*, 463–471.

Mintz, L. B., & O'Halloran, M. S. (2000). The Eating Attitudes Test: Validation with DSM-IV eating disorder criteria. *Journal of Personality Assessment, 74*, 489–503.

Mintz, L. B., O'Halloran, M. S., Mulholland, A. M., & Schneider, P. A. (1997). Questionnaire for eating disorder diagnoses: Reliability and validity of operationalizing DSM-IV criteria into a self-report format. *Journal of Counseling Psychology, 44*, 63–79.

Mizes, J. S. (1991). Construct validity and factor stability of the Anorectic Cognitions Questionnaire. *Addictive Behaviors, 16*, 89–93.

Mizes, J. S., Christiano, B., Madison, J., Post, G., Seime, R., & Varnado, P. (2000). Development of the Mizes Anorectic Cognitions Questionnaire—Revised: Psychometric properties and factor structure in a large sample of eating disorder patients. *International Journal of Eating Disorders, 28*, 415–421.

Mizes, J. S., & Klesges, R. C. (1989). Validity, reliability, and factor structure of the Anorectic Cognitions Questionnaire. *Addictive Behaviors, 14*, 589–594.

National Heart, Lung, and Blood Institute. (1998). *Clinical guidelines on the identification, evaluation, and treatment of overweight and obesity in adults.* Bethesda, MD: National Institutes of Health.

Neumark-Sztainer, D., & Story, M. (1998). Dieting and binge-eating among adolescents: What do they really mean? *Journal of the American Dietetic Association, 98*, 446–451.

Niv, N., Kaplan, Z., Mitrani, E., & Shiang, J. (1998). Validity study of the EDI-2 in Israeli population. *Israel Journal of Psychiatry and Related Sciences, 35*, 287–292.

O'Brien, K. M., & Vincent, N. K. (2003). Psychiatric comorbidity in anorexia and bulimia nervosa: Nature, prevalence, and causal relationships. *Clinical Psychology Review, 23,* 57–74.

Ogden, J. (1993). The measurement of restraint: Confounding success and failure? *International Journal of Eating Disorders, 13,* 69–76.

Ohzeki, T., Ontahara, H., Hanaki, K., Motozumi, H., & Shiraki, K. (1993). Eating attitudes test in boys and girls aged 6–18 years: Decrease in concerns with eating in boys and the increase in girls with their ages. *Psychopathology, 26,* 117–121.

Olivardia, R. (2001). Mirror, mirror on the wall, who's the largest of them all?: The features and phenomenology of muscle dysmorphia. *Harvard Review of Psychiatry, 9,* 254–259.

Olivardia, R., Pope, H. G., Mangweth, B., & Hudson, J. J. (1995). Eating disorders in college men. *American Journal of Psychiatry, 152,* 1279–1285.

Phillips, K. A., O'Sullivan, R. L., & Pope, H. G. (1997). Muscle dysmorphia. *Journal of Clinical Psychiatry, 58,* 361.

Polivy, J., Herman, C. P., & Garner, D. M. (1988). Cognitive assessment. In D. M. Donovan & G. A. Marlatt (Eds.), *Assessment of addictive behaviors* (pp. 274–295). New York: Guilford Press.

Pope, H. G., Jr., Katz, D. L., & Hudson, J. I. (1993). Anorexia nervosa and "reverse anorexia" among 108 male bodybuilders. *Comprehensive Psychiatry, 34,* 406–409.

Pope, H. G., Phillips, K. A., & Olivardia, R. (2000). *The Adonis complex: The secret crisis of male body obsession.* New York: Free Press.

Rebert, W. M., Stanton, A. L., & Schwarz, R. M. (1991). Influence of personality attributes and daily moods on bulimic eating patterns. *Addictive Behaviors, 16,* 497–505.

Ricciardelli, L. A., & McCabe, M. P. (2001). Children's body image concerns and eating disturbance: A review of the literature. *Clinical Psychology Review, 21,* 325–344.

Ricciardelli, L. A., & McCabe, M. P. (2004). A biopsychosocial model of disordered eating and the pursuit of masculinity in adolescent boys. *Psychological Bulletin, 130,* 179–205.

Ricciardelli, L. A., & Williams, R. J. (1997). A two-factor model of dietary restraint. *Journal of Clinical Psychology, 53,* 123–131.

Ricciardelli, L. A., Williams, R. J., & Kiernan, M. J. (1999). Bulimic symptoms in adolescent girls and boys. *International Journal of Eating Disorders, 26,* 217–221.

Shiffman, S., & Stone, A. A. (1998). Introduction to the special section: Ecological momentary assessment in health psychology. *Health Psychology, 17,* 3–5.

Simmons, J. R., Smith, G. T., & Hill, K. K. (2002). Validation of eating and dieting expectancy measures in two adolescent samples. *International Journal of Eating Disorder, 31,* 461–473.

Smith, M. C., & Thelen, M. H. (1984). Development and validation of a test for bulimia. *Journal of Consulting and Clinical Psychology, 52,* 863–872.

Sobell, L. C., & Sobell, M. B. (1992). Timeline Follow-Back: A technique for assessing self-reported alcohol consumption. In R. Z. Litten & J. P. Allen (Eds.), *Measuring alcohol consumption: Psychosocial and biochemical methods* (pp. 41–72). Totowa, NJ: Humana Press.

Spangler, D. L., & Stice, E. (2001). Validation of the Beliefs About Appearance Scale. *Cognitive Therapy and Research, 25,* 813–827.

Spitzer, R. L., Delvin, M., Walsh, B. T., Hasin, D., Wing, R., Marcus, M. D., Stunkard, A., Wadden, T., Yanovski, S., Agras, S., Mitchell, J., & Nonas, C. (1992). Binge eating disorder: A multisite field trial of the diagnostic criteria. *International Journal of Eating Disorders, 11,* 191–203.

Spitzer, R. L., Yanovski, S., Wadden, T., Wing, R., Marcus, M. D., Stunkard, A., Delvin, M., Mitchell, J., Hasin, D., & Horne, R. L. (1993). Binge eating disorders: Its further validation in a multisite study. *International Journal of Eating Disorders, 13,* 191–203.

Steiger, H. (1989). Anorexia nervosa and bulimia in males: Lessons from a low-risk population. *Canadian Journal of Psychiatry, 34,* 419–424.

Stice, E. (2001). A prospective test of the dual-pathway model of bulimic pathology: Mediating effects of dieting and negative affect. *Journal of Abnormal Psychology, 110,* 124–135.

Stice, E., Ozer, S., & Kees, M. (1997). Relation of dietary restraint to bulimic symptomatology: The effects of the criterion confounding of the Restraint Scale. *Behaviour Therapy and Research, 35,* 145–152.

Stice, E., Telch, C. F., & Rizvi, S. L. (2000). Development and validation of the Eating Disorder Diagnostic Scale: A brief self-report measure of anorexia, bulimia, and binge-eating disorder. *Psychological Assessment, 12,* 123–131.

Stunkard, A. J., & Messick, S. (1985). The Three-Factor Eating Questionnaire to measure dietary restraint, disinhibition, and hunger. *Journal of Psychosomatic Research, 29,* 71–83.

Sunday, S. R., Halmi, K. A., & Einhorn, A. (1995). The Yale–Brown–Cornell Eating Disorder Scale: A new scale to assess eating disorder symptomatology. *International Journal of Eating Disorders, 18,* 237–245.

Thelen, M. H., Farmer, J., Wonderlich, S., & Smith, M. (1991). A revision of the Bulimia Test: The BULIT-R. *Psychological Assessment, 3,* 119–124.

Thelen, M. H., Mintz, L. B., & Vander Wal, J. S. (1996). The Bulimia Test—Revised: Validation with DSM-IV criteria for bulimia nervosa. *Psychological Assessment, 8,* 219–221.

Thombs, D. L., Rosenberg, J. M., Mahoney, C. A., & Daniel, E. L. (1996). Weight-loss expectancies, relative weight, and symptoms of bulimia in young women. *Journal of College Student Development, 37,* 405–414.

Thompson, J. K., & Gardner, R. M. (2002). Measuring perceptual body image among adolescents and adults. In T. F. Cash & T. Pruzinsky (Eds.), *Body image: A handbook of theory, research, and clinical practice* (pp. 135–141). New York: Guilford Press.

Thompson, J. K., & van den Berg, P. (2002). Measuring body image attitudes among adolescents and adults. In T. F. Cash & T. Pruzinsky (Eds.), *Body image: A handbook of theory, research, and clinical practice* (pp. 142–154). New York: Guilford Press.

van Strien, T. (1996). On the relationship between dieting and "obese" and bulimic eating patterns. *International Journal of Eating Disorders, 19,* 83–92.

van Strien, T., Frijters, J. E., Bergers, G. P. A., & Defares, P. B. (1986). Dutch Eating Behavior Questionnaire for assessment of restrained, emotional and external eating behavior. *International Journal of Eating Disorders, 5,* 295–315.

van Strien, T., Frijters, J. E., van Staveren, W. A., Defares, P. B., & Deurenberg, P. (1986). The predictive validity of the Dutch Restrained Eating Scale. *International Journal of Eating Disorders, 5,* 747–755.

Vincent, M. A., McCabe, M. P., & Ricciardelli, L. A. (1999). Factorial validity of the Bulimia Test—Revised in adolescent boys and girls. *Behaviour Research and Therapy, 37,* 1129–1140.

Welch, G., Hall, A., & Norring, C. (1990). The factor structure of the Eating Disorder Inventory in a patient setting. *International Journal of Eating Disorders, 6,* 767–769.

Welch, G., Hall, A., & Walkey, F. H. (1988). The factor structure of the Eating Disorder Inventory. *Journal of Clinical Psychology, 44,* 51–56.

Wells, J. E., Coope, P. A., Gabb, D. C., & Pears, R. K. (1985). The factor structure of the Eating Attitudes Test with adolescent schoolgirls. *Psychological Medicine, 15,* 141–146.

Wilfley, D. E., Schwartz, M. B., Spurrell, E. B., & Fairburn, C. G. (1997). Assessing the specific psychopathology of binge eating disorder patients: Interview or self-report. *Behaviour Research and Therapy, 35,* 1151–1159.

Williams, G. J., & Power, K. G. (1995). *Manual of the Stirling Eating Disorder Scales.* London: Psychological Corporation.

Williams, G. J., Power, K. G., Miller, H. R., Freeman, C. P., Yellowlees, A., Dowds, T., Walker, M., & Parryjones, W. L. (1994). Development and validation of the Stirling Eating Disorder Scales. *International Journal of Eating Disorders, 16,* 35–43.

Williamson, D. A., Davis, C. J., Goreczny, A. J., McKenzie, S. J., & Watkins, P. C. (1989). The Eating Questionnaire—Revised: A symptom checklist for bulimia. In P. A. Keller & L. G. Ritt (Eds.), *Innovations in clinical practice: A source book* (pp. 321–326). Sarasota, FL: Professional Resource Press.

Williamson, D. A., Lawson, O. J., Brooks, E. R., Wozniak, P. J., Ryan, D. H., Bray, G. A., & Duchmann, E. G. (1995). Association of body mass with dietary restraint and disinhibition. *Appetite, 25,* 31–41.

Wilson, G. T., Fairburn, C. C., Agras, W. S., Walsh, B. T., & Kraemer, H. (2002). Cognitive-behavioral therapy for bulimia nervosa: Time course and mechanisms of change. *Journal of Consulting and Clinical Psychology, 70,* 267–274.

Wilson, G. T., & Vitousek, K. (1999). Self-monitoring in the assessment and treatment of eating disorders. *Psychological Assessment, 11,* 480–489.

CHAPTER 11

Assessment of Gambling-Related Disorders

HOWARD J. SHAFFER
CHRISTOPHER R. FREED

> Treatment depends upon diagnosis, and even the matter of timing is often misunderstood. One does not complete a diagnosis and then begin treatment; the diagnostic process is also the start of treatment. Diagnostic assessment is treatment; it also enables further and more specific treatment.
> —MENNINGER (1963, p. 385)

From substance abuse (Lesieur & Blume, 1987) to shopping (Christenson et al., 1994), crime (Hodge, McMurran, & Hollin, 1997), exercising (Morris, Steinberg, Sykes, & Salmon, 1990), eating carrots (Cerny & Cerny, 1992), and drinking water to intoxication (Pickering & Hogan, 1971; Rowntree, 1923), social observers and scientists have applied the notion of addiction to many and varied human activities (Orford, 1985). The contemporary use of addiction[1] is almost exclusively applied to substance use behavior patterns that evidence adverse consequences, often including the emergence of neuro-adaptation (i.e., tolerance and withdrawal). Earlier applications of the term "addiction" were much less onerous (e.g., reading, dancing, listening to jazz). It was not until scientists began to consider the matter of nonchemical addictions (e.g., Marks, 1990) that the construct of addiction became more plastic, complex, and ubiquitous. Consequently, clinicians confronted with the assessment and diagnosis of nonchemical excessive behavior patterns faced a more complex and challenging task. Nevertheless, by addressing nonchemical patterns of excess, clinicians raised important questions about the nature of addiction. Investigators observed, for example, that in the absence of psychoactive substance use, excessive behavior patterns such as pathological gambling could stimulate the development of neuroadaptation (e.g., Wray & Dickerson, 1981). Since neuroadaption can occur among both nonchemically and chemically dependent people, it is difficult to determine whether this circumstance results from (1) the drug taking, (2) the experiences associated with drug taking, or (3) a combination of both. Investigators studying gambling as a nonchemical dependence disorder (i.e., addiction) have the benefit of examining a pattern of excessive behavior that is not compounded by the influence of mind-altering drugs. Consequently, it is possible that study of nonchemical addictions will provide more insight into the complex nature of addiction than has the study of drug abuse and dependence.

Our purpose in this chapter is to examine the variety of assessment and diagnostic issues associated with the process of identifying and classifying intemperate or excessive gambling patterns. Since the study and treatment of gambling disorders is a nascent field, this chapter is organized into two parts. The first part introduces and explores the concept of gambling disorders from a public health perspective, including an epidemiological examination of gambling and gambling disorders. The second part presents conceptual and practical matters associated with assessing and diagnosing gambling disorders. Popular diagnostic and screening instruments are compared. Finally, we discuss the assessment and diagnostic challenges that face clinicians attempting to evaluate disordered gambling.

Although we review in this chapter a variety of conceptual and practical issues associated with assessment and diagnosis of gambling in particular, we do not address the array of important, but more general, interpersonal and clinical issues associated with the conduct of psychotherapy and addictive behaviors. Readers are encouraged to see the variety of more comprehensive works on this topic (e.g., Barron, 1998; Donovan & Marlatt, 1988; Hamilton, 1995; Havens, 1982, 1989; Imhof, 1991; Imhof, Hirsch, & Terenzi, 1984; Khantzian, Halliday, & McAuliffe, 1990; Kleinman, 1988; Ladouceur, Sylvain, Letarte, Giroux, & Jacques, 1998; Ladouceur & Walker, 1998; Levin, 1987; Maltsberger & Buie, 1974; McAulliffe & Ch'ien, 1986; Milkman & Sederer, 1990; Milkman & Shaffer, 1985; Miller & Rollnick, 1991; Najavits, 2002; Shaffer, 1994, 1997b; Shaffer & Robbins, 1991, 1995; Shaffer & Simoneau, 2001; Weiner, 1975). Because gambling studies and treatment are a new addition to the array of more established addictive behaviors, this chapter remains focused on the conceptual and practice issues that face clinicians attempting to assess and treat this disorder.

Gambling also is related to a variety of physical disorders of consequence. For example, people with gambling problems can suffer from repetitive movement disorders, orthopedic distress, sexual dysfunction, gastrointestinal problems, and cardiovascular difficulties or other physical maladies (e.g., Daghestani, 1987; Jarrell, 1988; Karch, Graff, Young, & Ho, 1988; Pasternak & Fleming, 1999). Although the assessment of these and related neurobiological disorders represents an integral part of the evaluative process associated with excessive gambling, we nevertheless are going to limit our discussion throughout this chapter to the assessment of gambling as a psychosocial disorder.

GAMBLING DISORDERS:
FROM CONCEPT TO PUBLIC HEALTH CONCERN

Background

Humans have gambled since the beginning of recorded history. The lifespan of gambling is matched in breadth by the domains that have explored it. For example, gambling activities have been understood from moral, mathematical, economic, social, psychological, cultural and, more recently, biological perspectives (e.g., Bergh, Sodersten, & Nordin, 1997; Comings, 1998; Quinn, 1891; Rose, 1986; Rosecrance, 1985; Shaffer & Korn, 2002; Shaffer, Stein, Gambino, & Cummings, 1989; Skinner, 1969; Taber, 1987). In addition, a remarkable growth of gambling-related research took place during the last decade of the 20th century (Eber & Shaffer, 2000). In the United States, this growing interest raised concerns that gambling might be the cause of extraordinary social costs (e.g., bankruptcy, suicide, crime); these developments prompted former President Clinton to establish the National Gambling Impact Study Commission (National Gambling Impact Study Commission Act, 1996). This Commission, in turn, requested that (1) the National Research Council (NRC) conduct a scientific review of pathological gambling, and that (2) the National Opinion Research Center (NORC) provide new data on the extent of gambling-related problems in America. The NRC published its findings (1999), and the NORC revised and released its findings twice (Gerstein et al., 1999a, 1999b), perhaps because of political pressures that surrounded the National Gambling Impact Study Commission and its report (1999). Finally, the debate was extended when Representative Frank Wolf (R-VA-10th) called upon the General Accounting Office (GAO) to review independently the findings proffered by both of these bodies and the National Gambling Impact Study Commission (General Accounting Office, 2000). We include some findings from these reports later in this chapter.

During the latter part of the 20th century, political and scholarly considerations of gambling and its potential impact emerged in greater numbers than ever before (e.g., Eber & Shaffer, 2000). One exception was gambling as a public health issue. While public health perspectives were gaining strength with respect to other addictive behaviors (e.g., Curry & Kim, 1999; Institute of Medicine, 1990; Marlatt, 1998; Single, 1995; Tucker, Donovan, & Marlatt, 1999; Zinberg, 1974, 1975, 1984), this viewpoint remained peculiarly absent (Korn, 2000; Korn & Shaffer, 1999; Korn & Skinner, 2000; Productivity Commission, 1999) from the contemporary dialogue on gambling-related problems. For example, in 1998, a comprehensive search of MEDLINE, HealthSTAR, Current Contents, and Web of Science databases revealed less than 20 gambling-related articles in public health journals or peer-reviewed journals that had gambling-related titles and were of public health relevance (Korn & Shaffer, 1999). Until Korn and Shaffer published their monograph on gambling and the health of the public, professionals simply had not applied public health strategies and perspectives to gambling-related problems.

Because of this paucity of work on health-related issues, very little research has focused on the assessment and treatment of gambling and gambling-related disorders. Korn and Shaffer (1999) suggested that by understanding gambling and its potential impacts on the public's health, policymakers and practitioners could minimize gambling's negative impacts and appreciate its potential benefits. Furthermore, they proposed that the classic public health model for communicable disease, which examines the interaction among host, agent, environment and vector, also could be instructive for gambling. Korn and Shaffer suggested that a multidimensional public health framework could stimulate a better understanding of gambling phenomena, elucidate the determinants of disordered gambling and point to a range of interventions. In addition to organizing a public health framework, this architecture also serves to organize the assessment and treatment of gambling-related disorders.

For gambling, the "host" is the individual who chooses to gamble and who might be at risk for developing problems depending upon his or her neurobiology, psychology, and behavior patterns. The "agent" represents the specific gambling activities in which players engage (e.g., lotteries, slot machines, casino table games, bingo, horse race betting). The "vector" can be thought of as money, credit, or something else of value. The "environment" is both the microenvironment of the gambling venue, family, and local community, and the socioeconomic, cultural, social policy, and political context within which gambling occurs (e.g., whether it is legal, how available it is, and whether it is socially sanctioned or promoted). Like most public health matters, there is a complex relationship among multiple determinants. This confluence can produce a variety of possible outcomes ranging from desirable to undesirable. Applied to gambling, this public health paradigm invites consideration of a broad array of prevention, harm reduction, and treatment strategies directed toward various elements of the model. Figure 11.1 summarizes a public health perspective on gambling, its potential consequences, and opportunities for multilevel interventions.

Contemporary public health perspectives are not limited to the biological and behavioral dimensions related to gambling and health; they also can address social and economic determinants such as income, employment, and poverty. A public health viewpoint can lead to the design of more comprehensive and effective strategies for preventing, minimizing, and treating gambling-related problems. In addition, a public health perspective encourages public policymakers to distinguish acceptable from unacceptable risks. It encourages an epidemiological examination of gambling and gambling-related disorders to better understand the distribution and determinants of gambling, as well as the factors that influence a transition to disordered states.

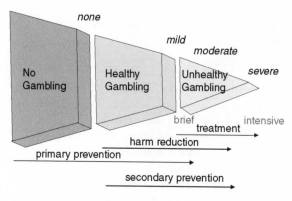

Public Health Interventions

FIGURE 11.1. Public health perspective on gambling and gambling-related problems.

History of Gambling Disorders

The formal study of gambling disorders began during the mid-1970s, when a research team (Kallick, Suits, Dielman, & Hybels, 1979) undertook the daunting task of describing the nature and scope of gambling activities in the United States on behalf of the U.S. Commission on a National Policy Toward Gambling. One of their objectives was to determine the extent of "compulsive" gambling. While this national survey was being conducted, Robert Custer was offering the American Psychiatric Association Task Force a description of compulsive gambling for use in the third edition of the *Diagnostic and Statistical Manual of Mental Disorders* (DSM-III) (Kallick et al., 1979).

The results of Robert Custer's and others' advice and guidance to the American Psychiatric Association on the subject of gambling first surfaced in the DSM-III (American Psychiatric Association, 1980). The diagnosis of pathological gambling joined pyromania, kleptomania, and intermittent and isolated explosive disorders as an impulse disorder in the DSM-III. Since 1980, many researchers and instrument developers have opted to use the DSM-III or subsequent DSM-based instruments (e.g., DSM-III-R, DSM-IV) to assess and measure the presence, prevalence, and severity of pathological gambling.

Addiction, Impulse, or Syndrome?

Despite its current inclusion in DSM-IV-TR (American Psychiatric Association, 2000) as an impulse disorder, many clinicians consider excessive gambling to be an addiction. Should pathological gambling be considered an addiction? The difficulty of this question has more to do with the nature of addiction than with the essence of pathological gambling. To render an informed opinion on this matter, we must be able to define "addiction," which is a lay term often used by scientists and clinicians. "Dependence" is a more scientific construct, occasionally used by laypeople. While there are many working definitions of "addiction," the essence of the construct has remained elusive to nosologists. Consequently, addiction remains an imprecise lay concept that has not yet been welcomed into diagnostic manuals such as DSM-IV or the *International Classification of Diseases and Related Health Problems* (ICD). Recognizing the problem, Vaillant (1982) suggested that instead of seeking a strict operational definition, we should think of alcoholism (or other addictions) the way we perceive mountains and seasons: We know these things when we see them.

Contemporary conceptualizations of addiction might be inadequate. Addiction workers have come to think of addictive behavior as having three primary components: (1) some element of craving or compulsion; (2) loss of control; and (3) continuing the behavior in question in spite of associated adverse consequences. While these dimensions provide a useful atlas for understanding the elements of addiction, we must remember that the map is not the territory (Shaffer & Robbins, 1991), and a diagnosis is not the disease (Szasz, 1991). When clinicians and scientists identify a behavior pattern as an addiction, even if they can identify it reliably, how do they know that it is indeed an addiction as opposed to mania, misbehavior, poor judgment, or an impulse disorder? We can add to this question: When is pathological gambling, pathological gambling? Furthermore, does this pattern of behavior justify consideration as an addiction?

For scientists, the concept of addiction represents a troublesome tautology that has contributed to keeping an addiction classification from entering the diagnostic nomenclature. Therefore, the notion of addiction remains a lay concept—and a very popular one indeed. The tautology operates like this: When observers notice adverse consequences, stimulated by repetitive behavior patterns, apparently occurring against the actor's better judgment, they often infer the presence of addiction. "The problem is that there is no independent way to confirm that the 'addict' cannot help himself and therefore the label is often used as a tautological explanation of the addiction. The habit is called an addiction because it is not under control but there is no way to distinguish a habit that is uncontrollable from one that is simply not controlled" (Akers, 1991, in Davies, 1996, p. S41).

Even if we consider the substance use disorders and pathological gambling as the leading categorical candidates for addiction status in a new diagnostic classification system, the process of assessment and the diagnostic manuals will remain inadequate if social consequences and self-report direct the nosological schema. As organized currently, diagnostic manuals such as DSM-IV increase the likelihood that clinicians can repeatedly classify disorders such as pathological gambling correctly. However, these systems fail to address the construct validity of what is being classified, because the "addictive" disorders (e.g., pathological gambling and substance use disorders) are assumed to exist by inference from the consequences of behaviors in question (e.g., Barron, 1998). Diagnostic systems that rest upon a mix of self-report and corroborating perspectives do not resolve the problem. Individuals struggling with intemperate behavior suffer the burden of the fundamental attribution error (Ross, 1977). This cognitive error leads actors to the perception that an external object stimulated their excessive behavior (e.g., addictive drugs, or addictive gambling); conversely, observers tend to think the cause of intemperance is a relatively stable underlying trait (e.g., addictive personality). Both perspectives are biased and can compromise clinical assessment.

For addiction to emerge as a viable scientific construct, whether psychoactive drug use or pathological gambling is the concern, investigators must establish a "gold standard" against which the presence or absence of the disorder can be judged. To achieve gold status, the benchmark must be independent of the disorder being judged. As with many psychiatric disorders, pathological gambling does not have an independent gold standard. Absent a gold standard, pathological gambling suffers from the "myth of mental illness" stigma (Szasz, 1987, 1991): "The psychiatric community seems determined to ground its medical legitimacy on principles that confuse diagnoses with diseases" (Szasz, 1991, p. 1574). If pathological gambling represents an uncontrollable impulse and not an uncontrolled habit, then there must be independent validation of the irrepressible impulse or the impaired regulatory mechanisms[2] (Kipnis, 1997). Pathological gambling cannot be limited to intemperate bettors who lose more than they win, because these gamblers also represent a group that plays sufficiently for statistical probability to take its toll. If pathological gambling represents a primary disorder orthogonal both to its consequences and the laws of probability, then clinicians and scientists should be able to identify the disorder without knowing the winning or losing status of the player.

An independent gold standard likely will come from neurogenetic or biobehavioral attributes. Early neuroscience research is encouraging. Dopaminergic and serotinergic functions have been found to be altered among pathological gamblers (Bergh et al., 1997; DeCaria, Begaz, & Hollander, 1998). Biogenetic vulnerabilities also have been identified among pathological gamblers (e.g., Comings, 1998), and there is evidence to suggest that there might be genetic markers for novelty-seeking behavior among normals that can predispose people to take "chances" (Benjamin et al., 1996; Ebstein et al., 1996).

There is no simple solution to the matter of what is an addiction. For pathological gambling to find a legitimate home in the psychiatric nomenclature as a primary disorder, people will need to view it as the consequence of (1) overwhelming and uncontrollable impulses, (2) compromised biobehavioral regulatory mechanisms, or (3) a combination of both. Anything short of this will leave people thinking that intemperate gambling is simply the result of people not controlling their "habits." Currently, however, even DSM-IV reflects ambivalence about the psychiatric status and construct validity of pathological gambling by including it in a "cautionary statement." We examine this issue further in the second part of this chapter.

In spite of the critical scientific views regarding the nature of addiction and pathological gambling, people increasingly believe they are suffering from an uncontrollable impulse to gamble. These people are beginning to seek treatment in greater numbers. New public education and awareness programs have lowered the threshold for identifying problems among excessive gamblers. This trend, coupled with emerging treatment opportunities for gambling-related problems, is bringing more people into treatment and teaching them that they have an addiction. With few outcome studies available, the efficacy of treatments for disordered gambling remains to be determined. Nevertheless, human suffering deserves our attention and response. Therefore, the *clinical* issue—as opposed to the scientific and conceptual debate—is not now, nor has it ever been, whether pathological gambling is an addiction or the result of a biobehavioral vulnerability. From a clinical perspective, this issue involves establishing a working formulation that clinicians and patients can share (Perry, Cooper, & Michels, 1987; Shaffer, 1986a). These clinical devices permit clinicians to select treatment methods that offer patients a favorable prognosis given knowledge of the problem and the patient.

For science, improving our understanding of pathological gambling and addiction rests in the development of better theory. Improved theory can guide better research. From a community perspective, as our understanding of addiction and pathological gambling improves, the vehicle for more effective social policy emerges. From the treatment side, there is little or no value to understanding any individual as addicted or mentally disordered unless it permits clinicians to choose a treatment plan that will maximize the well-being of the patient. The value of the concept of pathological gambling or the classification of any addictive behavior, then, is dependent upon the extent to which an *individual sufferer* benefits from its application. While the art and science of diagnosis are dependent upon comparisons among groups, we encourage clinicians to apply their choice of treatments prescriptively. Prescriptive or differential treatment requires consideration of three interactive domains: (1) the health care provider (e.g., medical management strategy); (2) the patient (e.g., compliance rules and expectations of care and concern); and (3) society (e.g., social mores and attributions of responsibility). Together, these domains define the "sickness" that is to be treated (Kleinman, 1988). The relationship between pathological gambling and addiction ultimately rests upon sociocultural acceptability. After all, "it is best to think of any affliction—a disease, a disability . . . —as a text and of 'society' as its author" (A. Blum, 1985, p. 221).

Is Pathological Gambling a Primary and Unique Disorder?

The research methods associated with promulgating basic estimates of gambling prevalence have not changed much during the past 20 years (Shaffer,

Hall, & Vander Bilt, 1997). Despite exceptions, the NRC (1999) noted the overall weakness of research methods in the area of gambling studies. Shaffer et al. (1997) reported that regardless of the quality of these studies, weak and strong methods seem to produce comparable estimates of disordered gambling prevalence. Nevertheless, as we have discussed, two critically important conceptual and methodological issues face the study of gambling and related psychiatric disorders. First, is pathological gambling a primary and unique disorder or a multidimensional syndrome? Second, are existing estimates of disordered gambling prevalence accurate in the absence of a gold standard? These concerns commingle, and their confluence affects how we understand and assess gambling disorders. For example, while clinicians might be heeding exclusion criteria for purposes of treatment planning, for the most part, researchers simply have ignored the implications of exclusion criteria (Boyd et al., 1984) during the conduct of prevalence research. One of the research consequences of ignoring exclusion recommendations is that prevalence estimates of pathological gambling might be overestimated; that is, if other primary disorders, such as manic episodes, are not identified by survey instruments and then excluded by the investigator, the evidence will yield inflated prevalence estimates of gambling disorders. In addition, between DSM-III and DSM-IV-TR, the American Psychiatric Association shifted the exclusion criteria from antisocial personality disorder to mania. This change reflects an ongoing struggle to develop a clear definition of pathological gambling in the absence of a gold standard. Much remains unknown about the nature of the overlap and interaction among antisocial personality, manic episodes, and pathological gambling. Future research that measures the prevalence of related psychiatric disorders along with pathological gambling will provide important insight into these questions. Ultimately, the field of gambling studies is in need of research that can provide additional construct validity.

If pathological gambling represents a primary and unique disorder, then it can emerge in the absence of other comorbidity and cause sequelae independent of any other condition. However, if it is a secondary disorder, subordinate to other dysfunctional behavior, then pathological gambling only will exist as a consequence of another condition (e.g., manic episode, antisocial personality, alcohol abuse, obsessive–compulsive disorder, or adolescence; Jessor & Jessor, 1977). In this case, pathological gambling is not a unique disorder, but rather a cluster of symptoms associated with one or many other disorders. Although worldwide prevalence estimates of disordered gambling have identified a relatively robust phenomenon, investigators have not established with ample certainty that this phenomenon represents a *unique* construct.

Symptoms or Syndrome?

The symptoms associated with pathological gambling reflect a complex syndrome instead of a single disorder. The comorbidity/co-occurrence of pathological gambling with other diagnostic entities probably is an artifact of DSM-IV-TR, misdirecting observers away from the likelihood that it is a syndrome. Overlapping symptoms can represent a common underlying factor. However, when a variety of symptoms are associated with a disorder, but not all the symptoms are always present, a syndrome is in evidence.

Constructing pathological gambling as a syndrome suggests that it has both common and unique components. A syndrome's common component (e.g., depression) is shared with other disorders (e.g., substance use disorders), while its unique component (e.g., betting increasing amounts of money) is specific to pathological gambling. The shared component, which accounts for the comorbidity evidence, reflects broad individual differences that can vary along multiple dimensions (e.g., intensity and duration); the unique component distinguishes pathological gambling from other disorders and is specific only to it (e.g., Widiger & Clark, 2000).

Although it has unique elements, pathological gambling shares many signs and symptoms with other disorders (e.g., anxiety, depression, impulsivity); consequently, we suggest that disordered gambling is best thought of as a syndrome. From this perspective, the most effective treatments for gambling problems will reflect a multimodal "cocktail" approach combined with patient–treatment matching. These multidimensional treatments will include various combinations of psychopharmacology, psychotherapy, and financial, educational, and self-help interventions: These various treatment elements are both additive and interactive, a circumstance necessary to deal with the multidimensional nature of gambling disorders.

Since syndromes are multidimensional, these disorders typically do not respond favorably to a single treatment modality. Whether we view disordered gambling as primary or secondary, unique or syndromal, intemperate gambling inflicts human suffering. If pathological gambling is a primary disorder, it often will require professional assistance; if it is a disorder secondary to another problem, it still requires specialized modalities focusing on gambling issues in addition to the problems related to the primary disorder. Future research will help clarify these theoretical, research, and clinical issues.

Considering the Absence of a Gold Standard

The extant body of prevalence research reveals that estimates of disordered gambling appear relatively stable and robust despite various statistical maneuvers and wide variation in research study quality and characteristics (Shaffer et al., 1997). Although these results encourage confidence about the *reliability* of this phenomenon, estimate stability should not be interpreted as a proxy for *validity*. Validity represents the extent to which a measure accurately reflects the true state of nature (Blacker & Endicott, 2000) and the purpose for which the measure is being applied. A valid measure should yield important information that extends beyond the score (Blacker & Endicott, 2000). Validity is often determined by comparing the measure to a criterion of accuracy, or a gold standard. However, psychiatric disorders rarely have independent criteria to serve as a gold standard. Consequently, validity is established by using indices that are external to the measure under evaluation but which reflect the same underlying construct (i.e., construct validity; Cronbach & Meehl, 1955). Yet, as with many other psychiatric disorders, clinicians and patients alike infer the presence of gambling disorders by identifying the presence of adverse consequences. Effectively, pathological gambling is an independent variable responsible for its consequences; clinicians determine the presence of this independent variable by the characteristics of its dependent variables. Although common in psychiatric diagnosis, this is not consistent with the scientific method. Independent variables must be identified and determined by factors unrelated to their consequences; anything less represents a tautology. Consequently, to determine whether clinical assessments provide a "valid" approximation of disordered gambling, we must first consider what the constructs of disordered gambling and validity mean within the context of contemporary scientific theory.

Validity is relative idea that is only as serviceable as the current theory that provides it safe haven (Cochrane & Holland, 1971; Cronbach & Meehl, 1955; Dohrenwend, 1995; Malagady, Rogler, & Tryon, 1992; Robins, Helzer, Ratcliff, & Seyfried, 1982). When considering the validity of gambling disorders, clinicians, scientists and public policymakers must ask the primary question: valid for what? A construct can have considerable validity and utility, only to lose these attributes in a technological instant when a new finding shifts our understanding. Instead of simply assuming that a "true" disorder awaits our capacity to identify it accurately, we believe that a dynamic interplay of factors influences every clinical assessment: which measurement instrument, with which population, with which clinical procedure, at which historical point in time, under the direction of which clinician. All of these factors influence the outcome of a clinical assessment.

Absent an independent "gold standard" for determining pathological gambling, we do not know whether any screening device or clinical assessment activity over or under-estimates the rate of gambling disorders. This problem of anchoring reveals itself often as scientists attempt to determine how best to frame prevalence estimates. To illustrate, while discussing the results of her New York replication study, Volberg (1996a, p. 50) suggests that "the cutoff point for the DSM-IV Screen (5+ = pathological gambling) is too severe and should be moved back to include individuals with less severe gambling difficulties . . . . [This adjustment] would allow the screen to capture individuals whose pathology is well developed but perhaps not yet extreme."

Despite these concerns about validity and the absence of a gold standard, as we show later, estimates of disordered gambling prevalence tend to be similar. Regardless of the investigator, methods, or study venue, the rates of this disorder tend to be comparable across similar population segments. This observation suggests that the rates of disordered gambling are either a robust and reliable phenomenon or a scientific artifact.

Reconsidering Clinical Diagnoses as the "Gold Standard"

In the absence of a gold standard, some investigators of gambling prevalence have assumed that clinicians provide the proxy gold standard against which the accuracy of screening instruments can be measured (e.g., Lesieur & Blume, 1987; Volberg, 1996a; WEFA Group, ICR Survey Research Group, Lesieur, & Thompson, 1997). For example, Volberg (1996a, p. 3) uses the term "probable pathological gambling" rather than "pathological gambling." She notes, "the term *probable* distinguishes the results of prevalence surveys, where classification is based on responses to questions in a telephone interview, from a clinical diagnosis." Drawing a similar conclusion, the WEFA Group et al. (1997) state that "because only a clinical evaluation using DSM-IV can diagnose pathological gambling, we have used the term 'probable' pathological gambling" (p. 5-2). "Since the survey is not a clinical diagnosis, we cannot say that respondents can be 'diagnosed' as pathological gamblers, rather we use the term 'probable' pathological gamblers" (p. 5-5).

However, clinicians who perform diagnostic evaluations are not as reliable as many people have assumed. Meehl (1954, 1973) and others (e.g., Rosenhan, 1973; Ziskin, 1970) demonstrated long ago that clinicians are extremely vulnerable to biases in clinical judgment. Faraone and Tsuang (1994) emphasized the fact that psychiatric diagnoses should not be considered a gold standard, and that it is important to assess the adequacy of these diagnoses. Therefore, the assumption that gamblers should be grouped into a tentative class, for example, probable pathological gamblers, partly because clinicians have not yet determined the accuracy of that categorical assignment, is faulty. There is little evidence suggesting that clinicians are more accurate instruments for classification than screening instruments. In fact, Lee Robins noted that "clinical practice is not an adequate standard against which to measure the validity of a research instrument'" (cited in Malagady et al., 1992, p. 63). We suggest that all diagnostic classification—whether clinician- or instrument-based—be held as tentative, and not as the final word (e.g., Kleinman, 1987; Shaffer, 1986a).

The Epidemiology of Gambling and Gambling Disorders

An epidemiological review of gambling and gambling-related disorders revolves around the distribution and determinants of gambling and the factors that can influence its transition to disordered states. The distribution and onset of gambling and its associated disorders across population segments comprise the study of prevalence and incidence. Prevalence represents the number of people with a specific disorder at a point or period in time. Incidence represents the number of people who acquire the disorder during a point or period in time. As this volume goes to press, there are more than 200 existing studies of prevalence related to gambling and its consequences, but there are few incidence studies (e.g., Shaffer & Hall, 2002; Slutske, Jackson, & Sher, 2003;

Winters, Stinchfield, Botzet, & Slutske, in press). Furthermore, there are few studies of the contextual determinants of gambling and disordered gambling. Most of the research on the causes of disordered gambling has focused on psychological factors at the expense of social environment (Eber & Shaffer, 2000).

A Brief History of Disordered Gambling Prevalence Studies

As we mentioned earlier, during the mid-1970s, on behalf of the U.S. Commission on a National Policy Toward Gambling, Kallick et al. (1979) undertook the first formal study of the extent of "compulsive" gambling in the United States. This study was the first to assess gambling and its potentially adverse consequences formally. Since they lacked an instrument with which to measure compulsive gambling, Kallick and her colleagues created an 18-item scale. This measure was based upon concepts from the extant literature that seemed related to compulsive gambling. This first research instrument became known as the ISR (Institute for Social Research) scale. Only one other researcher subsequently used Kallick et al.'s gambling scale (Culleton & Lang, 1985). Nevertheless, the process of attempting to measure accurately the construct of disordered gambling had commenced, and the era of gambling-related epidemiological research was under way.

Kallick et al. (1979) designed the ISR test to be used in population-based samples by researchers. The DSM-III and subsequent diagnostic manuals have offered clinicians a guide to determining whether an individual who presents with gambling-related problems has a diagnosable disorder. In 1987, in an effort to develop a "consistent, quantifiable, structured instrument that can be administered easily by nonprofessional as well as professional interviewers" (Lesieur & Blume, 1987, p. 1184), Henry Lesieur and Sheila Blume developed The South Oaks Gambling Screen (SOGS). They used the DSM-III-R criteria to guide both the development and validation of the SOGS. The SOGS rapidly became the instrument of choice among researchers estimating disordered gambling prevalence. Now, there are more than 27 instruments for identifying gambling disorders, with many more in development. Despite the apparent differences among the array of existing instruments, most measures continue to assess gambling disorders by evaluating the consequences of gambling rather than independent events that might be associated with gambling-related problems. This assessment strategy is problematic since it effectively employs dependent variables (i.e., the consequences) to infer the presence of an independent variable (e.g., pathological gambling).

Several observers of the disordered gambling prevalence field have reviewed prevalence instruments and methodological issues in gambling research (e.g., Culleton, 1989; Lesieur, 1994; Lesieur & Rosenthal, 1991; Shaffer et al., 1997; Volberg, 1996b; Walker & Dickerson, 1996). The intended use of these assessment instruments differs. For example, Culleton

(1989) raised the question of the appropriateness of applying a screening test (e.g., the SOGS) to a population-based sample to establish a prevalence rate. He believes the SOGS fails to account for the increase in false positives when used within a population with low base rates of gambling pathology. New evidence suggests that Culleton might be correct (e.g., American Psychiatric Association, Task Force for the Handbook of Psychiatric Measures, 2000; Ladouceur et al., 2000; Shaffer et al., 1997), and that the SOGS might inflate the rate of gambling problems. Culleton recommends estimating prevalence using the Cumulative Clinical Signs Method (CCSM), a shortened version of the Inventory of Gambling Behavior (Zimmerman, Meeland, & Krug, 1985). Culleton considers the CCSM to be the best instrument for addressing the misclassification of false positives and for generating a precise prevalence estimate. Despite this recommendation, only two prevalence studies have used the CCSM (Culleton & Lang, 1985; Transition Planning Associates, 1985).

Culleton's concern with estimating the prevalence of low base rate behaviors represents a fundamental issue for investigators. Culleton introduced the important matter of positive predictive value to the gambling literature. Screening instruments appear most capable of identifying the problem of interest given a positive score (i.e., have high positive predictive value) when measuring a phenomenon that is common among the sample population; the accuracy of any screening instrument diminishes when investigators apply it to a sample whose base rate of the disorder is low. Even when an instrument has excellent criterion validity, "the actual predictive value of the instrument could be much more limited, depending on the prevalence of the disorder of interest" (Goldstein & Simpson, 1995, p. 236).

The history of the disordered gambling research field reflects an assortment of scientific attempts to measure a singular phenomenon. Although various instruments are available to assess the prevalence of disordered gambling, each instrument is best understood by viewing it through an evaluative lens that can focus on the context of its origin, driving motivation, relationship to funding, and its inherent strengths and weaknesses.

Prevalence Estimates of Gambling and Disordered Gambling

Since scientists first examined the prevalence of gambling in the United States, increasing numbers of people have gambled. As more people have experienced gambling, both licit and illicit, interest in excessive gambling has grown from clinical, public policy, and scientific perspectives. During the past 25 years, the public has sensed that gambling problems have been increasing. Public policymakers have pushed repeatedly for the review of gambling and its adverse consequences. In response, scientists have increasingly studied the prevalence of gambling-related disorders (e.g., Eber & Shaffer, 2000). A review of prevalence data points to the need for medical professionals to make screening for disordered gambling a more consistent part of their assessment protocol.

Shaffer, Hall, and Vander Bilt demonstrated that an assortment of different algorithms used to calculate the rate of disordered gambling in North America provided quite stable and similar estimates (Shaffer & Hall, 2001; Shaffer et al., 1997; Shaffer, Hall, & Vander Bilt, 1999). Results of many international studies are consistent with this observation. However, differences in reporting standards have made comparisons difficult. Consequently, Shaffer and Hall (1996) suggested a universal system for reporting prevalence rates. In addition to avoiding pejorative and misleading language, and to reflect the underlying continuum of gambling, this system also is consistent with a public health perspective on populations. Within this system, level 0 represents the prevalence of nongamblers; level 1 represents respondents who do not report any gambling-related symptoms (i.e., not experiencing any gambling problems). Level 2 represents respondents who are experiencing subclinical levels of gambling problems, and level 3 represents respondents who meet diagnostic criteria for having a gambling disorder. It is important to note that level 2 gamblers can move in two directions: They can progress to a more disordered state (i.e., level 3), or they can move to a less disordered state (i.e., level 1). New research suggests that gambling problems are less stable than previously hypothesized (e.g., Slutske et al., 2003). For example, gamblers progress to level 3 less than expected and move toward level 1 more than the conventional wisdom would predict (Shaffer & Hall, 2002).

Table 11.1 summarizes the prevalence rates for lifetime and past-year gambling among adults from the general population in the United States and Canada. Table 11.2 revises these estimates using three methods (i.e., median, 5% outliers, and Andrews Wave M-estimator) to trim outliers and provide a more precise estimate of disordered gambling (Shaffer & Hall, 2001). Table 11.3 compares national estimates throughout the world.[3]

Approximately half of prevalence estimates reside in unpublished reports, and these documents have not been subjected to critical peer review. However, prevalence estimates from published and unpublished reports do not differ significantly (Shaffer & Hall, 2001; Shaffer et al., 1997; Shaffer, Hall, et al., 1999). Furthermore, the inconsistent quality of the various studies that generate prevalence rates seems not to influence the magnitude of these estimates (Shaffer et al., 1997). Perhaps most notable about this evidence is the relative consistency of the prevalence rates that have been observed by different investigators, in different venues, using different measures and methods. This observation reveals that the prevalence of disordered gambling is a relatively stable phenomenon.

Trends in Population Segments

In this section, we consider the nature of gambling exposure and review the studies associated with trends related to population segment prevalence rates. We begin with the empirical studies that illuminate the issue of trends among youth and adults.

TABLE 11.1. Mean Gambling Prevalence Estimates and 95% Confidence Intervals for Four Study Populations

Estimate time frame	Adult	Adolescent[a]	College	Treatment/ Prison
Level 3 lifetime	1.92 (1.52–2.33)	3.38 (1.79–4.98)	5.56 (3.54–7.59)	15.44 (11.58–19.31)
Level 2 lifetime	4.15 (3.11–5.18)	8.40 (5.61–11.18)	10.88 (4.86–16.89)	17.29 (11.05–23.53)
Level 1 lifetime	93.92 (92.79–95.06)	90.38 (86.49–94.29)	83.13 (74.71–91.55)	67.61 (58.10–77.11)
Level 3 past year	1.46 0.92–2.01)	4.80 3.21–6.40)	—	—
Level 2 past year	2.54 1.72–3.37)	14.60 8.32–20.89)	—	—
Level 1 past year	96.04 94.82–97.25)	82.68 76.12–89.17)		

[a]Although mean past-year estimates are higher than mean lifetime estimates for adolescents, there is considerable overlap between the confidence intervals of these measures; adolescents' past-year gambling experiences are likely to be comparable to their lifetime gambling experiences. Differences between instruments that provide past-year estimates and those that provide lifetime estimates among adolescents most likely account for these discrepancies.

TABLE 11.2. Trimmed Gambling Prevalence Estimates

Estimate time frame	Statistic	Adult	Adolescent	College	Treatment/ prison
Level 3 lifetime	Mean	1.92	3.38	5.56	15.44
	Median	1.80	3.00	5.00	14.29
	5% trimmed mean	1.78	3.33	5.14	15.07
	Andrews's wave M-estimator	1.73	2.74	4.64	13.49
Level 2 lifetime	Mean	4.15	8.40	10.88	17.29
	Median	3.50	8.45	6.50	15.64
	5% trimmed mean	3.76	8.35	9.83	17.01
	Andrews's wave M-estimator	3.31	8.22	6.51	16.59
Level 3 past year	Mean	1.46	4.80	—	—
	Median	1.20	4.37	—	—
	5% trimmed mean	1.27	4.77	—	—
	Andrews's wave M-estimator	1.10	4.65	—	—
Level 2 past year	Mean	2.54	14.60	—	—
	Median	2.20	11.21	—	—
	5% trimmed mean	2.25	13.83	—	—
	Andrews's wave M-estimator	2.15	11.26	—	—

TABLE 11.3. International Estimates of Lifetime and Past-Year Disordered Gambling Prevalence Rates

	U.S./ Canada[a]	Sweden[b]	Switzerland[c]	New Zealand[d]	Britain[e]	South Africa[f]	Hong Kong[g]	Spain[b]	Norway[i]	Australia[j]
Level 3 lifetime	1.9	1.2	—	1.0	—	—	1.8	1.4–1.7	—	—
Level 2 lifetime	4.2	2.7	—	1.9	—	—	4.0	1.6–5.2	—	—
Level 1 lifetime	93.9	96.1	—	97.1	—	—	94.1	93.1–97.0	—	—
Level 3 past year	1.5	0.6	0.8	0.5	0.7	1.4	—	—	0.2	2.1
Level 2 past year	2.5	1.4	2.2	0.8	—	1.4	—	—	0.5	2.8
Level 1 past year	96.0	98.0	97.0	98.7	—	97.2	—	—	99.3	95.1

Note. Since all studies used either the SOGS or DSM criteria, cases within each study endorsing five or more criteria from those instruments were categorized as level 3, cases endorsing three to four criteria were categorized as level 2, and the rest of each study sample (i.e., nongamblers and nonproblem gamblers) were categorized as level 1. lifetime levels include results from the SOGS and DSM criteria not otherwise specified. Past-year levels include results specified as past year or within last 6 months. [a]Shaffer and Hall (2001b); [b]Volberg, Abbott, Roennberg, and Munck (2001); [c]Bondolfi, Osiek, and Ferrero (2002); [d]Abbott (2001); [e]Sproston, Erens, and Orford (2000); [f]Collins and Barr (2001); [g]Wong and So (2003); [h]Becona (1996); [i]Gotestam and Johansson (2003); [j]Productivity Commission (1999).

Adolescents and Adults

In one of the rare longitudinal studies that monitored gambling-related behaviors, Winters, Stinchfield and Kim (1995) observed that the prevalence of Minnesota adolescents with gambling disorders did not increase, despite a shift away from informal games toward more legalized games. Wallisch studied Texas adolescents between 1992 and 1995. She observed that rate of gambling remained steady and the prevalence of gambling disorders actually diminished (Wallisch, 1993, 1996). With few longitudinal studies to illuminate this issue, Shaffer and Hall (2001a) and Shaffer, Hall, and Vander Bilt (1999) examined this question using meta-analysis and found that the rate of disordered gambling had indeed increased during the last three decades of the 20th century, but only among adults from the general population.

Estimates of gambling disorders among young people suggest that they experience this problem at approximately 2.5–3.0 times the rate of their adult counterparts. Despite this observation, the NRC (1999) concluded that variation in methods, instrumentation, and conceptualization might influence these findings, so that it is not yet possible to draw confident conclusions about the rate of gambling disorders among youth. Table 11.1 reflects this problem, revealing that mean past-year rates are higher than lifetime rates. This observation results in part from the considerable variation in estimates and suggests that there might be a cohort effect, memory distortion, or other methodological difficulties associated with screening young people. New research also suggests that SOGS-based youthful prevalence rates might simply be inflated (Ladouceur et al., 2000), though this problem still does not adequately explain how past-year rates can exceed lifetime rates.

Shaffer et al. noted that while more people started to gamble as legalized gambling proliferated, the *rate* of gambling disorders increased only among adults from the general population (Shaffer et al., 1997; Shaffer, Hall, et al., 1999). Consistent with the few local studies that had monitored young people's gambling behavior, the rate of disorder was not increasing among youth or patients with psychiatric or substance use disorders (Shaffer & Hall, 2001; Shaffer et al., 1997; Shaffer, Hall, et al., 1999). Shaffer et al. argued that, for adults, legalized gambling provided an increasingly acceptable opportunity to try a new activity. However, for young people, gambling continued to remain illicit. For psychiatric patients, the social sanctions and proscriptions were less influential than those for adults from the general population. As gambling became legalized, therefore, adults from the general populace were the population segment most responsive to these changes.

Regional state replications have started to emerge (e.g., Volberg, 1996a; Volberg & Moore, 1999). The evidence regarding trends is mixed: Some reports show an increase in gambling disorders, and others shows a decrease. It is possible that observed increases in past-year level 3 gambling reflect a cohort-related artifact. For example, regions implementing replication studies initially might have had either higher or lower rates of level 3 gambling than the regions that do not conduct replication projects. Shaffer and Hall (2001) tested this hypothesis to gain insight into the possibility of a confounding effect. They compared the prevalence estimates obtained from the first available statewide adult population studies from states that later conducted replication studies with estimates derived from states without replication studies. Although initial prevalence estimates were consistently lower from the replication states, the paucity of these studies yielded insufficient statistical power to identify significant differences between replication and nonreplication states.

Some observers have noted that the magnitude of contemporary gambling suggests that North America is experiencing an "epidemic" of gambling (e.g., American Academy of Pediatrics, 1998). Taken together, the extant evidence suggests that adults from the general population are evidencing a gradually increasing rate of gambling disorders. If this trend continues unabated, it might become appropriate to characterize disordered gambling in the general adult population as pandemic. For now, however, to clarify this kind of characterization, prospective epidemiological studies are needed.

To date, the many and consistent findings derived from studies of adults from the general population suggest that—with the exception of tracking the impact of public policy modifications—the era of general population prevalence research might be coming to a close and the next phase of epidemiological research beginning. This next phase of epidemiological investigation needs to focus on more vulnerable and special-needs population segments (Shaffer, LaBrie, LaPlante, Nelson, & Stanton, 2004), for example, women, older adults, Native Americans, and selected ethnocultural and lower socioeconomic-level groups. The following section reviews some of the completed studies on special population segments.

Vulnerable and Special-Needs Population Segments

As we described earlier, the social gradient (e.g., poverty and the psychoeconomics of gambling) disproportionately influences disordered gambling patterns across population segments (Lopes, 1987). People with lower socioeconomic status experience gambling and other socioeconomically related problems at rates higher than those associated with high socioeconomic standing (Lapage, Ladouceur, & Jacques, 2000; Sebastian, 1985; Shaffer, Freed, & Healea, 2002). This factor pervades considerations of gambling among vulnerable population segments. Given the early phase and preliminary nature of research on population segments, ironically, the current value of segment-specific research is generic. Nevertheless, future research directed toward specific population segments holds important potential for the next wave of epidemiological gambling research (Fisher, 2000; Shaffer et al., 2002).

In the following discussion, we examine some vulnerable and special-needs populations. This discussion is not exhaustive. We illustrate the potential of sector-specific prevalence research by briefly reviewing a selection of population segments. As research on the distribution and determinants of gambling matures, scientists likely will identify other population segments as vulnerable.

WOMEN

Epidemiological research suggests that disordered gambling is more prevalent among men than among women (National Research Council, 1999; Shaffer et al., 1997); adolescent boys are about four times more likely to be pathological gamblers than adolescent girls. Some have speculated that women gamble to "escape" more often than men, who gamble for the "action" (e.g., Custer & Milt, 1985). However, there is little experimental evidence to support this psychological conclusion. More likely, gender differences reflect complex issues surrounding the attitudes and opportunities about recreational activities and the social milieu within which these occur (e.g., Bettencourt & Miller, 1996; Kiesler & Sproull, 1985).

CASINO EMPLOYEES

During the 1990s, as gambling opportunities expanded around the world, some observers expressed concern that the rate of gambling-related disorders also was increasing because of this growing exposure. This idea of social environmental "exposure" has its roots in McGuire's (1964) "resistance to persuasion" and "social inoculation" model. This theory suggests that exposure to gambling, or to activities and materials that promote it, reflects a sequence of social contacts that conceptually act like "germs" or "toxins" that can lead to adverse health consequences. However, few studies provided empirical evidence about the nature of gambling exposure or its association with the prevalence of gambling disorders.

Casino employees represent a unique and conceptually important segment of the population. They experience full access and exposure to gambling; that is, casino workers have increased proximity to, and knowledge of, gambling compared to the public. If gambling is the cause of adverse health and disordered gambling, then occupational experience is central to determining its impact. During the middle part of the 19th century, when epidemiology was taking root as a science, John Snow argued that if a trade truly causes adverse health consequences, then it should "be extremely so to the workmen engaged in those trades" (Lillenfield, 2000, p. 5). The same is true of gaming industry employees today. If gambling is the cause of adverse health consequences, then those with the greatest gambling exposure should experience more health problems than those with less exposure (Shaffer, LaBrie, & LaPlante, 2003). Alternatively, workers might have sought employment in the gaming industry because of their gambling interests.

Shaffer, Vander Bilt, and Hall (1999) revealed that casino employees have higher levels of gambling, smoking, drinking, and mood disorder compared to the general population. These findings encouraged the development and implementation of prospective research designs to monitor the movement of gamblers through the various transitional stages that might be associated with gambling disorders (Shaffer & Hall, 1996; Shaffer et al., 1997). Gambling problems, like the abuse of alcohol, tobacco, opiates, and cocaine, are more dynamic than the conventional wisdom suggests (Shaffer & Hall, 1996; Shaffer et al., 1997). Shaffer, LaBrie, Scanlan, and Cummings (1994) proposed that there are transitional stages from which people move toward either more healthy states or more disordered states during their involvement with gambling (Shaffer & Hall, 2002; Shaffer et al., 1997). Furthermore, it is likely that concurrent psychiatric and alcohol or other substance use problems can influence transitions to more or less disordered states (e.g., Briggs, Goodin, & Nelson, 1996; Crockford & el-Guebaly, 1998; Galdston, 1951; Kessler et al., 1996; Lesieur, Blume, & Zoppa, 1986; Lesieur et al., 1991; Shaffer, Hall, et al., 1999). The NRC (1999) noted, "There is no direct empirical evidence supporting either the possibility that pathological gamblers can or cannot return to and remain in a state of social or recreational gambling" (p. 20). However, since a small percentage of people with chemical addictions can return to recreational use, it is likely that the same is true of pathological gamblers (Blaszczynski, McConaghy, & Frankova, 1991; Rosecrance, 1988). Our understanding about these movements or transitions toward more healthy gambling states has remained largely theoretical and controversial; however, new empirical research supports the idea that gambling problems are more plastic than previously thought (Shaffer & Hall, 2002; Slutske et al., 2003; Winters et al., in press). For example, level 3 gamblers can return to more healthy states, and within a relatively short time. The first multiyear prospective study of casino employees (Shaffer & Hall, 2002) revealed that people troubled with gambling, drinking, or both shifted these behavior patterns regularly; in addition, these shifts tended toward reduced levels of disorder rather than the increasingly serious intensity often suggested by a traditional view of "addictive" behavior patterns.

YOUNGER AND OLDER ADULTS

While younger people have evidenced higher rates of gambling-related problems compared with their adult counterparts (e.g., Poulin, 2000), recent attention has shifted toward older adults and their increased risk for gambling problems. As gambling has expanded and older adults have sought more varied recreational activities, gambling junkets have became more common. Recently, for example, investigators reported that older adults gamble to relax, to pass time, to get away for the day, to avoid boredom, and to have inexpensive meals (McNeilly & Burke, 2000). The prevalence of disordered gambling in this population segment is not yet determined. It is interesting to note that the reasons for gambling among elderly persons are likely very similar to those among adolescents.

THE HOMELESS

The first studies of homeless treatment seekers reveal that, like other psychiatric population segments, community service recipients (Lapage et al., 2000) in general and the homeless in particular evidence elevated rates of gambling disorders (Shaffer et al., 2002). Evaluating 171 consecutive homeless, substance abuse treatment seekers, Shaffer et al. reported past-year prevalence rates at intake of level 2 and 3 gambling disorders (i.e., 12.8 and 5.4, respectively) that were significantly higher among this population than among the general adult population.

SELECTED ETHNOCULTURAL POPULATIONS

Though there has been no systematic evaluation of the effects of culture on gambling and problem gambling, there is evidence of cultural variation in prevalence rates in the literature. For example, higher than average rates of gambling and gambling problems are found among African American, Native American, and Latin American adolescents (Stinchfield, Nadav, Winters, & Latimer, 1997). Other studies point to group differences in gambling that likely have ethnocultural roots. In Florida, for example, problem gamblers are disproportionately Latin American (Cuadrado, 1999). Likewise, Asian groups in the United States have shown higher rates of gambling disorders compared to other groups (Zane & Huh-Kim, 1998). Gambling, including illegal gambling, continues to be popular in Chinese communities in the United States, with many willing to work extra shifts to afford this recreational activity (Kinkead, 1992). There is evidence of gambling's popularity in Asian countries as well, for example, in Singapore, where gambling is associated with substance abuse and other detrimental behaviors (Teck-Hong, 1992).

Native American people deserve attention because evolving gaming policy has a potentially positive economic impact on Native American communities by generating revenue and providing additional employment opportunities. Native Americans also might be particularly vulnerable to the negative impacts of gambling for a variety of complex health and social reasons. For example, a survey comparing people being treated for alcohol dependence in a Veterans Administration hospital in South Dakota found that aboriginal patients score in the probable gambling addiction range three times as often as Caucasians and twice as often as persons admitting to difficulty with gambling (Elia & Jacobs, 1993). In general, aboriginal people evidence higher rates of problem and pathological gambling (e.g., Hewitt, 1994; Volberg & Abbott, 1997; Wardman, el-Guebaly, & Hodgins, 2001; Zitzow, 1996), poorer mental health status as well as higher rates of substance-related problems compared with the general population (National Steering Committee, 1999; Office of Public Health, 1999).

Comorbidity

The various versions of DSM that have included pathological gambling as a distinct disorder also have drawn attention to the possibility that other disorders may coexist with pathological gambling. For example, DSM-IV notes that pathological gamblers "may be prone to developing general medical conditions that are associated with stress. . . . Increased rates of Mood Disorders, Attention-Deficit Hyperactivity Disorder, Substance Abuse or Dependence, and Antisocial, Narcissistic, and Borderline Personality Disorders have been reported in individuals with Pathological Gambling" (American Psychiatric Association, 1994, p. 616).

Clinicians often report that, like casino employees with gambling problems, patients who seek treatment for pathological gambling have a variety of social problems caused by gambling. However, treatment seekers are very different from people who have gambling problems but do not seek treatment. Treatment seekers typically have a greater variety and intensity of psychological problems compared to their counterparts who do not seek treatment (e.g., Crockford & el-Guebaly, 1998; Kessler et al., 1997; Regier et al., 1990; Shaffer, Vander Bilt, et al., 1999). Among the group of gamblers who seek treatment, are the comorbid problems the cause or consequence of pathological gambling?

Comorbidity reflects the coexistence of gambling with other disorders. This confluence makes it difficult to determine whether (1) gambling behavior causes a "gambling disorder," (2) other disorders cause intemperate gambling or the problems that often accompany excessive gambling, or (3) both sets of problems reflect another underlying disorder. To illustrate, where X represents a comorbid condition, and PG represents level 3 gambling disorders, there are seven primary relationships that can describe the association between disordered gambling and psychiatric comorbidity (Shaffer & Korn, 2002):

- X contributes to, is a risk factor for, or causes PG.
- X protects against or "treats" the occurrence of or progression to PG.
- PG contributes to, is a risk factor for, or causes X.
- PG protects against or "treats"[4] the occurrence of or progression to X.
- X and PG co-occur/coexist but are coincidental and completely independent.
- X and PG share common determinants (i.e., biological, psychological, behavioral or social).
- X and PG combined are actually components of some "larger" entity, disorder or syndrome.

Despite this organizing map of the complex relationships that can exist between gambling and comorbid disorders, "research on psychiatric comorbidity in pathological gambling is still very much in its infancy. While an overlap of symptoms belonging to a variety of diagnostic disorders is common, a more systematic analysis . . . reveals a much more tentative picture" (Crockford & el-Guebaly, 1998, p. 48). To consider these complicating factors in more depth, we examine the comorbidity of gambling and other mental disorders in the following section.

The Prevalence of Related Mental Disorders

A variety of mental disorders occur at disproportionately high levels among persons with gambling disorders. Despite this observation, there is a paucity of empirical research about the comorbidity of gambling and other psychological disorders. Currently, several groups are working to improve our understanding of gambling and other psychiatric disorders. For example, the new and not yet completed National Comorbidity Survey (NCS) includes a gambling module (Kessler, personal communication, 2000). The following discussion provides a brief overview of the available research on gambling and comorbid mental disorders.

Crockford and el-Guebaly (1998) published a seminal review article on comorbid conditions and gambling, and Black and Moyer (1998) described the clinical features of these conditions. In an important study from the St. Louis 1981 Epidemiologic Catchment Area (ECA) study, the authors reported,

> Recreational gamblers and problem gamblers had higher rates of most psychiatric disorders than nongamblers after adjustment for race, sex, and age effects. The association between gambling and antisocial personality disorder was strongest— recreational gamblers and problem gamblers were at increased odds of meeting the diagnostic criteria for this disorder (odds ratios = 2.3 and 6.1, respectively). Using age-of-onset information, we found that problems with depression and phobias usually preceded gambling among problem gamblers with comorbid depression and phobias (Cunningham-Williams, Cottler, Compton, & Spitznagel, 1998, p. 1094).

Cunningham-Williams et al. observed that 0.9% of their 1981 Diagnostic Interview Schedule–DSM-III screened sample evidenced a lifetime rate of pathological gambling, and another 9.2% reported at least one gambling-related symptom. Like the seminal Kallick et al. (1979) prevalence research conducted more than 25 years ago, this 20-year-old data yielded an estimate of the most serious level of disordered gambling that is very similar to contemporary rates generated from international studies.

SUBSTANCE USE DISORDERS

Most studies examining the relationship between gambling and other psychiatric conditions have focused on substance use and mood disorders (e.g., Feigelman, Wallisch, & Lesieur, 1998). Crockford and el-Guebaly report "that between 25% and 63% of pathological gamblers meet criteria for a substance use disorder in their lifetime. Correspondingly, 9% to 16% of patients with a substance use disorders are also found to be probable pathological gamblers" (Crockford & el-Guebaly, 1998, p. 44). Crockford and el-Guebaly found that alcohol is the most commonly abused substance; a high rate of nicotine use is also very common among pathological gamblers. When individuals abuse more than one substance, the prevalence and severity of their pathological gambling is increased compared to individuals who abuse only one drug. Like Shaffer et al. (1997), Crockford and el-Guebaly note that there is considerable variation among study estimates of the comorbidity of substance abuse and gambling, as well as the quality of these study methods.

Fromme, Katz, and D'Amico (1997) demonstrated that alcohol intoxication reduced the perception of negative consequences of risk taking. In addition, alcohol intoxication encourages drinkers to perceive the potential benefits associated with risk taking more reliably than the negative consequences (Fromme, Katz, & Rivet, 1997). Emerging evidence suggests common genetic risk factors for alcohol dependence and pathological gambling; however, the risk for alcohol dependence accounts for a significant but only modest proportion of the genetic and environmental risk for subclinical and DSM-III-R pathological gambling disorders (Slutske et al., 2000).

Research from the ECA study reveals that the rate of lifetime prevalence of pathological gambling among drug users from the community is no different than the rate of this disorder among those in drug treatment settings (Cunningham-Williams, Cottler, Compton, Spitznagel, & Ben-Abdallah, 2000). The rate of level 2 and level 3 gambling among these groups is 22 and 11%, respectively (Cunningham-Williams et al., 2000). These authors also reported that while most psychiatric disorders were not associated with gambling disorders, antisocial personality disorder was more prevalent among persons with gambling disorders than among recreational gamblers (Cunningham-Williams et al., 2000). Finally, another study of eight drug treatment settings in five northeastern states found a similar rate of pathological gambling (13%); this research also identified impulsivity and antisocial characteristics as important determinants associated with pathological gambling (Langenbucher, Bavly, Labouvie, Sanjuan, & Martin, 2001).

GAMBLING, SUICIDE, AND MORTALITY

Clinical observations have associated gambling problems with suicidal thoughts and attempts. However, between 1980 and 1997, since pathological gambling entered the psychiatric nosology, no U.S. death certificate has listed gambling as the underlying cause of death (i.e., 0 deaths for 312.3, the ICD-9 code for impulse-control disorder, which includes pathological gambling [312.31]) (Centers for Disease Control, 2001).[5] Nevertheless, there have been many attempts in the scientific and lay literature to establish gambling as an *indirect* cause of death (e.g., McCleary et al., 1998; Phillips, Welty, & Smith, 1997). The idea that gambling is a cause of suicide emerges primarily from (1) anecdotes about successful suicides that are preceded by episodes of losing at gambling (e.g., Lakshmanan, 1996), (2) higher rates of reported depression among persons with gambling disorders, and (3) case studies (e.g., Blaszczynski & Farrell, 1998; Jason, Taff, & Boglioli, 1990). A definitive answer about the relationship between gambling and suicide will only emerge by conducting large-scale epidemiological research that avoids indirect inference and instead focuses specifically on gamblers and suicide as the unit of analysis. Even with such research, the presence of co-occurring disorders can make the results confusing and difficult to interpret.

With respect to mortality, a study of casino-related deaths in Atlantic City between 1982 and 1986 showed that, of the total number of fatalities, 83% were cardiac sudden deaths. Perhaps the stress of gambling activities can induce sudden cardiac death (Jason et al., 1990). Nevertheless, scientific studies have not yet established that problem or pathological gamblers die at different rates compared with their non-problem-gambling counterparts. Absent this research, it is not yet possible to conclude that there is a relationship between gambling and mortality. In their review of the NRC and the National Gambling Impact Study Commission findings, the General Accounting Office (2000) arrived at the same conclusion (National Gambling Impact Study Commission, 1999; National Research Council, 1999).

MOOD DISORDERS

As we discussed earlier, there is evidence to suggest that the prevalence of dysthymia, depression (unipolar and bipolar), suicidal ideation, and suicide attempts is inflated among persons with gambling disorders. However, Lesieur and Blume (1990) noted that among patients treated for mood disorders, there was not an elevated prevalence of pathological gambling. This observation runs counter to the often-observed relationship between these disorders. Consequently, an accurate rate of comorbidity might best be provided by a follow-up study. Taber, McCormick, Russo, Adkins, and Ramirez (1987) observed that about 18% of persons with gambling disorders experienced continued depression "despite abstinence from gambling and improvement in their work and family lives—a percentage of depressive disorders similar to that seen in patients with substance use disorders" (Crockford & el-Guebaly, 1998, p. 46).

ANXIETY DISORDERS

Anxiety often appears as a hallmark of gamblers who seek treatment; however, this anxiety typically is more representative of anxious depression than anxiety disorders. Clinicians have described the signs and symptoms of anxiety (i.e., fear and stress) as common prior to a person becoming a gambler, while betting and playing (i.e., gambling as escape from these unpleasant emotions), as a DSM-IV diagnostic criterion for pathological gambling, and as a subjective state during treatment and recovery. However, clinical anxiety disorders are a complex grouping of specific mental disorders ranging from general anxiety disorder (GAD), panic attacks, and obsessive–compulsive disorder (OCD) to post traumatic stress disorder (PTSD). For these clinical conditions, "little is known about the association of anxiety disorders and problem gambling" (National Research Council, 1999, p. 138). After a careful review of the literature, Crockford and el-Guebaly (1998, p. 47) concluded, "Despite an increased prevalence being reported in 3 studies, there would appear to be insufficient data to support the theory that anxiety disorders are comorbid with pathological gambling. In particular, there is little support for the comorbidity with obsessive–compulsive disorder (OCD)."

PERSONALITY DISORDERS

Despite little empirical evidence to estimate the comorbidity of personality and gambling disorders, clinicians regularly describe a high level of narcissistic personality disorder among pathological gamblers. Two important general population studies found that problem gambling was associated with antisocial personality disorder (ASPD) and that pathological gambling always was secondary to ASPD study (Cunningham-Williams et al., 1998, 2000). Blaszczynski and Steel (1998) examined 82 of 100 consecutive treatment seekers interested in assistance with their gambling related problems. Of the 82 treatment seekers, 76 (93%) met diagnostic criteria for at least one personality disorder. "Multiple overlapping personality disorders per subject (Adams, Barry, & Fleming, 1996) [were] more the rule than the exception . . . On average, subjects met criteria for 4.6 DSM-III personality disorders" (Blaszczynski & Steel, 1998, pp. 60, 65). In addition, the number of personality disorders was significantly related to SOGS scores in a positive direction. "The results of this study indicate that pathological gamblers as a group exhibit rates of personality disorders that are comparable to those found in general psychiatric patient populations" (p. 65). Recently, Langenbucher et al. (2001) supported these results, adding support for the relationship between ASPD and pathological gambling among treatment-seeking cohorts.

IMPULSE DISORDERS AND OTHER DISORDERS

Currently, DSM-IV-TR places pathological gambling within the impulse disorders category (American Psychiatric Association, 2000). Kleptomania, pyromania, and trichotillomania also reside in this class of impulse disorders. It is reasonable to expect that pathological gambling would covary with these disorders of similar origin. However, despite occasionally examining impulsiveness, researchers have not comparatively investigated gambling and the other diagnoses from the DSM impulse disorders category. Instead, apparently influenced by the addiction model, investigators have elected to compare and contrast gambling with substance use disorders. Consequently, there is a paucity of evidence to inform us about the comorbidity of pathological gambling and the other impulse disorders.

Similarly, Crockford and el-Guebaly (1998) concluded that there is little evidence to suggest a comorbid relationship between gambling disorders and eating or sexual addictions. In addition, they noted that despite clinical descriptions of dissociative-like symptoms among pathological gamblers, "it would seem highly unlikely that this would be probable" (p. 48). Compulsive shopping, or oniomania, has been identified as having similar etiology and comorbidity patterns to pathological gambling, with a very similar prevalence rate (i.e., 1.1%) (Lejoyeux, Ades, Tassain, & Solomon, 1996). Scientists have suggested that pathological gambling and other excessive behavior patterns have a common etiology that is characterized by a reward deficiency syndrome (K. Blum et al., 2000). These investigators suggest that addiction is "a biogenetic disease" and that "vulnerability to addiction (as well as impulsive and compulsive behaviors) is genetically transmitted. It is not necessary to establish that all addiction is caused by genetic vulnerability. Heavy exposure to alcohol and other drugs may set in motion perturbators of neurochemistry and receptors which may have similar end results" (p. 2). This common neurobiological vulnerability has linked the prevalence of pathological gambling to increased rates of Tourette's syndrome (Comings, 1998).

Neurobiological, neuropsychological, and clinical studies (e.g., Rugle & Melamed, 1993) provide growing evidence that there is an increase in attention-deficit/hyperactivity disorder (ADHD) among pathological compared with nonpathological gamblers (Comings et al., 1999; Hollander, Buchalter, & DeCaria, 2000; National Research Council, 1999; Specker, Carlson, Christenson, & Marcotte, 1995; Wise, 1995). Research has identified preliminary evidence that noradrenaline is associated with attention problems (e.g., ADHD) and that dopamine level shifts might be associated with pathological gambling (Bergh et al., 1997).

ASSESSMENT AND DIAGNOSIS:
FROM CONCEPT TO PRACTICE

As gambling-related disorders have emerged as a public health concern, this attention has encouraged increasing attention from treatment providers. New treatments for gambling disorders are appearing. Assessment is the first and an ongoing element of the treatment process. Although it is seemingly straightforward, assessment reflects a complex and difficult set of multidimensional activities. For example, the assessment process provides a foundation for developing an alliance with patients, a blueprint for treatment planning, and a reference point for treatment monitoring and aftercare. Assessment is a broad concept that represents screening, evaluation, and diagnostic activities.

Typically, screening involves a brief assessment of people who are not in treatment but have interest in whether a particular disorder might apply to them. Consequently, they participate in a series of questions (i.e., a survey) or laboratory test (e.g., cholesterol screen) to determine whether they might have a disorder. Once screened positive, this segment of the population is typically referred to a clinician for more extensive evaluation. This assessment might yield a diagnosis (i.e., the identification of a stereotypical disorder). Conceptually, one important issue for clinicians to consider is whether they are assessing problems or people (Shaffer, 1986a). For example, is the evaluative task to identify excessive gambling patterns and the consequences of these activities, or is it to understand the nature and dynamics of the excessive gambler?

Cornerstones of Assessment and Diagnosis

The task of assessing and diagnosing addiction in general and gambling disorders in particular is complex and difficult. This circumstance is the result of the multiplicity of approaches that coexist in the clinical environment. Indeed, clinicians might become overwhelmed by the quantity of seemingly relevant data or, conversely, select only data they subjectively deem important. The concept of addiction complicates assessment and diagnosis. Although pathological gambling is often framed as dichotomous—one has it or one does not, addiction is not a dichotomous concept. Nevertheless, diagnosticians make dichotomous decisions (i.e., blind or sighted, alcoholic or nonalcoholic) even though the phenomena of pathological gambling and disordered gambling are not readily agreed upon.

The absence of a theory of practice in the addictions contributes to the ambiguities that surround the task of addiction assessment. Practitioners often fail to distinguish between addiction theories and theories of abstinence and controlled use. Long ago, Shaffer and Gambino (1979) suggested that practitioners are left only with their ideas about the nature of addiction, the course of treatment, and the goals of intervention, without a sound practice theory to guide clinical work. The development of a practice theory will be most likely achieved when practitioners recognize the need to incorporate their values and goals into explicit and precise theories of practice (Gambino & Shaffer, 1979; Shaffer & Gambino, 1979).

Conceptual Clinical Camps:
Technical Rationality to Clinical Reflection

In the absence of explicit practice theories, the doctrine of "technical rationality" emerged and influenced the clinical practice activities of psychotherapists and counselors until the first half of the 20th century. Technical rationality rests on two assumptions: (1) clinical practice activities are "made rigorous by the application of scientific theory and technique" (Schon, 1983, p. 21), and (2) professional treatment providers are diagnostically superior to their amateur counterparts because of a precise application of scientific principles to practice. Adherents to technical rationality consequently believe "real" knowledge exists in the utilization of the scientific principle. Indeed, "the application of these principles to clinical practice should follow only after basic substantive information has been sufficiently mastered" (Shaffer, 1986a, p. 386).

The popularity of technical rationality waned as the scientific establishment failed to solve important social problems during the mid-20th century.

Indeed, professional treatment providers began to consider assessment approaches that were based less on scientific theory and more on tacit knowledge (Polanyi, 1967). The ability to know tacitly—as we do when we recognize a person's face or a change of seasons—continues to stimulate interest in how treatment providers and clinicians solve the problems confronted by their patients and clients (e.g., Vaillant, 1982). A practitioner's reflection before, during, and after his or her work serves to focus activities on the particular task. Problem-solving capacities also are enhanced. The reflective process allows practitioners to consider alternative perspectives and to confirm hypotheses generated by technical rationality and tacit knowledge. "Reflection in action, then, serves to integrate the scientific method with those techniques more representative of the arts" (Shaffer, 1986a, p. 387).

There are benefits to both a technically rational and a tacit assessment strategy. Clinicians will benefit from learning and attending to each clinical approach; by integrating the tacit information with technical knowledge, it is possible to optimize the assessment process; that is, by paying attention to their intuitive and emotional reactions and then processing these feeling through a technically sound rationale, clinicians will become more effective at assessing and diagnosing gambling disorders in particular and addictive behaviors in general. Nevertheless, it also is important for clinicians to remain aware of the paradigmatic forces that shape both their tacit and their technical knowledge.

The concept of a paradigm has been applied to clinical practice as an implicit worldview that shapes how clinicians understand the phenomenon to be assessed or treated (Shaffer, 1986b, 1987, 1991, 1997a, 1999b; Shaffer & Robbins, 1991). An operating paradigm acts as an implicit blueprint that guides clinical work. This paradigm (i.e., a preexisting template) encourages clinicians to view patients and their problems from a perspective that organizes information by focusing attention, while simultaneously blinding clinicians to alternative views. A paradigm tacitly guides clinicians as to which questions should be asked and which data are important.

Clinical and Psychodynamic Formulations

Two different strategies are available for clinicians to protect themselves from assessment errors and to resolve the issues associated with tacit assumptions. First, a clinical formulation provides a framework for understanding the nature and extent of the problem (Shaffer, 1986a). This understanding is static and time-limited to the moment of evaluation—like a photograph. To complete a *clinical formulation*, clinicians must address three key areas: (1) determine whether the gambling problem is caused by psychological, biological, or a combination of these causes; (2) ascertain whether the gambler is fundamentally psychotic, neurotic, or character disordered; and (3) determine whether the gambler requires immediate (i.e., crisis), no, or some intermediate level of intervention. Armed with responses to these three sets of issues, clinicians have an understanding of the gambler's problems. However, understanding these problems is insufficient to understand the gambler as a person.

A *psychodynamic formulation* (Perry et al., 1987; Shaffer, 1986a; Shaffer & Robbins, 1991) provides an ongoing, plastic, and evolving understanding of gamblers as persons and how they got to be the way they are. This is a shifting understanding that ebbs and flows as new information becomes available. Like a clinical formulation, a psychodynamic formulation requires clinicians to address three key areas:

1. How do we understand the patient as a human being?
2. How did they get to be the way they are, socially, emotionally, biologically, and so on?
3. What is their character and defensive structure like?

In addition, Perry et al. (1987) suggest that a dynamic formulation should include a prediction of how conflicts are likely to affect treatment and the therapeutic relationship.

> In many respects a dynamic formulation and a clinical diagnosis share a common purpose. Although both hold intellectual, didactic, and research interests, their primary function is to provide a succinct conceptualization of the case and thereby guide a treatment plan. Like a psychiatric diagnosis, a psychodynamic formulation is specific, brief, focused, and therefore limited in its intent, scope, and wisdom. (p. 543)

Although using clinical and psychodynamic formulation assessment strategies protects treatment providers from assessment errors, treatment providers and clinicians alike should recognize the importance of revising and repeating assessment activities throughout the treatment process. Just as Menninger suggested that the diagnostic process is the beginning of treatment, an ongoing assessment process permits clinicians to identify "triggers" that might influence the likelihood of relapse. These triggers include, but are not limited to, intoxicant use and abuse, family problems, social relationships, work related stress and changes and financial pressure or windfalls. Maintaining a clinical posture of ongoing assessment also provides clinician and client with an opportunity to reinforce the positive changes patients make during the recovery process by reflecting upon where the client "has been" and how their shifting behavior and emotional patterns are moving them toward treatment objectives. These treatment issues are addressed in more detail in Chapter 10 of the second edition of *Relapse Prevention* (Marlatt & Donovan, 2005).

Diagnostic Criteria

There are two primary sets of criteria to guide the diagnosis of gambling disorders: the *Diagnostic and Statistical Manual of Mental Disorders*, published by the American Psychiatric Association (1994) and the *International Classification of Diseases* (ICD-10), published by the World Health Organization (2001). Like DSM, the ICD-10 includes pathological gambling as a disorder of impulse, classifying it within the habit and impulse section of the adult personality and behavior disorders. Although the following considerations fundamentally apply to both the DSM and ICD diagnostic schemas, to expedite the discussion, the following discussion focuses on DSM-IV.

DSM-IV Criticisms and Concerns

THE CLASSIFICATION OF PATHOLOGICAL GAMBLING

While DSM-IV has contributed greatly to the assessment and diagnosis of gambling disorders, the instrument is not without its flaws. For example, DSM-IV classifies pathological gambling within the category of "Impulse-Control Disorders Not Elsewhere Classified" (American Psychiatric Association, 1994). Other disorders included in this category are intermittent explosive disorder, kleptomania, pyromania, trichotillomania, and impulse-control disorder not otherwise specified. Classifying pathological gambling as an impulse-control disorder represents the first attempt to fit intemperate gambling nosologically into the psychiatric diagnostic schema. Grouping pathological gambling with impulse disorders such as kleptomania and pyromania suggests that pathological gambling is the result of the same underlying irrepressible impulse that is common to the impulse disorders with which it is classified. DSM-IV, however, does not describe the discrepancies between pathological gambling and these other impulse disorders. Impulse-control disorders such as kleptomania and pyromania are very uncomfortable experiences. Those affected by these disorders feel overwhelmed by an impulse to act and often report a sense of relief after having acted. This discomfort is egodystonic; that is, the experience is ego alien: Sufferers do not want to steal or set fires, but they do it to relieve an overwhelming impulse to act. On the contrary, while in action, pathological gamblers often find their gambling enjoyable, or ego-syntonic. Typically, only after the gambling is terminated or losses are incurred do pathological gamblers begin to feel distress and dysthymia (Shaffer, 1999b).

If pathological gambling is similar to kleptomania and pyromania—and driven by similar irrepressible impulses rather than an irrepressible habit, then there must be validation of the impulse or impaired regulatory mechanisms (Kipnis, 1997). This similarity, however, has not been examined. With very few exceptions (e.g., Bergh et al., 1997; K. Blum et al., 2000; Christenson et al., 1994; Ebstein et al., 1996; Lejoyeux et al., 1996; Ninan et al., 2000; Orford, 1985), investigators have not focused on sets of impulse disorders for commonalities. Instead, most investigators compare gambling disorders with substance use disorders, leaving observers to wonder about the proper place of gambling disorders within the diagnostic classification system.

SOCIAL VERSUS PATHOLOGICAL GAMBLING

DSM-IV differentiates between social and pathological gambling. "Social gambling" is defined as that which "typically occurs with friends or colleagues and lasts for a limited period of time, with predetermined acceptable losses" (American Psychiatric Association, 2000, p. 673). Despite such a strict definition, it remains plausible that a social gambler might meet at least five of the criteria for pathological gambling (Table 11.4).

Indeed, a social gambler can limit gambling time and commit to "acceptable" losses, and still remain preoccupied with gambling, that is, rely on gambling as an escape from weekly stressors, while remaining unsuccessful in efforts to cut back—which can breed restlessness and irritability—as a result of desires to "break even" preceding a less than successful gambling session.

In addition, Criterion A states that pathological gambling is identified by "persistent and recurrent maladaptive gambling behavior as indicated by five or more" (American Psychiatric Association, 2000, p. 674) of the criteria listed. However, there is no discussion of the weight given to the severity of each criterion; similarly, there is no mention of the relationships that might exist among various criteria. In other words, if someone presents for assessment satisfying eight of the 10 criteria for pathological gambling, is his or her diagnosis more or less problematic compared with someone who satisfies only four criteria—even if one of these four is so significant that it problematically

---

TABLE 11.4. DSM-IV Diagnostic Criteria for Pathological Gambling

A. Persistent and recurrent maladaptive gambling behavior as indicated by five (or more) of the following:

  (1) is preoccupied with gambling (e.g., is preoccupied with reliving past gambling experiences, handicapping or planning the next venture, or thinking of ways to get money with which to gamble)
  (2) needs to gamble with increasing amounts of money in order to achieve the desired excitement
  (3) has repeated unsuccessful efforts to control, cut back, or stop gambling
  (4) is restless or irritable when attempting to cut down or stop gambling
  (5) gambles as a way of escaping from problems or of relieving a dysphonic mood (e.g., feelings of helplessness, guilt, anxiety, depression)
  (6) after losing money gambling, often returns another day to get even ("chasing" one's losses)
  (7) lies to family members, therapists, or others to conceal the extent of involvement with gambling
  (8) has committed illegal acts such as forgery, fraud, theft, or embezzlement to finance gambling
  (9) has jeopardized or lost a significant relationship, job, or educational or career opportunity because of gambling
  (10) relies on others to provide money to relieve a desperate financial situation caused by gambling

B. The gambling behavior is not better accounted for by a Manic Episode.

Note. From American Psychiatric Association (2000). Copyright 2000 by the American Psychiatric Association. Reprinted by permission.

supersedes all other criteria (e.g., repeated unsuccessful efforts to stop or cut down on their gambling)? Indeed, researchers (e.g., Radden, 1995) address such psychiatric nosology issues and further cite a growing unease associated with DSM-IV in terms of its susceptibility to yield misleading results if singularly applied to all clinical and research populations.

THE CAUTIONARY STATEMENT

In a cautionary note, the DSM-IV states that

> inclusion here, for clinical and research purposes, of a diagnostic category such as Pathological Gambling or Pedophilia does not imply that the condition meets legal or other nonmedical criteria for what constitutes mental disease, mental disorder, or mental disability. The clinical and scientific considerations involved in categorization of these conditions as mental disorders may not be wholly relevant to legal judgments, for example, that take into account such issues as individual responsibility, disability determination, and competency (American Psychiatric Association, 1994, p. xxvii).

By merely mentioning[6] pathological gambling in this cautionary note, the editors of DSM-IV purposely or inadvertently have removed the full standing of this problem as a psychiatric disorder—rightly or wrongly—with all of its exculpatory power.

Indeed, are the Cautionary Statement and its reference to pathological gambling simply that, a warning to clinicians and scientists that not all diagnostic categories might meet nonmedical criteria for what constitutes mental disorders? Alternatively, is the Cautionary Statement simply an affirmation by DSM-IV editors that the manual is still a work in progress and, as such, reflects ambivalence toward the classification of pathological gambling as a mental disorder? If the latter is true, then the editors also compromise a comprehensive utilitarian application of DSM-IV. Specifically, if the manual cannot commit to its classification of pathological gambling, what does this imply about its commitment to the classification of other mental disorders (e.g., alcohol and cocaine dependence)? Moreover, we can only speculate as to what makes these disorders more acceptably classified than pathological gambling.

Despite such uncertainties, the Cautionary Statement smartly recognizes that classification of mental disorders such as pathological gambling might not be *wholly relevant* to legal judgments (American Psychiatric Association, 2000). We interpret *wholly relevant*, in this context, to mean that it is indeed *partly relevant*. As such, the term *wholly relevant* provides DSM-IV protection from legal challenges that the disorder is without exculpatory power. Simultaneously, it allows clinicians and scientists to make treatment and research decisions with discretion on an individual basis. Without the obligation to match all patients and research subjects with all criteria for pathological gambling, DSM-IV and the Cautionary Statement provide clinicians and researchers with freedom to identify criteria that match an individual's gambling behavior. However, while clinical freedom often translates into better treatment of problem and pathological gamblers, it also can confuse and complicate assessment and other clinical activities. DSM-IV is truly a work in progress, with a host of diagnostic issues that can be addressed in DSM-V (Widiger & Clark, 2000).

Making a Diagnosis

Taking a History: The Games People Play

Although we do not believe that using a specific object of addiction (e.g., heroin, cocaine, keno, lottery, or shopping) represents the necessary and sufficient cause to produce addictive behavior,[7] there is reason to examine the epidemiological relationship between gambling disorders and the specific games on which people wager. By understanding the biopsychosocial influences of specific games, scientists can gain insight into determinants that facilitate or inhibit the development of gambling disorders. A research synthesis examined the extent of participation in seven different common gambling activities among general population adults, adolescents, adults in treatment and prison populations, and college students. Shaffer et al. (1997) found that, as expected, adolescents participate significantly more than adults in gambling activities that are most socially accessible and do not require authorization; that is, adolescents are gambling more than adults on games of skill, noncasino card games, and sports betting. Adolescents can participate in these three activities with a group of school friends, with their families, or with their friends' families. Similarly, college students are betting more than adults in the general population on noncasino card games and games of skill; these represent activities that are popular within a college setting. Not surprisingly, adults in the general population are gambling more than adolescents on casino games, the lottery, and pari-mutuel wagering. Though there are exceptions, vendors of these adult activities generally require authorization from a licensing bureau or certification board. Although there is evidence that adolescents are engaging in these three activities despite their illegal status, the vast majority of individuals who participate in these "legal" forms of gambling are adults.

Deciphering relationships among specific gaming activities and gambling disorders requires sophisticated interviewing skills that focus on the nature of the relationships that exist between individuals and the object of their addiction, that is, their gambling activity of choice. For example, persons with gambling disorders often believe that they have the capacity to influence random events with a special gambling "skill." This characteristic has become known as the illusion of control (e.g., Thompson, Armstrong, & Thomas, 1998). They also fall prey to the gambler's fallacy by failing to recognize certain events (e.g., repeatedly flipping a coin or weekly lottery drawings) as statistically independent (e.g., Ladouceur & Walker, 1998). Not all gamblers relate to every game similarly, which makes the assessment challenge even more complex.

The field of gambling research would do well to emulate lines of inquiry within the substance abuse research field, which has discovered many important and illuminating differences among various substances and their substance-specific physiological, psychological, and socioeconomic influences on their users. For example, Khantzian (1975, 1985, 1997) observed that alcohol has special "releasing" properties that tend to disinhibit users. Cocaine has antidepressant stimulating properties. Khantzian suggested that certain personality types are more attracted to each of these drug classes to produce a self-medicating effect. Similarly, Jacobs (1989) hypothesized that certain gambling activities (e.g., video poker machines) could produce dissociative effects that might differentially attract individuals with certain personality attributes. Much remains to be learned about the relationship between people and the games they choose to play (Table 11.5). For example, while most games serve to stimulate and energize players, some games might satiate others. Do some games stimulate dissociative experiences more than others, and is this characteristic different for different players? Are players of certain personality types attracted to specific games, and does this "game matching" place them at increased risk for developing gambling disorders?

As we noted before, understanding gambling-related problems rests upon an understanding of the confluence of the game or games played, the setting within which people play the game, and the expectations that the player

TABLE 11.5. Prevalence of Gambling Activity by Population Segment

	Adults (%)	Adolescents (%)	College (%)
Lifetime prevalence of gambling	81.19	77.55	85.04
Casino games—lifetime	32.32	7.74	40.59
Casino games—past year	14.95	12.56	60.83
Lottery—lifetime	61.25	34.89	50.29
Lottery—past year	49.05	30.16	60.18
Sports gambling—lifetime	26.83	38.17	28.45
Sports gambling—past year	14.76	30.69	30.5
Pari-mutuel—lifetime	25.11	10.88	27.17
Pari-mutuel—past year	7.13	11.24	8.9
Financial markets—lifetime	13.11	—	16.65
Financial markets—past year	5.81	—	4.2
Non-casino card games—lifetime	28.16	53.46	47.37
Non-casino card games—past year	15.89	39.61	36.1
Games of skill—lifetime	18.57	40.43	39.93
Games of skill—past year	10.25	31.61	23.93

brings to the gambling experience. Consequently, to assess gambling disorders properly during an evaluative interview, we suggest that clinicians inquire and examine the particular game, the conditions under which the game is played (e.g., with whom, where, and when), and any expectations associated with playing the game. Clinicians must ask clients about the frequency, amount, place, and nature of their gambling experiences. They also must ask clients to recall their experience of each gambling event, for example, how it made them feel to gamble (win, lose, etc.). Clinicians will find that some clients play only specific games and not others (e.g., casino games, horseracing, or the lottery); similarly, certain settings energize clients, while others will not (e.g., casinos, racetracks, restaurants, bars, etc.). For each game, clinicians must inquire about the extent of play and how the game influences the client. In addition to information gathered during a clinical interview, screening instruments can help determine the extent and severity of a gambling disorder.

Screening Instruments

The following discussion briefly reviews some of the major contemporary screening instruments used to identify gambling-related disorders in clinical and general populations. New screening devices are introduced on a regular basis. There are now more than 27 instruments for identifying gambling disorders, with many more in development (Shaffer et al., 1997). Although a comprehensive analysis of these instruments is beyond the scope of this chapter, the following discussion considers a representative sampling of common screening devices to facilitate a reader's entry into this literature.

SOUTH OAKS GAMBLING SCREEN

During 1987, in an effort to develop a "consistent, quantifiable, structured instrument that can be administered easily by nonprofessional as well as professional interviewers," Lesieur and Blume (1987, p. 1184) developed the SOGS. They used DSM-III-R criteria (American Psychiatric Association, 1987) to guide both the development and validation of the SOGS, which rapidly became the instrument of choice among researchers estimating disordered gambling prevalence.

SOGS-RA

The SOGS-RA, a modified version of the original SOGS instrument, is designed for use with adolescents; it uses 12 scored items and a past-year time frame (Winters, Stinchfield, & Fulkerson, 1993). The SOGS-RA can be scored in two different ways: the "narrow criteria" and the "broad criteria" (Winters et al., 1995). These two methods are scored as follows: For the narrow criteria, "no problem" = 0–1; "at risk" = 2–3; "problem" = 4+. For the broad criteria, "no problem" = no history of gambling, or gambling less than daily and score of 0; "at risk" = weekly gambling and score of 1, or less than weekly gambling and score of 2+; "problem" = weekly gambling and score of 2+, or daily gambling and any score.

DSM-IV-J

DSM-IV-J (J = Juvenile) is closely modeled after the adult version of DSM-IV. Developed by Fisher (1992), DSM-IV-J is designed to detect pathological gambling among juveniles. Two criteria differ most between DSM-IV and DSM-IV-J with respect to pathological gambling. Criterion 7 in DSM-IV (American Psychiatric Association, 1994)—has committed illegal acts such as forgery and fraud, theft, or embezzlement to finance gambling—reads in DSM-IV-J as "Committed illegal/unsocial acts, such as misuse of school dinner/fare money, and theft from the home or elsewhere in order to finance gambling" (Fisher, 1992, p. 267). Criterion 9 in DSM-IV (American Psychiatric Association, 1994) refers to having "jeopardized or lost a significant relationship, job, or educational or career opportunity because of gambling." In DSM-IV-J, Criterion 9 reads: "Fell out with family or close friends and jeopardized education because of gambling" (Fisher, 1992, p. 267).

MASSACHUSETTS GAMBLING SCREEN

The Massachusetts Gambling Screen (MAGS; Shaffer et al., 1994) assesses gambling disorders from a series of no–yes questions on two subscales. It was the first screening instrument to provide multiple measures of gambling problems: the MAGS classification key or the DSM-IV classification key. The MAGS classification system avoids dichotomous classification, recognizing that some people are moving toward more healthy states despite the presence of symptoms. The MAGS was developed for two primary reasons: (1) to yield an index of pathological or nonpathological gambling from a 5- to 10-minute interview or survey, and (2) to document the first psychometric translation of DSM-IV criteria for pathological gambling into a set of either research or clinical interview questions. The MAGS is the only screening device for gambling problems to use weighted responses. The MAGS was developed originally using data collected from a survey of 856 adolescents in suburban Boston high schools but has been used with a variety of populations since its release.

NATIONAL OPINION RESEARCH CENTER SCREEN
FOR GAMBLING PROBLEMS

The National Opinion Research Center (NORC) developed the NORC DSM-IV Screen for Gambling Problems (NODS). Because this instrument is associated with one of the few national studies of gambling impact, there has been considerable interest in this device. Like the MAGS, the NODS avoids dichotomous classification. According to the NODS typology, there are low-risk, at-risk, problem, and pathological gambler categories. The NODS has been used with adults.

Despite being offered as a DSM-IV–based screen, the NODS classification system represents more categories than the dichotomy that DSM-IV currently offers. Furthermore, the NODS depicts gambling as an impulse disorder by suggesting that the quantity of betting is diagnostic. Specifically, the NODS employs an arbitrary monetary criterion of $100 to screen or gate respondents for further questioning. In the original study, investigators administered the NODS only to those respondents who reported gambling losses of $100 dollars or more in one day of gambling, "as well as to those respondents who denied this, but acknowledged that they had been behind at least $100 across an entire year of gambling at some point in their lives" (Gerstein et al., 1999b, p. 19). While there is a relationship between how much someone gambles and gambling problems, this criterion is not sufficient to develop a formulation or diagnosis. The financial losses criterion is similar to suggesting that clinicians judge kleptomania by the number or value of the objects stolen, or trichotillomania simply by the number of hair strands pulled. DSM-IV does not include such financial criteria.

COMPOSITE INTERNATIONAL DIAGNOSTIC INTERVIEW

Like the MAGS, the Composite International Diagnostic Interview (CIDI; World Health Organization, 1990) assesses mental disorders according to DSM-IV definitions and criteria. A recent revision of this subject-oriented self-report instrument now includes a standardized assessment of gambling disorders. The CIDI gambling assessment examines how often respondents have bet or gambled for money, as well as the extent of monetary loss and/or gain, specific gambling activities, settings, and treatment history. Throughout the completion of the questionnaire, respondents are asked to think about all the times they have made a bet of any sort, "from betting on sports in an office pool to playing cards with friends, buying lottery tickets, playing bingo, speculating on high risk stocks, playing pool or golf for money, playing slot machines, betting on horse races, and any other kind of betting or gambling" (World Health Organization, 2001, p. 1).

GAMBLERS ANONYMOUS 20 QUESTIONS

Gamblers Anonymous (GA) offers 20 questions that screen for a gambling problem. Representing one of the original gambling screens, these questions, according to GA, "help the individual decide if he or she is a compulsive gambler and wants to stop gambling" (Gamblers Anonymous, 2001). As an early screening instrument that served as a model for many that followed, Table 11.6 presents the GA 20 questions. While there is little psychometric evidence to guide the classification of disorders using this instrument, according to GA,

TABLE 11.6. Gamblers Anonymous 20 Questions

1. Did you ever lose time from work or school due to gambling?

2. Has gambling ever made your home life unhappy?

3. Did gambling affect your reputation?

4. Have you ever felt remorse after gambling?

5. Did you ever gamble to get money with which to pay debts or otherwise solve financial difficulties?

6. Did gambling cause a decrease in your ambition or efficiency?

7. After losing did you feel you must return as soon as possible and win back your losses?

8. After a win did you have a strong urge to return and win more?

9. Did you often gamble until your last dollar was gone?

10. Did you ever borrow to finance your gambling?

11. Have you ever sold anything to finance gambling?

12. Were you reluctant to use "gambling money" for normal expenditures?

13. Did gambling make you careless of the welfare of yourself or your family?

14. Did you ever gamble longer than you had planned?

15. Have you ever gambled to escape worry or trouble?

16. Have you ever committed, or considered committing, an illegal act to finance gambling?

17. Did gambling cause you to have difficulty in sleeping?

18. Do arguments, disappointments or frustrations create within you an urge to gamble?

19. Did you ever have an urge to celebrate any good fortune by a few hours of gambling?

20. Have you ever considered self-destruction or suicide as a result of your gambling?

Note. Copyright 2001 by Gamblers Anonymous. Reprinted by permission.

compulsive gamblers commonly answer "yes" to at least seven of these 20 questions.

Comparing Screening Instruments

Five studies have provided the opportunity to compare a variety of screening instruments. This set of five comparisons included both college student and adult population samples for both lifetime and past-year time frame prevalence estimates. In these studies, the SOGS provided higher rates than the DSM criteria by factors ranging from 1.4 to 2.67, with a mean factor of approximately 2. The SOGS-RA broad criteria have been compared with the SOGS-RA narrow criteria in three studies; in these studies, the broad criteria provided higher rates than the narrow criteria by a mean factor of approximately 2.5. The MAGS has been compared with DSM-IV criteria in three studies; in two of these studies, the MAGS rate exceeded the DSM-IV rate, and in one of these studies, the DSM-IV rate exceeded the MAGS rate. The mean ratio of MAGS to DSM-IV was approximately 1. Table 11.7 summarizes these and other comparisons.

TABLE 11.7. Comparing Screening Instruments across Studies with Multiple Measures of Level 3 Gambling Rates

Study	Sample	Time frame	Instr. 1	Instr. 1 rate	Instr. 2	Instr. 2 rate	Ratio
Oster & Knapp (1994)	College	Lifetime	SOGS	11.2	DSM-III-R	5.1	SOGS = 2.20 DSM-III-R
Oster & Knapp (1994)	College	Lifetime	SOGS	8.0	DSM-III-R	5.7	SOGS = 1.40 DSM-III-R
Ferris & Stirpe (1995)	Adults	Lifetime	SOGS	0.97	DSM-IV	0.485	SOGS = 2.00 DSM-IV
Oster & Knapp (1994)	College	Lifetime	SOGS	11.2	DSM-IV	4.2	SOGS = 2.67 DSM-IV
Volberg (1996b)	Adults	Past year	SOGS	1.4	DSM-IV	0.875	SOGS = 1.60 DSM-IV
Volberg (1996a)	Adolescents	Lifetime	SOGS	3.4	Multifactor method	2.8	SOGS = 1.21 MM
Volberg (1993b)	Adolescents	Lifetime	SOGS	1.5	Multifactor method	.9	SOGS = 1.67 MM
Wallisch (1993)	Adolescents	Lifetime	SOGS	3.7	Multifactor method	5.0	SOGS = 0.74 MM
Govoni et al. (1996)	Adolescents	Past year	SOGS-RA "narrow" criteria	10.3	SOGS-RA "broad" criteria	21.1	Broad = 2.05 narrow
Winters et al. (1995)	Adolescents	Past year	SOGS-RA "narrow" criteria	2.9	SOGS-RA "broad" criteria	8.2	Broad = 2.83 narrow

Study	Population	Timeframe					Comparison
Winters et al. (1995)	Adolescents	Past year	SOGS-RA "narrow" criteria	3.5	SOGS-RA "broad" criteria	9.5	Broad = 2.71 narrow
Shaffer et al. (1994)	Adolescents	Past year[a]	MAGS	8.5	DSM-IV	6.4	MAGS = 1.33 DSM-IV
Vagge (1996)	Adolescents	Past year	MAGS	4.3	DSM-IV	4.2	MAGS = 1.02 DSM-IV
Shaffer & Hall (1996)	Adolescents	Past year	MAGS	7.0	DSM-IV	8.0	MAGS = .875 DSM-IV
Ladouceur & Mireault (1988)	Adolescents	Lifetime	PGSI[b]	3.6	DSM-III	1.7	PGSI = 2.118 DSM-III
Govoni et al. (1996)	Adolescents	Past year	SOGS	8.1	SOGS-RA "narrow" criteria	10.3	Narrow = 1.27 SOGS
Govoni et al. (1996)	Adolescents	Past year	SOGS	8.1	SOGS-RA "broad" criteria	21.1	Broad = 2.60 SOGS
Steinberg (1997)	Adolescents	Past year	MAGS	3.2	SOGS-RA "broad" criteria	8.7	Broad = 2.72 MAGS

[a]The rates from Shaffer et al. (1994) are calculated among respondents who have gambled in their Lifetime.
[b]Pathological Gambling Signs Index.

Critical Consideration of Screening Instruments

Dickerson suggests that the reliability of the SOGS is not well established, and that respondents with identical scores could have entirely different characteristics. For example, using the SOGS might result in an overestimation of pathological gambling prevalence (Dickerson, 1994; Volberg & Boles, 1995; Walker & Dickerson, 1996).

Lesieur (1994) evaluated the criticisms of the SOGS in his critique of epidemiological surveys. He suggests that most epidemiological surveys *underestimate* the extent of disordered gambling as a result of methodological flaws such as not including the homeless or hospitalized populations, and not "catching" gamblers at home in a telephone survey. Lesieur is correct on methodological grounds; however, investigators have failed to recognize that scientists can identify over- or underestimates of prevalence screening instruments only when a "gold standard" also exists to identify the attribute of interest.

The central question is not (1) whether any particular screening instrument provides an overestimate or an underestimate, or (2) whether the methodological weaknesses of research protocols offset the unique measurement characteristics of a screening instrument. Similarly, it would be incorrect to conclude that any screening device yields a lower or higher estimate of disordered gambling until scientists are sure that comparison instruments do not *over-* or *underestimate* the prevalence of disordered gambling (Shaffer et al., 1997). Rather, the principal question is: With what independent standard can we compare any estimate of prevalence? Only by evaluating a screening instrument against an independent and valid standard can we decide about the precision of its measurements.

Unfortunately, most screening devices are incestuous, having been derived from each other and then used to test the development of their progeny. The result is a psychometric tautology. Since DSM was used as the standard for the development of the SOGS, the confusion around this issue—and the completion of the tautology—was evident when Volberg suggested that "in the case of the DSM-IV Screen we must use the SOGS as the 'gold standard' since this is the primary method that has been used to identify problem and pathological gamblers since the late 1980s" (Volberg, 1997, p. 34). Like many other psychiatric disorders, there is no epidemiological "gold standard" in the area of disordered gambling prevalence (American Psychiatric Association, Task Force for the Handbook of Psychiatric Measures, 2000).

Obstacles to Assessment and Diagnosis

We began this review of assessment and diagnosis by suggesting that addictive behavior and gambling disorders represent a difficult-to-understand class of human behavior. By recognizing that clinicians have the tendency to assess only what they look for and diagnose what they know (e.g., Rosenhan, 1973), we can see that understanding the complexity of issues associated with excessive gambling are magnified. When clinicians are armed with the information in this chapter, their chances of "seeing" the full range of problems are increased. Nevertheless, when clinicians experience emotions and reactions to their patients that are not part of the treatment contract, they are feeling countertransference (Imhof, 1991; Imhof et al., 1984; Maltsberger & Buie, 1974; Weiner, 1975).

Countertransferential experiences can be both positive (e.g., feelings of attraction) and negative (e.g., feelings of disdain). These feelings often are exaggerated: Patients seem more likeable or troublesome than the situation reflects. Too often during the treatment of addictive behavior patterns, these feelings are negative—and clinicians justify their negative feelings by invoking psychological theories. For example, clinicians might blame their patients for failing to thrive in treatment or for not being sufficiently motivated to change. Similarly, clinicians could assume that *all* people with gambling problems commit crimes. These are expressions of countertransference hate (Maltsberger & Buie, 1974; Shaffer, 1994); often, formulations emerge to protect a clinician's emotional state. These events are troubling and potentially hazardous to the therapeutic alliance. At the very least, this state of affairs can compromise the conduct of assessment and diagnosis. Clinical supervision often provides even the most experienced clinicians with an important system of checks and balances that can protect them from themselves. However, only about 50% of addiction treatment specialists experience regular clinical supervision (e.g., Shaffer, Walsh, Howard, Hall, & Wellington, 1995), and gambling treatment workers likely have even less. Consequently, we encourage clinicians to schedule clinical supervision and to review the conduct of their clinical assessment activities regularly. As Miller (2000) noted, very small interventions can yield extremely large effects on human behavior; an empathic, caring, and respectful clinical posture will elicit the most useful information and yield the most meaningful assessment and diagnoses possible.

CONCLUSIONS

Gambling-related disorders have emerged as an important public health concern. Growing public health attention has generated increasing notice from treatment providers. New treatments for gambling disorders are appearing. Assessment is the first and an ongoing element of the treatment process. Seemingly straightforward, assessment is a thorny and difficult activity. The assessment process provides a foundation for developing an alliance with patients, a blueprint for treatment planning, and a reference point for treatment monitoring and aftercare. This chapter has focused on the important conceptual and practical problems that clinicians and scientists face when they attempt to assess the presence, prevalence, and extent of gambling problems. These difficulties surface because gambling studies is an emerging and youthful field; the conceptual underpinnings of disordered gambling are less than certain. Rational and tacit components contribute to our understanding of intemperate gambling. Similarly, the validity of screening instruments also is uncertain given the paucity of scientific evidence, the uncertainty of the underlying constructs, and the pervasive prevalence of co-occurring disorders.

These conceptual concerns emphasize the importance of using clinical and psychodynamic formulations to guide the treatment process. In addition, given the conceptual uncertainty associated with the construct of pathological gambling and the adverse effects of countertransference hate that can emerge from tacit influences, we encourage clinicians to schedule clinical supervision regularly. Finally, we suggest that the assessment and diagnosis of gambling disorders—like other behavioral problems—is culturally relative; society serves as the ultimate arbiter of sickness and whether a pattern of behavior is acceptable.

ACKNOWLEDGMENTS

Portions of this chapter derive, in part, from a series of publications. We want to extend thanks and acknowledge the important contributions of Milton Burglass, Matthew Hall, Janice Kauffman, David Korn, Debi LaPlante, Sarah Nelson, Joni Vander Bilt, Gabriel Eber, and Richard LaBrie to this chapter.

Preparation of this chapter was supported, in part, by support from the Center for Substance Abuse Treatment (CSAT), the Addiction Technology Transfer Center of New England, the Institute for the Study of Pathological Gambling and Related Disorders, and the National Center for Responsible Gaming (NCRG).

NOTES

1. Addiction represents a repetitive health disorder that alters the way in which one experiences the world. This shift can be affective (feelings), cognitive (thoughts), behavioral (actions), or a combination of these (Shaffer, 1996, 1997a). The natural history of addiction reveals that individuals initially see their experience as positive, but over time, as their behavior continues, problems often begin to emerge, though they may not be aware of them (Shaffer, 1997b; Shaffer & Robbins, 1995). The behavior can become excessive and habitual. When repetitive compulsive behaviors emerge and seem well established, a feeling of loss of control often develops. Despite adverse consequences to self, family, or community, addictive behavior continues. The person struggling with addiction can experience powerful craving triggered by specific stimuli. Addiction most commonly is associated with mood-altering chemicals, such as alcohol or other drugs, but can include other problem activities including gambling, exercise, and shopping. Finally, people with addiction often demonstrate signs and symptoms reflecting neuroadaptation (i.e., tolerance and withdrawal).

2. Pathological gambling is now classified in DSM-IV as an impulse disorder. From this perspective, it represents an irrepressible impulse—the hallmark of an impulse disorder. Unlike most characterizations of addiction as primarily ego-syntonic, cli-

nicians consider impulse disorders such as obsessive–compulsive disorders as primarily ego-dystonic.

3. While these tables refer to "level 1 gamblers," it should be noted that in these tables, this group includes both nongamblers and gamblers without any gambling-related symptoms.

4. When pathological gambling "treats" the occurrence of a coexisting disorder or the progression of these problems, gambling serves as a "self-medication" (e.g., Khantzian, 1985).

5. The absence of pathological gambling as the underlying cause of death on the death certificate does not mean that no one has died of factors associated with pathological gambling. Medical examiners, who must identify the immediate cause and contributing causes of death on the death certificate, for any number of reasons, might be unaware of pathological gambling or unwilling to list it as an underlying cause of death.

6. Readers also might consider the social and public policy impact of having only one conceptual counterpart, pedophilia, included in this cautionary note.

7. We encourage interested readers to review other relevant works (Shaffer, 1986b, 1996, 1997a, 1999a, 1999b) for a more complete discussion of this matter.

REFERENCES

Abbott, M. W. (2001). *Problem and non-problem gamblers in New Zealand: A report on phase two of the 1999 National Prevalence Survey* (Report No. 6 of the New Zealand Gaming Survey). Wellington: New Zealand Department of Internal Affairs.

Adams, W. L., Barry, K. L., & Fleming, M. F. (1996). Screening for problem drinking in older primary care patients. *Journal of the American Medical Association, 276*(24), 1964–1967.

American Academy of Pediatrics. (1998, August 3). *Teen gambling epidemic linked to risky behavior.* Retrieved November 14, 1999, from www.aap.org/advocacy/archives/auggam/htm.

American Psychiatric Association. (1980). *Diagnostic and statistical manual of mental disorders* (3rd ed.). Washington, DC: Author.

American Psychiatric Association. (1987). *Diagnostic and statistical manual of mental disorders* (3rd ed., rev.). Washington, DC: Author.

American Psychiatric Association. (1994). *Diagnostic and statistical manual of mental disorders* (4th ed.). Washington, DC: Author.

American Psychiatric Association. (2000). *Diagnostic and statistical manual of mental disorders* (4th ed., text rev.). Washington, DC: Author.

American Psychiatric Association, Task Force for the Handbook of Psychiatric Measures. (2000). *Handbook of psychiatric measures.* Washington, DC: American Psychiatric Association.

Barron, J. (Ed.). (1998). *Making diagnosis meaningful: Enhancing evaluation and treatment of psychological disorders.* Washington, DC: American Psychological Association.

Becona, E. (1996). Prevalence surveys of problem and pathological gambling in Europe: The cases of Germany, Holland and Spain. *Journal of Gambling Studies, 12*(2), 179–192.

Benjamin, J., Lin, L., Patterson, C., Greenberg, B. D., Murphy, D. L., & Hamer, D. H.

(1996, January). Population and familial association between the D4 dopamine receptor gene and measures of novelty seeking. *Nature Genetics, 12*, 81–83.

Bergh, C., Sodersten, E. P., & Nordin, C. (1997). Altered dopamine function in pathological gambling. *Psychological Medicine, 27*, 473–475.

Bettencourt, B. A., & Miller, N. (1996). Gender differences in aggression as a function of provocation: A meta-analysis. *Psychological Bulletin, 119*(3), 422–447.

Black, W. B., & Moyer, T. (1998). Clinical features and psychiatric comorbidity of subjects with pathological gambling behavior. *Psychiatric Services, 49*, 1434–1439.

Blacker, D., & Endicott, J. (2000). Psychometric properties: Concepts of reliability and validity. In American Psychiatric Association, Task Force for the Handbook of Psychiatric Measures (Ed.), *Handbook of psychiatric measures* (pp. 7–14). Washington, DC: American Psychiatric Association.

Blaszczynski, A., & Farrell, E. (1998). A case series of 44 completed gambling-related suicides. *Journal of Gambling Studies, 14*(2), 93–109.

Blaszczynski, A., McConaghy, N., & Frankova, A. (1991). Control versus abstinence in the treatment of pathological gambling: A two to nine year follow-up. *British Journal of Addiction, 86*, 299–306.

Blaszczynski, A., & Steel, Z. (1998). Personality disorders among pathological gamblers. *Journal of Gambling Studies, 14*(1), 51–71.

Blum, A. (1985). The collective representation of affliction: Some reflections on disability and disease as social facts. *Theoretical Medicine, 6*, 221–232.

Blum, K., Braverman, E. R., Holder, M. M., Lubar, J. F., Monastra, V. J., Miller, D., et al. (2000). Reward deficiency syndrome: A biogenetic model for the diagnosis and treatment of impulsive, addictive, and compulsive behaviors. *Journal of Psychoactive Drugs, 32*(Suppl.), 1–112.

Bondolfi, G., Osiek, C., & Ferrero, F. (2002). Pathological gambling: An increasing and underestimated disorder. *Schweizer Archiv für Neurologie und Psychiatrie, 153*(3), 116–122.

Boyd, J. H., Burke, J. D., Gruenberg, E., Holzer, C. E., Rae, D. S., George, L. K., et al. (1984, October). Exclusion criteria of DSM-III: A study of co-occurrence of hierarchy-free syndromes. *Archives of General Psychiatry, 41*, 983–989.

Briggs, J. R., Goodin, B. J., & Nelson, T. (1996). Pathological gamblers and alcoholics: Do they share the same addiction? *Addictive Behaviors, 21*(4), 515–519.

Centers for Disease Control. (2001). *Compressed mortality database*. Retrieved March 9, 2001, from wonder.cdc.gov.

Cerny, L., & Cerny, K. (1992). Can carrots be addictive?: An extraordinary form of drug dependence. *British Journal of Addiction, 87*, 1195–1197.

Christenson, G. A., Faber, R. J., de Zwaan, M., Raymond, N. C., Specker, S. M., Edern, M. D., et al. (1994). Compulsive buying: Descriptive characteristics and psychiatric comorbidity. *Journal of Clinical Psychiatry, 55*(1), 5–11.

Cochrane, A. L., & Holland, W. W. (1971). Validation of screening procedures. *British Medical Bulletin, 27*, 3–8.

Collins, P., & Barr, G. (2001). *Gambling and problem gambling in South Africa: A national study*. National Center for the Study of Gambling, Cape Town, University of Cape Town.

Comings, D. E. (1998). The molecular genetics of pathological gambling. *CNS Spectrums, 3*(6), 20–37.

Comings, D. E., Gonzalez, N., Wu, S., Gade, R., Muhleman, D., Saucier, G., et al.

(1999). Studies of the 48 bp repeat polymorphism of the DRD4 gene in impulsive, compulsive, addictive behaviors: Tourette syndrome, ADHD, pathological gambling, and substance abuse. *American Journal of Medical Genetics, 88*(4), 358–368.

Crockford, D. N., & el-Guebaly, N. (1998). Psychiatric comorbidity in pathological gambling: A critical review. *Canadian Journal of Psychiatry—Revue Canadienne de Psychiatrie, 43*(1), 43–50.

Cronbach, L. J., & Meehl, P. E. (1955). Construct validity in psychological tests. *Psychological Bulletin, 52*(4), 281–302.

Cuadrado, M. (1999). A comparison of Hispanic and Anglo calls to a gambling help hotline. *Journal of Gambling Studies, 15*(1), 71–81.

Culleton, R. P. (1989). The prevalence rates of pathological gambling: A look at methods. *Journal of Gambling Studies, 5*(1), 22–41.

Culleton, R. P., & Lang, M. H. (1985). *The prevalence rate of pathological gambling in the Delaware Valley in 1984* (Report to People Acting To Help, Philadelphia). Camden, NJ: Forum for Policy Research and Public Service, Rutgers University.

Cunningham-Williams, R. M., Cottler, L. B., Compton, W. M., & Spitznagel, E. L. (1998). Taking chances: Problem gamblers and mental health disorders—Results from the St. Louis Epidemiologic Catchment Area study. *American Journal of Public Health, 88,* 1093–1096.

Cunningham-Williams, R. M., Cottler, L. B., Compton, W. M., Spitznagel, E. L., & Ben-Abdallah, A. (2000). Problem gambling and comorbid psychiatric and substance use disorders among drug users recruited from drug treatment and community settings. *Journal of Gambling Studies, 16*(4), 347–376.

Curry, S. J., & Kim, E. L. (1999). Public health perspective on addictive behavior change interventions: Conceptual frameworks and guiding principles. In J. A. Tucker, D. M. Donovan, & G. A. Marlatt (Eds.), *Changing addictive behavior* (pp. 221–250). New York: Guilford Press.

Custer, R. L., & Milt, H. (1985). *When luck runs out: Help for compulsive gamblers and their families.* New York: Warner Books.

Daghestani, A. N. (1987). Impotence associated with compulsive gambling. *Journal of Clinical Psychiatry, 48*(3), 115–116.

Davies, J. B. (1996). Reasons and causes: Understanding substance users' explanations for their behavior. *Human Psychopharmacology, 11,* S39–S48.

DeCaria, C. M., Begaz, T., & Hollander, E. (1998). Serotonergic and noradrenergic function in pathological gambling. *CNS Spectrums, 3*(6), 38–47.

Dickerson, M. (1994, June). *Alternative approaches to the measurement of the prevalence of pathological gambling.* Paper presented at the Ninth National Conference on Gambling and Risk Taking, Las Vegas, NV.

Dohrenwend, B. P. (1995). "The problem of validity in field studies of psychological disorders" revisited. In M. T. Tsuang, M. Tohen, & G. E. Zahner (Eds.), *Textbook in psychiatric epidemiology* (pp. 3–20). New York: Wiley-Liss.

Donovan, D. M., & Marlatt, G. A. (Eds.). (1988). *Assessment of addictive behaviors.* New York: Guilford Press.

Eber, G. B., & Shaffer, H. J. (2000). Trends in bio-behavioral gambling studies research: Quantifying citations. *Journal of Gambling Studies, 16*(4), 461–467.

Ebstein, R. P., Novick, O., Umansky, R., Priel, B., Osher, Y., Blaine, D., et al. (1996, January). Dopamine D4 receptor (D4DR) exon III polymorphism associated with the human personality trait of novelty seeking. *Nature Genetics, 12,* 78–80.

Elia, C., & Jacobs, D. F. (1993). The incidence of pathological gambling among Native Americans treated for alcohol dependence. *International Journal of the Addictions, 28*(7), 659–666.

Faraone, S. V., & Tsuang, M. T. (1994). Measuring diagnostic accuracy in the absence of a "gold standard." *American Journal of Psychiatry, 151*(5), 650–657.

Feigelman, W., Wallisch, L. S., & Lesieur, H. R. (1998). Problem gamblers, problem substance users, and dual problem individuals: An epidemiological study. *American Journal of Public Health, 88*(3), 467–470.

Ferris, J., & Stirpe, T. (1995). *Gambling in Ontario: A report from a general population survey on gambling-related problems and opinions.* Toronto: Addiction Research Foundation.

Fisher, S. (1992). Measuring pathological gambling in children: The case of fruit machines in the U.K. *Journal of Gambling Studies, 8*(3), 263–285.

Fisher, S. (2000). Measuring the prevalence of sector-specific problem gambling: A study of casino patrons. *Journal of Gambling Studies, 16*(1), 25–51.

Fromme, K., Katz, E., & D'Amico, E. (1997). Effects of alcohol intoxication on the perceived consequences of risk taking. *Experimental and Clinical Psychopharmacology, 5*(1), 14–23.

Fromme, K., Katz, E. C., & Rivet, K. (1997). Outcome expectancies and risk-taking behavior. *Cognitive Therapy and Research, 21*(4), 421–442.

Galdston, I. (1951). The psychodynamics of the triad, alcoholism, gambling, and superstition. *Mental Hygiene, 35*, 589–598.

Gambino, B., & Shaffer, H. J. (1979). The concept of paradigm and the treatment of addiction. *Professional Psychology, 10*, 207–223.

Gamblers Anonymous. (2001). *Twenty questions.* Retrieved July 16, 2001, from www.gamblersanonymous.org/20questions.html.

Gerstein, D., Murphy, S., Toce, M., Hoffmann, J., Palmer, A., Johnson, R., et al. (1999a). *Gambling Impact and Behavior Study: Report to the National Gambling Impact Study Commission.* Chicago: National Opinion Research Center.

Gerstein, D., Murphy, S., Toce, M., Hoffmann, J., Palmer, A., Johnson, R., et al. (1999b). *Gambling Impact and Behavior Study: Final report to the National Gambling Impact Study Commission.* Chicago: National Opinion Research Center.

Goldstein, J. M., & Simpson, J. C. (1995). Validity: Definitions and applications to psychiatric research. In M. T. Tsuang, M. Tohen, & G. E. Zahner (Eds.), *Textbook in psychiatric epidemiology* (pp. 229–242). New York: Wiley-Liss.

Götestam, K. G., & Johansson, A. (2003). Characteristics of gambling and problematic gambling in the Norwegian context: A DSM-IV-based telephone interview study. *Addictive Behaviors, 28*, 189–197.

Govoni, R., Rupcich, N., & Frisch, G. (1996). Gambling behavior of adolescent gamblers. *Journal of Gambling Studies, 12*(3), 305–317.

Hamilton, B. (1995). *Getting started in AA.* Center City, MN: Hazelden.

Havens, L. (1982). The choice of clinical methods. *Contemporary Psychoanalysis, 18*, 16–42.

Havens, L. (1989). *A safe place: Laying the groundwork of psychotherapy.* Cambridge, MA: Harvard University Press.

Hewitt, D. (1994). *Spirit of bingoland: A study of problem gambling among Alberta native people.* Edmonton: Nechi Training Research and Health Promotions Institute.

Hodge, J. E., McMurran, M., & Hollin, C. R. (Eds.). (1997). *Addicted to crime?* West Sussex, UK: Wiley.

Hollander, E., Buchalter, A. J., & DeCaria, C. M. (2000). Pathological gambling. *Psychiatric Clinics of North America, 23*(3), 629–642.

Imhof, J. E. (1991). Countertransference issues in alcoholism and drug addiction. *Psychiatric Annals, 21*(5), 292–306.

Imhof, J. E., Hirsch, R., & Terenzi, R. E. (1984). Countertransferential and attitudinal considerations in the treatment of drug abuse and addiction. *Journal of Substance Abuse Treatment, 1*(1), 21–30.

Institute of Medicine. (1990). *Broadening the base of treatment for alcohol problems: Report of a study by a committee of the Institute of Medicine, Division of Mental Health and Behavioral Medicine.* Washington, DC: National Academy of Science.

Jacobs, D. F. (1989). A general theory of addictions: Rationale for and evidence supporting a new approach for understanding and treating addictive behaviors. In H. J. Shaffer, S. Stein, B. Gambino, & T. N. Cummings (Eds.), *Compulsive gambling: Theory, research and practice* (pp. 35–64). Lexington, MA: Lexington Books.

Jarrell, H. R. (1988). Vegas neuropathy. *New England Journal of Medicine, 319*(22), 1487.

Jason, J. R., Taff, M. L., & Boglioli, L. R. (1990). Casino-related deaths in Atlantic City, New Jersey: 1982–1986. *American Journal of Forensic Medicine and Pathology, 11*(2), 112–123.

Jessor, R., & Jessor, S. L. (1977). *Problem behavior and psychosocial development: A longitudinal study of youth.* New York: Academic Press.

Kallick, M., Suits, D., Dielman, T., & Hybels, J. (1979). *A survey of American gambling attitudes and behavior* (Research Report Series, Survey Research Center, Institute for Social Research). Ann Arbor: University of Michigan Press.

Karch, S. B., Graff, J., Young, S., & Ho, C. (1988). Response times and outcomes for cardiac arrests in Las Vegas casinos. *American Journal of Emergency Medicine, 16*(3), 249–253.

Kessler, R. C., Crum, R. M., Warner, L. A., Nelson, C. B., Schulenberg, J., & Anthony, J. C. (1997). Lifetime co-occurrence of DSM-III-R alcohol abuse and dependence with other psychiatric disorders in the National Comorbidity Survey. *Archives of General Psychiatry, 54*, 313–321.

Kessler, R. C., Nelson, C. B., McGonagle, K. A., Edlund, M. J., Frank, R. G., & Leaf, P. J. (1996). The epidemiology of co-occurring addictive and mental disorders: Implications for prevention and service utilization. *American Journal of Orthopsychiatry, 66*(1), 17–31.

Khantzian, E. J. (1975). Self selection and progression in drug dependence. *Psychiatry Digest, 36*, 19–22.

Khantzian, E. J. (1985). The self-medication hypothesis of addictive disorders: Focus on heroin and cocaine dependence. *American Journal of Psychiatry, 142*(11), 1259–1264.

Khantzian, E. J. (1997). The self-medication hypothesis of substance use disorders: A reconsideration and recent applications. *Harvard Review of Psychiatry, 4*(5), 231–244.

Khantzian, E. J., Halliday, K. S., & McAuliffe, W. E. (1990). *Addiction and the vulnerable self: Modified dynamic group therapy for substance abusers.* New York: Guilford Press.

Kiesler, S., & Sproull, L. (1985). Pool halls, chips, and war games: Women in the culture of computing. *Psychology of Women Quarterly, 9*(4), 451–462.

Kinkead, G. (1992). *Chinatown: Portrait of a closed society.* New York: HarperCollins.

Kipnis, D. (1997). Ghosts, taxonomies, and social psychology. *American Psychologist, 52*(3), 205–211.

Kleinman, A. (1987). Culture and clinical reality: Commentary on culture-bound syndromes and international disease classifications. *Culture, Medicine and Psychiatry, 11*, 49–52.

Kleinman, A. (1988). *The illness narratives: Suffering, healing and the human condition.* New York: Basic Books.

Korn, D. A. (2000). Expansion of gambling in Canada: Implications for health and social policy. *Canadian Medical Association Journal, 163*(1), 61–64.

Korn, D. A., & Shaffer, H. J. (1999). Gambling and the health of the public: Adopting a public health perspective. *Journal of Gambling Studies, 15*(4), 289–365.

Korn, D. A., & Skinner, H. A. (2000). Gambling expansion in Canada: An emerging public health issue. *Canadian Public Health Association Health Digest, 24,* 10.

Ladouceur, R., Bouchard, C., Rheaume, N., Jacques, C., Ferland, F., Leblond, J., et al. (2000). Is the SOGS an accurate measure of pathological gambling among children, adolescents and adults? *Journal of Gambling Studies, 16*(1), 1–24.

Ladouceur, R., & Mireault, C. (1988). Gambling behaviors among high school students in the Quebec area. *Journal of Gambling Studies, 4*, 3–13.

Ladouceur, R., Sylvain, C., Letarte, H., Giroux, I., & Jacques, C. (1998). Cognitive treatment of pathological gamblers. *Behaviour Research and Therapy, 36*(12), 1111–1119.

Ladouceur, R., & Walker, M. (1998). The cognitive approach to understanding and treating pathological gambling. In A. S. Bellack & M. Hersen (Eds.), *Comprehensive clinical psychology* (pp. 588–601). New York: Pergamon.

Lakshmanan, I. A. R. (1996, March 9). A woman's life lost to gambling: Suicide highlights betting's dark side. *Boston Globe,* pp. 13, 20.

Langenbucher, J., Bavly, L., Labouvie, E., Sanjuan, P. M., & Martin, C. S. (2001). Clinical features of pathological gambling in an addictions treatment cohort. *Psychology of Addictive Behaviors, 15*(1), 77–79.

Lapage, C., Ladouceur, R., & Jacques, C. (2000). Prevalence of problem gambling among community service users. *Community Mental Health Journal, 36*(6), 597–601.

Lejoyeux, M., Ades, J., Tassain, V., & Solomon, J. (1996). Phenomenology and psychopathology of uncontrolled buying. *American Journal of Psychiatry December, 153*(12), 1524–1529.

Lesieur, H. R. (1994). Epidemiological surveys of pathological gambling: Critique and suggestions for modification. *Journal of Gambling Studies, 10*(4), 385–398.

Lesieur, H. R., & Blume, S. B. (1987). The South Oaks Gambling Screen (SOGS): A new instrument for the identification of pathological gamblers. *American Journal of Psychiatry, 144*(9), 1184–1188.

Lesieur, H. R., & Blume, S. B. (1990). Characteristics of pathological gamblers identified among patients on a psychiatric admissions service. *Hospital and Community Psychiatry, 41*, 1009–1012.

Lesieur, H. R., Blume, S. B., & Zoppa, R. M. (1986). Alcoholism, drug abuse, and gambling. *Alcoholism: Clinical and Experimental Research, 10*(1), 33–38.

Lesieur, H. R., Cross, J., Frank, M., Welch, M., White, C. M., Rubenstein, G., et al. (1991). Gambling and pathological gambling among university students. *Addictive Behaviors, 16*(6), 517–527.

Lesieur, H. R., & Rosenthal, R. J. (1991). Pathological gambling: A review of the literature (prepared for the American Psychiatric Association Task Force on DSM-IV Committee on Disorders of Impulse Control Not Elsewhere Classified). *Journal of Gambling Studies, 7*(1), 5–39.

Levin, J. D. (1987). *Treatment of alcoholism and other addictions.* Northvale, NJ: Aronson.

Lillenfield, D. E. (2000). John Snow: The first hired gun? *American Journal of Epidemiology, 152*(1), 4–12.

Lopes, L. L. (1987). Between hope and fear: The psychology of risk. In L. Berkowitz (Ed.), *Advances in experimental social psychology* (Vol. 20, pp. 255–295). San Diego: Academic Press.

Malagady, R. G., Rogler, L. H., & Tryon, W. W. (1992). Issues of validity in the Diagnostic Interview Schedule. *Journal of Psychiatric Research, 26*(1), 59–67.

Maltsberger, J. T., & Buie, D. (1974). Countertransference hate in the treatment of suicidal patients. *Archives of General Psychiatry, 30,* 625–633.

Marks, I. (1990). Behavioural (nonchemical) addictions. *British Journal of Addiction, 85,* 1389–1394.

Marlatt, G. A. (Ed.). (1998). *Harm reduction: Pragmatic strategies for managing high-risk behaviors.* New York: Guilford Press.

Marlatt, G. A., & Donovan, D. M. (Eds.). (2005). *Relapse prevention* (2nd ed.). New York: Guilford Press.

McAulliffe, W. E., & Ch'ien, J. M. N. (1986). Recovery training and self help: A relapse-prevention program for treated opiate addicts. *Journal of Substance Abuse Treatment, 3,* 9–20.

McCleary, R., Chew, K., Feng, W., Merrill, V., Napolitano, C., Males, M., et al. (1998). *Suicide and gambling: An analysis of suicide rates in U.S. counties and metropolitan areas.* Irvine: University of California Irvine, School of Social Ecology.

McGuire, W. J. (1964). Inducing resistance to persuasion. In L. Berkowitz (Ed.), *Advances in experimental social psychology* (Vol. 1, pp. 191–229). New York: Academic Press.

McNeilly, D. P., & Burke, W. J. (2000). Late life gambling: The attitudes and behaviors of older adults. *Journal of Gambling Studies, 16*(4), 393–415.

Meehl, P. E. (1954). *Clinical versus statistical prediction; a theoretical analysis and a review of the evidence.* Minneapolis: University of Minnesota Press.

Meehl, P. E. (1973). *Psychodiagnosis; selected papers.* New York: Norton.

Menninger, K. (1963). *The vital balance: The life process in mental health and illness.* New York: Viking Press.

Milkman, H. B., & Sederer, L. I. (Eds.). (1990). *Treatment choices for alcoholism and substance abuse.* Lexington, MA: Lexington Books.

Milkman, H. B., & Shaffer, H. J. (Eds.). (1985). *The addictions: Multidisciplinary perspectives and treatments.* Lexington, MA: Lexington Books.

Miller, W. R. (2000). Rediscovering fire: Small interventions, large effects. *Psychology of Addictive Behaviors, 14*(1), 6–18.

Miller, W. R., & Rollnick, S. (Eds.). (1991). *Motivational interviewing: Preparing people to change addictive behavior.* New York: Guilford Press.

Morris, M., Steinberg, H., Sykes, E. A., & Salmon, P. (1990). Effects of temporary withdrawal from regular running. *Journal of Psychosomatic Research, 34*(5), 493–500.

Najavits, L. (2002). *Seeking safety.* New York: Guilford Press.

National Gambling Impact Study Commission. (1999). *National Gambling Impact Study Commission report.* Washington, DC: Author.

National Gambling Impact Study Commission Act. (1996). Pub. L. No. 104-169.

National Research Council. (1999). *Pathological gambling: A critical review.* Washington, DC: National Academy Press.

National Steering Committee. (1999). *First Nations and Inuit Regional Health Survey.* St. Regis, Quebec: Author.

Ninan, P. T., McElroy, S. L., Kane, C. P., Knight, B. T., Casuto, L. S., Rose, S. E., et al. (2000). Placebo-controlled study of fluvoxamine in the treatment of patients with compulsive buying. *Journal of Clinical Psychopharmacology, 20*(3), 362–366.

Office of Public Health. (1999). *Trends in Indian health.* Rockville, MD: Indian Health Services.

Orford, J. (1985). *Excessive appetites: A psychological view of addictions.* New York: Wiley.

Oster, S., & Knapp, T. J. (1994, June 2). *Casino gambling by underage patrons: Two studies of a university student population.* Paper presented at the Ninth International Conference on Gambling and Risk-Taking, Las Vegas, NV.

Pasternak, A. V., & Fleming, M. F. (1999, November/December). Prevalence of gambling disorders in a primary care setting. *Archives of Family Medicine, 8,* 515–520.

Perry, S., Cooper, A. M., & Michels, R. (1987). The psychodynamic formulation: Its purpose, structure, and clinical application. *American Journal of Psychiatry, 144,* 543–550.

Phillips, D. P., Welty, W. R., & Smith, M. M. (1997). Elevated suicide levels associated with legalized gambling. *Suicide and Life-Threatening Behavior, 27*(4), 373–378.

Pickering, L. K., & Hogan, G. R. (1971). Voluntary water intoxication in a normal child. *Journal of Pediatrics, 78,* 316–318.

Polanyi, M. (1967). *The tacit dimension.* New York: Doubleday.

Poulin, C. (2000). Problem gambling among adolescent students in the Atlantic provinces of Canada. *Journal of Gambling Studies, 16*(1), 53–78.

Productivity Commission. (1999). *Australia's gambling industries: Final report* (No. 10). Canberra: AusInfo.

Quinn, J. P. (1891). *Fools of fortune.* Chicago: Anti-Gambling Association.

Radden, J. (1995). Recent criticism of psychiatric nosology: A review. *Philosophy, Psychiatry, and Psychology, 1*(3), 193–200.

Regier, D. A., Farmer, M. E., Rae, D. S., Locke, B. Z., Keith, S. J., Judd, L. L., et al. (1990). Comorbidity of mental disorders with alcohol and other drug abuse: Results from the Epidemiologic Catchment Area (ECA) Study. *Journal of the American Medical Association, 264*(19), 2511–2518.

Robins, L. N., Helzer, J. E., Ratcliff, K. S., & Seyfried, W. (1982). Validity of the Diagnostic Interview Schedule, version II: DSM-III diagnoses. *Psychological Medicine, 12,* 855–870.

Rose, I. N. (1986). *Gambling and the law* (1st ed.). Hollywood, CA: Gambling Times.

Rosecrance, J. (1985). Compulsive gambling and the medicalization of deviance. *Social Problems, 32,* 275–284.

Rosecrance, J. (1988). *Gambling without guilt: The legitimation of an American pastime*. Pacific Grove, CA: Books/Cole.

Rosenhan, D. L. (1973). On being sane in insane places. *Science, 179,* 250–258.

Ross, L. (1977). The intuitive psychologist and his shortcomings: Distortions in the attribution process. In L. Berkowitz (Ed.), *Advances in experimental social psychology* (Vol. 10, pp. 173–220). New York: Academic Press.

Rowntree, L. G. (1923). Water intoxication. *Archives of Internal Medicine, 32*(2), 157–174.

Rugle, L., & Melamed, L. (1993). Neuropsychological assessment of attention problems in pathological gamblers. *Journal of Nervous and Mental Disorders, 18*(2), 107–112.

Schon, D. A. (1983). *The reflective practitioner*. New York: Basic Books.

Sebastian, J. G. (1985). Homelessness: A state of vulnerability. *Family and Community Health, 8*(3), 11–24.

Shaffer, H. J. (1986a). Assessment of addictive disorders: The use of clinical reflection and hypotheses testing. *Psychiatric Clinics of North America, 9*(3), 385–398.

Shaffer, H. J. (1986b). Conceptual crises and the addictions: A philosophy of science perspective. *Journal of Substance Abuse Treatment, 3,* 285–296.

Shaffer, H. J. (1987). The epistemology of "addictive disease": The Lincoln–Douglas debate. *Journal of Substance Abuse Treatment, 4*(2), 103–113.

Shaffer, H. J. (1991). Toward an epistemology of "addictive disease." *Behavioral Sciences and the Law, 9*(3), 269–286.

Shaffer, H. J. (1994). Denial, ambivalence and countertransference hate. In J. D. Levin & R. Weiss (Eds.), *Alcoholism: Dynamics and treatment* (pp. 421–437). Northdale, NJ: Aronson.

Shaffer, H. J. (1996). Understanding the means and objects of addiction: Technology, the Internet, and gambling. *Journal of Gambling Studies, 12*(4), 461–469.

Shaffer, H. J. (1997a). The most important unresolved issue in the addictions: Conceptual chaos. *Substance Use and Misuse, 32*(11), 1573–1580.

Shaffer, H. J. (1997b). The psychology of stage change. In J. H. Lowinson, P. Ruiz, R. B. Millman, & J. G. Langrod (Eds.), *Substance abuse: A comprehensive textbook* (3rd ed., pp. 100–106). Baltimore: Williams & Wilkins.

Shaffer, H. J. (1999a). On the nature and meaning of addiction. *National Forum, 79*(4), 10–14.

Shaffer, H. J. (1999b). Strange bedfellows: A critical view of pathological gambling and addiction. *Addiction, 94*(10), 1445–1448.

Shaffer, H. J., Freed, C. R., & Healea, D. (2002). Gambling disorders among homeless persons with substance use disorders seeking treatment at a community center. *Psychiatric Services, 55*(9), 1112–1117.

Shaffer, H. J., & Gambino, B. (1979). Addiction paradigms II: Theory, research, and practice. *Journal of Psychedelic Drugs, 11,* 299–304.

Shaffer, H. J., & Hall, M. N. (1996). Estimating the prevalence of adolescent gambling disorders: A quantitative synthesis and guide toward standard gambling nomenclature. *Journal of Gambling Studies, 12*(2), 193–214.

Shaffer, H. J., & Hall, M. N. (2001). Updating and refining meta-analytic prevalence estimates of disordered gambling behavior in the United States and Canada. *Canadian Journal of Public Health, 92*(3), 168–172.

Shaffer, H. J., & Hall, M. N. (2002). The natural history of gambling and drinking problems among casino employees. *Journal of Social Psychology, 142*(4), 405–424.

Shaffer, H. J., Hall, M. N., & Vander Bilt, J. (1999). Estimating the prevalence of disordered gambling behavior in the United States and Canada: A research synthesis. *American Journal of Public Health, 89,* 1369–1376.

Shaffer, H. J., & Korn, D. A. (2002). Gambling and related mental disorders: A public health analysis. In J. E. Fielding, R. C. Brownson, & B. Starfield (Eds.), *Annual Review of Public Health* (Vol. 23, pp. 171–212). Palo Alto: Annual Reviews.

Shaffer, H. J., LaBrie, R., & LaPlante, D. (2003). Laying the foundation for quantifying regional exposure to social phenomena: Considering the case of legalized gambling as a public health toxin. *Psychology of Addictive Behaviors, 18*(1), 40–48.

Shaffer, H. J., LaBrie, R. A., LaPlante, D. A., Nelson, S. E., & Stanton, M. V. (2004). The road less traveled: Moving from distribution to determinants in the study of gambling epidemiology. *Canadian Journal of Psychiatry, 49*(8), 504–516.

Shaffer, H. J., LaBrie, R., Scanlan, K. M., & Cummings, T. N. (1994). Pathological gambling among adolescents: Massachusetts Gambling Screen (MAGS). *Journal of Gambling Studies, 10*(4), 339–362.

Shaffer, H. J., & Robbins, M. (1991). Manufacturing multiple meanings of addiction: Time-limited realities. *Contemporary Family Therapy, 13,* 387–404.

Shaffer, H. J., & Robbins, M. (1995). Psychotherapy for addictive behavior: A stage-change approach to meaning making. In A. M. Washton (Ed.), *Psychotherapy and substance abuse: A practitioner's handbook* (pp. 103–123). New York: Guilford Press.

Shaffer, H. J., & Simoneau, G. (2001). Reducing resistance and denial by exercising ambivalence during the treatment of addiction. *Journal of Substance Abuse Treatment, 20*(1), 99–105.

Shaffer, H. J., Stein, S., Gambino, B., & Cummings, T. N. (Eds.). (1989). *Compulsive gambling: Theory, research and practice.* Lexington, MA: Lexington Books.

Shaffer, H. J., Vander Bilt, J., & Hall, M. N. (1999). Gambling, drinking, smoking and other health risk activities among casino employees. *American Journal of Industrial Medicine, 36*(3), 365–378.

Shaffer, H. J., Walsh, J. S., Howard, C., Hall, M. N., & Wellington, C. (1995). *Science and substance abuse education: A needs assessment for curriculum design* (SEDAP Technical Report No. 082595-300). Boston: Division on Addictions, Harvard Medical School.

Single, E. (1995). Defining harm reduction. *Drug and Alcohol Review, 14,* 287–290.

Skinner, B. F. (1969). *Contingencies of reinforcement: A theoretical analysis.* Englewood Cliffs, NJ: Prentice-Hall.

Slutske, W. S., Eisen, S., True, W. R., Lyons, M. J., Goldberg, J., & Tsuang, M. (2000). Common genetic vulnerability for pathological gambling and alcohol dependence in men. *Archives of General Psychiatry, 57*(7), 666–673.

Slutske, W. S., Jackson, K. M., & Sher, K. J. (2003). The natural history of problem gambling from age 18 to 29. *Journal of Abnormal Psychology, 112*(2), 263–274.

Specker, S. M., Carlson, G. A., Christenson, G. A., & Marcotte, M. (1995). Impulse control disorders and attention deficit disorder in pathological gamblers. *Annals of Clinical Psychiatry, 7*(4), 175–179.

Sproston, K., Erens, B., & Orford, J. (2000). *Gambling behaviour in Britain: Results from the British Gambling Prevalence Survey*. London: National Centre for Social Research.

Steinberg, M. A. (1997). *Connecticut high school problem gambling surveys 1989 and 1996*. Guilford, CT: Connecticut Council on Problem Gambling.

Stinchfield, R., Nadav, C., Winters, K., & Latimer, W. (1997). Prevalence of gambling among Minnesota public school students in 1992 and 1995. *Journal of Gambling Studies, 13*(1), 25–48.

Szasz, T. (1987). *Insanity: The idea and its consequence*. New York: Wiley.

Szasz, T. (1991). Diagnoses are not diseases. *Lancet, 338*, 1574–1576.

Taber, J. I. (1987). Compulsive gambling: An examination of relevant models. *The Journal of Gambling Behavior, 3*, 219–223.

Taber, J. I., McCormick, R. A., Russo, A. M., Adkins, B. J., & Ramirez, I. F. (1987). Follow-up of pathological gamblers after treatment. *American Journal of Psychiatry, 144*, 757–761.

Teck-Hong, O. (1992). The behavioral characteristics and health conditions of drug abusers: Some implications for workers in drug addiction. *International Social Work, 35*(1), 7–17.

Thompson, S. C., Armstrong, W., & Thomas, C. (1998). Illusions of control, underestimations, and accuracy: A control heuristic explanation. *Psychological Bulletin, 123*(2), 143–161.

Transition Planning Associates. (1985). *A survey of pathological gamblers in the state of Ohio*. Philadelphia: Author.

Tucker, J. A., Donovan, D. M., & Marlatt, G. A. (Eds.). (1999). *Changing addictive behavior*. New York: Guilford Press.

U.S. General Accounting Office. (2000). *Impact of gambling: Economic effects more measurable than social effects* (Report to the Honorable Frank R. Wolf No. GGD-00–78). Washington, DC: Author.

Vagge, L. M. (1996). *The development of youth gambling* (Unpublished honors thesis). Cambridge, MA: Harvard–Radcliffe Colleges.

Vaillancourt, F. (1979). *A survey of American gambling attitudes and behavior* (Research report series, Survey Research Center, Institute for Social Research). Ann Arbor, MI: University of Michigan Press.

Vaillant, G. E. (1982). On defining alcoholism. *British Journal of Addiction, 77*, 143–144.

Volberg, R. A. (1993). *Gambling and problem gambling among adolescents in Washington state* (Report to the Washington State Lottery). Albany, NY: Gemini Research.

Volberg, R. A. (1996a). *Gambling and problem gambling in New York: A 10-year replication study, 1986 to 1996*. New York: New York Council on Problem Gambling.

Volberg, R. A. (1996b). Prevalence studies of problem gambling in the United States. *Journal of Gambling Studies, 12*(2), 111–128.

Volberg, R. A. (1997). *Gambling and problem gambling in Oregon*. Northampton, MA: Gemini Research.

Volberg, R. A., & Abbott, M. W. (1997). Gambling and problem gambling among indigenous peoples. *Substance Use and Misuse, 32*(11), 1525–1538.

Volberg, R. A., Abbott, M. W., Roennberg, S., & Munck, I. M. (2001). Prevalence and risks of pathological gambling in Sweden. *Acta Psychiatrica Scandinavica, 104*(4), 250–256.

Volberg, R. A., & Boles, J. (1995). *Gambling and problem gambling in Georgia* (Report to the Georgia Department of Human Resources). Roaring Spring, PA: Gemini Research.

Volberg, R. A., & Moore, W. L. (1999). *Gambling and problem gambling in Washington state: A replication study, 1992 to 1998* (Report to the Washington State Lottery). Northampton, MA: Gemini Research.

Walker, M. B., & Dickerson, M. G. (1996). The prevalence of problem and pathological gambling: A critical analysis. *Journal of Gambling Studies, 12*(2), 233–249.

Wallisch, L. S. (1993). *Gambling in Texas: 1992 Texas survey of adolescent gambling behavior.* Austin: Texas Commission on Alcohol and Drug Abuse.

Wallisch, L. S. (1996). *Gambling in Texas: 1992 Texas survey of adult and adolescent gambling behavior.* Austin: Texas Commission on Alcohol and Drug Abuse.

Wardman, D., el-Guebaly, N., & Hodgins, D. (2001). Problem and pathological gambling in North American Aboriginal populations: A review of the empirical literature. *Journal of Gambling Studies, 17*(2), 81–100.

WEFA Group, ICR Survey Research Group, Lesieur, H., & Thompson, W. (1997). *A study concerning the effects of legalized gambling on the citizens of the state of Connecticut.* State of Connecticut Department of Revenue Services, Division of Special Revenue, Newington, CT.

Weiner, I. B. (1975). *Principles of psychotherapy.* New York: Wiley.

Widiger, T. A., & Clark, L. A. (2000). Toward DSM-V and the classification of psychopathology. *Psychological Bulletin, 126*(6), 946–963.

Winters, K. C., Stinchfield, R., & Fulkerson, J. (1993). Patterns and characteristics of adolescent gambling. *Journal of Gambling Studies, 9*(4), 371–386.

Winters, K. C., Stinchfield, R. D., Botzet, A., & Slutske, W. S. (in press). Pathways of youth gambling problem severity. *Psychology of Addictive Behaviors.*

Winters, K. C., Stinchfield, R. D., & Kim, L. G. (1995). Monitoring adolescent gambling in Minnesota. *Journal of Gambling Studies, 11*(2), 165–183.

Wise, R. A. (1995). Addictive drugs and brain stimulation reward. *Annual Review of Neuroscience, 18,* 319–340.

Wong, I. L. K., & So, E. M. T. (2003). Prevalence estimates of problem and pathological gambling in Hong Kong. *American Journal of Psychiatry, 160*(7), 1353–1354.

World Health Organization. (1990). *Composite International Diagnostic Interview* (CIDI, version 1.0). Geneva: Author.

World Health Organization. (2001). *Composite International Diagnostic Interview.* Geneva: Author.

Wray, I., & Dickerson, M. (1981). Cessation of high frequency gambling and "withdrawal" symptoms. *British Journal of Addiction, 76,* 401–405.

Zane, N. W. S., & Huh-Kim, J. (1998). Addictive behaviors. In L. C. Lee & N. W. S. Zane (Eds.), *Handbook of Asian American psychology* (pp. 527–554). Thousand Oaks, CA: Sage.

Zimmerman, M. A., Meeland, T., & Krug, S. E. (1985). Measurement and structure of pathological gambling behavior. *Journal of Personality Assessment, 49,* 76–81.

Zinberg, N. E. (1974). *High states: A beginning study* (Drug Abuse Council Publication No. SS-3). Washington, DC: Drug Abuse Council.

Zinberg, N. E. (1975). Addiction and ego function. *Psychoanalytic Study of the Child,* *30,* 567–588.

Zinberg, N. E. (1984). *Drug, set, and setting: The basis for controlled intoxicant use.* New Haven, CT: Yale University Press.

Ziskin, J. (1970). *Coping with psychiatric and psychological testimony* (2nd ed.). Beverly Hills, CA: Law and Psychology Press.

Zitzow, D. (1996). Comparative study of problematic gambling behaviors between American Indian and non-Indian adolescents within and near a northern plains reservation. *American Indian and Alaskan Native Mental Health Research, 7*(2), 14–26.

CHAPTER 12

Assessment of Sexual Offenders

A Model for Integrating Dynamic Risk Assessment and Relapse Prevention Approaches

JENNIFER G. WHEELER
WILLIAM H. GEORGE
KARI A. STEPHENS

No area to which relapse prevention (RP) has been applied is as controversial as sexual offending. Recently, "priest abuse" revelations have unfolded in the media, detailing widespread patterns of pedophilic offenses committed and covered up by Catholic clergy for decades. The national climate for discourse about sexual offending, while remaining sensationalistic and prurient, has grown increasingly harsh. Incarceration is deemed the best societal response to sex offending. Public confidence in the ability of psychological treatments to prevent sex offender relapse seems at a nadir.

Further manifestation of coarsening public sentiment is evidenced by the growing list of states implementing "sexual predator" laws, legitimating postincarceration civil commitment of sex offenders. Furthermore, sex offenders are the only type of felon for which the public insists on "community notification." All 50 states have now adopted a version of "Megan's Law," requiring that convicted offenders enroll in a sex offender registry and that communities be notified upon an offender's release. In summary, the application of RP to the treatment of sexual offenders is laden with intense public concern and scrutiny.

Twenty years have elapsed since RP was first applied to sex offender treatment (Pithers, Marques, Gibat, & Marlatt, 1983). This transfer of theory and techniques from the addictions field was deemed promising and greeted with considerable enthusiasm. It provided a fresh way to conceptualize sex offender treatment, posttreatment recovery, and postincarceration adjustment. Since its introduction, RP has become the most widely used treatment for sexual offenders (Laws, Hudson, & Ward, 2000). As a result of this popularity, RP sex offender treatment has also been subject to considerable scrutiny and debate (e.g., Hanson, 2000; Laws, 1996, 1999a, 1999b, 2003; Thornton, 1997). Despite theory- and evidence-based criticisms (e.g., Hanson, 2000; Laws, 1995; Thornton, 1997; Ward & Hudson, 1996a; see Laws, 2003, for review), and revisions or reformulations (Hudson, Ward, & Marshall, 1992; Ward & Hudson, 1996b, 1998, 2000; Ward, Louden, Hudson, & Marshall, 1995; see Laws, 2003, for review), RP remains the most influential conceptual framework for sex offender treatment.

The overarching goal of this chapter and Chapter 11 in the second edition of *Relapse Prevention* (Wheeler, George, & Stoner, 2005) is to describe an enhancement to the RP model for sex offender treatment that will "update" the model with some recent and important developments in the field. One key development is the emergence of "risk assessment" as a dominant conceptual framework for managing sex offenders in correctional, treatment, and community settings. Another important development has been the migration of other cognitive-behavioral techniques into sex offender treatment. For instance, the skills training "modules" of dialectical behavior therapy (Linehan, 1993) have received attention for their potential application to sexual offending (e.g., Hover, 1999; Hover & Packard, 1998, 1999; Quigley, 2000; Shingler, 2004). In the context of these two developments, we propose an approach called recidivism risk reduction therapy (3RT) that integrates the problem/need-targeting advantages of the risk assessment paradigm with the skills training/treatment module advantages of RP and other cognitive-behavioral strategies. We believe that this integration of risk assessment with strategically applied treatment modules offers an updated approach and an enhanced model of RP for sexual offenders.

In the present chapter, we review extant methods for identifying important elements of the sexual offense cycle and approaches for assessing sex offenders' risk factors for recidivism. First, we provide an overview of the application of RP to sexual offenders, including the challenges of using RP terminology to describe the offense cycle. Second, we describe more recent developments in sex offender risk assessment and distinguish forensic and therapeutic assessments of sexual offenders. Finally, we provide suggestions and recommendations for assessing "dynamic risk factors" in the context of planning and providing sex offender treatment.

Elsewhere, Wheeler, George, and Stoner (2005) describe the theoretical underpinnings of the 3RT model, discuss how dynamic risk factors can be conceptualized as skills deficits, and provide specific techniques for targeting dynamic risk factors in sex offender treatment. This chapter and Chapter 11 of the second edition of *Relapse Prevention* (Marlatt & Donovan, 2005) attempt to demonstrate how our proposed 3RT model might enhance the RP model by more effectively evaluating and targeting dynamic risk factors associated with sexual offense recidivism.

THE APPLICATION OF RELAPSE PREVENTION TO SEXUAL OFFENDING

Parallels between sexual offending and addiction are easily drawn. Both are associated with high costs for individuals and society. Both provide immediate short-term gratification but cause long-term negative consequences. Furthermore, both are often associated with impulsiveness, compulsiveness, secrecy, and/or denial. Because of these similarities, some writers have advocated a sex addiction model necessitating a disease-oriented 12-step approach to treatment (Carnes, 2001; Tays, Earle, Wells, Murray, & Garrett, 1999). However, this approach may have potentially more downsides than benefits (George & Marlatt, 1989). In our judgment, the key similarity between sexual offending and addiction lies in the persistence of relapse.

Although RP was adapted from the addictions field, the rationale for its application to sex offenders is not based on the idea that sexual offending is an "addiction." Instead, the rationale for this application is based on the shared problem of maintaining successful abstinence following treatment. And, as with addiction, successful cessation of sexual offending (that was achieved as a consequence of adjudication, incarceration, supervision, and/or treatment) is often followed by the sexual offenders' subsequent failure to maintain their "abstinence" successfully. It is this struggle to maintain the success of treatment (i.e., to remain successfully abstinent from the problem behavior) that makes RP relevant to the treatment of sexual offenders. And as with addiction, the desired outcome of sexual offender treatment goes beyond the point of stopping the problematic behavior in the present, by teaching skills and techniques for preventing the problem behavior from recurring in the future.

Identifying the "Relapse Cycle" of Sexual Offenders

The goal of RP is to prevent the offender from committing another sexual offense. Thus, the offending behavior is conceptualized as a harmful behavior that supplants and/or supersedes healthier ways of coping with distress and/or responding to sexual urges. For any given offender, the offending behavior is understood to follow an ideographic progression of thoughts, feelings, and behaviors; this is typically referred to as his relapse cycle. Accordingly, an early objective of treatment is to assess the offender's individualized relapse cycle; that is, the unique stream of cognitive, behavioral, and environmental events that have previously been associated with his offending behavior and therefore are likely to be associated with future offenses.

The relapse cycle is understood to embody interlocking RP constructs that facilitate a relapse—in this case, the commission of a new offense. Similar to the original RP model, these constructs include observable and unobservable factors.

Observable Factors in the Relapse Cycle

1. *Chronic lifestyle imbalances and/or acute triggering events.* These phenomena activate the "chain" of maladaptive thoughts and behaviors preceding a sexual offense (e.g., employment instability; conflict with an intimate partner).

2. *Seemingly unimportant decision (SUD).* Such decisions made by the offender create or support an environment conducive to committing a sexual offense (e.g., ruminating about a negative interaction with his partner; putting himself in a place where he has access to a potential victim).

3. *Lapse.* The "lapse" has been defined for sexual offending as "offense precursor activities" (e.g., Laws, 2003), such as using pornography,[1] indulging deviant masturbatory fantasies, or cruising for potential victims.

4. *High-risk situations (HRSs).* In these situations are requisite factors, both internal and external, that have been historically associated with the offender's decision to commit a sexual offense (e.g., feeling sexually aroused; being alone with a potential victim).

5. *Relapse.* For sexual offending, the "relapse" has been defined as the occurrence of a new sexual offense.

Unobservable Factors in the Relapse Cycle

In addition to these "observable" events in the offense cycle, the progression from a lapse to a relapse may be mitigated by internal events (i.e., cognitive and/or affective), including the abstinence violation effect (AVE) and the problem of immediate gratification (PIG).

1. *The abstinence violation effect.* The AVE is a cognitive and affective event that is hypothesized to occur following a lapse. Simply put, the AVE refers to an individual's recognition that he or she has broken a self-imposed rule: By engaging in a single act of prohibited behavior, his or her commitment to abstinence has been violated.[2] According to the RP model, an individual's response to this violation can determine whether the lapse turns into a full-blown relapse (Marlatt & George, 1984; Marlatt & Gordon, 1985), and therefore plays a critical role in the relapse cycle.

2. *The problem of immediate gratification.* The PIG refers to the process of attending only to the positive aspects of a prohibited behavior, while ignoring the negative consequences. The PIG can occur before or after a lapse; therefore it can increase the risk of a high-risk situation leading to a lapse, in addition to increasing the risk of a lapse becoming a full-blown relapse (see Marlatt, 1989).

The Identification of Relapse Prevention Constructs in a Sexual Offense Cycle: A Hypothetical Example

Joe Offender[3] had a fight with his girlfriend, Lucy, who stormed out of the house. Joe continued thinking about their fight (e.g., "Who is she to treat me like that?" and "I deserve a break from all of her sh**"). He soon left the house to seek out his friends at the local tavern, where he spent several hours drinking and exchanging negative stories about wives and girlfriends. After returning home from the tavern, Joe learned that Lucy was not due home for a few hours, leaving him home alone with her 12-year-old daughter, Tina. Intoxicated, he went to Tina's room to see if she needed help with her homework. Joe found Tina lying on her bed in a t-shirt and underwear, and he found himself becoming sexually aroused. He entered Tina's room, sat next to her on the bed, and said he needed to talk with her about something important. He proceeded to tell her about the fight he had had earlier with Lucy, including details about his and Lucy's sexual relationship. Joe told Tina how sad and lonely he felt, and suggested that a hug would make him feel better. During the hug, Joe told Tina how much he cared about her, what a pretty girl she was, and how good it felt to hug her. He then touched her genitals.

In this example, several RP constructs are easily identified. Specifically, from an RP perspective, Joe's conflict with Lucy would be conceptualized as a triggering event that led to self-indulgent thoughts and actions. His efforts at self-soothing (i.e., drinking and "commiserating" with his friends) led to further cognitive distortions about his partner (if not women in general), fueling his subjective perception of an imbalanced lifestyle and his associated sense of entitlement. These distortions and justifications would be conceptualized a cognitive antecedents that support Joe's "internal environment" for sexual reoffending. Later, Joe's decision to "check in on" Tina would be conceptualized as an SUD that helped create an "external environment" for reoffending (e.g., identifying and isolating himself with a potential victim). When Joe found himself sexually aroused by Tina, he accelerated this HRS by entering her room and sitting down with her. He proceeded to set up his victim for reoffending by grooming verbally (by talking about his sexual relationship), emotionally (by portraying himself as rejected by Lucy but consoled by Tina), and physically (by requesting a hug). Finally, Joe's progression from hugging to fondling might be conceptualized as a function of the PIG, since it is likely that Joe focused only on the positive aspects of sexual contact with Tina, ignoring the negative aspects of this behavior.

Once the cognitive, behavioral, and other environmental factors have been identified and defined in the context of an offense "cycle," points for intervention are easily identified and techniques can be implemented to help the offender learn how to interrupt this pattern and prevent future reoffenses. In the this example, Joe might learn alternative responses to going to the tavern when he is feeling angry or skills to manage more effectively his deviant sexual arousal (see Wheeler et al., 2005, for more specific information regarding treatment interventions).

Limitations of Applying Relapse Prevention Terminology to Sexual Offending

Despite the apparent utility of defining these events in terms of a "relapse cycle," it is important to note that some elements of the relapse cycle are not as clearly defined in the RP model for sexual offenders. This is due to the fact that the original RP model was modified for its application to the treatment of sexual offenders, and these modifications resulted in challenges to defining the relapse cycle in this population. In the following section, we summarize the modifications and the subsequent limitations they have presented with regard to understanding the sexual offense cycle.

Lapse and Relapse

In the vignette, which behavior(s), if any, should be regarded as a "lapse" and which behavior(s), if any, should be regarded as a "relapse"? The definitions of the terms "lapse" and "relapse" have proved problematic for applying RP to sex offending (Pithers et al., 1983; George & Marlatt, 1989). In the original RP model, the term "relapse" is usually defined as a return to pretreatment rates of the target behavior, and the term "lapse" is defined as a single recurrence of the problem behavior. These definitions, and the relationship between the two, are at the heart of any RP application. Thus, the specific objectives of RP techniques are to prevent a lapse from occurring and, if a lapse does occur, to prevent it from escalating into a relapse.

Unlike most other RP applications, the traditional RP definition of lapse for sexual offenders involves serious victimization of another person. To reflect the philosophy that even a single act of sexual victimization is unacceptable, the definitions of "lapse" and "relapse" were arbitrarily shifted to encompass behaviors that occur earlier in the cycle. "Relapse" was redefined as any new sexual offense, while "lapse" was redefined as "any occurrence of willful and elaborate fantasizing about sexual offending or any return to sources of stimulation associated with the offense pattern, but short of the performance of the offense behavior" (George & Marlatt, 1989, p. 6). This redefinition of the "lapse" necessarily designates it as a preoffense behavior, which could include fleeting thoughts and dreams, fantasizing about offending, acquiring offense-related pornography, masturbating to offense fantasies, cruising for a potential victim, selecting the victim, grooming a victim, and setting up the assault—any offense-related behavior that precedes the sexual offense itself. However, there is evidence to suggest that this semantic redesignation of these terms is not consistent with the phenomenological experiences of the offenders themselves, and that offenders naturalistically regard offense behavior (rather than preoffense behavior) as a "lapse" (Ward,

Hudson, & Marshall, 1994; Wheeler, 2003). Such evidence supports the use of ideographic assessments to evaluate each offender's pattern of offending and his subjective regard for each of the events in his cycle, and to resist presumptions or expectations that all offenders regard the same preoffense behaviors similarly.

The Abstinence Violation Effect

An important cognitive–emotional event in the relapse cycle, the AVE, is hypothesized to occur following a lapse. But in the modified relapse model for sexual offenders, it is less clear at which point the AVE is reputed to occur. A semantically consistent position would suggest that the AVE should occur following what has been defined as the "lapse" (e.g., a willful, deviant sexual fantasy; Pithers, 1990; Pithers, Kashima, Cumming, Beal, & Buell, 1988), and would influence the progression of this "lapse" to a "relapse" (the sex offense; Pithers, 1990; Ward & Hudson, 1996a). In contrast, a theoretically consistent position would suggest that the AVE should occur following a violation of a commitment to abstinence from the prohibited behavior (a sex offense) and would influence the progression of this violation to the pretreatment pattern of behavior (repeated sexual offending).

As described in the most recent conceptualizations of RP for sexual offenders, the AVE is hypothesized to occur following both a lapse (e.g., a willful deviant sexual fantasy; Pithers, 1990; Stoner & George, 2000; Ward & Hudson, 1998) and a relapse (a sexual offense; Stoner & George, 2000; Ward & Hudson, 1998, 2000). Central to the hypothesis that the AVE can occur following a lapse (e.g., a willful deviant sexual fantasy) is the assumption that the offender has made a commitment to abstain from not only the prohibited behavior (sexual offending), but also the redefined lapse behavior (e.g., willful deviant sexual fantasies). However, to date, there is little empirical support for such an assumption, whereas there is some empirical evidence to suggest that sexual offenders' experience of the AVE is more theoretically consistent with the original RP model (i.e., it follows sexual offending, and not preoffense fantasies or behaviors), rather than semantically consistent with the RP model as it was redefined (Ward et al., 1994; Wheeler, 2003). Such evidence further supports the use of ideographic assessments to evaluate each offender's pattern of offending and his affective and attributional responses to each of the events in his cycle, and to resist presumptions or expectations that any particular behavior should elicit an AVE response in all sexual offenders.

An additional consideration for the application of the AVE to sex offenders is the implicit assumption that the offender experiences a genuine motivation to refrain from offending. This assumption may or may not be true for some offenders, particularly when they have entered treatment only because they were caught for their crimes. Additional assessment and research may be needed to appreciate the relevance of offenders' commitment to abstinence and readiness to change. Issues such as therapeutic alliance and readiness to change are receiving increased attention in recent literature (see Derrickson, 2000; Sarran, Fernandez, & Marshall, 2003; Tierney & McCabe, 2002, 2004). For example, it has been suggested that sex offender treatment might be benefit from the initial assessment of each offender's readiness to change (e.g., McConnaughty, Prochaska, & Velicer, 1983; Miller & Tonigan, 1996; Rollnick, Heather, Gold, & Hall, 1992; see Prochaska & DiClemente, 1984; 1992; Prochaska, DiClemente, & Norcross, 1992) and—if readiness is low— the subsequent implementation of motivational interviewing techniques (Miller & Rollnick, 1991) to enhance the efficacy of RP treatment for sexual offenders (Dandsescu & Christopher, 2003).

The Problem of Immediate Gratification

Another problematic aspect of the applying the original RP model to sexual offenders is the conflict between the problem of immediate gratification (PIG) that is inherent to sexual fantasizing/arousal, and the negative affective response that is putatively associated with the AVE (see Hudson et al., 1992; Ward, Hudson, & Siegert, 1995; Ward & Hudson, 1996a). There is some evidence to suggest that for sexual offenders, the progression from lapse to relapse may be more influenced by the PIG than by other factors (Wheeler, 2003). Accordingly, the assessment of the potential role of the PIG (e.g., considering positive outcome expectancies) may need to assume a more important role in RP for sexual offenders.

High-Risk Situations and Covert Antecedents

As with other RP applications, an important objective for sexual offenders is to identify the triggers in their external and internal environments that facilitate their progression through relapse "cycle." These triggers include high-risk situations (HRSs), which refer to the circumstances that acutely threaten the offender's sense of control over offending. These HRSs include both interpersonal circumstances (e.g., being confronted with individuals who resemble former victims) and intrapersonal states (e.g., feeling lonely, depressed, angry, or bored). Once an offender is aware of his idiographic HRS profile, he is taught to strategically avoid HRSs and/or to develop skills that help him cope with such situations and thereby reduce the risk these situations otherwise present.

Covert antecedents are represented not by acute discrete situations but by chronic processes—specifically, processes associated with experiencing life as high in stressful demands and low in gratifications. This chronic imbalance between "wants" and "shoulds" can spawn unacknowledged urges for gratification and eventually manifest itself as SUDs that lead the offender toward HRSs. Therefore, another goal embedded in RP sex offender treatment is to identify lifestyle imbalance and promote a healthier lifestyle, in which obligatory stressors are balanced against or offset by safe, nonproblematic indulgences. Attaining a healthier "want–should" equilibrium can halt the progression through the relapse cycle from a chronic sense of deprivation, leading to urges and cravings, followed by SUDS that deliver the offender to a HRS, that would ultimately culminate in lapse and relapse.

Summary of Relapse Prevention for Sexual Offenders

In the last two decades, RP has become the most popular and perhaps most effective approach to the treatment of sexual offenders (e.g., Hanson et al., 2002; Marques, Day, Nelson, & West, 1994; Laws et al., 2000; Knopp, Freeman-Longo, & Stevenson, 1992). The sex offender RP application has also undergone important criticism (Ward & Hudson, 1996a, 1996b; Ward, Hudson, et al., 1995; Wheeler, 2003; Wheeler, George, & Marlatt, in press). One concern is the necessary but perhaps confusing semantic redesignation of the terms "lapse" and "relapse," and the questions that this raises about the role of the AVE in facilitating the progression of a lapse to a relapse. Another concern is whether the PIG is being adequately emphasized in current RP format given the relative weighting of pleasurable experiences that may be associated with sexual offending (e.g., arousal, orgasm) over the negative lapse reactions emphasized by the theoretical underpinnings of the AVE.

In addition to problems applying RP terminology to sexual offending, another major criticism of the RP model is that, unlike its predecessor in the addictions field, RP for sex offenders has assumed the role of the primary treatment modality rather than an adjunct to successful treatment. Although RP may be useful for identifying problematic thoughts, behaviors and possible points of intervention, it was not intended to be the primary approach to change those aspects of an offender's lifestyle that result in his sexual offense cycle (i.e., maladaptive coping skills, self-regulation deficits, problematic thinking styles, and/or ineffective interpersonal skills). Nor was RP developed for application to individuals whose "commitment" to abstaining from harmful behavior has been artificially imposed (i.e., by incarceration and/or supervision). For these reasons, RP has been criticized as a necessary but insufficient approach to the treatment of sexual offenders (e.g., Laws, 2003; Ward & Hudson, 2000).

RECENT DEVELOPMENTS IN SEX OFFENSE RESEARCH: RISK ASSESSMENT

In addition to the previously described limitations of the RP model for sex offenders, another limitation of RP for sex offenders is that the model was originally developed and applied to sexual offenders, without the benefit of our current knowledge about risk factors for sexual offense recidivism. Risk assessment is a fast-growing area in the criminal justice system and forensic mental health settings. For sexual offenders, their evaluators, and treatment providers, risk assessment has assumed a particularly important role, because these types of assessments are being used to guide critical decisions involving sentencing, civil commitment, conditional release, family reunification, community tracking, and treatment eligibility. Data indicate that not all sexual offenders are equally at risk to commit a sexual reoffense; sexual offense recidivism rates typically range between 10 and 15% for most offenders over a 5-year follow-up period (Hanson & Bussiere, 1998). However, there appear to be some subgroups of sexual offenders that reoffend at much higher rates (see Harris et al., 2003), underscoring the importance of conducting ideographic assessments of each offender's risk to reoffend.

Actuarial Risk Assessment

For many years, clinicians relied primarily on their own judgments to make decisions about an offender's likelihood to reoffend. Because this method was demonstrated to be subjective, unreliable, and ineffective (see Hanson & Bussiere, 1998), the exclusive use of clinical judgment in risk assessment is no longer regarded as empirically defensible (Bonta, 2002). More recently, a growing body of evidence has provided increased support for the use of actuarial risk assessments to guide forensic decision making. Specifically, certain demographic and historical factors—such as age, marital status, and history of juvenile delinquency—have been reliably associated with an increased risk to reoffend (see Hanson & Bussiere, 1998; Hanson & Morton-Bourgon, 2004; Hanson & Thornton, 2000; Harris et al., 2003, for review). Accordingly, risk assessment instruments have been developed that vary in terms of the population to which they can be validly applied (e.g., sexual vs. "general" criminal offenders), the problem behavior they address (e.g., sexual vs. nonsexual offenses), and the types of actuarial data they consider (e.g., static vs. dynamic factors). If utilized appropriately, such instruments can significantly improve the clinician's ability to distinguish offenders at high versus low recidivism risk (Hanson, 1998; Hanson & Bussiere, 1998) and have demonstrated moderate to large effects in improving the clinician's predictive accuracy (see Hanson & Morton-Bourgon, 2004, for a recent meta-analytic review).

Static and Dynamic Risk Factors

Risk assessment instruments may consider two types of actuarial data: static and dynamic risk factors. *Static risk factors* are aspects of an offender's history that are permanent, or "fixed" (e.g., childhood maladjustment, prior offenses), and are therefore not amenable to change. For example, some factors that have been identified as being associated with increased risk of sexual reoffending include an offender's age (less than 25 years old), any prior nonsexual violence conviction, any unrelated victims, any stranger victims; or any male victims. These factors are typically associated with a more deviant developmental trajectory, and indicate a more diversified and chronic propensity to engage in criminal behavior. However, given that these factors are not amenable to change, their assessment is not directly relevant for the purposes of developing an ideographic treatment plan but may be required for other aspects of offender management, such as for allocating resources according to risk level or for conducting forensic evaluations (see Heilbrun, 2003, for further discussion on the difference between forensic and therapeutic assessment of sex offenders).

Unlike static risk factors, *dynamic risk factors* are aspects of an offender's behavior or environment that may be associated with increased likelihood to reoffend but are potentially subject to change (e.g., substance use, antisocial attitudes). A variable is identified as a dynamic risk factor if any change in this variable is associated with an increase or decrease in recidivism risk. Dynamic risk factors can be further classified as either stable or acute. *Stable risk factors* have the potential for change but usually endure for months or even years (e.g., alcohol dependence). Accordingly, if a stable dynamic factor can be reduced or eliminated, this may affect longer term change in an individual's reoffense risk. *Acute risk factors* have rapidly changing states occurring across the course of a few days, or even hours or minutes (e.g., intoxication). These factors may be an indicator that a reoffense is likely to occur, but they are less useful than static or stable dynamic factors for evaluating an individual's risk to reoffend over a longer period of time.

With regard to sexual offenders, dynamic risk factors for sexual offense recidivism appear to be associated with one of two broad categories: maladaptive sexual behavior and an antisocial orientation (Hanson & Morton-Bourgon, 2004; Hanson & Bussiere, 1998; Hanson & Harris, 2001; Hanson & Harris, 2000a; Hudson, Wales, Bakker, & Ward, 2002; Quinsey, Lalumiere, Rice, & Harris, 1995; Roberts, Doren, & Thornton, 2002). For example, a recent meta-analysis found that certain measures of sexual deviancy (e.g., sexual interests and preferences, sexual preoccupations) and/or an antisocial orientation (e.g., antisocial personality and/or traits, general self-regulation problems, hostility, substance abuse, rule violations) significantly predicted sexual offense recidivism (Hanson & Morton-Bourgon, 2004; Hanson & Harris, 2000a). Other significant dynamic risk factors in this analysis included intimacy deficits (e.g., emotional identification with children, conflicts in an intimate relationship) and attitudes tolerant of sexual offending (Hanson & Morton-Bourgon, 2004). Although research on dynamic factors is an ongoing process, these preliminary findings provide a basic framework for integrating dynamic risk factors into extant approaches to sex offender treatment.

INCORPORATING RISK ASSESSMENT
INTO SEX OFFENDER TREATMENT:
RECIDIVISM RISK REDUCTION THERAPY

Although RP was designed to reduce problem behavior by prescribing idiographic assessment and skills training practices, current RP applications with sex offenders only indirectly emphasize the identification and targeting of dynamic risk factors. Furthermore, there is evidence to suggest that in its current form, RP for sexual offenders could benefit from further refinements and modifications to address the specific needs of sex offenders more effectively (Laws, 2003; Ward et al., 1994; Stoner & George, 2000; Wheeler, 2003). Specifically, RP could be enhanced by integrating dynamic risk factors into the treatment paradigm and generally approaching sex offender treatment from a more risk-based perspective (Andrews, 1989).[4] Therefore, we propose an enhanced treatment model that is grounded in the RP approach but incorporates an emphasis on directly identifying offenders' dynamic risk factors and targeting these in treatment.

With these considerations in mind, we propose that sex offender treatment providers and programs (henceforth referred to as SOTPs) adopt a new risk-based, primary approach to the assessment and treatment of sexual offenders that we refer to as *Recidivism Risk Reduction Therapy* (3RT). This 3RT approach is not a specific "fixed" treatment model. Instead, 3RT can include a variety of group-format approaches, and draw upon extant assessment and treatment techniques to target dynamic risk factors in conjunction with RP treatment. In RP groups, offenders will have the opportunity to practice new 3RT skills, while specifically addressing the risk areas associated with their sexual offense cycle (Please refer to the second edition of *Relapse Prevention* [Marlatt & Donovan, 2005]). Consistent with the recommendation that treatment plans should be based on ideographic rather than prototypical treatment plans (e.g., Heilbrun, Nezu, Keeney, Chung, & Wasserman, 1998), 3RT treatment plans would be developed based on an assessment of each individual offender's risk-based treatment needs.

An important question to address is how 3RT and RP might coexist with one another. One way of considering how the 3RT approach would be integrated with extant RP treatment approaches is to consider "stable" versus "acute" dynamic risk factors for recidivism (Hanson & Harris, 2001). The goal of 3RT is to reduce maladaptive thoughts and behaviors associated with risk to sexually reoffend and to replace these with more adaptive skills and behaviors. Thus, 3RT might be conceptualized as a treatment for "stable" dynamic risk factors, with a goal of facilitating longer term changes in offenders' behavior. RP techniques, on the other hand, give primary consideration to the offender's thoughts and behaviors in the days, hours, or even minutes preceding a sexual offense. Thus, RP might be conceptualized as a treatment approach to managing the offender's "acute" dynamic risk factors. A comprehensive dynamic risk assessment protocol would provide data relevant to both 3RT and RP treatment planning and delivery, and behavioral observations made during both 3RT and RP treatment would provide valuable information for monitoring the progress of both stable and acute risk–needs areas.

Assessing Dynamic Risk Factors in the Context of Treatment Planning and Delivery

As described in the previous section, our understanding of sex offender recidivism and risk factors for reoffending has been enhanced considerably in the last decade as a result of improvements to risk assessment technology and recidivism research methodology. The predominant theme that has emerged from this research is that sexual offense recidivism is associated with two broad categories of dynamic risk factors: sexual deviance and an antisocial orientation. In 3RT, these two broad categories of dynamic risk are the foundation for developing treatment groups designed to target specific risk–needs. Depending on the particular risk–needs, a particular offender would be assigned to a treatment group designed to target those risk–need areas (Wheeler et al., 2005).

Therefore, the first step in 3RT is to conduct an ideographic assessment of each offender's dynamic risk needs. This assessment might be conducted in the context of an "intake" evaluation, in which historical, observational, and other assessment data (e.g., psychological testing) are gathered for the purposes of developing a treatment plan. It is likely that much of the information that is typically gathered in SOTP intake and/or treatment progress assessment would provide much of the required data regarding offenders' dynamic risk–needs. However, in some cases, additional assessment approaches may be needed.

In the following sections, we draw attention to assessment techniques that may be useful in evaluating the presence–absence of those risk factors most recently reported as significant predictors of sexual offense recidivism (Hanson & Morton-Bourgon, 2004).[5] When possible, we have included assessment techniques from multiple approaches, including (1) psychological tests or other objective measures; (2) structured interviews (e.g., Hanson & Harris, 2000b, 2001, 2002); (3) collateral sources (e.g., file review; prior evaluations); and (4) behavioral observations of offenders' risk–needs (e.g., behavior in group; institutional infractions). This is not meant to be an exhaustive or an exclusive list of dynamic risk factors or approaches to assessment; nor is it our intention to endorse specifically a particular assessment and/or its psychometric properties as the "gold standard" of measuring a particular risk item. Rather, we have provided these suggestions simply to illustrate how extant psychological assessments, structured interviews, and other data-gathering techniques might be applied to identify sex offenders' dynamic risk factors in the context of providing treatment.

The reader is reminded that the very process of identifying dynamic risk factors for recidivism is, in and of itself, a dynamic process; that is, the empirical analysis of dynamic risk factors and their relationship to sexual offense recidivism is ongoing (e.g., Beech, Fisher, & Beckett, 1999; Hudson et al., 2002; Hanson & Harris, 2000a, 2002; Hanson & Morton-Bourgon, 2004; Thornton, 2002). Although some empirical themes have remained relatively consistent, other risk factors have emerged as more or less significant in various reports (e.g., Hanson & Harris, 1998, 2000a, 2002; Hanson & Morton-Bourgon, 2004). Therefore, the 3RT model was developed to be a flexible, modular approach that can be easily modified and adapted as new research becomes available. Similarly, we have suggested multiple approaches to assessment, in consideration of the fact that some techniques may be more useful at treatment intake and/or termination (e.g., psychological testing, structured interviews), while others may be more useful for ongoing monitoring of treatment progress (e.g., behavioral observations, brief screening measures).[6] Finally, we have limited the scope of this chapter to the assessment of sexual offenders for therapeutic purposes (i.e., treatment planning and delivery) and are not referring to forensic evaluations (i.e., to provide an opinion to a third party regarding risk to reoffend or civil commitment; see Heilbrun, 2003, for further discussion of the difference between forensic and therapeutic assessment of sex offenders).

Antisocial Risk Needs

Although sex offenders are regarded as special subpopulation of criminals, research indicates that they have many of the same "criminogenic needs" (see Andrews & Bonta, 2003) as offenders in the general criminal population. Furthermore, when a sex offender does reoffend, he is more likely to commit a nonsexual offense than a sexual offense. Thus, dynamic factors associated with the development and maintenance of an unstable, antisocial lifestyle are important treatment needs for sexual offenders. This problem area reflects a generally unstable life that facilitates and indulges the use of the deception, manipulation, and secrecy; fosters resentment of others, and a sense of entitlement and self-indulgence; supports noncompliance with rules and authority; and provides opportunities and reinforcement for behavioral disinhibition. Although not unique to sex offenders, some or all of these factors may be necessary preconditions to the perpetration of a sexual offense. Conversely, the development of a stable lifestyle that supports individual responsibility and accountability, prosocial attitudes and relationships, and compliance with rules and structure could serve to curtail such antisocial behaviors, attitudes, and relationships.

For the purposes of this chapter, the dynamic risk factors associated with the development and maintenance of an imbalanced, non-"mainstream," defiant, or otherwise antisocial lifestyle, are collectively referred to as the sex offender's antisocial risk–needs, and offenders who endorse risk–needs in this area would be assigned to a 3RT—Antisocial Risk–Needs Group (or 3RT-A) to target those problem areas. The goal of 3RT-A is to help offenders' identify their antisocial risk needs; monitor and self-regulate antisocial thoughts, behaviors, and relationships; and develop alternative approaches to functioning more effectively in a prosocial environment (please refer to Wheeler et al., 2005, for a more detailed description of 3RT-A treatment goals).

MALADAPTIVE SOCIAL FUNCTIONING/ANTISOCIAL TRAITS

Research suggests that offenders who have antisocial personality traits (including attitudes and behaviors), who lack prosocial peers, and/or who lead generally unstable, irresponsible, and chaotic lifestyles are more likely to sexually recidivate than offenders who do not have antisocial personality traits (Hanson & Harris, 2000a; Hanson & Morton-Bourgon, 2004). "Antisocial" deficits reflect an overall tendency to get one's own needs met at the expense of others and/or failure to consider the harmful consequences of his behaviors, and are likely to impair one's ability to have prosocial relationships, engage in prosocial activities, and maintain a stable, "mainstream," lifestyle.

With regard to conducting an assessment of antisocial traits for the purposes of evaluating dynamic risk needs, the following might be considered:

- A structured interview of dynamic risk factors (e.g., the STABLE and ACUTE scoring guides, Hanson & Harris, 2002)
- Antisocial Features scale of the Personality Assessment Inventory (PAI; Morey, 1991)
- Item descriptions from the *Diagnostic and Statistical Manual of Mental Disorders, 4th Edition, Text Revision* (DSM-IV-TR; American Psychiatric Association, 2000)
- Item descriptors Level of Service Inventory—Revised (Andrews & Bonta, 1995)
- Item descriptions from the Hare Psychopathy Checklist—Revised (PCL-R; Hare, 1991)

It is likely that structured interview data (e.g., Hanson & Harris, 2002) and file reviews will yield much of the important data regarding these deficits. Specifically, collateral documents and interview data might include propensity for violence/aggression, a pattern of deceitfulness, reckless behaviors, antisocial peer influences and activities, employment/financial history, and criminal activity.

In addition to the assessment sources indicated earlier, behavioral observations of offenders' behavior in the treatment setting may provide useful data for assessing this risk area in an ongoing fashion (Hanson & Harris, 2002; Spizman, 2004). Observable examples of antisocial personality in the treatment setting might include deceitfulness (e.g., lying to the therapist or group members), impulsivity (e.g., angry outbursts in group; inability to conform to group norms; property destruction), irritability/aggressiveness (e.g., toward the therapist or group members), disregard for others (e.g., ignoring group decisions; monopolizing resources on the living unit; disrespectful/disparaging comments toward therapist or group members), irresponsibility (e.g., skipping/frequently late for group; failing to complete assignments), and/or lack of remorse (e.g., rationalizing his hurtful behaviors toward group members). These observational data may be useful not only to assess the presence of this risk area, but also to monitor behavioral change throughout treatment, as an indicator of treatment progress.

GENERAL SELF-REGULATION DEFICITS

A history of lifestyle instability may be associated with "nonprosocial" factors that are not necessarily "antisocial," but nonetheless preclude one's ability to function in a prosocial environment and associated with increased risk to sexually reoffend (Hanson & Harris, 2000a; Hanson & Morton-Bourgon, 2004). Examples would include cognitive impairments (e.g., learning deficits, developmental disabilities), negative emotionality (e.g., depression, anxiety, irritability), behavioral dyscontrol (e.g., aggressiveness, general impulsivity), delayed social development (e.g., financial/residential dependence on others), problem-solving deficits (e.g., deficits in planning, judgment, reasoning ability) or substance abuse disorders (including any substance abuse and/or intoxication at the time of the offense). Other broad indicators of lifestyle instability may also be present, such as difficulties maintaining steady employment and/or peer relationships; a functional analysis should reveal whether such lifestyle instability was a function of the offender's decision to reject a prosocial lifestyle (that would reflect more "antisocial" traits) or whether he simply lacked the requisite skills to maintain a prosocial lifestyle (the would reflect other, more general self-regulation deficits).

General self-regulation deficits might be assessed using the following measures:

- A structured interview of dynamic risk factors (e.g., the STABLE scoring guide, Hanson & Harris, 2002)
- Mental Status Exam
- Clinical, Treatment, and Interpersonal scales of the PAI (Morey, 1991)
- Brief Symptom Inventory (BSI; Derogatis, 1975)
- Item descriptors from the LSI-R (Andrews & Bonta, 1995)
- Shipley Institute of Living Scale (SILS; 1967) or other screening measure of cognitive functioning
- Delis–Kaplan Executive Function System (D-KEFS)

Like antisocial traits, data to assess the presence of general self-regulation deficits will likely be available through structured interviews and file reviews.

Collateral documents may reveal a history of academic problems, employment instability, failure to fulfill financial obligations, mental health or behavioral treatment, or chronic problems with substance abuse.

In some cases, general self-regulation deficits will be better conceptualized as "responsivity needs" (Andrews, 1989), such as when they are not associated with a pattern of sexual offending but are likely to impact effective treatment delivery (e.g., a history of panic attacks). These deficits are best conceptualized as dynamic risk needs when they are directly associated with sexual offending (e.g., association with children or teenagers secondary to delayed social development) or an otherwise offense-supportive lifestyle (i.e., instability/irresponsibility).

RULE VIOLATION/NONCOMPLIANCE

Given that an offender's supervisor (or treatment provider) is an authority figure who promotes a more prosocial lifestyle, an offender's failure to comply with the expectations of this authority and/or fulfill his prosocial responsibilities may be behavioral indicators of an "antisocial" orientation. Problems in this area may also reflect skill deficits and/or maladaptive attitudes that are associated with a generally "nonprosocial" lifestyle, such as failing to communicate openly and honestly; failing to take responsibility for his choices and actions; placing blame outside of himself; failing to use effective coping strategies (and instead using avoidance coping); or failing to effectively identify problems and their possible solutions. For these reasons, the risk–need area of "rule violations" is conceptualized in 3RT as an "antisocial" risk–need and targeted in 3RT-A group(s).

Formal assessment of Rule Violations/Noncompliance might include the following:

- A structured interview of dynamic risk factors (e.g., the STABLE scoring guide, Hanson & Harris, 2002)
- Treatment scales of the PAI (Morey, 1991)
- Treatment index items on the Multiphasic Sex Inventory (MSI; Nichols & Molinder, 1999);
- Readiness to change questionnaires (see Miller, 1999, for references) that are easily modified for use with sex offenders

Noncompliance with supervision or treatment is easily and effectively assessed through the use of behavioral observation and collateral data. Hanson and Harris (2002) have described numerous indicators of this risk area to be considered, such as an offender's apparent disengagement (e.g., "just going through the motions" of treatment; not invested in making therapeutic change), manipulation (trying to "play the system" by being "buddy-buddy," lying, asking for favors, staff-splitting, etc.), or more obvious indicators of noncompliance (e.g., failing to keep scheduled appointments). When these behaviors are observed by SOTPs, they would be documented as an indication of the presence of this risk factor and/or for the purposes of monitoring behavioral change as an indicator of treatment progress. Collateral data sources include records of supervision violations, institutional infractions, and/or prior history of treatment failure/noncompliance.

Another means of observing an offender's tendency toward rule violations is his commitment to/respect for the environmental conditions and limitations associated with his offense cycle. Accordingly, an offender's knowledge about and understanding of his own offense cycle (e.g., triggers, HRSs) may be a useful tool for assessing his compliance with self-imposed rules. For example, willingness to put himself in a situation that would place him at increased risk to reoffend (e.g., putting himself in an HRS as a "test" of his self-control, or to "prove" that the offender is "cured") suggests that the offender is rationalizing a poor decision for the purposes of getting his immediate needs met. Thus, ongoing assessment of the offender's sexual offense cycle may be a useful way to assess his awareness of and respect for HRSs, and compliance with rules and conditions of treatment/supervision.

"Erotopathic" Risk Needs

In addition to sex offenders' general "criminogenic needs," risk assessment research has also identified dynamic risk factors that appear to be particularly characteristic of sexual offenders; specifically, factors associated with their deviant sexual interests and attitudes, deficits in sexual self-regulation, and impairments associated with intimate relationships (Hanson & Morton-Bourgon, 2004). When examined together, these dynamic risk factors appear to be broadly associated with the confluence of two inter- and intrapersonal behavioral trajectories: (1) the offender's failure to successfully develop and maintain stable, intimate relationships with appropriate partners; (2) his development and maintenance of deviant sexual interests, attitudes, preferences and behaviors. For the purposes of 3RT, we have clustered these two trajectories and labeled them collectively as an offender's *"erotopathic" risk–needs.* This problem area refers to the offender's maladaptive sexual/love "schema" and its associated behaviors and relationships, including the development/maintenance of emotionally detached and/or abusive relationships and avoidance of relationships/interactions that threaten his detachment; a preference for "relationships" with partners he can control (e.g., with minors, or through the use of force) and avoidance of relationships/partners that challenge his control; and/or the paired association between his sexual gratification and real or imagined situations in which he is in ultimate control and avoidance of situations in which his or her "sexual ideal" is threatened. Conversely, the development of satisfying and prosocial intimate/sexual relationships could serve to curtail future acts of sexual offending.

Offenders who endorse risk–needs in this area would be assigned to a 3RT-Erotopathic Risk Needs group (3RT-E) to target those problem areas.

The goal of 3RT-E is to help offenders identify their erotopathic risk–needs; monitor and self-regulate his maladaptive sexual thoughts, behaviors, and relationships; and develop alternative approaches to functioning more effectively in satisfying intimate relationships with appropriate partners (see Wheeler et al., 2005, for a more detailed description of 3RT-A treatment goals).

SEXUAL SELF-REGULATION DEFICITS

Sexual self-regulation can include numerous cognitive and behavioral problems associated with the maladaptive use of sex, including sexual offense behavior. For example, deficits in sexual self-regulation could include sexually deviant interests or behaviors, sexual preoccupation, use of sex as coping, hyper- and/or indiscriminant sexuality, sexual secrecy/deceit, "overcontrolled" sexual behaviors, or self-perceived sexual inadequacy. In particular, three areas of "deviant sexual interest" have been recently associated with increased risk for sexual offense recidivism (Hanson & Morton-Bourgon, 2004), including sexual interest in and/or arousal to children, paraphiliac interests (e.g., exhibitionism, voyeurism, cross-dressing), and sexual preoccupation (paraphiliac or nonparaphiliac).

Structured assessments of sexual self-regulation deficits might include the following:

- A structured interview of dynamic risk factors (e.g., the STABLE scoring guide, Hanson & Harris, 2002)
- Multiphasic Sex Inventory–II (MSI-II; Nichols & Molinder, 1999)
- Clarke Sexual History Questionnaire for Males—Revised (SHQ-R; Langevin & Paitche, 2003)
- Abel and Becker Sexual Interest Cardsort (SIC; Holland, Zolondek, Abel, Jordan, & Becker, 2000)
- Penile plethysmograph (PPG) assessment

Deviant sexual interests and sexual preoccupations may be reported in the context of an intake interview or from file review data. Offenders might be asked to keep a diary or behavioral log of their sexual thoughts and behaviors, that might later be a useful tool for evaluating sexual preoccupation (e.g., intrusive thoughts, excessive masturbation or use of pornography; visiting strip clubs or prostitutes) and/or the use of sexual thoughts and behaviors as a coping mechanism for distress (i.e., to "self-soothe").

Deviant sexual interest may also be assessed using objective physiological measures of sexual arousal to deviant stimuli (i.e., penile plethysmography, or PPG). Arousal to deviant stimuli has demonstrated a significant association with sexual offense recidivism, and will be considered separately here. In addition to providing objective data on deviant sexual interest, phallometric assessment can provide information regarding deviant sexual *preferences*; that is, the stimuli that induces the greatest amount of sexual arousal, relative to other sexual stimuli. Although most sexual offenders (including most of those who sexually offend against children) indicate that their ideal, or preference, is to have consensual sexual relations with an adult, other groups of offenders indicate that, although they may have consensual sex with adults, they *prefer* to have sexual relations that are regarded as "deviant" (defined in the dominant culture as sexual relations that are victimizing and therefore illegal). These deviant preferences include (but are not limited to) prepubescent children, postpubescent adolescents below the age of consent, and adults who resist or do not consent to sexual activity. Deviant sexual preferences, including any deviant preference and a specific sexual preference for children, have been identified as significant predictors of sexual offense recidivism (Hanson & Morton-Bourgon, 2004), supporting the use of PPG assessment in the context of treatment planning and delivery. For offenders who endorse this risk area, repeated PPG assessments may be useful tools for ongoing treatment planning and modification, and as an objective method for evaluating a treatment progress.

ATTITUDES SUPPORTIVE OF SEXUAL CRIMES

Although typically considered separately from sexual deviance with regard to categorizing risk factors (e.g., Hanson & Morton-Bourgon, 2004), attitudes supportive of sexual crimes are regarded as relevant to an offender's erotopathic risk needs in the context of 3RT. Hanson and Morton-Bourgon (2004) reported that, although not all such attitudes were significant, many of these types of attitudes were significant predictors of sexual offense recidivism. Examples of sex-offense supportive attitudes might include victim-blaming, failure to take responsibility, minimization of negative impact on the victim, hostility toward women, adversarial sexual beliefs, sexual objectification of children/females, sexual conservatism, benevolent sexism, misinterpretation of sexual/social cues, sexual entitlement, or identification with child molesters

Although there are limitations to the "objective" assessment of non-observable behavior (i.e., attitudes and beliefs), there are many measures available for this purpose. An offender's sex offense supportive attitudes might be assessed using the following:

- A structured interview of dynamic risk factors (e.g., the STABLE scoring guide, Hanson & Harris, 2002)
- MSI-II (Nichols & Molinder, 1999)
- RAPE and/or MOLEST scales (Bumby, 1996)
- Abel and Becker Cognitions Scale (Abel, Gore, Holland, Camp, Becker, & Rather, 1989)
- Hanson Sexual Attitude Questionnaire (SAQ; Hanson, Gizzarelli, & Scott, 1994)

INTIMACY DEFICITS

Although typically considered separately from deviant sexual interests with regard to risk assessment (e.g., Hanson & Morton-Bourgon, 2004), for the purposes of 3RT, intimacy deficits are considered as relevant to sexual deviance, in the context of an offender's "erotopathic risk needs." Although various "intimacy deficits" have been described previously as potential predictors of recidivism, Hanson and Morton-Bourgon (2004) reported that the following two areas emerged as significant predictors of sexual reoffending: emotional identification with children and conflicts with intimate partners. Other examples of intimacy deficits to be addressed in 3RT-E could include lack of intimate partners, avoidance of adult intimate partners, infidelity, partner violence, lack of concern/empathy for intimate partners/victims, jealousy/mistrust/insecurity in intimate relationships, use of behavioral extremes to control partner behavior, relationships with young/vulnerable "partners."

Intimacy deficits, specifically those related to impairments in adult romantic functioning, might be assessed using the following measures:

- Clinical and Interpersonal scales of the PAI (Morey, 1991)
- MSI-II (Nichols & Molinder, 1999)
- Interpersonal Reactivity Index (IRI; Davis, 1980)
- Hostility Toward Women Scale (HTWS; Lonsway & Fitzgerald, 1995)

With regard to conflicts with intimate partners, data regarding relationship patterns and interactions can be gathered from intake interviews and file reviews (see Hanson & Harris, 2002). The attitudes and behaviors that underlie an offender's history of conflicts may also be apparent in group treatment setting. For example, an offender might regularly communicate his disregard for the observations/opinions of the therapist or other group members, or maintain a generally adversarial approach to discussing and resolving problems.

Responsivity Needs

The "responsivity principle" of offender treatment (Andrews, 1989) indicates that treatment plans should be developed and implemented with consideration for approaches that have demonstrated effectiveness with managing offense-related behaviors (e.g., cognitive-behavioral therapies), and that account for the offender's ideographic needs that may impact the effectiveness of treatment delivery. For example, include cognitive impairments (e.g., learning deficits, developmental disabilities), mental or behavioral health issues (e.g., post-traumatic stress disorder, paranoia, suicidality), cultural issues (e.g., cultural values/attitudes about sexual behavior; religious beliefs; "healthy paranoia" about psychological treatment), or other factors unique to that individual (e.g., hearing impairment, seizure disorder, veteran status) that may be important to consider in formulating treatment plans.

Responsivity needs might be assessed using the following approaches:

- A clinical interview
- File review
- Clinical, Treatment, and Interpersonal scales of the PAI (Morey, 1991); or other objective personality/clinical assessment
- Brief Symptom Inventory (BSI; Derogatis, 1975)
- Shipley Institute of Living Scale (SILS; 1967) or other screening measure of cognitive functioning
- Delis–Kaplan Executive Function System (D-KEFS)

Responsivity needs may also emerge during the course of treatment (e.g., diagnosis with a major medical illness or physical injury requiring treatment accommodation). In some cases, the issues will be better conceptualized as "general self-regulation" deficits, when they are associated with a pattern of sexual offending (e.g., when an offender acts out sexually during manic episodes; when a developmentally delayed offender seeks out children as social/cognitive "peers" then acts out sexually with them).

Dynamic Risk Assessment: A Hypothetical Example

We return to our hypothetical sex offender, Joe Offender, to demonstrate how dynamic risk assessment data might be gathered in the context of a SOTP's intake and treatment planning protocols.[7] We'll assume Joe was caught for the above mentioned crime, and sentenced to a prison term that included participation in a 12–24-month institution-based sex offender treatment program. Prior to beginning treatment, Joe participated in a complete intake assessment, conducted by the SOTP assessment team. This assessment consisted of the following:

- A *structured clinical interview* to gather data about Joe's psychosocial and psychosexual history, antisocial and erotopathic risk–need areas (e.g., the STABLE and ACUTE scoring guides; Hanson & Harris, 2002), and his current emotional, cognitive, and behavioral functioning
- A *file review* to gather additional data regarding Joe's antisocial and erotopathic risk needs and responsivity issues
- Administration of psychological "testing," including the SILS (Shipley, 1967), PAI (Morey, 1991), SIC (Holland et al., 2000), MSI-II (Nichols & Molinder, 1999), SAQ (Hanson et al., 1994), and RAPE and MOLEST scales (Bumby, 1986), IRI (Davis, 1980), and

HTWS (Lonsway & Fitzgerald, 1995), to gather additional data about Joe's antisocial and erotopathic risk–need areas and possible responsivity issues

- *A phallometric assessment* to gather objective physiological data about Joe's deviant sexual interests and preferences

After Joe's intake assessment protocol was completed, the SOTP assessment team provided a brief summary report to Joe's therapist, summarizing the relevant dynamic risk data, highlighting Joe's antisocial and erotopathic risk needs areas and responsivity issues (see Appendix 12.1 for a sample summary). Joe's therapist then used this summary report to guide Joe's ideographic treatment plan, to target his stable risk factors in 3RT group(s) and his acute risk factors in RP treatment (see Wheeler et al., 2005, for more information on treatment planning and delivery).

Summary of Assessment Considerations for 3RT

In 3RT, the goal of assessment is to identify each offender's particular constellation of dynamic risk factors, so that an ideographic treatment plan can be developed to target his particular risk–needs. In previous sections, we have outlined recently identified dynamic factors as significant predictors of sexual offense recidivism (Hanson & Morton-Bourgon, 2004). For each risk factor, we have provided suggested methods for assessment, including formal measures, structured interviews, and behavioral observations.

It is likely that much of the data gathering we have described is already conducted as a standard component of treatment intake and delivery, and for the purposes of monitoring treatment progress. The 3RT assessment model simply reflects a paradigm shift, such that extant procedures are reconceptualized as serving the critical function of assessing offenders' dynamic risk–needs, so that these needs can be effectively addressed in treatment. Ideally, 3RT assessment protocols would be compatible with existing protocols and would not place a prohibitive additional burden on SOTP resources. In fact, given the overt relationship between these assessment techniques and treatment monitoring, it is likely that the modular and risk-based 3RT model would lend itself to preformatted templates for intake assessments, progress notes, and treatment summaries, thereby minimizing (if not reducing) therapists' workload.

As with any situation necessitating assessment of an individual's cognitive and behavioral functioning, some techniques may require advanced qualifications or specialty training (e.g., PPG, PCL-R, or MMPI-2), while other techniques may be implemented by staff members who are generally familiar with principles of clinical interviewing and actuarial assessment (e.g., the STABLE scoring guide, Hanson & Harris, 2002). The flexibility of the 3RT model allows SOTP to custom-tailor assessment protocols to meet the demands of the risk–need (i.e., which factors must be assessed and for what purpose) with the resources that are available to conduct the assessment (e.g., more assessment resources may be allocated at intake for the purposes of treatment planning, while therapists would play a primary role in gathering observational data during treatment).

CONCLUSIONS

In this chapter, we have outlined some problems with the current model of RP, a primary treatment for sex offenders, and proposed a new primary approach called 3RT, which refers to a combination of techniques for assessing sex offenders' dynamic risk factors for recidivism and later targeting these factors for intervention. Current identified risk domains include antisocial and "erotopathic" risk factors; however, 3RT can be continually modified and enhanced as we increase our understanding about sex offenders' dynamic risk factors for recidivism.

The introduction of a new, primary approach to the assessment treatment of sexual offenders responds to a long-standing criticism that RP (which was originally developed as an adjunctive enhancement to a successful course of treatment) has evolved into a primary treatment approach for this population. With the introduction of 3RT techniques to address sexual offenders' long-standing cognitive, behavioral, emotional, and interpersonal problems (insofar as these problems are associated with recidivism risk), RP techniques could be implemented for their original purpose: to facilitate the prolonged success of offenders' commitment to abstaining from sexual offending.

Much has changed in the 20 years since the first application of RP to sex offenders (Marshall & Laws, 2003). In accord with its initial enthusiastic reception, RP has become a very popular SOTP treatment approach, and there is evidence to support its effectiveness. However, as critics have noted, its popularity has been problematic because many SOTP now rely on RP as the primary treatment strategy rather than as being adjunctive to offense cessation intervention. Professionals responsible for managing and treating sex offenders have come to embrace the importance of actuarial risk assessment as a central pivot point in predicting reoffense, prioritizing treatment access, and tailoring treatment protocols.

In response to these trends and observations, we are offering an enhanced and updated RP approach for sex offenders to maximize reoffense prevention, called Recidivism Risk Reduction Therapy (3RT). This approach incorporates risk assessment principles and tailored intervention protocols to target the precise recidivism reduction focal points for each offender. In this chapter, we have summarized methods for conducting ideographic assessments of each offender's dynamic risk–needs, for the purpose of assigning him to a 3RT group and monitoring his treatment progress. In our chapter in the second edition of *Relapse Prevention* (Wheeler et al., 2005), we provide specific 3RT techniques and interventions for targeting dynamic risk factors in sex offenders, and for integrating 3RT approaches with existing RP-based treatment programs. The 3RT approach can be employed sequentially or concurrently with traditional RP sex offender protocols. It is expected that, like RP, 3RT will be subjected to future empirical evaluation.

APPENDIX 12.1. SAMPLE DYNAMIC RISK ASSESSMENT SUMMARY REPORT

Dynamic Risk Assessment Summary for Joe Offender

Erotopathic Risk Needs

SEXUAL SELF-REGULATION

Mr. Offender frequently indulges in impersonal sexual activities (pornographic videos, Internet sites and chat rooms, and strip clubs). He reports that he is preoccupied with thoughts about sex and that he has a "strong sex drive." He described using sexual thoughts and behaviors to "feel better" when he is feeling depressed or is faced with stressful life events. He reports a history of engaging in sexual acts as an instrumental behavior in his social relationships (i.e., "on a dare") and engaging in impersonal sexual activity (e.g., surfing the Internet for porn sites) when he feels bored, lonely, or depressed. He also reports a history of acting out sexually when under the influence of alcohol, including being intoxicated at the time of the offense. He has a history of deviant sexual interests, including sex with inanimate objects (women's underwear) and with postpubescent minor females. His phallometric assessment indicated that he had numerous deviant sexual interests, including arousal to minor females, adult females, and the use of force. His sexual preference appeared to be for consensual sex with an adult female.

ATTITUDES SUPPORTIVE OF SEXUAL CRIMES

Mr. Offender provided a clear indication that he feels entitled to sex when he is aroused. He also attributed the "cause" of his offense to the fact that he was intoxicated and that his victim was "sexy." He endorsed many items and made several statements consistent with attitudes supportive of engaging in sexual contact with postpubescent minors (e.g., his belief girls are "horny" at this age). Specifically, he demonstrated a tendency to place blame on his victim for the sexual activity and a belief that some young people are sexually "precocious." He provided no evidence of rape-supportive attitudes.

INTIMACY DEFICITS

Mr. Offender has a history of conflictual relationships with his lovers/intimate partners. The nature of these conflicts typically involves the degree of his female partners' social, financial, occupational independence from him; and differences in their approach to sex and intimacy (e.g., he would prefer to have a more "dominant" role in his intimate relationships than he has had). He also has a history of identifying with teenage girls, but not younger children. He appears to have a pattern of rationalizing his sexual behavior (i.e., having sexual relationships with very young girls), but he does

not seem to have a general pattern of indifference towards others outside of his sexual relationships.

Antisocial Risk Needs

MALADAPTIVE SOCIAL FUNCTIONING

Mr. Offender does not have a significant pattern of antisocial attitudes or behaviors. He has finished his college degree and has had a successful career as a bar and restaurant manager. However, his social activity is limited primarily to gathering with his drinking companions at a local tavern and commiserating about their romantic partners.

General Self-Regulation Deficits

Mr. Offender has a history of identifying with teenagers, including purchasing alcohol and marijuana for teenagers who hang out where he works (a restaurant). He described himself as "I never grew up emotionally," and "I just like to hang out and have a good time, and young people seem to like that about me." He reported a history of significant alcohol use for the 6 months prior to the index offense, including being intoxicated at the time of the offense. His problem-solving ability is limited (specifically, he had difficulty generating alternate solutions to common problems); this appears to be a function of fears about trying new behaviors, rather than a cognitive deficit.

History of Rule Violations

Mr. Offender has no significant history of rule violations. However, there was some evidence during this evaluation process that at times he was disengaged and/or manipulative with regard to taking responsibility for his behavior. He had limited insight about the problematic nature of his sexual thoughts and behaviors, and became notably defensive with regard to the circumstances of the index offense (e.g., suggesting that the victim "ratted him out" only after she got mad at him for an unrelated incident a few days later). However, this appeared to be limited to his distortions and justifications for his sexual behavior, rather than a pervasive pattern of noncompliance or rule-testing.

Responsivity Needs Identified for Joe Offender

COGNITIVE AND LEARNING ISSUES

Mr. Offender had some difficulties with regard to problem-solving ability (specifically, he had difficulty generating alternate solutions to common problems); this appears to be a function of fears about trying new behaviors, rather than a cognitive deficit. His has no history of learning problems.

MENTAL AND BEHAVIORAL HEALTH

Mr. Offender has a history of transient depressive symptoms in response to stress. Since these "episodes" are associated with his offense behavior, these will be conceptualized as dynamic risk needs (general self-regulation deficits; use of sex as a coping mechanism).

CULTURAL ISSUES

Mr. Offender is a white, Europeam American male. He identified his family of origin as "typical Irish-catholic," but denied current affiliation with any organized religion.

OTHER

Mr. Offender mentioned his status as a war veteran several times during the interview, became notably irritable when discussing "draft dodgers," and indicated that his peer group has historically been comprised of other veterans. He did not endorse any symptoms suggesting chronic posttraumatic effects from his experience, but his military history may nonetheless be an important consideration for enhancing the effectiveness of treatment (e.g., assignment to a group that includes other veterans).

ACKNOWLEDGMENTS

Preparation of this chapter was supported in part by a grant from the National Institute on Alcohol Abuse and Alcoholism (AA13565) to William H. George. Gratitude is expressed to Ken Schafer and Rebecca Schacht for their assistance.

NOTES

1. Depending on the client and the orientation of the therapist, use of any type of pornography (including adult consensual sex) may be regarded as a preoffense behavior and therefore determine a lapse. There is, however, a potential role for viewing pornography as a form of harm reduction. For a discussion of the harm reduction approach, see Wheeler, George, and Stoner (2005).
2. The "rule" that has been broken is not necessarily abstinence. Moderation is also considered a legitimate goal within the RP model for substance use.
3. This example is entirely fictional. Any resemblance between this example and actual persons/events is purely coincidental.
4. Andrews (1989) has enumerated three risk-based treatment principles for working with criminal offenders. These principles provide a structure for prioritizing treatment candidates and tailoring the treatment process.
5. In addition to identifying significant risk factors, this meta-analysis provided data on nonsignificant factors that had previously received attention for their potential role in sexual offending (e.g., history of child sexual abuse; low self-esteem). Please refer to the original report for more specific data on significant versus nonsignificant dynamic risk factors.
6. It should be noted that structured approaches to sex offender assessment have been described elsewhere (e.g., Hanson & Harris, 2000, 2001, 2002; Thornton, 2002); although they were developed to assess many dynamic factors that have not yet demonstrated an empirical relationship to recidivism (Hanson & Morton-Bourgon, 2004), these models may nonetheless be useful guides for conducting structured risk assessments.
7. For the purposes of this chapter, the hypothetical evaluation of Joe Offender was conducted for therapeutic purposes (i.e., to develop his treatment plan), and not fo-

rensic purposes (i.e., to provide an opinion to a third party regarding his risk to reoffend; see Heilbrun, 2003, for further discussion on the difference between forensic and therapeutic assessment). A forensic sex offender risk assessment would include scores and risk estimates derived from other actuarial instruments, such as the Minnesota Sex Offender Screening Tool—Revised (MnSOST-R; Epperson, Kaul, & Hesselton, 1998), the Violence Risk Appraisal Guide (VRAG) and the Sex Offender Risk Appraisal Guide (SORAG; Quinsey, Harris, Rice, & Cormier, 1998), including information from the Hare Psychopathy Checklist—Revised (PCL-R; Hare, 1991); the Static-99 (Hanson & Thornton, 2000) that includes the Rapid Risk Assessment for Sex Offence Recidivism (RRASOR; Hanson, 1997), and the Sexual Violence Risk-20 (SVR-20; Boer, Hart, Kropp, & Webster, 1997).

REFERENCES

Abel, G. G., Gore, D. K., Holland, C. L., Camp, N., Becker, J. V., & Rather, J. (1989). The measurement of the cognitive distortions in child molesters. *Annals of Sex Research, 2*, 135–153.

American Psychiatric Association. (2000). *Diagnostic and statistical manual of mental disorders* (4th ed., text rev.). Washington, DC: Author.

Andrews, D., & Bonta, J. (1995). *LSI-R: The Level of Service Inventory—Revised*. Toronto, Canada: Multi-Health Systems.

Andrews, D. A. (1989). Recidivism is predictable and can be influenced: Using risk assessments to reduce recidivism. *Forum on Corrections Research, 1*(2), 11–18.

Andrews, D. A., & Bonta, J. (2003). *The psychology of criminal conduct* (3rd ed.). Cincinnati: Anderson.

Beech, A., Fisher, D., & Beckett, R. (1999). *STEP 3: An evaluation of the prison sex offender treatment programme*. Report available from Home Office Information Publications Group, Research and Statistics Directorate, Room 201, Queen Anne's Gate, London, SW1H9 AT, UK.

Bonta, J. (2002). Offender risk assessment: Guidelines for selection and use. *Criminal Justice and Behavior, 29*, 355–379.

Boer, D. P., Hart, S. D., Kropp, P. R., & Webster, C. D. (1997). *Manual for the Sexual Violence Risk–20*. Vancouver, BC: British Columbia Institute Against Family Violence.

Bumby, K. M. (1996). Assessing the cognitive distortions of child molesters and rapists: Development and validation of the MOLEST and RAPE scales. *Sexual Abuse: Journal of Research and Treatment, 8*, 37–53.

Carnes, P. (2001). *Out of the shadows: Understanding sexual addiction*. Minneapolis: Hazelden Information Education.

Dandescu, A., & Christopher, M. (2003). *Improving treatment readiness and motivation for sex offender treatment: A pilot study*. Poster presented at the 22nd annual meeting of the Association for the Treatment of Sexual Abusers, St. Louis, MO.

Davis, M. H. (1980). A multidimensional approach to individual differences in empathy. *JSAS: Catalog of Selected Documents in Psychology, 10*, 85.

Delis, D. C., Kaplan, E., & Kramer, J. H. (2001). *Delis–Kaplan Executive Function System*. San Antonio, TX: Psychological Corporation.

Derogatis, L. R. (1975). *Brief Symptom Inventory*. Minneapolis, MN: Pearson Assessments.

Derrickson, D. L. (2000). Working alliance and readiness to change in incarcerated sex offenders. *Dissertation Abstracts International: Section B: The Sciences and Engineering, 60*(8-B), 4215.

Epperson, D. L., Kaul, J. D., & Hesselton, D. (1998). *Minnesota Sex Offender Screening Tool—Revised (MnSOST-R): Development, performance, and recommended risk level cut scores.* St. Paul, MN: Iowa State University & Minnesota Department of Corrections.

George, W. H., & Marlatt, G. A. (1989). Introduction. In D. R. Laws (Ed.), *Relapse prevention with sex offenders* (pp. 1–31). New York: Guilford Press.

Hanson, R. K. (1997). *The development of a brief actuarial risk scale for sexual offense recidivism* (User Report No. 97004). Ottawa: Department of the Solicitor General of Canada.

Hanson, R. K. (1998). What do we know about sex offender risk assessment? *Psychology, Public Policy, and Law, 4,* 50–72.

Hanson, R. K. (2000). What is so special about relapse prevention? In D. R. Laws, S. M. Hudson, & T. Ward (Eds.), *Remaking relapse prevention with sex offenders: A sourcebook* (pp. 27–38). Thousand Oaks, CA: Sage.

Hanson, R. K., & Bussiere, M. T. (1998). Predicting relapse: A meta-analysis of sexual offender recidivism studies. *Journal of Consulting and Clinical Psychology, 66,* 348–362.

Hanson, R. K., Gizzarelli, R., & Scott, H. (1994). The attitudes of incest offenders: Sexual entitlement and acceptance of sex with children. *Criminal Justice and Behavior, 21*(2), 187–202.

Hanson, R. K., Gordon, A., Harris, A. J., Marques, J. K., Murphy, W., Quinsey, V. L., & Seto, M. C. (2002). First report of the Collaborative Outcome Data Project on the effectiveness of psychological treatment for sex offenders. *Sexual Abuse: A Journal of Research and Treatment, 14*(2), 169–194.

Hanson, R. K., & Harris, A. J. R. (1998). *Dynamic predictors of sexual recidivism* (User Report No. 1998-01). Ottawa: Department of the Solicitor General of Canada.

Hanson, R. K., & Harris, A. J. R. (2000a). Where should we intervene? Dynamic predictors of sexual offense recidivism. *Criminal Justice and Behavior, 27*(1), 6–35.

Hanson, R. K., & Harris, A. J. R. (2000b). *The Sex Offender Needs Assessment Rating (SONAR): A method for measuring change in risk levels* (User Report No. 2000-01). Ottawa: Department of the Solicitor General of Canada.

Hanson, R. K., & Harris, A. J. R. (2001). A structured approach to evaluating change among sexual offenders. *Sexual Abuse: A Journal of Research and Treatment, 13*(2), 105–122.

Hanson, R. K., & Harris, A. (2002). *STABLE Scoring Guide: Developed for the Dynamic Supervision Project: A collaborative initiative on the community supervision of sexual offenders* (May 30, 2002 Version). Ottawa: Department of the Solicitor General of Canada.

Hanson, R. K., & Morton-Bourgon, K. (2004). *Predictors of sexual recidivism: An updated meta-analysis* (User Report No. 2004-02). Ottawa: Public Safety and Emergency Preparedness Canada. Available online at www.psepc.gc.ca

Hanson, R. K., & Thornton, D. (1999). *Static-99: Improving actuarial risk assessments for sex offenders* (User report 1999-02). Ottawa: Public Safety and Emergency Preparedness Canada. Available at www.psepc.gc.ca

Hanson, R. K., & Thornton, D. (2000). Improving risk assessments for sex offenders:

A comparison of three actuarial scales. *Law and Human Behavior, 24*(1), 119–136.

Hare, R. D. (1991). *The Hare Psychopathy Checklist—Revised*. Toronto, Ontario: Multi-Health Systems.

Harris, G. T., Rice, M. E., Quinsey, V. L., Lalumiere, M. L., Boer, D., & Lang, C. (2003). A multisite comparison of actuarial risk instruments for sex offenders. *Psychological Assessment, 15,* 413–425.

Heilbrun, K. (2003). Principles of forensic mental health assessment: Implications for the forensic assessment of sexual offenders. *Annals of the New York Academy of Sciences, 989,* 167–184.

Heilbrun, K., Nezu, C. M., Keeney, M., Chung, S., & Wasserman, A. L. (1998). Sexual offending: Linking assessment, intervention, and decision making. *Psychology, Public Policy, and Law, 4,* 138–174.

Holland, L. A., Zolondek, S. C., Abel, G. G., Jordan, A. D., & Becker, V. B. (2000). Psychometric analysis of the Sexual Interest Cardsort Questionnaire. *Sexual Abuse: A Journal of Research and Treatment, 12*(2), 107–122.

Hover, G. (1999). Using DBT skills with incarcerated sex offenders. *ATSA Forum, 11*(3).

Hover, G. R., & Packard, R. L. (1998, October). *The effects of skills training on incarcerated sex offenders and their ability to get along with their therapist*. Poster presented at the 27th Annual Conference Research and Treatment Conference of the Association for the Treatment of Sexual Abusers, Vancouver, British Columbia.

Hover, G. R., & Packard, R. L. (1999, September). *The treatment effects of dialectical behavior therapy with sex offenders*. Paper presented at the 18th Annual Conference of the Association for the Treatment of Sexual Abusers, Lake Buena Vista, Florida.

Hudson, S. M., Wales, D. S., Bakker, L., & Ward, T. (2002). Dynamic risk factors: The Kia Marama evaluation. *Sexual Abuse: A Journal of Research and Treatment, 14*(2), 103–119.

Hudson, S. M., Ward, T., & Marshall, W. L. (1992). The abstinence violation effect in sex offenders: A reformulation. *Behavior Research and Therapy, 30*(5), 435–441.

Knopp, F. H., Freeman-Longo, R., & Stevenson, W. F. (1992). *Nationwide survey of juvenile and adult sex offender treatment programs and models*. Brandon, VT: Safer Society.

Langevin, R., & Paitche, D. (2003). *Clarke Sex History for Males, Revised*. North Tonawanda, NY: Multi-Health Systems.

Laws, D. R. (1995). Central elements in relapse prevention procedures with sex offenders. *Psychology, Crime, and Law, 2,* 41–53.

Laws, D. R. (1996). Relapse prevention or harm reduction? *Sexual Abuse: A Journal of Research and Treatment, 8,* 243–247.

Laws, D. R. (1999a). Relapse prevention: The state of the art. *Journal of Interpersonal Violence, 14*(3), 285–302.

Laws, D. R. (1999b). Harm reduction or harm facilitation?: A reply to Maletzky. *Sexual Abuse: A Journal of Research and Treatment, 11*(3), 233–241.

Laws, D. R. (2003). The rise and fall of relapse prevention. *Australian Psychologist, 38*(1), 22–30.

Laws, D. R., Hudson, S. M., & Ward, T. (2000). The original model of relapse prevention with sex offenders. In D. R. Laws, S. M. Hudson, & T. Ward (Eds.), *Re-*

making relapse prevention with sex offenders: A sourcebook (pp. 2–24). New York: Guilford Press.

Lilienfeld, S. O., Purcell, C., & Jones-Alexander, J. (1997). Assessment of antisocial behavior in adults. In D. M. Stoff, J. Brieling, & J. D. Maser (Eds.), *Handbook of antisocial behavior* (pp. 60–74). New York: Wiley.

Linehan, M. M. (1993). *Skills training manual for treating borderline personality disorder.* New York: Guilford Press.

Lonsway, K. A., & Fitzgerald, L. F. (1995). Attitudinal antecedents of rape myth acceptance: A theoretical and empirical reexamination. *Journal of Personality and Social Psychology, 68*(4), 704–711.

Marlatt, G. A. (1989). Feeding the PIG: The problem of immediate gratification. In D. R. Laws (Ed.), *Relapse prevention with sex offenders.* New York: Guilford Press.

Marlatt, G. A., & Donovan, D. M. (Eds.). (2005). *Relapse prevention* (2nd ed.). New York: Guilford Press.

Marlatt, G. A., & George, W. H. (1984). Relapse prevention: Introduction and overview of the model. *British Journal of Addictions, 79,* 261–273.

Marlatt, G. A., & Gordon, J. R. (Eds.). (1985). *Relapse prevention: Maintenance strategies in the treatment of addictive behavior.* New York: Guilford Press.

Marques, J. K., Day, D. M., Nelson, C., & West, M. A. (1994). Effects of cognitive-behavioral treatment on sex offender recidivism. *Criminal Justice and Behavior, 21*(1), 28–54.

Marshall, W. L., & Laws, D. R. (2003). A brief history of behavioral and cognitive-behavioral approaches to sexual offender treatment: Part 2. The modern era. *Sexual abuse: A Journal of Research and Treatment, 15,* 93–120.

McConnaughty, B. A., Prochaska, J. O., & Velicer, W. F. (1983). Stages of change in psychotherapy: Measurement and sample profiles. *Psychotherapy: Theory, Research, and Practice, 20,* 368–375.

Miller, W. R. (1999). *Enhancing motivation for change in substance abuse treatment: Treatment improvement protocol series.* Rockville, MD: U.S. Department of Health and Human Services: Substance Abuse and Mental Health Services Administration.

Miller, W. R., & Rollnick, S. (1991). *Motivational interviewing.* New York: Guilford Press.

Miller, W. R., & Tonigan, J. S. (1996). Assessing drinkers' motivation for change: The Stages of Change Readiness and Treatment Eagerness Scale (SOCRATES). *Psychology of Addictive Behaviors, 10,* 81–89.

Millon, T. (2004). *Millon Clinical Multiaxial Inventory—III.* Bloomington, MN: NCS/Pearson Assessments.

Morey, L. C. (1991). *Personality Assessment Inventory.* Point Huron, MI: Sigma.

Nichols, H. R., & Molinder, I. (1999). *Multiphasic Sex Inventory II Manual.* (Available from Nichols & Molinder, 437 Bowes Drive, Tacoma, WA 98466).

Pithers, W. D. (1990). Relapse prevention with sexual aggressors: A method for maintaining therapeutic gain and enhancing external supervision. In W. M. Marshall, D. R. Laws, & H. E. Barbaree (Eds.), *Handbook of sexual assault: Issues, theories, and treatment of the offender* (pp. 363–389). New York: Plenum Press.

Pithers, W. D., Kashima, K. M., Cumming, G. F., Beal, L. S., & Buell, M. M. (1988). Relapse prevention of sexual aggression. In R. A. Prentky & V. L. Quinsey (Eds.), Human sexual aggression: Current perspectives. *Annals of the New York Academy of Sciences, 528,* 244–260.

Pithers, W. D., Marques, J. K., Gibat, C. C., & Marlatt, G. A. (1983). Relapse prevention with sexual aggressives: A self-control model of treatment and maintenance of change. In J. G. Greer & I. R. Stuart (Eds.), *The sexual aggressor* (pp. 124–239). New York: Van Nostrand Reinhold.

Prochaska, J. O., & DiClemente, C. C. (1984). *The transtheoretical approach: Crossing traditional boundaries of therapy.* Homewood, IL: Dow Jones/Irwin.

Prochaska, J. O., & DiClemente, C. C. (1992). Stages of change in the modification of problem behaviors. In M. Hersen, R. Eisler, & P. M. Miller (Eds.), *Progress in behavior modification* (Vol. 28, pp. 184–214). Sycamore, IL: Sycamore.

Prochaska, J. O., DiClemente, C. C., & Norcross, J. C. (1992). In search of how people change: Applications to addictive behaviors. *American Psychologist, 47,* 1102–1114.

Quigley, S. M. (2000). Dialectical behavior therapy and sex offender treatment: An integrative model. *Dissertation Abstracts International: Section B: The Sciences and Engineering, 60*(9-B), 4904.

Quinsey, V. L., Harris, G. T., Rice, M. E., & Cormier, C. A. (1998). *Violent offenders: Appraising and managing risk.* Washington, DC: American Psychological Association.

Quinsey, V. L., Lalumiere, M. L., Rice, M. E., & Harris, G. T. (1995). Predicting sexual offenses. In J. C. Campbell (Ed.), *Assessing dangerousness: Violence by sexual offenders, batterers, and child abusers* (pp. 114–137). Thousand Oaks, CA: Sage.

Roberts, C. F., Doren, D. M., & Thornton, D. (2002). Dimensions associated with assessments of sex offender recidivism risk. *Criminal Justice and Behavior, 29,* 569–589.

Rollnick, S., Heather, N., Gold, R., & Hall, W. (1992). Development of a short "readiness to change" questionnaire for use in brief, opportunistic interventions among excessive drinkers. *British Journal of Addiction, 87,* 743–754.

Shipley, W. C. (1967). *Shipley Institute of Living Scale.* Los Angeles: Western Psychological Association.

Spence, J. T., & Helmreich, R. L. (1972). The Attitudes Toward Women Scale: An objective instrument to measure attitudes toward the rights and roles of women in contemporary society. *Psychological Documents, 2,* 153.

Spizman, P. (2004, February). *Working with dynamic risk factors.* Paper presented at the Annual Meeting of the Washington Association for the Treatment of Sexual Abusers, Blaine, WA.

Stoner, S. A., & George, W. H. (2000). Relapse prevention and harm reduction: Areas of overlap. In D. R. Laws, S. M. Hudson, & T. Ward (Eds.), *Remaking relapse prevention with sex offenders: A sourcebook* (pp. 56–75). Thousand Oaks, CA: Sage.

Tays, T. M., Earle, R. H., Wells, K., Murray, M., & Garret, B. (1999). Treating sex offenders using the sex addiction model. *Sexual Addiction and Compulsivity, 6,* 281–288.

Thornton, D. (1997). *Is relapse prevention really necessary?* Paper presented at the meeting of the Association of the Treatment of Sexual Abusers, Arlington, VA.

Thornton, D. (2002). Constructing and testing a framework for dynamic risk assessment. *Sexual Abuse: A Journal of Research and Treatment, 14*(2),139–153.

Tierney, D. W., & McCabe, M. (2002). Motivation for behavior change among sex offenders: A review of the literature. *Clinical Psychology Review, 22*(1), 113–129.

Tierney, D. W., & McCabe, M. P. (2004). The assessment of motivation for behaviour change among sex offenders against children: An investigation of the utility of the Stages of Change Questionnaire. *Journal of Sexual Aggression, 10*(2), 237–249.

Ward, T., & Hudson, S. M. (1996a). Relapse prevention: A critical analysis. *Sexual Abuse: A Journal of Research and Treatment, 8*, 177–200.

Ward, T., & Hudson, S. M. (1996b). Relapse prevention: Future directions. *Sexual Abuse: A Journal of Research and Treatment, 8*, 249–256.

Ward, T., & Hudson, S. M. (1998). A model of the relapse process in sexual offenders. *Journal of Interpersonal Violence, 13*, 700–725.

Ward, T., & Hudson, S. M. (2000). A self-regulation model of relapse prevention. In D. R. Laws, S. M. Hudson, & T. Ward (Eds.), *Remaking relapse prevention with sex offenders: A sourcebook* (pp. 79–101). New York: Guilford Press.

Ward, T., Hudson, S. M., & Marshall, W. L. (1994). The abstinence violation effect in child molesters. *Behaviour Research and Therapy, 32*, 431–437.

Ward, T., Hudson, S. M., & Siegert, R. J. (1995). A critical comment on Pither's relapse prevention model. *Sexual Abuse: A Journal of Research and Treatment, 7*(2), 167–175.

Ward, T., Louden, K., Hudson, S. M., & Marshall, W. L. (1995). A descriptive model of the offense chain for child molesters. *Journal of Interpersonal Violence, 10*, 452–472.

Wheeler, J. G. (2003). The abstinence violation effect in a sample of incarcerated sexual offenders: A reconsideration of the terms lapse and relapse. *Dissertation Abstracts International: Section B: The Sciences and Engineering, 63*(8–B), 3946.

Wheeler, J. G., George, W. H., & Marlatt, G. A. (in press). The Abstinence Violation Effect: A reconsideration of the terms lapse and relapse for sexual offenders. *Sexual Abuse: Journal of Research and Treatment.*

Wheeler, J. G., George, W. H., & Stoner, S. A. (2005). Enhancing the relapse prevention model for sex offenders: Adding recidivism reduction therapy to target offenders' dynamic risk needs. In G. A. Marlatt & D. M. Donovan (Eds.), *Relapse prevention* (2nd ed.). New York: Guilford Press.

CHAPTER 13

Assessment of Sexually Risky Behaviors

WILLIAM H. GEORGE
TINA M. ZAWACKI
JANE M. SIMONI
KARI A. STEPHENS
KRISTEN P. LINDGREN

AIDS is one of the worst public health crises in moden history. Since the start of the epidemic in the United States, at least 800,000 people have been infected with HIV; 480,060 people have died of AIDS; and over 40,000 are newly infected each year (Centers for Disease Control and Prevention, 2002). Globally, approximately 40 million people are living with HIV (UNAIDS/WHO, 2003). Because sexual transmission is a key route to new infections, there is an urgent need for a psychometrically sound measure to assess sexual behaviors.

In recent decades, largely because of the HIV/AIDS crisis, interest in assessing sexual behavior has soared. This renewed attention continues despite recurrent political efforts to curtail such research (Kaiser, 2003, 2004). In particular, much of the important research in human sexuality, HIV/AIDS, health psychology, and health promotion and disease prevention now addresses unsafe sexual practices or sexually risky behaviors (SRBs). By definition, SRBs, such as vaginal intercourse without a condom, lead to increased rates of sexually transmitted infections (STIs) such as the life-threatening HIV/AIDS.

Sexual behaviors need not be deemed addictive to pose formidable assessment challenges. Like many addictions, however, sexual behaviors are not readily accessible for measurement. There are few useful biological markers. Customs of privacy and confidentiality dictate modesty. Concerns about public impressions and potential stigmatization foster secrecy. In the West, sex is traditionally politically charged and morally scripted. All these factors contribute to the difficulty in accurately assessing SRBs.

Critics have duly noted the psychometric and methodological challenges of accurately assessing SRBs (Catania, Gibson, Chitwood, & Coates, 1990; Catania, Binson, Van Der Straten, & Stone, 1995). Unfortunately, and somewhat surprisingly, scant research attention has focused on the systematic development of SRB assessment protocols that are conceptually and psychometrically rigorous. Most glaringly absent are cohesive lines of inquiry dedicated to instrument development, validation, and cross-validation culminating in clear "best choices" or "best practices" for SRB assessment instrumentation. Instead, novice SRB investigators encounter a morass of project-specific SRB instruments, with little guidance in how to distill a short list of possibilities. They, like their veteran counterparts, often resort to developing their own project-driven instruments. The valid assessment of SRBs is necessary in order to determine actual rates of risky behavior, its correlates, its determinants, and the efficacy of interventions designed to curtail it.

Our purpose in this chapter is to offer a brief overview of SRB assessment and a practical guide to formulating and appraising SRB instruments. After first defining SRB, we (1) briefly consider the state of the field of SRB assessment; (2) overview the psychometric properties of sound SRB assessment measures; and (3) discuss guidelines for culturally appropriate assessment of SRB. Throughout our coverage, we offer suggestions for researchers struggling with the issue of SRB assessment.

WHAT ARE SEXUALLY RISKY BEHAVIORS?

Because an exchange of bodily fluids is necessary to transmit HIV, SRBs are defined as behaviors that allow for such exchange. Besides breast milk, the only body fluids that can contain a concentration of HIV sufficient enough for transmission are blood, semen, and vaginal fluids. The most efficient route for sexual transmission of HIV infection is unprotected (i.e., condomless) anal intercourse, both penetrative and receptive (Jemmott & Jemmott, 2000; Kelly & Kalichman, 2002). Penetrative anal sex incurs risk by exposing penile mucous membranes—as well as small lacerations that may exist on the penis—to HIV potentially contained in a receptive partner's rectal blood. Receptive anal sex partners run the risk of absorbing potentially HIV-infected semen through the vascular anal cavity.

Vaginal intercourse is considered less risky than anal intercourse, because it typically involves fewer lacerations and less bleeding. Nonetheless, as with anal sex, both penetrative and receptive vaginal intercourse partners are potentially exposed to HIV, either via semen penetrating vaginal walls or via vaginal fluids entering the genital tissue of the penis. Women are two to four times more likely than their male partners to contract HIV through vaginal sex (Haverkos & Battjes, 1992).

There is much debate surrounding the risk level of oral sexual practices (e.g., oral–genital receptive sex [Caceres & van Griensven, 1994; Newton, 1996; Page-Shafer et al., 2002], although it is biologically tenable that oral mucous membranes can absorb HIV). Relatively stronger support—although extremely mixed and controversial—has been found for penile–oral transmission (Samuel et al., 1993; Schacker, Collier, Hughes, Shea, & Corey, 1996) compared to vaginal–oral transmission (Chu, Conti, Schable, & Diaz, 1994; Cohen, Marmor, Wolfe, & Ribble, 1993).

The most common SRB assessment targets include the frequency of anal, vaginal, and oral sex without the barrier protection of a condom (or dental dam in the case of female-receptive oral sex). Empirical research has substantiated that assessing unprotected sexual behavior (e.g., occasions of anal-receptive intercourse without a condom) tends to yield more accurate risk data than assessing general sexual behaviors (e.g., occasions of anal intercourse; Mantell, DiVittis, & Auerbach, 1997). The risk of infection increases with the practice of these behaviors with a large number of partners.

In addition to assessing respondents' unprotected sexual behavior and number of partners, it is also useful to assess the characteristics of their sexual partners. Relevant data include the partner's HIV status, past and current HIV risk due to SRB and injection drug use, and whether the partnership is exclusive. Assessing exclusivity of the relationship is important, because individuals may engage in different practices with different partners.

THE STATE OF THE FIELD

Numerous research teams have developed questions for measuring engagement in SRBs. The proliferation of questions has paralleled the rapid propagation of research studies, intervention projects, and investigative teams funded to scrutinize the role of SRBs in the HIV/AIDS crisis. Unfortunately, the majority of these questions were developed with project-specific objectives in mind rather than with a unifying objective of establishing a sound and generalizable SRB assessment protocol. Consequently, most available items and questionnaires are inadequate for general research purposes, because they are without supporting reliability and validity data, or because they are excessively long. In a review of the psychological, psychiatric, and medical literature since 1990 regarding the reliability and validity of self-report SRB measures, Weinhardt, Forsyth, Carey, Jaworski, and Durant (1998) underscored the lack of a "gold standard" measure. Their summary of 30 studies highlighted the unstandardized nature of SRB assessment both in terms of methodology and conceptual framework. Measures varied widely with respect to item contents, administration technique (i.e., survey, face-to-face interview, computer assisted self-interview [CASI]); reporting range (3 weeks up to several years); number of assessment items (3–398), and length of assessment (6–90 minutes). Nevertheless, a subset of commonly assessed variables includes number of sexual partners and frequency of protected and unprotected oral, anal, and vaginal sex (presented in Figure 13.1). In summary, it remains a challenge for researchers to select an empirically validated self-report SRB measure. Because there is a notable scarcity of standardized measures, as well as instruments tailored for specific populations, this chapter emphasizes information that can guide researchers in the construction and modification of methodologically sound measures of SRBs.

Please think carefully about your life and activities over the past 3 months. Think about places you have been, people you have met, and things you have done in the past 3 months. Please answer the following questions about your sexual behavior during the past 3 months. For each item below, write a number in the space for your most accurate estimate. If the situation did not occur, write a zero (0) in the blank. Please do not leave spaces empty.

Over the past 3 months, what was your . . .

1. Number of different *female* sex partners   _____
2. Number of different *male* sex partners   _____

Now think of any sexual activities with female partners. Listed below are various sexual activities that may have occurred. Please mark in each space how often each has occurred in the past 3 months.

3. Number of times you had vaginal intercourse *with* latex condoms   _____
4. Number of times you had vaginal intercourse *without* latex condoms   _____
5. Number of times you had anal intercourse with a woman
   with latex condoms   _____
6. Number of times you had anal intercourse with a woman
   without latex condoms   _____

Next, think of any sexual activities with male partners. Listed below are various sexual activities that may have occurred. Please mark in each space how often each has occurred in the past 3 months.

7. Number of times you had oral sex with a man *with* latex condoms   _____
8. Number of times you had oral sex with a man *without* latex condoms   _____
9. Number of times you had anal intercourse, you inserted,
   with latex condoms   _____
10. Number of times you had anal intercourse, you inserted,
    without latex condoms   _____
11. Number of times you had anal intercourse, partner inserted,
    with latex condoms   _____
12. Number of times you had anal intercourse, partner inserted,
    without latex condoms   _____

Data from Kelly (1995); Scandell et al. (2003).

FIGURE 13.1. Sample Sexual Behavior Questionnaire.

PROPERTIES OF PSYCHOMETRICALLY SOUND MEASURES FOR ASSESSING SEXUALLY RISKY BEHAVIORS

The accurate assessment of any human behavior through survey methods involves the following complex and challenging set of steps: (1) Researchers must write items that adequately reflect the objectives of the research program; (2) items need to be delivered to participants in a clearly comprehensible fashion; (3) participants must accurately recall the behavior of interest; and (4) participants must be able to report the requested information via the response options presented to them. All of these challenges exist in assessing SRBs, along with the added concern that participants may choose to alter their reports in a socially desirably direction because of the private and culturally stigmatized nature of sexual behavior. Nonetheless, well-designed self-report instruments can provide useful data. This section provides a guide to researchers in the design of psychometrically sound measures of SRBs, but is not meant to serve as a comprehensive primer on survey design. Several excellent resources on behavior measurement provide in-depth discussions and recommendations on general issues of measure development (e.g., Carmines & Zeller, 1979; Devellis, 2003); here, we focus on a circumscribed subset of design issues that are particularly relevant to the measurement of SRBs.

Validity of Measure Items

In order to provide meaningful data, an assessment measure must be valid; that is, it must assess what it purports to assess. The different types of validity include content, face, criterion, and construct. An instrument that has *content validity* assesses all the pertinent domains, as determined by a review of the literature, a panel of experts, or some predetermined theory. For a measure of SRBs, the domains should include, for example, number and risk characteristics of partners, types of sexual behavior (i.e., anal, vaginal, and oral intercourse), and consistency of condom use. *Face validity* refers to the extent to which an instrument *appears* to measure what it is supposed to measure: Is the item's intent patently obvious? With respect to SRBs, the utility of high face validity is dubious, because it may enhance socially desirable responding. *Criterion validity* is based on how well a respondent's scores on a particular measure correlate with some performance indicator assessed either at the same time (*concurrent validity*) or in the future (*predictive validity*). SRB researchers have attempted to corroborate the accuracy of self-reported sexual behavior with HIV and other STI testing (Coates, Stall, Catania, Dolcini, & Hoff, 1989; Winkelstein et al., 1987), as well as with partner reports (Coates et al., 1988). When used individually, neither of these approaches provides an ideal validity check. For example, HIV and other STIs do not occur in every individual who engages in a SRB, and partner reports of sexual behavior are susceptible to the same inaccuracies as participant self-reports. Corroborating a measure with multiple sources increases confidence in its validity but can be prohibitively difficult and expensive to accomplish.

Because it is so difficult to establish an index of validity, researchers must be particularly careful to minimize measurement error in self-report instruments. Underreporting is the primary threat to the validity of self-reported SRBs because of their sensitive and socially undesirable nature (Bradburn & Sudman, 1979; Herold & Way, 1988). Researchers can maximize self-disclosure of sensitive behaviors by providing private survey conditions (Jones & Forrest, 1992; O'Reilly, Hubbard, Lessler, Biemer, & Turner, 1994) and highlighting the normative nature of behaviors in questionnaire instructions and item wording. A detailed review of the literature on questionnaire item wording is beyond the scope of this chapter; however, many behavioral research references provide in-depth guidance for designing survey questions (see Converse & Presser, 1986; Krosnick & Fabrigar, 2001).

Level of Behavioral Specificity of Risk Assessment

It is important to select or construct an instrument that measures SRBs at the level of precision required to answer the project's research or intervention goals. Different types of objectives require different levels of behavioral specificity. Table 13.1 provides examples of items that measure the same SRBs at different behavioral specificity levels.

TABLE 13.1. Examples of SRB Assessment Items at Different Levels of Behavioral Specificity

Level of Behavioral Specificity	Example item	Research purpose
Risk screening	Do you always use condoms during sexual intercourse? ____ No ____ Yes	Screening participants in and out of studies Skip patterns leading to more specific questions
Risk event assessment	Think of the last time you had sexual intercourse. Did you use a condom? ____ No ____ Yes	Assessing covariates of SRB Within-subjects comparisons of SRB and non-SRB events
Risk level assessment	When you have had vaginal intercourse during the past 3 months, on how many occasions did you use a condom? _____ occasions	Assessing covariates of SRB Evaluating interventions to decrease SRB frequency

Risk Screening

At the least precise level of behavioral specificity, risk screening produces a dichotomous index of whether a respondent has engaged in any risk behavior during a given time period. This type of assessment is appropriate, for example, when the objective is to determine eligibility of potential research participants for a risk reduction intervention or to exclude individuals with any level of risk, such as in the screening of potential blood donors. Because risk-screening questions typically occur very early in the interaction of participants and researchers, often before rapport can be established, they may underestimate actual SRB. Murphy, Roheram-Borus, Srinivasan, Hunt, and Mitnick (1997) found a way to increase the reporting of stigmatizing SRBs. Instead of asking participants to respond to each item in a series of risky behaviors, they instructed participants to read through a list of risk behaviors and then indicate whether they had engaged in *any* of them (without indicating which ones specifically).

Risk Event Assessment

The most precise level of behavioral specificity is provided by risk event assessment, which produces detailed information about a single sexually risky incident. This approach is ideal for in-depth studies of situational covariates of risk behaviors or for within-subject analyses contrasting safe sex events with risky sex events (Weinhardt et al., 1998).

Risk Level Assessment

Assessing the frequency of engaging in SRBs provides a measure of level of risk. This level of specificity is appropriate for studies aiming to determine covariates of risk behaviors, such as substance use (e.g., Hines, Snowden, & Graves, 1998; Mahoney, 1995), and in intervention studies aiming to decrease frequency of risk behaviors; hence, this is the most common level of behavioral specificity used in HIV research.

Response Formats

The type of response format is likely to vary with the level of behavioral specificity. Table 13.2 illustrates how the same behavior can be assessed using different response formats.

True–False or Yes–No

If risk screening is the survey's purpose, then dichotomous items are likely to be sufficient. Within a more in-depth assessment procedure, affirmative re-

TABLE 13.2. SRB Response Formats and Example Items

Types	Example items
True–false or yes–no	I always use a condom during anal-receptive intercourse. _____ True _____ False
Multiple-choice	On the occasions that you have anal-receptive intercourse, how frequently do you use condoms? _____ Never _____ On less than half of the occasions _____ On about half of the occasions _____ On more than half of the occasions _____ Every time
Open-ended	Describe a time in the last 2 months when you had anal-receptive intercourse and _did not_ use a condom.

sponses to these types of items are commonly used to skip respondents in and out of more specific question branches.

Multiple-Choice

A multiple-choice response format requires participants to select from a list of prespecified options. It is important to include response options that adequately reflect the range of participants' potential answers. Pilot research with focus groups and with open-ended survey questions is recommended to develop comprehensive closed-ended response options. One hazard of using this type of question is that the response options that researchers provide can systematically influence participants' answers. For example, when researchers provide numeric response choices to participants (e.g., 1 or 2 times, 3 or 4 times, 5 or 6 times, more than 7 times), participants may interpret the middle response options as the normal or average level of that behavior and avoid using the high end of the scale (Schwartz, 1999). To address this problem, researchers can provide response choices with very large ranges, so that higher numbers of incidents do not appear as extreme. For example, when given response options ranging from 1 to 20 for the question "How many different sexual partners do you have in a typical month?", some participants are likely to avoid selecting a number near 20—and hence underestimate their number of sexual partners—because it appears to be an extremely high number on the given scale. However, if the response options ranged from 1 to 1000, numbers near 20 no longer seem as extreme, and some participants may be less likely to underestimate their number of sexual partners. For comprehensive reviews on systematic bias in closed-ended questions and guidelines for avoiding errors, see Converse and Presser (1986) and Krosnick and Fabrigar (2001).

Open-Ended

Open-ended items allow participants to respond in their own words. One advantage of this item type is that participants can provide valuable information that the researchers did not anticipate, at a level of detail that closed-ended questions do not allow. With this added richness comes the challenge of coding diverse answers into a relatively small number of categories for data analysis. This involves a time-consuming, labor-intensive process of developing a coding scheme for each item, having multiple raters read and categorize each response, and determining the level of agreement among the raters. This type of question is best used to investigate motivations or contextual factors involved in risky sex rather than to assess specific sexual risk-taking behaviors.

Item Scaling

Respondents can be asked to report the occurrence of risk-taking behaviors using a number of formats or item scales, the most common of which are relative frequency and raw counts.

Relative Frequency

Relative frequencies of risky sex indicate what percentage of a respondent's total sexual encounters involved risky activity. For example, a percentage for unprotected vaginal intercourse can be estimated directly by the participant who answers a question such as "When you have had vaginal intercourse during the past 3 months, on what percent of the occasions did you *not use* a condom?" Participants can either provide a percentage or select one from a range of options (as presented in Table 13.2).

Raw Counts

Raw count measures request that participants report the precise number of times they engaged in an SRB during a specific time frame. Raw count measures commonly assess unprotected sex with a series of two questions, such as "In the past 3 months, how many times did you have anal intercourse?" followed by "How many of these times did you use a condom?" The number of unprotected anal intercourse occasions can be tallied as the total number of anal intercourse occasions minus the number of occasions on which condoms were used. Raw count data also can be transformed into relative frequency data by dividing the number of occasions of unprotected sex by total occasions of intercourse.

Raw count data have emerged as the most effective indices of HIV risk for several reasons. From a biological perspective, one's risk of HIV infection increases as a function of the number of times one is exposed to the virus; thus, each individual occasion of unprotected sex increases the risk of HIV transmission (if all other factors, such as viral load, are held constant). Recent reviews and critiques of the HIV-risk assessment literature support the superiority of raw count data in terms of both precision and external validity (Fishbein & Pequegnat, 2000; Jaccard, McDonald, Wan, Dittus, & Quinlan, 2002; Schroder, Carey, & Vanable, 2003). For example, using relative frequency measures, participants who have vastly different raw counts of unprotected sex can be assigned the identical relative frequency of unprotected sex (e.g., 50 of 200 or 5 of 20 intercourse occasions both equal 25%). In this way, relative frequency measures do not provide the level of measurement required for effective risk assessment and intervention. It is therefore recommended that researchers assess raw counts of unprotected sex, using a series of questions such as those presented in Figure 13.1.

Susser, Desvarieux, and Wittkowski (1998) recommend that raw counts of numbers of unprotected sex acts be adjusted to account for differences in the risk of transmission among vaginal, oral-receptive, and anal sex acts. Based on epidemiological research, they have developed the Vaginal Episode Equivalent (VEE) index. Based on raw count data, VEE = (number of risky vaginal acts) + (number of risky anal acts * 2) + (number of risky receptive oral acts * 0.1).

Time Frame for Risk Behavior

Researchers need to aim for a methodological balance when selecting a time frame for assessing sexual risk-taking behaviors. Common sense, general research on survey methodology, and research specific to HIV-risk assessment all concur that recall of behavior over briefer intervals is likely to be more accurate. However, shorter time frames can reduce the range of reported behaviors. Several studies suggest that a 3-month retrospective period allows for accurate yet representative reporting of sexual risk-taking behaviors (Carey, Carey, Maisto, Gordon, & Weinhardt, 2001; Jaccard et al., 2002; Kauth, St. Lawrence, & Kelly, 1991). Because of memory distortions that are possible even within a 3-month time frame, researchers should incorporate recall aids into their protocols to enhance accurate responding. Simple forgetting, as well as participants' common use of heuristics to compute counts of events (such as reporting in increments of 10 and recalling vivid events as occurring more recently than they actually did [i.e., telescoping]), can reduce the accuracy of reports of SRB (Croyle & Loftus, 1993; Weinhardt et al., 1998). Several excellent resources exist for designing surveys that enhance participants' accurate recall (e.g., Croyle & Loftus, 1993; Loftus, Klinger, Smith, & Fiedler, 1990).

Mode of Administration

The mode of administration of the instrument is particularly important to consider in assessing SRB because of participants' concerns about both their privacy and the credibility of the research. The nature of the sample and of the questions to be asked, as well as the size of the project's budget, determine the choice of administration mode. The relative strengths and weaknesses of common administration modes are briefly summarized in Table 13.3.

Self-Administered Questionnaire

The strongest advantages of self-administered questionnaires (SAQs) in HIV research are the privacy and potential anonymity they offer, which result in greater disclosure of sexual behaviors. Their ease of administration and low cost also make them an attractive option. A disadvantage, however, is that respondents are more likely to leave questions unanswered, because SAQs are completed without direct supervision by the researcher (Turner, Miller, & Moses, 1989). Researchers also lose the opportunity to probe responses for further details, and complex branching patterns are difficult for respondents to follow. SAQs also require literacy, potentially leading to sample bias, because this means excluding the considerable proportion of the world population that is illiterate, mainly concentrated among people of lower socioeconomic status.

Telephone Interview

The largest U.S. surveys of sexual risk-taking behavior have used telephone interview techniques; *in-person* interviews of comparable size would have been nearly prohibitively expensive to conduct. Unlike SAQs, telephone interviews allow the administrator to explain unfamiliar terms; to probe ambiguous, inconsistent, or refused responses; and to lead respondents through complex question branching. Although telephone respondents are allowed a relatively high level of privacy because there is no face-to-face interaction with the interviewer, privacy still may be undermined if other people are within earshot of the participant. The researcher can advise the participant to answer the questions in a private place, but ultimately the researcher has little to no control over the respondent's environment. As in all telephone-based data collection, the researcher is prone to be mistaken for a telemarketer. In addition, researchers calling to inquire about sexual behaviors can be mistaken for obscene or prank callers. The legitimacy of telephone interviewers can be bolstered by sending potential participants letters in advance to prepare them for the call and to explain its purpose. A disadvantage less easily solved is that many high-risk individuals may be excluded from telephone interviews because they do not have access to a telephone.

TABLE 13.3. Mode of Sexually Risky Behavior Assessment Administration

Assessment mode	Advantages	Disadvantages
Self-administered questionnaire (SAQ)	Potential anonymity Enhanced confidentiality Ease of administration Low cost	No or low researcher involvement Skipped and misunderstood items Limited potential to probe responses Limited question branching and skip patterns Literacy dependent
Telephone interview (TI)	Researcher involvement Ability to explain unfamiliar terms Ability to probe responses and nonresponses Complex question branching and skip patterns More privacy than IPI Less interpersonal reaction than IPI	Loss of control over respondent's environment Misidentification of researcher as telemarketer Misidentification of researcher as prank caller Many high-risk individuals have no phone
In-person interview (IPI)	Interviewer/respondent rapport Enhanced credibility of study Opportunity to probe responses and nonresponses Opportunity to explain terms Minimizes nonresponding	Less privacy than SAQ, IPI, TI, A-CASI Respondent reactivity to interviewer Interviewer nonstandardization Potentially biased interpretation of responses by interviewer Underreporting of SRBs by respondent
Audio computer-assisted self-administered interviewing (A-CASI)	More privacy than TI and IPI Lower literacy requirement than SRQ Some ability to probe ambiguous, inconsistent, or nonresponse Some ability to explain unfamiliar terms Complex question branching and skip patterns Less respondent reactivity to interviewer than TI or IPI Direct data entry Higher levels of reported SRB than IPI	Can be costly Participant resistance to computer technology

In-Person Interview

In-person interviews provide the most intimate interviewer–respondent interaction, which is the source of both their advantages and disadvantages. Whereas this method allows the interviewer to build a rapport with the participant that may increase self-disclosure, it also allows for the development of a negative interpersonal reaction that could inhibit disclosure. Interviewers are able to assess participants visually for cues that they are confused by a question or that they need reassurance of their privacy. In this way, interviewers can enhance the credibility of the overall study and minimize nonresponding to specific questions. However, closely tracking and responding to each participant's responses introduces an element of nonstandardization that could lead to systematic differences in participants' responses. For example, if women consistently required reassurance in order to answer a certain question, in effect, a different item was administered to women than to men. The interviewer can transcribe into written form information that participants provide verbally in interviews. This filtering of responses through the interviewer, however, may lead to inaccurate interpretation of responses. The drawback that is of most concern in in-person assessment is that it leads to more overreporting of protected sex and underreporting of unprotected sex than more anonymous assessment techniques (Siegel, Krauss, & Karns, 1994; Boekeloo, Schiavo, Rabin, Conlon, Jordon, & Mundt, 1994). This bias is particularly worrisome given that *in-person* interviewing is among the most common assessment modalities in research and intervention settings (Scandell, Klinkenberg, Hawkes, & Spriggs, 2003).

Audio Computer-Assisted Self-Interview

Audio computer-assisted self-interviews (A-CASI) involves having respondents use laptop computers to listen to questions through headphones and enter their responses via labeled keys or touch-screen technology. This approach is fast replacing telephone surveys as the best compromise between SAQs and *in-person* interviews. Because questions are administered without the interviewer being able to hear them, this method preserves the privacy of SAQs. Clearly labeling or color-coding the computer keys and touch screen technology can minimize literacy requirements. Nonresponse is decreased because questions are often presented one per computer screen, and survey software can be programmed so that when participants press the "skip" key, they are shown a message reminding them that their answers are very important. Survey software also can be programmed to incorporate complex branching patterns and to allow for limited probing of responses. The use of A-CASIs can be enormously time-saving to a research project because data is entered directly into a database when participants make their responses on the computer. Moreover, studies have found that respondents using A-CASI report higher levels of sexual behaviors than do respondents using in-person interviews (e.g., Newman, Des Jarlais, Turner, Gribble, Cooley, & Paone, 2002).

Interviewer Sensitivity

Because of the private and often culturally stigmatized nature of sexual behavior, the demeanor of assessment administrators—even if their role is limited to handing out a survey—is critical to creating an environment in which respondents can feel comfortable giving honest and frank answers. Staff may encounter sexual language, attitudes, and behaviors that are different from their own and may conflict with their own cultural or religious values. Although the effects of interviewer characteristics on reporting of sexual behavior are inadequately understood, matching the gender of staff and respondent is one simple step that can increase disclosure of sexual behavior (Catania, Moskowitz, Ruiz, & Cleland, 1996). In addition, staff training should encourage interviewers to acknowledge and examine their own opinions and judgments about sexual behaviors and to respect the differences of others. In particular, if staff are required to give respondents HIV-risk reduction information, it is essential that they are trained to be comfortable, nonjudgmental, and knowledgeable when discussing sexual behavior (Kelly, 1995). The interaction of interviewers with respondents should be carefully scripted, so that respondents are treated as similarly as possible and every assessment measure is administered in a uniform fashion.

CULTURALLY APPROPRIATE ASSESSMENT OF SEXUALLY RISKY BEHAVIORS

People of color constitute the majority of those currently living with HIV/AIDS. African American and Latino individuals are especially vulnerable and are disproportionately represented among new cases. Thus, although cultural considerations are important when selecting or formulating any assessment instrument, attention to cultural concerns is crucial when evaluating SRBs among communities of color. Failure to attend adequately and sensitively to the cultural relevance of SRB instrumentation is far from inconsequential. Such failures can culminate in research findings and impressions that, once established, can prove difficult to dislodge and erroneously portray SRB trends and HIV prevalence patterns in communities that are already oppressed and disempowered. Such failures can also damage already fragile relationships between communities of color and research or service institutions.

Consequently, the importance of cultural relevance cannot be overemphasized (Wilson & Miller, 2003). For example, some issues related to sexuality, and to AIDS in particular, may be highly stigmatized in communities of color. Research efforts that are insufficiently attentive to this cultural pattern may yield low response rates and underestimates of key variables, while simultaneously insulting and alienating community members. An in-depth consideration of cultural factors would exceed the scope of the current chapter. Nevertheless, several general guidelines and key recommendations are obligatory.

Researchers should never assume that instrumentation developed and standardized with majority samples can be transferred directly, without modification, to use with communities of color. Such an assumption negates the importance of cultural factors. Even when there are no language differences, experienced researchers—who preferably are knowledgeable about the community being investigated—must vet the instrument's instructions, item content, psychometric structure, and scoring protocols.

When using established instruments, researchers should seek to cross-validate the instrumentation with the sample of interest. Both quantitative (e.g., surveys, experiments) and qualitative (e.g., key informant interviews, focus groups) methods should be employed in assessing cross-validation. The obvious goal is to ensure that the instrument validly extends SRB assessment to the culturally distinct community of interest.

Language issues must be identified and remedied (e.g., dialect, accent, slang). With slang, the remedy may merely involve word substitutions that have been carefully selected by knowledgeable informants. In the case of different languages, the remedy may involve multiple and intensive iterations of painstaking translation and back-translation of the instrument.

In addition to SRBs, researchers should prepare to measure constructs pertinent to potential cultural cofactors that could mediate or moderate the relationship between SRBs and other variables. These constructs might include an individual's acculturation level, ethnic identity, or the regularity of racist victimization, which have established assessment protocols.

The demographic characteristics and cultural sensitivity of frontline research personnel must be considered. Personnel, as a result of their demographic makeup or discomfort with cross-cultural interactions, can torpedo a potential participant's receptivity, goodwill, and data quality. It is imperative that research personnel be seen and experienced by the community as credible and trustworthy agents.

Researchers must engage community leaders and organizations. Some communities view researchers as being akin to invading forces from distant powers, dispatched to pillage data from the colonies and abscond with the spoils back to the fortress. Therefore, it is vital that researchers engage trusted community organizations and leaders to enlist their imprimatur and support in launching research projects that will investigate and—no doubt—affect community members.

It is important to identify and consider culturally specific stigma issues. While there is generally stigma about STIs, this can be magnified in communities of color. For instance, in many African American communities, stigma about homosexuality is severe, affecting disclosures among men having sex with men and especially men living on the "down low," who also maintain heterosexual activities and lifestyle (Malebranche, 2003; Myers, Javanbakht,

Martinez, & Obediah, 2003). Alternatively, in many Asian American communities, concerns about family shame and "loss of face" can squelch research participation and disclosures (Nemoto, Operario, Takenaka, Iwamoto, & Le, 2003).

Once findings are analyzed and compiled, researchers must interpret the data with openness to culturally informed theory revision. Insights gleaned from community engagement, consideration of cultural dynamics, and measurement of cultural constructs may have implications for preexisting theories. These insights can challenge these theories and foster revisions leading toward more comprehensive and externally valid models.

Finally, it is important that researchers contribute to the communities in which they conduct research. For instance, researchers should identify and provide culturally meaningful individual rewards and community services (Fullilove et al., 1993). This philosophy is antithetical to the historical pillage-and-run analogy of research in nonmajority cultural communities.

CONCLUSIONS

STIs pose a significant threat to human health and well-being around the globe. Until such infections are eradicated, SRB will remain an important assessment domain with regard to mental and physical health. Furthermore, because co-occurrence with substance use and abuse is common, SRB assessment will be relevant to the field of addictions assessment.

In this chapter, we have defined SRB and briefly described the current state of the field of SRB assessment. Thus far, efforts to assess SRBs have been plagued by a proliferation of project-specific instruments, with little convergence toward standardization. Insularity and fragmentation among research efforts in this field are rampant. Insufficient attention has been paid to the development of conceptually and psychometrically sound protocols capable of distilling clear "best choices" among available SRB instruments.

We have reviewed requisite psychometric properties and have emphasized the importance of considering culture in SRB assessment, presenting "best practices" in both the selection of SRB instruments and the development of new ones. These practices emphasize deliberation about several pragmatic and cultural concerns, and psychometric parameters. Together, these practices constitute a checklist or set of guidelines and suggestions for researchers and clinicians seeking to assess SRBs. Researchers and clinicians can make good choices about SRB assessment by considering validity, the level of behavioral specificity, response formats, item scaling, time frame for risk behavior, mode of administration, interviewer sensitivity, and cultural relevance and appropriateness. It is our hope that future work will conspire toward needed standardization, psychometric refinement, and cultural sensitivity. If so, subsequent generations of SRB instrumentation should yield "best choices" that increase the rigor of studies and the comparability of findings.

REFERENCES

Boekeloo, B. O., Schiavo, L., Rabin, D. L., Conlon, R. T., Jordan, C. S., & Mundt, D. J. (1994). Self-reports of HIV risk factors by patients at a sexually transmitted disease clinic: Audio vs. written questionnaires. *American Journal of Public Health, 84,* 754–760.

Bradburn, N. M., & Sudman, S. (1979). *Improving interview method and question-naire design.* San Francisco: Jossey-Bass.

Caceres, C. F., & van Griensven, G. (1994). Male homosexual transmission of HIV-1. *AIDS, 8,* 1051–1061.

Carey, M. P., Carey, K. B., Maisto, S. A., Gordon, C. M., & Weinhardt, L. S. (2001). Assessing sexual risk behaviour with the Timeline Followback (TLFB) approach: Continued development and psychometric evaluation with psychiatric outpatients. *International Journal of STDs and AIDS, 12,* 365–375.

Carmines, E. G., & Zeller, R. A. (1979). *Reliability and validity assessment.* Beverly Hills, CA: Sage.

Catania, J. A., Binson, D., Van Der Straten, A., & Stone, V. (1995). Methodological research on sexual behavior in the AIDS era. *Annual Review of Sex Research, 6,* 77–125.

Catania, J. A., Gibson, D. R., Chitwood, D. D., & Coates, T. J. (1990). Methodological problems in AIDS behavioral research: Influences on measurement error and partic-ipation bias in studies of sexual behavior. *Psychological Bulletin, 108,* 339–362.

Catania, J. A., Moskowitz, J. T., Ruiz, M., & Cleland, J. (1996). A review of national AIDS-related behavioral surveys. *AIDS, 10,* S183–S190.

Centers for Disease Control and Prevention. (2002). *HIV/AIDS Surveillance Report* (Vol. 13). Atlanta: Author.

Chu, S. Y., Conti, L., Schable, B. A., & Diaz, T. (1994). Female-to-female sexual con-tact and HIV transmission. *Journal of the American Medical Association, 272,* 433.

Coates, R. A., Calzavara, L. M., Soskolne, C. L., Read, S. E., Fanning, M. M., Shep-herd, F. A., et al. (1988). Validity of sexual histories in a prospective study of male sexual contacts of men with AIDS or an AIDS-related condition. *American Journal of Epidemiology, 128,* 719–728.

Coates, T. J., Stall, R., Catania, J. A., Dolcini, M. M., & Hoff, C. C. (1989). Priorities for AIDS risk reduction: Research and programmatic direction. *AIDS Clinical Review,* 29–52.

Cohen, H., Marmor, M., Wolfe, H., & Ribble, D. (1993). Risk assessment of HIV transmission among lesbians. *Journal of Acquired Immune Deficiency Syndrome, 6,* 1173–1174.

Converse, J. M., & Presser, S. (1986). *Survey questions: Handcrafting the standardized questionnaire.* Beverly Hills, CA: Sage.

Croyle, R. T., & Loftus, E. F. (1993). Recollection in the kingdom of AIDS. In R. Kessler & D. Ostrow (Eds.), *Methodological issues in AIDS behavioral research* (pp. 163–180). New York: Plenum Press.

Devellis, R. F. (2003). *Scale development: Theory and application* (2nd ed.). Thousand Oaks, CA: Sage.

Fishbein, M., & Pequegnat, W. (2000). Evaluating AIDS prevention interventions us-ing behavioral and biological outcome measures. *Sexually Transmitted Diseases, 27,* 101–110.

Fullilove, M. T., Fullilove, R. E., Smith, M., Winkler, K., Michael, C., Panzer, P. G., et al. (1993). Violence, trauma, and post-traumatic stress disorder among women drug users. *Journal of Traumatic Stress, 6,* 533–543.

Haverkos, H. W., & Battjes, R. J. (1992). Female-to-male transmission of HIV. *Journal of the American Medical Association, 268,* 1855–1856.

Herold, E. S., & Way, L. (1988). Sexual self-disclosure among university women. *Journal of Sex Research, 24,* 1–14.

Hines, A., Snowden, L. R., & Graves, K. L. (1998). Acculturation, alcohol consumption and AIDS-related risky sexual behavior among African American women. *Women and Health, 27,* 17–35.

Jaccard, J., McDonald, R., Wan, C. K., Dittus, P. J., & Quinlan, S. (2002). The accuracy of self-reports of condom use and sexual behavior. *Journal of Applied Social Psychology, 32,* 1863–1905.

Jemmott, J. B., III, & Jemmott, L. S. (2000). HIV behavioral interventions for adolescents in community settings. In J. L. Peterson & R. J. DiClemente (Eds.), *Handbook of HIV prevention: AIDS prevention and mental health* (pp. 103–127). New York: Kluwer/Plenum.

Jones, E. F., & Forrest, J. D. (1992). Underreporting of abortion in surveys of U.S. women: 1976 to 1988. *Demography, 29,* 113–126.

Kaiser, J. (2003, October 31). Biomedical politics. NIH roiled by inquiries over grants hit list. *Science, 303,* 758.

Kaiser, J. (2004, February 6). Sex studies "properly" approved. *Science, 303,* 741.

Kauth, M. R., St. Lawrence, J. S., & Kelly, J. A. (1991). Reliability of retrospective assessments of sexual HIV risk behavior: A comparison of biweekly, three-month, and twelve-month self-reports. *AIDS Education and Prevention, 3,* 207–214.

Kelly, J. A. (1995). *Changing HIV risk behavior: Practical strategies.* New York: Guilford Press.

Kelly, J. A., & Kalichman, S. C. (2002). Behavioral research in HIV/AIDS primary and secondary prevention: Recent advances and future directions. *Journal of Consulting and Clinical Psychology, 70,* 626–639.

Krosnick, J. A., & Fabrigar, L. R. (2001). *Designing great questionnaires: Insights from psychology.* New York: Oxford University Press.

Loftus, E. F., Klinger, M. R., Smith, K. D., & Fiedler, J. (1990). A tale of two questions: Benefits of asking more than one question. *Public Opinion Quarterly, 54,* 330–345.

Mahoney, C. A. (1995). The role of cues, self-efficacy, level of worry, and high-risk behaviors in college student condom use. *Journal of Sex Education and Therapy, 21,* 103–116.

Malebranche, D. J. (2003). Black men who have sex with men and the HIV epidemic: Next steps for public health. *American Journal of Public Health, 93,* 862–865.

Mantell, J. E., DiVittis, A. T., & Auerbach, J. D. (1997). *Evaluating HIV prevention interventions.* New York: Plenum Press.

Murphy, D., Roheram-Borus, M., Srinivasan, S., Hunt, W., & Mitnick, L. (1997). Recruiting a cohort for the HIV vaccine trial: Sensitivity and specificity of a screening for sexual and substance use acts. *AIDS and Behavior, 1,* 75–80.

Myers, H. F., Javanbakht, M., Martinez, M., & Obediah, S. (2003). Psychosocial predictors of risky sexual behaviors in African American men: Implications for prevention. *AIDS Education and Prevention, 15,* 66–79.

Nemoto, T., Operario, D., Takenaka, M., Iwamoto, M., & Le, M. N. (2003). HIV risk among Asian women working at massage parlors in San Francisco. *AIDS Education and Prevention, 15,* 245–256.

Newman, J. C., Des Jarlais, D. C., Turner, C. F., Gribble, J., Cooley, P., & Paone, D. (2002). The differential effects of face-to-face and computer interview modes. *American Journal of Public Health, 92,* 294–297.

Newton, P. (1996). Oral sex: Just how dangerous is it? *Southern Voice, 1,* 9.

O'Reilly, J. M., Hubbard, M. L., Lessler, J. T., Biemer, P. P., & Turner, C. F. (1994). Audio and video computer assisted self-interviewing: Preliminary tests of new technologies for data collection. *Journal of Official Statistics, 10,* 197–214.

Page-Shafer, K., Shiboski, C. H., Osmond, D. H., Dilley, J., McFarland, W., Shiboski, S. C., Klausner, J. D., Balls, J., Greenspan, D., & Greenspan, J. S. (2002). Risk of infection attributable to oral sex among men who have sex with men and in the population of men who have sex with men. *AIDS, 16,* 2350–2352.

Samuel, M. C., Hessol, N., Shiboski, S., Engel, R. R., Speed, T. P., & Winkelstein, W., Jr. (1993). Factors associated with human immunodeficiency virus seroconversion in homosexual men in three San Francisco cohort studies, 1984–1989. *Journal of Acquired Immune Deficiency Syndrome, 6,* 303–312.

Scandell, D. J., Klinkenberg, W. D., Hawkes, M. C., & Spriggs, L. S. (2003). The assessment of high-risk sexual behavior and self-presentation concerns. *Research on Social Work Practice, 13,* 119–141.

Schacker, T., Collier, A. C., Hughes, J., Shea, T., & Corey, L. (1996). Clinical and epidemiologic features of primary HIV infection. *Annals of Internal Medicine, 125,* 257–264.

Schroder, K. E. E., Carey, M. P., & Vanable, P. A. (2003). Methodological challenges in research on sexual risk behavior: II. Accuracy of self-reports. *Annals of Behavioral Medicine, 26,* 104–124.

Schwartz, N. (1999). Self reports: How the questions shape the answers. *American Psychologist, 54,* 93–105.

Siegel, K., Krauss, B. J., & Karus, D. (1994). Reporting recent sexual practices: Gay men's disclosure of HIV risk by questionnaire and interview. *Archives of Sexual Behavior, 23,* 217–230.

Susser, E., Desvarieux, M., & Wittkowski, K. M. (1998). Reporting sexual risk behavior for HIV: A practical risk index and a method for improving risk indices. *American Journal of Public Health, 88,* 671–674.

Turner, C. F., Miller, H. G., & Moses, L. E. (1989). *AIDS: Sexual behaviors and intravenous drug use.* Washington, DC: National Academy Press.

UNAIDS/WHO. (2003). *AIDS Epidemic Update, December 2003* (UNAIDS/03.39E. NLM classification: WC 503.41). Geneva: UNAIDS Information Centre.

Weinhardt, L. S., Forsyth, A. D., Carey, M. P., Jaworski, B. C., & Durant, L. E. (1998). Reliability and validity of self-report measures of HIV-related sexual behavior: Progress since 1990 and recommendations for research and practice. *Archives of Sexual Behavior, 27,* 155–180.

Wilson, B. D. M., & Miller, R. L. (2003). Integrating culture into HIV prevention research: A review. *AIDS Education and Prevention, 15,* 184–202.

Winkelstein, W., Jr., Samuel, M., Padian, N. S., Wiley, J. A., Lang, W., Anderson, R. E., et al. (1987). The San Francisco Men's Health Study: III. Reduction in human immunodeficiency virus transmission among homosexual/bisexual men, 1982–86. *American Journal of Public Health, 77,* 685–689.

Author Index

Subject Index